W9-CFQ-257

Human Diseases and Conditions

Second Edition

Advisors

A number of experts in the medical community provided invaluable assistance in the formulation of this encyclopedia. The advisory board performed a myriad of duties, from defining the scope of coverage to reviewing individual entries for accuracy and accessibility. To them our sincerest appreciation is extended.

LEAD ADVISOR

EUGENE W. STRAUS, M.D.
Emeritus Professor of Medicine
State University of New York Health Science Center at Brooklyn
Downstate Medical Center

LARRY I. LUTWICK, M.D.
Professor of Medicine
State University of New York, Downstate Medical School
Director of Infectious Diseases
Veterans Affairs New York Harbor Health Care System, Brooklyn Campus

STEPHAN L. KAMHOLZ, M.D., M.A.C.P., F.C.C.P.
Chairman, Department of Medicine
North Shore University Hospital and Long Island Jewish Medical Center
David J. Greene Professor of Medicine
New York University School of Medicine
Adjunct Professor of Medicine
Albert Einstein College of Medicine
State University of New York Downstate College of Medicine

PETER H. ROCHELEAU, M.D.

HUMAN DISEASES AND CONDITIONS

Second Edition
Volume 4
S–Z

Miranda Herbert Ferrara

Project Editor

CHARLES SCRIBNER'S SONS
A part of Gale, Cengage Learning

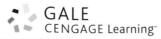

GALE
CENGAGE Learning

Detroit • New York • San Francisco • New Haven, Conn • Waterville, Maine • London

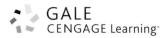

Human Diseases and Conditions,
Second Edition

Project Editor: Miranda Herbert Ferrara

Assistant Project Editor: Brigham Narins

Editorial: Kristin Key, Amy Kwolek, Shirelle Phelps,
Jeffrey Wilson

Production Technology Support: Luann Brennan

Manuscript Editor: Melodie Monahan

Proofreader: John K. Krol

Indexer: Katy Balcer

Product Design: Pamela A. E. Galbreath

Imaging: John Watkins

Graphic Art: Molly A. Moore Blessington,
Frank Forney, GGS Information Services, Inc.,
Corey Light

Rights Acquisition and Management: Jackie Jones,
Kelly Quin, Robyn Young

Composition: Evi Abou-El-Seoud,
Mary Beth Trimper

Manufacturing: Wendy Blurton

Product Manager: Hélène Potter

Publisher: Jay Flynn

© 2010 Charles Scribner's Sons, a part of Gale, Cengage Learning

ALL RIGHTS RESERVED. No part of this work covered by the copyright herein may
be reproduced, transmitted, stored, or used in any form or by any means graphic,
electronic, or mechanical, including but not limited to photocopying, recording,
scanning, digitizing, taping, Web distribution, information networks, or information
storage and retrieval systems, except as permitted under Section 107 or 108 of the 1976
United States Copyright Act, without the prior written permission of the publisher.

For product information and technology assistance, contact us at
Gale Customer Support, 1-800-877-4253.
For permission to use material from this text or product,
submit all requests online at **www.cengage.com/permissions.**
Further permissions questions can be emailed to
permissionrequest@cengage.com

Since this page cannot legibly accommodate all copyright notices, the credits
constitute an extension of the copyright notice.

While every effort has been made to ensure the reliability of the information
presented in this publication, Gale, a part of Cengage Learning, does not guarantee
the accuracy of the data contained herein. Gale accepts no payment for listing; and
inclusion in the publication of any organization, agency, institution, publication, service,
or individual does not imply endorsement of the editors or publisher. Errors brought to
the attention of the publisher and verified to the satisfaction of the publisher will be
corrected in future editions.

EDITORIAL DATA PRIVACY POLICY: Does this product contain information about
you as an individual? If so, for more information about our editorial data privacy policies,
please see our Privacy Statement at www.gale.cengage.com.

LIBRARY OF CONGRESS CATALOGING-IN-PUBLICATION DATA

Human diseases and conditions / Miranda Herbert Ferrara, editor. -- 2nd ed.
   p. cm
   Includes bibliographical references and index.
   ISBN 978-0-684-31238-5 (set) -- ISBN 978-0-684-31239-2 (v. 1) -- ISBN
978-0-684-31240-8 (v. 2) -- ISBN 978-0-684-31241-5 (v. 3) -- ISBN
978-0-684-31601-7 (v. 4) -- ISBN 978-0-684-31515-7 (ebook)
   1. Medicine, Popular--Encyclopedias. I. Ferrara, Miranda Herbert, 1950-

RC81.A2H75 2010
616.003--dc22   2009006533

Gale
27500 Drake Rd.
Farmington Hills, MI, 48331-3535

ISBN 13: 978-0-684-31238-5 (set)   ISBN 10: 0-684-31238-7 (set)
ISBN 13: 978-0-684-31239-2 (vol. 1)   ISBN 10: 0-684-31239-5 (vol. 1)
ISBN 13: 978-0-684-31240-8 (vol. 2)   ISBN 10: 0-684-31240-9 (vol. 2)
ISBN 13: 978-0-684-31241-5 (vol. 3)   ISBN 10: 0-684-31241-7 (vol. 3)
ISBN 13: 978-0-684-31601-7 (vol. 4)   ISBN 10: 0-684-31601-3 (vol. 4)

This title is also available as an e-book.
ISBN-13: 978-0-684-31515-7 ISBN 10: 0-684-31515-7
Contact your Gale, a part of Cengage Learning sales representative for ordering
information.

Printed in China by China Translation & Printing Services Limited
1 2 3 4 5 6 7 13 12 11 10 09

Editorial and Production Staff

Project Editor
Miranda Herbert Ferrara

Assistant Project Editor
Brigham Narins

Contributors
Margaret Alic • Linda Wasmer Andrews • William Arthur Atkins • Kate Barrett • Maria Basile
Elizabeth Bass • Raymond Brogan • Jennifer Brooks • Charles W. Carey, Jr. • Rosalyn Carson-DeWitt
Laura J. Cataldo • Joel Ciovacco • Allan Cobb • Kristine Conner • John A. Cutter • Helen Davidson
Tish Davidson • Paula Edelsack • L. Fleming Fallon, Jr. • Karl Finley • Rebecca J. Frey • Fran Hodgkins
Joan Huebl • Megan Huff • Judith S. Hurley • Mary Lou Jay • Evelyn B. Kelly • Monique Laberge
Johnna Laird • Lynn M. L. Lauerman • Marge Lurie • Jennifer Lynch • D'Arcy Lyness
Christopher Meehan • Elizabeth Merrick • Leslie Mertz • Sylvia K. Miller • Robert Nellis
Daphne Northrop • Ilene Raymond • Jordan P. Richman • Vita Richman • Karen Riley • Ruth Ross
Eugénie Seifer • Sharon Sexton • Hennie Shore • Shaynee Snider • Amy Sutton
Chitra Venkatasubramanian • Giselle Weiss • Theodore Zinn • Faye Zucker

Editorial
Kristin Key • Amy Kwolek • Shirelle Phelps • Jeffrey Wilson

Production Technology Support
Luann Brennan

Manuscript Editor
Melodie Monahan

Proofreader
John K. Krol

Indexer
Katy Balcer

Product Design
Pamela A. E. Galbreath

Imaging
John Watkins

Graphic Art
Molly A. Moore Blessington • Frank Forney • GGS Information Services, Inc. • Corey Light

Rights Acquisition and Management
Jackie Jones • Kelly Quin • Robyn Young

Composition
Evi Abou-El-Seoud • Mary Beth Trimper

Manufacturing
Wendy Blurton

Product Manager
Hélène Potter

Publisher
Jay Flynn

Contents

Contents

Contents

Contents

Please Read—Important Information

Human Diseases and Conditions, Second Edition, is a health reference product designed to inform and educate readers about a wide variety of diseases and conditions, nutrition and dietary practices, treatments and drugs, as well as other issues associated with general health. Cengage Learning believes the product to be comprehensive, but not necessarily definitive. It is intended to supplement, not replace, consultation with a physician or other healthcare practitioner. While Cengage Learning has made substantial efforts to provide information that is accurate, comprehensive, and up-to-date, Cengage Learning makes no representations or warranties of any kind, including without limitation, warranties of merchantability or fitness for a particular purpose, nor does it guarantee the accuracy, comprehensiveness, or timeliness of the information contained in this product. Readers should be aware that the universe of medical knowledge is constantly growing and changing, and that differences of opinion exist among authorities. Readers are also advised to seek professional diagnosis and treatment for any medical condition, and to discuss information obtained from this product with their healthcare provider.

S

SAD *See Seasonal Affective Disorder.*

Salmonellosis

Salmonellosis (sal-mo-nel-O-sis) is a gastrointestinal disease caused by bacteria called salmonella. This type of bacterium from infected animals is usually found in foods such as poultry, milk, and eggs.

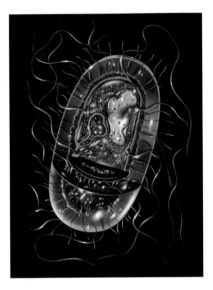

▲

The structure of a *Salmonella* bacterium. The DNA (inside the nucleus) is yellow. The cytoplasm is green. The part of the cell wall shown in brown secretes the toxins that cause symptoms in salmonellosis. *Custom Medical Stock Photo, Inc. Reproduced by permission.*

What Is Salmonellosis?

Salmonellosis is an illness caused by *salmonella* bacteria that affects the intestine, usually resulting in diarrhea. In some people, the infection spreads to the bloodstream and other areas of the body and can be life-threatening unless they receive prompt treatment.

Salmonellosis, named after the American scientist Daniel Salmon, is one of the most common causes of food poisoning in the United States. Each year, about 40,000 cases of salmonellosis are reported to the Centers for Disease Control and Prevention (CDC), and up to 4 million additional cases may go unreported. About 400 people in the United States die each year of complications related to salmonellosis. Infants, the elderly, and people whose immune system* are weakened are most vulnerable to severe infection.

How Do People Get Salmonellosis?

In the United States, people usually get salmonellosis from eating or drinking contaminated food, most often raw milk or undercooked poultry and poultry products such as eggs. Undercooked ground beef or other meat can also cause salmonellosis. In some cases, food can be contaminated by the people handling it. Salmonellosis can also be spread through the stools of some pets, especially reptiles and pets with diarrhea.

A different species of *Salmonella* bacteria causes typhoid fever, a serious disease common in developing countries in Latin America, Africa, and Asia. Typhoid fever is spread by food and water contaminated with the bacteria. Clean water, pasteurized* milk, and effective sewage systems have made typhoid fever rare in the United States and other developed countries.

* **immune system** (im-YOON SIS-tem) is the system of the body composed of specialized cells and the substances they produce that helps protect the body against disease-causing germs.

* **pasteurize** (PAS-cha-rise) to sterilize a substance, generally a liquid such as milk, by bringing it to high temperature and keeping it at that temperature long enough to destroy unhealthy organisms in it without changing its other characteristics.

* **dehydration** (dee-hi-DRAY-shun) is a condition in which the body is depleted of water, usually caused by excessive and unreplaced loss of body fluids, such as through sweating, vomiting, or diarrhea.

What Are the Symptoms of Salmonellosis?

The symptoms of salmonellosis include diarrhea, stomach cramps, pain, fever, headache, nausea, and vomiting. They occur within 12 to 48 hours of eating or drinking contaminated food.

How Is Salmonellosis Diagnosed and Treated?

Salmonellosis is diagnosed through stool cultures from people with symptoms of the infection. *Salmonella* infections usually run their course without treatment in a few days to a week after an unpleasant period of vomiting and diarrhea. Healthcare professionals suggest that people drink lots of fluids and eat a bland diet while they recover from salmonellosis. Sometimes the symptoms create other problems, such as dehydration*. In those cases, people may need to go to the hospital to receive replacement fluids through their veins (an "IV"). Antibiotics may be used if the infection spreads beyond the intestine, but salmonellosis is often resistant to drugs.

How Can Salmonellosis Be Prevented?

Thorough cooking (until poultry or meat, especially ground beef, is no longer pink and eggs are no longer runny) and regular hand washing (after using the bathroom and between handling raw meat and other foods) are the main ways to prevent salmonellosis. Only pasteurized dairy products that have been kept refrigerated should be used. Raw meat or eggs should be especially avoided.

▶ *See also* **Diarrhea • Food Poisoning • Gastroenteritis • Typhoid Fever**

Resources

Books and Articles

Brands, Danielle A. *Salmonella.* Philadelphia, PA: Chelsea House Publishers, 2006.

Hirschmann, Kris. *Salmonella.* San Diego, CA: Kidhaven Press, 2004.

Pascoe, Elaine. *Spreading Menace: Salmonella Attack and the Hunger Craving (Body Story).* San Diego, CA: Blackbirch Press, 2004.

Organizations

Centers for Disease Control and Prevention. 1600 Clifton Road, Atlanta, GA, 30333. Toll free: 800-311-3435. Web site: http://www.cdc.gov/nczved/dfbmd/disease_listing/salmonellosis_gi.html.

Food Safety and Inspection Service. 1400 Independence Avenue SW, Room 2137 South Building, Washington, DC, 20250. Toll free: 800-336-3747. Web site: http://www.fsis.usda.gov/FactSheets/Salmonella_Questions_&_Answers/index.asp.

National Institute of Allergy and Infectious Diseases. Office of Communications and Public Liaison, 6610 Rockledge Drive, MSC, 6612, Bethesda, MD, 20892-66123. Toll free: 866-284-4107. Web site: http://www3.niaid.nih.gov/healthscience/healthtopics/salmonellosis.

San Joaquin (Valley) Fever *See Coccidioidomycosis.*

Sarcoma

Sarcoma is a type of cancer that affects the body's connective tissue (bones, muscles, fat, blood vessels, nerves, and cartilage).

What Is Sarcoma?

Sarcoma is a type of cancer that affects the body's connective tissue*, those types of tissue that provide structural support to the various organs of the body. Connective tissue all comes from the same type of embryonic tissue, called mesoderm. Examples of connective tissue include the bones, muscles, fat, blood vessels, nerves, and cartilage.

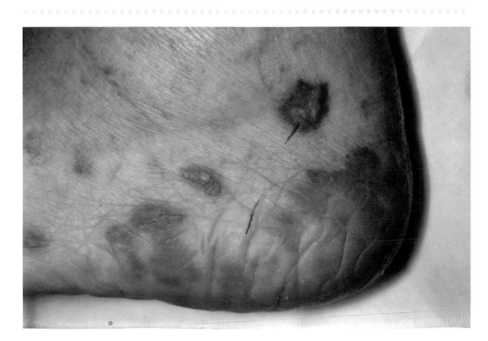

* **connective tissue** helps hold the body together, is found in skin, joints and bones.

Skin biopsy of Kaposi's sarcoma. Courtesy of the CDC.

* **AIDS** or acquired immunodeficiency (ih-myoo-no-dih-FIH-shen-see) syndrome, is an infection that severely weakens the immune system; it is caused by the human immunodeficiency virus (HIV).

What Are the Various Types of Sarcoma?

The general term "sarcoma" includes many specific types of cancer that can affect a wide variety of tissues and areas of the body. The following are examples:

- Liposarcoma: Develops from fat tissues, most often found in back of the abdomen, called the retroperitoneum
- Leiomyosarcoma: Develops from smooth muscle tissue (the type of muscle tissue over which individuals have no voluntary control), most commonly found in the uterus or the gastrointestinal tract
- Rhabdomyosarcoma: Develops within skeletal muscle, most commonly within the limbs, head, neck, and the genital organs and urinary tract
- Synovial sarcoma: Made up of cells that resemble those that line the joints; can be found anywhere in the body, not just in joints
- Angiosarcoma: Made up of cells that resemble those that compose the blood vessels (veins and arteries)
- Fibrosarcoma: Develops in cells called fibroblasts, which are responsible for scar formation
- Neurofibrosarcoma: Develops in the cells that surround nerve cells
- Osteosarcoma: A tumor of bone cells
- Chondrosarcoma: A tumor of cartilage cells

Who Gets Sarcoma?

In the United States, about 10,390 people are diagnosed with soft tissue sarcoma every year; 5,720 in men and 4,670 in women. About 3,680 people die of the disease yearly. About 900 people are diagnosed with osteosarcoma (bone cancer) yearly, with 400 of these diagnoses for people less than 30 years of age. In adults, only 1 percent of all cancers are due to sarcomas; in children, 20 percent of all cancers are due to sarcoma.

People have a higher risk of developing sarcoma if they have been exposed to radiation (including during the treatment of other forms of cancer), are subject to toxic exposures (e.g., during the production of various forms of plastics or due to wood preservatives), if there is a strong family history of these types of cancers, or if they have other conditions that seem to predispose to sarcoma, such as Li-Fraumeni syndrome, or von Recklinghausen's disease (neurofibromatosis). People with AIDS* have an increased risk of a rare cancer Kaposi's sarcoma.

What are the Symptoms of Sarcoma?

Sarcoma often has no recognizable symptoms until it has grown fairly large. Sometimes an individual notices an unusual lump or bump. Other times, the tumor eventually expands enough to press on nerves or muscles, causing numbness, pain, tingling, soreness, or problems with normal functioning. In the case of bone cancer (osteosarcoma), expansion of the tumor within the bone can cause the bone to weaken and fracture (referred to as a pathologic fracture).

How Is Sarcoma Diagnosed?

Sarcoma may be suspected based on the presence of characteristic symptoms, as well as due to knowledge of the individual's personal or family history. A physical examination may reveal the presence of a tumor within areas of soft tissue. Tests such as an x-ray, ultrasound*, computerized tomography* (CT scan), or MRI* may be performed in an effort to demonstrate the presence of a tumor. A biopsy may be performed in order to remove a small sample of a tumor, either with a very thin needle (fine needle aspiration), a hollow needle (core biopsy), through a tiny incision during laparoscopic surgery, or through a classical incision during an open operation. Examination of this tissue under a microscope allows identification of the specific type of cancer cell.

How Is Sarcoma Treated?

Sarcoma is treated in a number of different ways. Surgery may be used to remove tumors. If at all possible, amputation of limbs is avoided, although it may be necessary in certain advanced cases. Chemotherapy involves the use of drugs that are toxic to the cancer cells (but also often to normal cells as well). Radiation therapy uses x-rays to shrink tumors.

▶ *See also* **Cancer: Overview**

Resources

Books and Articles

Abeloff, Martin D., James O. Armitage, John E. Niederhuber, et al. *Abeloff's Clinical Oncology*, 4th ed. Philadelphia, PA: Elsevier, 2008.

Ferri, Fred, ed. *Ferri's Clinical Advisor 2008*. Philadelphia, PA: Mosby Elsevier, 2008.

Goldman, Lee, and Dennis Ausiello, eds. *Cecil Textbook of Internal Medicine*, 23rd ed. Philadelphia, PA: Saunders, 2008.

Organizations

American Cancer Society. P.O. Box 22538, Oklahoma City, OK, 73123. Toll free: 866-228-4327. Web site: http://www.aafp.org/afp/20040701/123.html.

National Cancer Institute. Public Inquiries Office, 6116 Executive Boulevard, Room 3036A, Bethesda, MD, 20892. Toll free: 800-4-CANCER. Web site: http://www.cancer.gov/cancertopics/wyntk/

* **ultrasound** also called a sonogram, is a diagnostic test in which sound waves passing through the body create images on a computer screen.

* **computerized tomography** (kom-PYOO-ter-ized toe-MAH-gruh-fee) or CT, also called computerized axial tomography (CAT), is a technique in which a machine takes many x-rays of the body to create a three-dimensional picture.

* **MRI** which is short for magnetic resonance imaging, produces computerized images of internal body tissues based on the magnetic properties of atoms within the body.

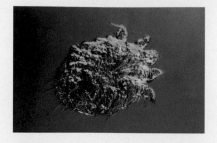

The itch mite *Sarcoptes scabiei* responsible for scabies. *Kent Wood/Photo Researchers, Inc.*

* **contagious** (kon-TAY-jus) means transmittable from one person to another, usually referring to an infection.

Sarcoma Foundation of American. 9884 Main Street, P.O. Box 458, Damascus, MD 20872. Toll free: 212/668-1000. Web site: http://www.curesarcoma.org/aboutSarcoma.htm.

SARS *See Severe Acute Respiratory Syndrome (SARS).*

Scabies

Scabies (SKAY-beez) is an itchy skin condition caused by mites that burrow under the skin.

Memories of Camp

Kelly returned from summer camp with many stories and a red, itchy rash. The skin on her wrists and thighs and between her fingers was covered with pimple-like bumps and she could see small S-shaped burrows under her skin. Kelly's neighbor, who is a dermatologist (der-ma-TOL-o-jist), or skin doctor, took one look and suspected scabies. When Kelly found out, she was embarrassed. She felt dirty even though she took a shower every day. She felt better when her neighbor told her that scabies does not discriminate. It affects young and old, boys and girls, and those who shower once a week or every day. He told her she must have picked it up at camp but that it was easy to get rid of.

What Causes Scabies?

Scabies is a skin condition caused by mites that dig under the skin. Mites are eight-legged animals related to spiders, scorpions, and ticks. They are so tiny that they require a microscope to be seen. The scientific name for the scabies mite, or "itch mite," is *Sarcoptes scabiei*. Its relatives cause mange (MAYNJ), an inflammation of the skin that results in hair loss, in dogs, pigs, horses, and cows.

Scabies is a common, contagious* skin condition that passes easily from person to person. Outbreaks of scabies, in which many people get infested at once, can occur in places such as nursing homes, childcare centers, and dormitories. The scabies mite cannot live very long away from the body. It can be spread by skin-to-skin contact or by clothing or bedding that has been used very recently by an infested person. Kelly acquired scabies from someone at camp, perhaps from borrowing a towel used recently by an infected person.

When Kelly first came into contact with the mites, females full of eggs burrowed under her skin and laid eggs. For a person who has never had scabies, it usually takes two to six weeks to develop symptoms, meaning itching and a rash, which is an allergic reaction to the mites. People who have had scabies before usually react within days.

How Is Scabies Diagnosed and Treated?

Kelly's neighbor, the dermatologist, suspected she had scabies based on her intense itching, the location of her rash, and how the rash looked. To make sure, he scraped at the skin between her fingers. He put the scrapings on a slide and when he looked at them with a microscope, he saw several mites and eggs.

Prescription drugs called scabicides (SKAY-bi-sydz), such as permethrin (per-METH-rin) and lindane (LIN-dayn), are usually used to kill scabies mites and eggs. Because scabies is so contagious, Kelly's neighbor instructed the whole family to bathe, then apply the scabicide lotion all over their bodies from chin to toes, and to wash all the recently used clothes, bedding, and towels in hot water. They were instructed to repeat the process in a week. The dermatologist also gave Kelly an antibiotic* ointment because she had some skin infections caused by scratching. Four weeks later, Kelly's skin was back to normal.

▶ See also **Parasitic Diseases: Overview • Skin Conditions**

Resources

Organizations

American Academy of Dermatology. PO Box 4014, Schaumburg, IL, 60168-4014. Toll free: 866-503-SKIN. Web site: http://www.aad.org/public/publications/pamphlets/common_scabies.html.

Centers for Disease Control and Prevention. 1600 Clifton Road, Atlanta, GA, 30333. Toll free: 800-311-3435. Web site: http://www.cdc.gov/ncidod/dpd/parasites/scabies/factsht_scabies.htm.

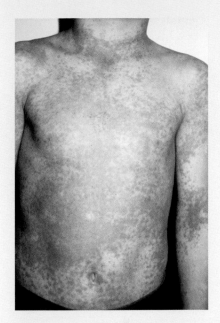

▲

The scarlet fever rash is caused by the streptococcus bacterium. *Biophoto Associate/Photo Researchers, Inc.*

* **antibiotic** (an-tie-by-AH-tiks) are drugs that kill or slow the growth of bacteria.

Scarlet Fever

Scarlet fever is a bacterial infection that causes a sore throat, rash, and chills.

Once Dreaded

The disease "scarlet fever" once was dreaded by many people. The bacteria that cause scarlet fever are easy to spread, and in the 1800s there were epidemics. Children younger than 10 years of age were especially at risk of serious complications, such as rheumatic fever, or death. Scarlet fever

---

POOR BETH

Louisa May Alcott's novel *Little Women* is based on the author's own growing-up years. It is the story of Jo March and her sisters, Meg, Amy, and Beth. Immensely popular since its publication in 1868, the novel bas been made into a movie at least five times.

In the book, Beth, beloved by family and friends for her sweet nature and musical talent, develops scarlet fever when the girls' mother is away caring for their father, who has been injured in the Civil War. Alcott captures the fear and tragedy that scarlet fever caused in the 1800s in a description of the dark days in the March household. Although at first Beth seems to recover, her illness progresses to rheumatic fever and she dies of congestive heart failure.

---

was also a mysterious disease because it would infect only some members of a family and not others. A good example of scarlet fever's effect can be found in the 1868 book *Little Women*.

By the early 2000s scarlet fever was not as deadly because antibiotics were available to fight the streptococcal bacteria that causes the infection.

A Sore Throat that Gets Worse

Scarlet fever is caused by exposure to someone who is infected with streptococcal bacteria. People with strep infection can spread it by sneezing or coughing. It can also be spread by sharing drinking glasses or eating utensils with people who are infected.

The first signs of scarlet fever usually appear within a week of exposure to the strep bacteria. A sore throat develops, which is called strep throat. But in some people, the particular kind of strep bacteria, known as Group A streptococcus, causes a toxic reaction. A skin rash appears within one or two days of the sore throat. It looks like a sunburn on the neck, chest, and underarms. Less often the rash can appear on the face or the groin. The skin feels rough, like sandpaper. Within a week, the rash usually starts to fade, and flaking and peeling of the skin occur.

Scarlet fever also causes a fever with temperatures of more than 101 degrees Fahrenheit. Glands around the jaw and neck swell and are painful. Chills, nausea, and vomiting can result.

In rare cases, scarlet fever also can result from a skin infection known as impetigo*.

Without medical treatment, strep throat and scarlet fever can be serious. A doctor who suspects a strep infection uses a cotton swab to get a bit of the bacteria from the throat for laboratory testing to confirm that it is streptococcal bacteria. Treatment with antibiotics for 10 days usually kills the bacteria.

* **parasitic** (pair-uh-SIH-tik) refers to organisms such as protozoa (one-celled animals), worms, or insects that can invade and live on or inside human beings and may cause illness. An animal or plant harboring a parasite is called its host.

* **infestations** refer to illnesses caused by multi-celled parasitic organisms, such as tapeworms, roundworms, or protozoa.

SCARLET FEVER IN HISTORY

The earliest description of scarlet fever and its symptoms was given by the German physiologist Daniel Sennert (1572–1637). In 1619 Sennert accurately observed and recorded the sequence of the disease's symptoms: the appearance of the rash, its decline, and scaling of the skin.

In the eighteenth century, epidemics of scarlet fever were reported throughout Europe and the United States. During this time, physicians developed their clinical understanding of the disease. The first clinical standards for differentiating scarlet fever from similar diseases were established by Armand Trousseau (1801–1867).

In 1887 the English physician Edmund Emmanuel Klein identified scarlet fever as being caused by streptococcus bacteria that were observed to grow on the tonsils and secrete a rash-producing toxin.

The American physician George Frederick Dick (1881–1967) and his wife Gladys R. H. Dick (1881–1963) isolated the toxin in the 1920s. After World War II, penicillin became available as an effective means of curing the disease.

▶ *See also* **Rheumatic Fever • Sore Throat/Strep Throat**

Resources

Books and Articles

Alcott, Louisa May. *Little Women, or, Meg, Jo, Beth, and Amy.* Boston: Roberts Brothers, 1868.

Organization

Centers for Disease Control and Prevention. 1600 Clifton Road, Atlanta, GA, 30333. Toll free: 800-311-3435. Web site: http://www. cdc.gov/ncidod/DBMD/diseaseinfo/scarletfever_g.htm.

Schistosomiasis

Schistosomiasis (shis-tuh-so-MY-uh-sis) is an illness caused by parasitic* worms. The worms must spend part of their life cycle growing in freshwater snails before they enter and cause infestations* in humans.

What Is Schistosomiasis?

Schistosomiasis is a parasitic disease that is not directly contagious from person to person. Five types of *Schistosoma* worm, also called blood flukes, can infest people and cause schistosomiasis. *S. mansoni, S japonicum,*

Schistosoma japonicum; (left) and *Schistosoma mansoni* (right). These parasites can enter the human body through the skin then develop into an adult worm in the bloodstream. *Custom Medical Stock Photo, Inc. Reproduced by permission.*

▶

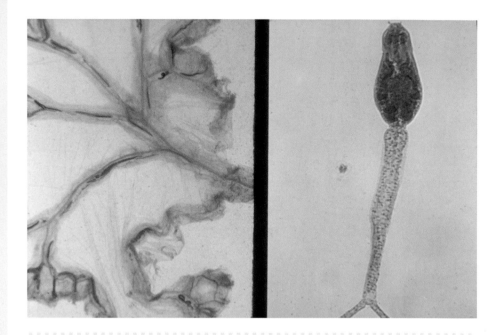

* **larva** (LAR-vuh) is the immature form of an insect or worm that hatches from an egg.

* **intestines** are the muscular tubes that food passes through during digestion after it exits the stomach.

S. mekongi, S. intercalatum, and *S. haematobium.* These parasites have a complex life cycle; they have to go through several separate stages on their way to adulthood, and both snails and humans play important roles in that cycle. Another name for the disease is bilharziasis (bil-har-ZYE-uh-sis) or "snail fever."

The worm starts life as an egg in a freshwater source such as a pond, lake, or stream. It hatches into a larva*. This larva, known as a miracidium (meer-uh-SID-ee-um), swims around until it locates a certain type of aquatic snail that lives in that water (the type of snail depends on the particular species of the parasite). The miracidium then penetrates the tissue of the snail. Once inside the snail, it passes through several stages of development, eventually multiplying into numerous larvae, called cercariae (sir-CARE-ee-ay), that leave the snail and swim through the water for up to two days. During that time, one or more may come into contact with a person who is bathing, wading, swimming, or washing clothes in the water. At that point, the parasite may burrow into bare skin and enter the bloodstream. Once it is in the person's blood, it matures into an adult worm.

The female adult worms lay their eggs within blood vessels. Where this occurs depends on the species of the worm. For instance, *S. japonicum* usually lays its eggs in vessels near the small intestine; *S. mansoni* usually lays them near the large intestine; and *S. haematobium* prefers blood vessels near the bladder. However, this pattern of behavior is not always followed, and eggs from the different species sometimes show up elsewhere in the human body. The eggs from all species gradually move to the urinary tract, liver, or intestines*, and finally leave the body in the person's urine or feces. If feces (excreted waste) or urine from an infested person contaminate a freshwater source such as a pond, the eggs can enter the water and begin the life cycle all over again.

How Common Is Schistosomiasis?

Schistosomiasis does not occur in the United States, but it does have a major impact on millions of people who live in developing countries around the world. According to the World Health Organization, 200 million people worldwide are infested with the worms, with perhaps 20 million of those having serious symptoms, and an estimated 200,000 dying every year as a result.

The disease is most common in tropical regions, where it is a leading cause of illness. *S. japonicum* occurs in China, the Philippines and other parts of the Far East; *S. mansoni* in certain regions of Africa, the Middle East, South America and the Caribbean; *S. haematobium* in Africa and the Middle East; *S. mekongi* in Cambodia and other parts of Southeast Asia; and *S. intercalatum* mainly in the Democratic Republic of Congo and other parts of West Africa. People from the United States who travel to these areas sometimes develop schistosomiasis if they swim or wade in tainted water, but they rarely get the severe, chronic* form of the disease.

What Are the Signs and Symptoms of Schistosomiasis?

A rash and itchy skin, particularly at the spot where the parasite burrowed into the body, may develop within a few days. Symptoms vary from person to person and may not even occur in some infected individuals. The symptoms also vary depending on the species of worm that has infected the person. The most common initial symptoms, however, appear about one to two months after the initial infestation and include muscle aches, fever, chills, and cough.

Certain other symptoms are associated with infections from different species. Infection with *Schistosoma mansoni*, for instance, sometimes causes such symptoms as nausea with blood in the vomit, lesions on the spinal cord, and/or an enlarged liver and spleen. *S. haematobium* infections can cause spinal cord lesions, frequent and/or painful urination, blood in the urine, and pain in the area of the anus and genital organs. Individuals infected with *S. japonicum* may experience nausea with blood in the vomit, a certain type of seizure known as focal epilepsy, and an enlarged liver and spleen. People who are infected with *S. japonicum* often also develop a fever, called Katayama fever, that can cause the body temperature to rise to 105 degrees Fahrenheit. The fever, which is sometimes also seen in *S. mansoni* infestations, may last several weeks, but it usually subsides on its own.

How Do Doctors Diagnose and Treat Schistosomiasis?

If the doctor suspects schistosomiasis, he or she examines a urine or stool (feces) sample taken from the patient to look for the worm's eggs. The doctor may need to examine several samples to identify the worms. He or she also may take a sample of blood for testing, although the blood

The United States and the World

Schistosomiasis is a leading cause of illness in tropical regions. About 200 million people worldwide are infected, and approximately 20 million of them suffer severe consequences of schistosomiasis. WHO estimates that about 85 percent of all the people infected with schistosomiasis live in sub-Saharan Africa. The infection leads to an estimated 200,000 deaths each year. U.S. residents can get schistosomiasis when traveling to other countries where the disease occurs.

In many parts of the world, people have no way of knowing whether a particular body of water is contaminated with blood fluke larvae. Medical professionals advise people to avoid any contact with fresh water in areas where *Schistosoma* are known to occur. Swimming in ocean water and chlorinated pools is generally considered safe.

* **chronic** (KRAH-nik) lasting a long time or recurring frequently.

* **biopsy** (BI-op-see) is a test in which a small sample of skin or other body tissue is removed and examined for signs of disease.

* **cirrhosis** (sir-O-sis) is a condition that affects the liver, involving long-term inflammation and scarring, which can lead to problems with liver function.

* **esophagus** (eh-SAH-fuh-gus) is the soft tube that, with swallowing, carries food from the throat to the stomach.

* **seizures** (SEE-zhurs) are sudden bursts of disorganized electrical activity that interrupt the normal functioning of the brain, often leading to uncontrolled movements in the body and sometimes a temporary change in consciousness.

* **paralysis** (pah-RAH-luh-sis) is the loss or impairment of the ability to move some part of the body.

test may not show evidence of the infestation unless it is done six to eight weeks after the patient's contact with the parasite. Occasionally, the doctor will order a tissue biopsy* to check for signs of the parasite in organs such as the liver.

Doctors may prescribe the drug praziquantel to treat the infestation. Patients usually need to take pills for only one to two days. For individuals who do not receive treatment and who continue to use the same tainted water source, the illness can last for years.

Can Schistosomiasis Cause Complications?

People who become repeatedly infested with schistosomiasis over many years can experience damage to the bladder, lungs, intestines, and liver. The disease is one of the leading causes of cirrhosis* in the world. In some cases, the resulting scarring of the liver is so severe that blood flowing through the organ becomes partly blocked, causing a condition known as portal hypertension. Severe portal hypertension can make veins in the esophagus* and stomach swell and bleed, sometimes to the point that the bleeding is fatal.

Other complications of the disease arise when the worm's eggs travel through the bloodstream to the spinal cord or brain, where they can cause seizures*, inflammation of the spinal cord, or paralysis*.

How Can Schistosomiasis Be Prevented?

Travelers visiting countries where schistosomiasis occurs should avoid wading, swimming, or bathing in any body of fresh water such as ponds, rivers, or lakes. Filtering or boiling drinking water for at least one minute kills parasites, including the *Schistosoma* worms. The Centers for Disease Control and Prevention recommends heating bathing water to 150 degrees Fahrenheit for at least five minutes to make sure it is free of potential parasites.

To reduce the spread of schistosomiasis, health officials focus on educating people who live in areas where the worms are found. They teach the public how the parasites spread and encourage people not to urinate or have bowel movements in rivers and ponds. In addition, some countries have mounted extensive campaigns to reduce the worm population in their streams. A program in Japan, for instance, used several means to eliminate *S. japonicum* from the country. One method was to encourage farmers to use horses instead of water buffalo when they were tending their rice paddies. The worms can enter these animals as they do humans, but horses are much less susceptible to the worms than water buffalo are.

A program in China includes several strategies. One of these involves the mass treatment of people and susceptible animals in certain regions with praziquantel. Another one involved the lowering of water levels in many streams and ponds to reduce the snails that are hosts during part of the worms' life cycle. Some earlier programs included the application of snail-destroying chemicals to streams, but scientists later discovered that many of those chemicals had unintended consequences, such as killing fish. China's schistosomiasis-reduction program was quite successful, but suffered a setback after extreme flooding along the Yangtze River in 1998 brought water levels up again. This rise in the water allowed the snails to repopulate and resulted in an outbreak in 2004 when about 850,000 people were infected. Control efforts in China continued as of 2008.

▶ *See also* **Intestinal Parasites • Parasitic Diseases: Overview • Zoonoses**

Resources

Organizations

Centers for Disease Control and Prevention. 1600 Clifton Road, Atlanta, GA, 30333. Toll free: 800-311-3435. Web site: http://www.cdc.gov/ncidod/dpd/parasites/schistosomiasis/default.htm.

World Health Organization. Avenue Appia 20, CH - 1211 Geneva 27, Switzerland. Telephone: +41 22 791 2111. Web site: http://www.who.int/topics/schistosomiasis/en.

Schizophrenia

Schizophrenia is a neurological disorder that is characterized by specific behaviors including: psychotic episodes, delusions, paranoia, and difficulty perceiving reality. Schizophrenia is treated with medication and psychotherapy.

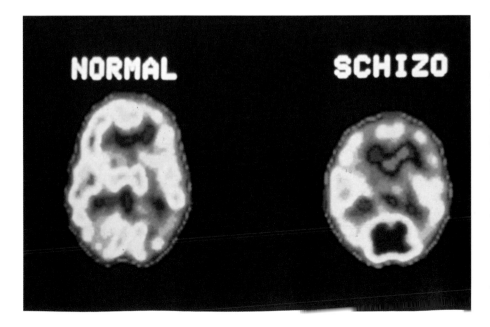

Positron emission tomography (PET) scans are computer-generated images of brain activity. When compared with PET scans of healthy people (left), the scans of people with schizophrenia (right) show disruptions in brain activity, changes in brain structures such as the ventricles, and decreased function in the frontal cortex. The red area in the brain on the right shows intense activity. *Photo Researchers, Inc.*

* **delusions** (de-LOO-zhuns) are false beliefs or judgment that remain even in the face of proof that they are not true.

* **paranoia** (pair-a-NOY-a) refers to either an unreasonable fear of harm by others (delusions of persecution) or an unrealistic sense of self-importance (delusions of grandeur).

* **genetic** (juh-NEH-tik) refers to heredity and the ways in which genes control the development and maintenance of organisms.

* **antipsychotic drugs** are medications that counteract or reduce the symptoms of a severe mental disorder such as schizophrenia.

Definition

Schizophrenia is a serious neurological disorder of unknown cause that is characterized by specific behaviors. Typical behavior seen in schizophrenia includes psychotic episodes, delusions*, paranoia*, and difficulty perceiving reality. Schizophrenia has a genetic* component, but many other factors are thought to be involved. Schizophrenia is treated with antipsychotic drugs* medication.

What Are Neurotransmitters?

The brain is a complex organ that functions through electrical and chemical signals. The substances that perform the chemical signaling are called neurotransmitters. There are many types of neurotransmitters, and they have distinct functions and locations for signaling within the brain. Neurotransmitters act on brain cells known as neurons. Neurons in different parts of the brain perform different functions and use neurotransmitters to communicate with each other. Neurotransmitters are passed from one neuron to another. The neuron receiving the chemical neurotransmitter signal has physical docks for the neurotransmitters known as neurotransmitter receptors. A neurotransmitter cannot perform its chemical signaling function without a receptor through which to act. Both proper levels of neurotransmitters and functional neurotransmitter receptors are necessary for successful signaling. Blocking a neurotransmitter from interacting with its receptor blocks that chemical signaling pathway. Blocking a neurotransmitter receptor is known as antagonizing the receptor.

Because areas of the brain need to interact with each other via these chemical signals, neuronal pathways are formed during fetal development that act as communication highways. Each neuronal pathway uses specific neurotransmitters to accomplish successful brain functioning. A disruption in the physical neuronal pathway such as the loss of neuron cells or the loss of communication between neurons may cause mental diseases such as schizophrenia. Additionally, an increase or decrease in the neurotransmitter chemical signals present in these pathways may also cause symptoms such as behavioral changes or neurological disorders and disease. Schizophrenia may be caused by both physical damage to certain groups of neurons in the brain and alteration of specific types of neurotransmitter signaling.

What Is Schizophrenia?

Schizophrenia involves a specific type of disordered thinking and behavior. It could be described as the splitting of the cognitive functions of the mind from the appropriate emotional responses. Family history of schizophrenia increases the chance of having the disease, but the exact way it is inherited is unknown. Only some schizophrenic patients have detectable anatomical brain abnormalities. The cause of schizophrenia had not been determined as of the early 2000s, yet drugs effective in its treatment had been identified. Schizophrenia is treated with antipsychotic drugs that primarily act on receptors in the brain for the neurotransmitters dopamine* and serotonin*. By inhibiting the activity of these receptors, antipsychotics are effective at decreasing some of the bizarre behavior typical of schizophrenia. Unfortunately this medication often also has severe negative side effects, mostly affecting movement.

How Many People Develop Schizophrenia?

Schizophrenia is estimated to afflict 1 percent of the world's population. Approximately 3 million people have schizophrenia in the United States. First-degree relatives (such as siblings and parents) of a person with the disease have approximately a 10 percent chance of developing it. Fraternal twins (twins that do not have identical genes*) have approximately a 10 to 12 percent chance, and children of two schizophrenic parents have about a 40 percent chance. However, the disease is not caused entirely by genetic factors. Because identical twins* have only a 30 to 50 percent tendency to have the same schizophrenic illness, scientists know other factors determine who develops the disease. Schizophrenia occurs equally in males and females. The disease may be seen at any age, but people who begin treatment are generally between 28 to 34 years of age. Schizophrenia is associated with low economic status, probably due to a lack of proper maternal healthcare during fetal development.

What Causes Schizophrenia?

The cause of schizophrenia is unknown. Some patients have physical changes associated with the disease, including wasting of specific areas of the brain, enlargement of the ventricles* (normal spaces in the brain), and loss of neurons. Neurotransmitter signaling is often changed too, specifically regarding the neurotransmitter pathways for dopamine and serotonin. The imbalance in the activities of these pathways is complex: Overactivity in some parts of the brain and decreased activity in other areas cause different symptoms. The symptoms of schizophrenia are divided into three types, the positive, negative, and cognitive.

What Are the Symptoms of Schizophrenia?

Positive Symptoms   Positive symptoms mark the presence of distinctive behaviors. There are many different positive symptoms of schizophrenia. Schizophrenic patients may experience strange or paranoid delusions. They may believe that they are being persecuted by others or having their minds controlled by others. Positive symptoms may include disturbing or frightening hallucinations. The most common hallucinations are auditory (heard), but visual hallucinations may also occur. Other positive symptoms include sensitivity to and fear regarding ordinary sights, sounds, or smells; agitation; tension; and insomnia*.

Negative symptoms   Negative symptoms mark the absence of normal social and interpersonal behaviors. There are various negative symptoms

* **dopamine** (DOE-puh-meen) is a neurotransmitter in the brain that is involved in the brain structures that control motor activity (movement).

* **serotonin** (ser-o-TO-nin) is a neurotransmitter, a substance that helps transmit information from one nerve cell to another.

* **genes** (JEENS) are the functional units of heredity that are that are composed of deoxyribonucleic acid (DNA) and help to determine a person' body structure and physical characteristics. Inherited from a person's parents, genes are segments of chromosomes found in the nuclei of the body's cells.

* **identical twins** are twins produced when a single egg from the mother is fertilized and divides to form two separate embryos of the same sex with nearly identical DNA.

* **ventricle** open cavities within the brain that contain the fluid that cushions and protects the central nervous system.

* **insomnia** abnormal inability to get adequate sleep.

* **bipolar disorder** a group of mood disorders that are characterized by alternating episodes of depression and mania.

* **antidepressant medications** are used for the treatment and prevention of depression.

* **psychiatrists** (sy-KY-uh-trist) are medical doctors who have completed specialized training in the diagnosis and treatment of mental illness. Psychiatrists can diagnose mental illnesses, provide mental health counseling, and prescribe medications.

of schizophrenia. Schizophrenic patients are often less able to experience appropriate emotions or express their emotions. This reduced expression is known as a blunted affect. Because they respond less and have less desire to interact with others, these patients often withdraw from others. Other negative symptoms may also include a lack of motivation, energy, and ability to experience pleasure. Schizophrenic patients speak less and avoid speaking to others.

Cognitive symptoms Schizophrenic patients may have confused thinking and speech, which makes it difficult for them to communicate effectively with others. Fractured (broken or fragmented) thoughts and communication are considered types of disorganized cognitive symptoms. Individuals with schizophrenia often seem to lose their train of thought and combine unrelated topics in a way that prevents a coherent conversation. Disorganized behaviors such as unnecessary, repetitive movements are also common. Schizophrenics often seem restless or hyperactive. They may have difficulty paying attention or maintaining an organized lifestyle.

How Is Schizophrenia Diagnosed?

Schizophrenics often first give what are known as prodromal signs, or signs preceding a psychotic episode. Schizophrenic prodromal signs may include social isolation, odd behavior, lack of personal hygiene, and blunted emotions. The prodromal phase is followed by one or more separate psychotic episodes. Physicians examining their behavior patterns first attempt to rule out disorders of mood that respond to antidepressants, such as bipolar disorder*. Sometimes schizophrenia is diagnosed through the patient's response to different therapeutic regimens. Schizophrenic symptoms are not affected by antidepressant medications*, but they are relieved by antipsychotics.

Once other disorders have been excluded the criteria for a diagnosis of schizophrenia is that a patient be continuously ill for at least six months and that there be one psychotic phase followed by one phase of odd behavior. During the psychotic phase, one or more of three groups of psychotic symptoms must be present. The three groups are delusions, hallucinations, and a disordered or incoherent thought pattern.

How Is Schizophrenia Treated?

Schizophrenic patients are diagnosed and treated by psychiatrists*. A licensed therapist may perform rehabilitation therapy to help a schizophrenic patient function during times when they are not in a psychotic episode. Treatment teams from supportive agencies may help with everyday living. Schizophrenia is treated with antipsychotic drugs used in the lowest effective doses. The antipsychotic drugs work mainly to antagonize (inhibit) dopamine and serotonin receptors in specific areas of the brain that are in dysfunction. Earlier antipsychotic medicines functioned primarily on dopamine receptors and had more side effects than later medications that also work on serotonin receptors. The older medications sometimes caused serious side effects such as severe, involuntary, repetitive movements of the face, arms, and legs (called tardive dyskinesia). The later medications do not have such troubling side effects. Positive symptoms of schizophrenia respond better to antipsychotic medications than the negative symptoms.

Although antipsychotic drug treatment is necessary for schizophrenic patients, it is not enough. Patients also require supportive psychotherapy*. Various psychosocial treatments are available for varying stages in the disease, and each patient requires a unique treatment regimen. Doctor and therapist appointments for medication management and psychological support are necessary in all stages of recovery, even when symptoms are under control. Peer support groups are also important. Assertive community treatment (ACT) programs are available for more severely affected patients. These programs may provide intensive services within a patient's home on a day-to-day basis. ACT teams can follow patients through all courses of their illness and assist them in normal living activities. Patients who are in the later stages of recovery and have few lingering symptoms may get involved with programs designed to help them achieve personal goals pertaining to work, education, and social interactions.

What Is the Prognosis for Schizophrenia?

The prognosis for schizophrenia varies according to each case. A diagnosis of schizophrenia does not necessarily mean that a person will experience a life-long illness. Over a period of 25 to 30 years approximately one-third of schizophrenic patients experience remission or even partial recovery. Some individuals lose their severe symptoms or learn to live acceptably with some minor symptoms. However, schizophrenia can be a severe and even dangerous disorder. A wide range of outcomes has been reported, including episodes of violence or severe incapacity. Quite a few schizophrenic patients are at risk for suicide. Suicide, accidents, and disease are common among patients with schizophrenia, along with an approximate 10-year decrease in life span. Typically, individuals have episodes of psychosis and episodes of remission*, with the outcome dependent on how effectively the medicine keep the patient in periods of remission and how well the patient is able to deal with the symptoms still associated with these periods.

What Special Concerns Exist for Schizophrenia?

One concern for these patients is that they may not go along with the treatment medical professionals say they need. Some patients may not remain in close contact with their treatment team, they may not take all their medications consistently, and they may not keep all their appointments. Schizophrenic patients are notorious for not being compliant with their necessary medications, either because they feel they have improved and no longer need medication or because they want to avoid the side effects it causes. Unfortunately, without proper and consistent drug intervention psychotic episodes are highly likely to recur.

* **psychotherapy** (sy-ko-THER-a-pea) is the treatment of mental and behavioral disorders by support and insight to encourage healthy behavior patterns and personality growth.

* **remission** is an easing of a disease or its symptoms for a prolonged period.

Resources

Books and Articles

DeLisi, Lynn E. *100 Questions and Answers about Schizophrenia: Painful Minds.* Sudbury, MA: Jones and Bartlett, 2006.

McIntosh, Kenneth, and Phyllis Livingston. *Youth with Juvenile Schizophrenia: The Search for Reality.* Philadelphia, PA: Mason Crest, 2008.

Saks, Elyn R. *The Centre Cannot Hold: A Memoir of My Schizophrenia.* London: Virago, 2007.

Torrey, E. Fuller. *Surviving Schizophrenia: A Manual for Families, Patients, and Providers,* 5th ed. New York: Collins, 2006.

Veague, Heather Barnett. *Schizophrenia.* New York: Chelsea House, 2007.

Organizations

National Alliance on Mental Illness. Colonial Place Three, 2107 Wilson Boulevard, Suite 300, Arlington, VA, 22201-3042. Toll free: 800-950-6264. Web site: http://www.nami.org.

National Hopeline Network Crisis and Suicide Prevention Center. Kristin Brooks Hope Center, 1250 Twenty-fourth Street NW, Suite 300, Washington, DC, 20037. Toll free: 800-784-2433. Web site: http://www.hopeline.com.

National Institute of Mental Health. Science Writing, Press, and Dissemination Branch, 6001 Executive Boulevard, Room 8184, MSC 9663, Bethesda, MD, 20892-9663. Toll free: 866-615-6464. Web site: http://www.nimh.nih.gov.

National Mental Health Association. 2000 N. Beauregard Street, 6th Floor, Alexandria, VA, 22311. Toll free: 800-969-6642. Web site: http://nmha.org.

National Mental Health Consumer Self Help Clearinghouse. 1211 Chestnut Street, Suite 1207, Philadelphia, PA, 19107. Toll free: 800-553-4539. Web site: http://www.mhselfhelp.org.

School Avoidance

School avoidance occurs when children and teens repeatedly stay home from school or are repeatedly sent home from school, due to emotional problems or because of aches and pains that are caused by emotions or stress and not by medical illness.

Ben's Story

Ben missed a lot of school because of his stomachaches. His stomach felt especially bad on Monday mornings. Often, while he was getting dressed for school, he felt as if he might throw up. His mother did not want him to go to school if he was sick. On days he stayed home, Ben got back into bed, and by lunchtime he felt much better. But by the next morning, he felt miserable all over again. He managed to get himself to school sometimes, but it was getting harder and harder. He would be embarrassed if he threw up on the bus. Ben's doctor had examined him and found him to be in excellent health despite his stomach pains. Still his stomachaches continued, and Ben's mother had started to worry about how many school days he was missing.

What Is School Avoidance?

School avoidance is a condition that occurs in up to 5 percent of schoolchildren and adolescents, with boys and girls equally affected. Sometimes school avoidance is called school "phobia*" (FO-bee-a) or school refusal. School avoidance is a pattern of missing school for symptoms that are caused by emotions or stress, rather than physical illness. School avoidance is different from truancy (TROO-an-see), which is a pattern of repeated unexcused absences from school. The student who is truant, or skips school, is neither at home nor at school. In school avoidance, the student stays home.

What Causes School Avoidance?

There are two main reasons students have school avoidance. One reason is that the student feels anxiety (ang-ZY-eh-tee), fear, or worry about some aspect of going to school or about leaving home. The other reason is that there is some benefit, or a secondary gain, to staying home from school.

Anxiety-related school avoidance   Most children have some anxiety about attending school for the first time, which is known as "separation anxiety." It is not surprising when separation anxiety occurs when a child is about to enter kindergarten or first grade. For many children this is the first time they are away from home or separated from their parents. But some children have separation anxiety that lasts beyond the expected age. Children who have recently been through other difficult separations, such as divorce or the death of a parent or the illness of a family member, may have an especially difficult time leaving home to go to school.

Children with school avoidance may have headaches, stomachaches, chest pain, or other symptoms brought on by the stress of separation. These pains are real, but they are caused by the body's response to stress and not by an illness. Usually, a checkup by the doctor finds the child or teen to be in good physical health. Students with anxiety-related school avoidance are often good students and like school, but because of their stress-related symptoms, they feel that they need to stay home.

Some students with school avoidance may have anxiety about school itself. They may worry about grades, about being bullied, about being called on in class by the teacher, or about having to undress for gym.

* **phobia** is an intense, persistent, unreasonable fear of (and avoidance of) a particular thing or situation.

Some schools have rules about when students may use the bathroom, and this may be a worry to children who may need to go more often. Dirty school bathrooms without enough privacy or issues about safety may be real concerns for some children.

In many cases, anxiety-related school avoidance begins with an upsetting event that happens at school, for example, being teased or experiencing something disturbing in class. Students who are shy and sensitive by nature and those who have an overprotective parent may be more likely to have anxiety-related school avoidance.

Secondary-gain school avoidance Not all children and teens with school avoidance are anxious or shy. Some may simply find that it is more comfortable staying home than attending school.which is called secondary-gain school avoidance. "Secondary gain" refers to the bonus or positive side of something unpleasant. For example, although it is unpleasant to be sick, it may be pleasant to watch television during the day and to have meals in bed. Another secondary gain of being sick might be not having to do homework or having the personal attention and care of a parent at home.

Secondary-gain school avoidance often starts with an illness that lasts for a few days and causes the student to miss school. The student may get behind in homework and begin to think about how hard it will be to catch up. To avoid the hard work ahead, the student may stretch out the illness a bit longer. Receiving the secondary gains of sympathy, the care and attention of parents, and the pleasure of watching daytime television can contribute to school avoidance. Lenient parents or parents who do not view school as important can contribute to secondary-gain school avoidance. Sometimes students exaggerate symptoms or claim to have symptoms they really do not have (such as a sore throat or leg pain) just to avoid school.

How Is School Avoidance Diagnosed?

School avoidance is diagnosed when a student has repeatedly missed school due to aches and pains or other symptoms, and a careful checkup by the doctor has found the student to be in good health. The doctor will check for school avoidance by evaluating the pattern of symptoms and asking about stresses. The doctor may explain how stress can cause certain physical symptoms and may have the student keep track of symptoms by writing them down.

Ben's doctor asked him about recent worries he had. Ben mentioned that since his parents had divorced the previous year and his dad had moved across town, he had started to worry about his mom being lonely. He had seen her cry a lot this year, and it made him sad. He said he missed his dad and wished they could be a family again, but without the arguing. Although he looked forward to the weekends he spent with his dad, he was sad that his mom had to spend weekends alone. Ben's doctor explained how people could get stomachaches from stress and sadness. She asked Ben to keep track of his stomachaches in a diary, and she told him to go to school anyway. She gave Ben and his mom the name of a therapist who would help Ben talk about his feelings and about how to adjust to all the changes in his family.

How Is School Avoidance Treated?

The first step in treating school avoidance is to help the student get back to school as soon as possible. The longer a student avoids school, the harder it is to return. Students with anxiety usually need reassurance that they are in good health. Students and their parents are helped by taking a "yes but" approach. Yes, the symptoms are real, but they are not a reason to miss school. Parents are guided about what symptoms are grounds to stay home and find ways to help their student attend school despite discomfort caused by aches and pains. The treatment often includes a plan for what to do when the student begins to feel ill at school. The plan may be for the student to go to the nurse's office to lie down for 5 to 10 minutes and then return to class, but not to go home. Psychotherapy and behavioral techniques to cope with school-related stress are often helpful.

Another part of treatment may involve working with school personnel to solve problems that are causing anxiety, such as bullying* or lack of privacy in bathrooms. Students who have separation anxiety or generalized worry may benefit from counseling to learn to cope with painful feelings or loss. The usual treatment for students with secondary-gain school avoidance is also to return to school right away. Clear limits, appropriate expectations, and support for regular school attendance are critical factors for successfully addressing the problem.

▶ *See also* **Anxiety and Anxiety Disorders • Conversion Disorder • School Failure • Somatoform Disorders • Stress and Stress-Related Illness**

Resources

Organizations

American Academy of Pediatrics. 141 Northwest Point Boulevard, Elk Grove Village, IL, 60007-1098. Telephone: 847-434-4000. Web site: http://www.aap.org/publiced/BK5_SchoolAvoid.htm.

* **bullying** is when a person repeatedly intimidates or acts aggressively toward those with less power or ability to defend themselves.

School Failure

School failure is the inability to meet the minimum academic standards of an educational institution.

School Failure Defined

School failure is a process in which a student slips farther and farther behind his peers and gradually disconnects from the educational system. The end result of school failure is dropping out before graduation. Many cases of school failure occur among students who have the ability and intelligence to succeed but who are unable or unwilling to apply these abilities in the school setting.

Students can begin the slide into failing patterns at any time during their school career, but school failure is more likely to occur at transitional stages, such as when graduating from elementary to middle school or after a family move to a new school system. Failing grades typically are symptoms of emotional, behavioral, or learning problems. In the United States, an estimated 10 to 15 percent of students fail at school.

Why Do People Fail in School?

People who fail in school may feel stupid, but emotional or mental health problems and unidentified learning disorders, rather than low intelligence, often are the causes of their inability to meet the standards of a school. There are several factors that can lead to school failure, among them depression, anxiety, problems in the family, and learning disabilities.

Depression   Depression is one of the most common causes of school difficulties. The condition makes people feel sad for long periods of time, have low energy, and lose interest in activities that normally give them pleasure. People with depression have continuing negative thoughts about themselves and the future, and they may experience changes in eating and sleeping patterns and in their ability to concentrate and make decisions. They may feel hopeless and may even think about suicide. Depression has been shown to be a leading cause of school failure in young people with learning disabilities. Depression can also cause school failure in students without learning disabilities.

Anxiety   Anxiety is a feeling of excessive worry about a possible danger or situation that is intense enough to interfere with a person's ability to concentrate and focus. Students can have genuine reasons to be anxious. People who have been bullied at school may worry that they will be bullied again. Students may legitimately fear personal violence on the way to or from school. They might worry about their families going through a divorce or about a parent who is ill. Ordinary adolescent worries about looking right and fitting in can be blown so far out of proportion that a student may try to be absent from school just to avoid a possibly embarrassing or uncomfortable situation. This is called "school avoidance." Anxiety in any of its forms can interfere with a student's performance in school.

Problems in the family   Students also may bring their problems at home to school with them. If a student's family is experiencing violence, unemployment, alcohol or drug use by a family member, problems with the law, or any other upsetting problems, the student may have difficulty concentrating on schoolwork. Many students who are having family problems might have trouble controlling their anger and frustration at school, and they may end up in trouble because of their behavior. Some students who are overburdened at home by circumstances that make it necessary for them to "parent" siblings, hold a job, or care for an ill or impaired parent may find it impossible to keep up in school. Many times students who face overwhelming family or personal problems keep these problems to themselves. School counselors can offer help and prevent student failure if they are made aware of the problem.

Learning disabilities Learning disabilities are conditions that interfere with gaining specific academic skills, such as reading or writing. Learning disorders can hinder a person's ability to concentrate or to process or remember information. When these difficulties are recognized early, certain teaching strategies can help a student overcome the learning disability. Unfortunately, many learning problems may go undiagnosed or may be diagnosed incorrectly as behavior problems. The frustration and depression that can result from undetected learning disabilities is a major cause of school failure or dropping out of school.

Other causes Many social factors can increase the risk of school failure. These include homelessness, poverty, frequent transfers from school to school, and the inability to speak English. Other circumstances such as truancy*, teenage pregnancy, and chronic illness* may also affect a student's ability to perform well in school.

Helping People at Risk of School Failure

Students at risk of school failure need to be identified as early as possible in their school careers if they are to receive the necessary help. This task usually falls to the teacher, school counselor, or parents, because many failing students are hostile to or disconnected from the educational system and will not or do not know how to ask for help. Bringing failing students back to school and fostering their success requires recognizing and understanding the reasons for school failure. Parents, teachers, counselors, and mental health professionals can offer help.

Parents can help by taking the following steps:

- Taking a genuine interest in their child's school life and attending school events
- Listening to and understanding their child's concerns about school
- Taking seriously sudden changes in behavior, sleeping, or eating
- Intervening for the student when unsafe situations are causing anxiety or school avoidance
- Setting and enforcing appropriate standards of school behavior
- Setting realistic goals for school attendance and academic improvement
- Eliminating barriers to homework completion and school attendance
- Working as a team with teachers and counselors to get children appropriate help

* **truancy** is staying out of school without permission.

* **chronic illness** (KRAH-nik) is an illness with symptoms that last a long time or that recur frequently.

■ Helping children identify their strengths and pinpointing career options that involve these strengths

■ Getting help in recognizing the reasons for school failure

Teachers can help by taking the following steps:

■ Developing learning plans that support the student's strengths

■ Referring the student for evaluations for possible learning disabilities

■ Providing referrals to programs that offer extra academic help or arranging peer tutoring

■ Teaching study skills and strategies to support learning

■ Encouraging students to participate in school activities, such as sports, plays, or clubs, so that they feel they are a part of the school

■ Arranging a mentor for the student

■ Promoting a tolerant, violence-free school environment

■ Communicating concerns or changes in school performance to parents right away

Mental health professionals can help by taking the following steps:

■ Screening for emotional problems and offering appropriate treatment

■ Listening to the student's concerns about family and school difficulties

■ Performing evaluations for learning disabilities or attention deficit hyperactivity disorder

■ Working with the school to formulate appropriate learning strategies for the student

■ Working with teachers and parents to help them eliminate barriers to school failure

▶ See also **Attention Deficit Hyperactivity Disorder (ADHD)** • **Learning Disabilities** • **School Avoidance**

Resources

Books and Articles

Espeland, Pamela, and Elizabeth Verdick. *Loving to Learn: The Commitment to Learning Assets.* Minneapolis, MN: Free Spirit, 2005.

How to Study for Success. Hoboken, NJ: Wiley, 2004.

Spevak, Peter A., and Maryann Karinch. *Empowering Underachievers: New Strategies to Guide Kids (8–18) to Personal Excellence,* rev. and expanded ed. Far Hills, NJ: New Horizon Press, 2006.

Organization

Center for Effective Collaboration and Practice. 1000 Thomas Jefferson Street, Suite 400, Washington, DC, 20007. Toll free: 888-457-1551. Web site: http://cecp.air.org/resources/schfail/prevsch.asp.

School Violence *See Violence.*

Sciatica

Sciatica (sy-AT-i-ka) is a form of lower back pain that usually moves from the buttocks down the back of the leg.

What Is Sciatica?

When something squeezes the sciatic nerve, the main nerve in the leg, people feel pain in the back of the lower body. That pain, frequently one-sided, but occasionally affecting both sides, called sciatica, usually moves down the buttocks to the leg below the knee, but it can go all the way down to the foot. Sciatica varies from mild, tingling pain to severe pain that leaves people unable to move. Some people with sciatica feel sharp pain in one part of the leg or hip and numbness in other parts. This pain gets worse after standing or sitting for a long time.

Sciatica is most common in people who are 30 to 70 years of age, and it affects about three times as many men as women. At risk are the following groups:

- people who are sedentary (not very active)
- people who exercise improperly
- people who smoke
- athletes
- people who lift, bend, and twist in awkward positions in their jobs
- pregnant women
- tall people

What Causes Sciatica?

There are many ways the sciatic nerve can become compressed, but the exact cause is often unknown. The most common causes of sciatica are a herniated disc or a tumor within the spine. Discs are the pads between the bones (called vertebrae) of the spine. They are filled with a gelatin-like substance that cushions the vertebrae from the impact of walking, running, lifting, and similar activities. A disc that has torn and has this gelatin-like material oozing out of it is said to be herniated.

Other common causes of sciatica include bony irregularities of the vertebrae such as spondylolisthesis*. Spinal stenosis* is a less common cause. In some cases, diabetes or alcoholism can cause sciatica.

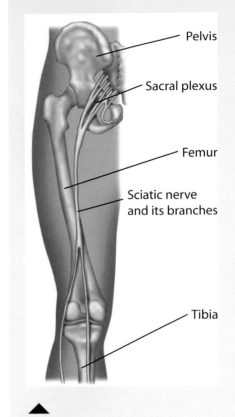

Pelvis

Sacral plexus

Femur

Sciatic nerve and its branches

Tibia

The sciatic nerve is the main nerve in the leg. It branches into the tibial and peroneal nerves. *Illustration by Frank Forney. Reproduced by permission of Gale, a part of Cengage Learning.*

* **spondylolisthesis** (spon-di-lo-lis-THEE-sis) is a condition in which one vertebra slips over the other.

* **spinal stenosis** (SPY-nal ste-NO-sis) is the narrowing of the spinal canal.

** **chronic** (KRAH-nik) lasting a long time or recurring frequently.*

How Is Sciatica Diagnosed and Treated?

Sciatica is diagnosed through a medical history and a physical examination. Sciatica often clears up within several days to a week. It is usually treated with bed rest for a day or two (only if people cannot bear the pain), local heat, massage, pain relievers, and muscle relaxants. Sciatica tends to return and can become chronic*. Chronic sciatica is treated by trying to alleviate the cause of the pain; people with this problem are advised to lose weight, improve their muscle tone and strength, and improve their posture. Surgery may be necessary in cases in which there is no relief from pain, disc disease, or spinal stenosis.

Surgical Treatment Techniques

Several surgical interventions are available for treating sciatica. The goal of surgery is to eliminate the source of pressure on the sciatic nerve.

Laser discectomy is the removal of herniated disc material using a laser technique. During this procedure laser energy is introduced under fluoroscopic guidance to remove tissue that has been pressing on nerves and causing pain or numbness.

Microdiscectomy is the removal of herniated disc material using a surgical microscope. Because this techniques involves a microscope, the incision remains small, which helps reduce disturbance of surrounding tissue.

Radiofrequency ablation uses radiofrequency energy to heat up and break bonds of small nerve tissue areas, creating small openings and decreasing pain for months and sometimes years.

Can Sciatica Be Prevented?

Sciatica or recurrence of sciatica can sometimes be prevented by standing, sitting, and lifting properly; exercising; and working in a safe environment. People can use chairs, desks, and equipment that support the back or help maintain good posture, and they can take precautions when lifting and bending.

▶ *See also* **Pain • Slipped (Herniated) Disk**

Resources

Books and Articles

Fishman, Loren, and Carol Ardman. *Sciatica Solutions: Diagnosis, Treatment, and Cure of Spinal and Piriformis Problems.* New York: Norton, 2007.

Organizations

National Institute of Arthritis and Musculoskeletal and Skin Diseases. 1 AMS Circle, Bethesda, MD, 20892-2520. Toll free: 877-226-4267. Web site: http://www.niams.nih.gov.

National Library of Medicine. 8600 Rockville Pike, Bethesda, MD, 20894, Web site: http://www.nlm.nih.gov/medlineplus/sciatica.html.

Scleroderma

Scleroderma is a slowly progressive disease characterized by deposits of fibrous connective tissue in the skin and often the internal organs.

What Is Scleroderma?

Scleroderma is a slowly progressive disease characterized by deposits of fibrous connective tissue in the skin and often the internal organs, by hand and foot pain during exposure to cold, and by tightening and thickening of the skin. Localized scleroderma primarily affects the skin, whereas more widespread scleroderma also affects such internal organs as the lungs, liver, and heart, kidneys, and those organs in the gastrointestinal* tract.

What Causes Scleroderma?

As of 2009, scientist were not sure what causes scleroderma. It was thought to be a type of autoimmune disease*. Ordinarily, the function of the immune system* is only directed against foreign agents such as viruses, bacteria, or fungi, which threaten the body's health. However, in the case of an autoimmune disease, the immune system accidentally becomes confused about what is "foreign" and what is "self." The immune system begins to marshal its resources to attack the organs and tissues of the body, causing damage and destruction. In the case of scleroderma, it appears that

* **gastrointestinal** (gas-tro-in-TES-tih-nuhl) means having to do with the organs of the digestive system, the system that processes food. It includes the mouth, esophagus, stomach, intestines, colon, and rectum and other organs involved in digestion, including the liver and pancreas.

* **autoimmune disease** (aw-toh-ih-MYOON) is a disease in which the body's immune system attacks some of the body's own normal tissues and cells.

* **immune system** (im-YOON SIS-tem) is the system of the body composed of specialized cells and the substances they produce that helps protect the body against disease-causing germs.

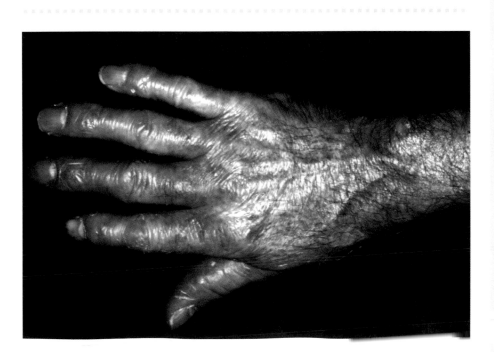

◄ Scleroderma, also known as systemic sclerosis, causes red, thickened, and tough looking skin. *Dr. P. Marazzi/Photo Researchers, Inc.*

* **chemotherapy** (KEE-mo-THER-a-pee) is the treatment of cancer with powerful drugs that kill cancer cells.

* **esophagus** (eh-SAH-fuh-gus) is the soft tube that, with swallowing, carries food from the throat to the stomach.

* **biopsies** (BI-op-seez) are tests in which small samples of skin or other body tissue are removed and examined for signs of disease.

the immune system's attack on connective tissue prompts an inflammatory response and the overproduction of collagen, which is an insoluble fibrous protein and the chief component of connective tissue. The accumulation of excess collagen causes the signs and symptoms of scleroderma.

Who Gets Scleroderma?

Scleroderma tends to strike people between 30 and 50 years of age. Women are four times as likely as men to develop this condition. Only about 4 to 12 individuals per 12 million people are diagnosed yearly, although more mild cases may occur without diagnosis. People of African descent are more likely to have the disease than people of European descent, and African-Americans are also more likely to have severe lung disease as a component of their condition. Other risk factors for the development of scleroderma include exposure to silica dust, paint thinners, and chemotherapy* agents.

What Are the Symptoms of Scleroderma?

Symptoms of scleroderma include thickening, tightening, and hardening of the skin, especially the skin of the fingers and hands; the appearance of hard deposits of calcium in the skin and connective tissues; inflammation of the esophagus*, the tube through which saliva, food, and fluids move from the mouth to the stomach; a spotty red rash on the hands and face; spasms of the blood vessels in the fingers and toes (Raynaud's phenomenon), resulting in blanching (whitening) of the skin and pain. If other organs are involved, the disease may cause various other symptoms. Lung involvement can result in shortness of breath, wheezing, cough, fatigue, and difficulty with exertion. Musculoskeletal involvement can result in joint pain, swelling, and stiffness, problems with mobility, and muscle inflammation and tenderness. Involvement of the gastrointestinal system can result in heartburn, gastroesophageal reflux (washing of acid from the stomach into the esophagus, which causes burning, pain, and damage to the esophagus), trouble swallowing, constipation, and liver problems. Inflammation of the heart can lead to congestive heart failure. Kidney involvement can result in severely high blood pressure and kidney failure.

How Is Scleroderma Diagnosed?

Scleroderma may be suspected based on the presence of characteristic symptoms, coupled with knowledge of the individual's personal or family history. A physical examination may reveal red, swollen, shiny, tight skin on the hands, as well as other signs of abnormal collagen production. A number of specific blood tests may be performed in order to demonstrate the presence of an autoimmune and connective tissue disorder. Tests may include antinuclear antibody testing, rheumatoid factor, erythrocyte sedimentation rate, and tests for a variety of other auto-antibodies (antibodies that are directed against the individual's body). Other blood tests may be performed in order to assess the functioning of various organs that may be affected. Biopsies* of affected organs may also help make the diagnosis, and specific imaging tests or function tests may demonstrate the effect that scleroderma is having on specific organ systems.

How Is Scleroderma Treated?

As of 2009, there was no cure for scleroderma. Treatments aimed at calming the overactive immune system and suppressing inflammation throughout the body. Medications used may include nonsteroidal anti-inflammatory agents, steroid drugs, and immunosuppressant agents such as those used to prevent organ rejection after transplant (methotrexate, cyclophosphamide, D-penicillamine). Medications that can dilate blood vessels may be used to treat Raynaud's phenomenon. Other treatments are focused on the specific affected organ systems. In very advanced cases of scleroderma, when lung or kidney damage is severe, lung or kidney transplant may be recommended.

▶ *See also* **Collagen Vascular Diseases**

Resources

Books and Articles

Ferri, Fred, ed. *Ferri's Clinical Advisor 2008*. Philadelphia, PA: Mosby Elsevier, 2008.

Firestein, Gary S., Ralph C. Budd, Edward D. Harris, et al. *Kelley's Textbook of Rheumatology*, 8th ed. Philadelphia, PA: Saunders, 2008.

Goldman, Lee, and Dennis Ausiello, eds. *Cecil Textbook of Internal Medicine*, 23rd ed. Philadelphia, PA: Saunders, 2008.

Mayes, Maureen D. *The Scleroderma Book: A Guide for Patients and Families*. New York: Oxford University Press, 2005.

Organizations

American College of Rheumatology. 1800 Century Place, Suite 250, Atlanta, GA, 30345. Telephone: 404-633-3777. Web site: http://www.rheumatology.org/public/factsheets/diseases_and_conditions/scleroderma.

National Institute of Arthritis and Musculoskeletal and Skin Diseases. 1 AMS Circle, Bethesda, MD, 20892. Toll free: 800-422-6237. Web site: http://www.niams.nih.gov/Health_Info/Scleroderma/default.asp.

Scoliosis

Scoliosis (sko-lee-O-sis) is a lateral, or side-to-side, curvature of the spine that most often occurs gradually during childhood or adolescent years.

Spinal column and pelvis in an adolescent girl with scoliosis. *Illustration by Frank Forney. Reproduced by permission of Gale, a part of Cengage Learning.*

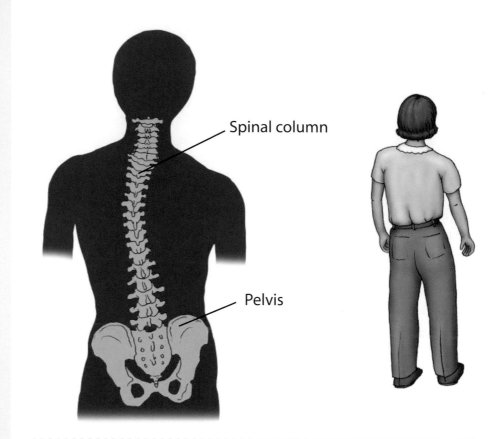

What Is Scoliosis?

The word "scoliosis" comes from the Greek word meaning curvature. Everyone's backbone curves to a significant degree when viewed from the side, which is necessary for proper movement and walking. When viewed from the front or back, however, the spine should appear as a straight line (or very nearly so). With scoliosis, the spine curves (from side to side) when viewed from the front or back, and this side-to-side curve may be S-shaped, which develops when another part of the spine develops a counterbalancing secondary curve. Depending on the degree of curvature, this condition may cause other physical problems, such as pain and breathing difficulties. The regions of the spine most commonly involved are the thoracic (tho-RAS-ik), or chest, region, and the lumbar (LUM-bar), or lower back, region.

Scoliosis is a fairly common condition. It has been estimated that about 3 out of every 100 people have this disorder to some degree. Girls are about five times more likely than boys to develop scoliosis.

Causes, Known and Unknown

The most common form of scoliosis is called idiopathic (id-ee-o-PATH-ik), which means that the cause is unknown. Usually, scoliosis becomes apparent just prior to or during adolescence, when the body's rate of growth speeds up markedly. The curvature stops increasing after people have reached their mature height.

Rarely, scoliosis is a congenital (present at birth) abnormality of the vertebrae (VER-te-bray), or spinal bones, and continues to develop throughout childhood. Poliomyelitis* (po-lee-o-my-uh-LYE-tis) has caused scoliosis in some people by paralyzing or weakening the spinal muscles on one side of the body.

Occasionally, an injury such as a disk prolapse (slipped disk) or a sprained ligament* in the backbone can cause temporary scoliosis. When this happens, the curvature may be accompanied by back pain and sciatica*.

People who have scoliosis often have family members with the same condition. In 2007 a gene linked to adolescent idiopathic scoliosis was identified by researchers at Texas Scottish Rite Hospital for Children which confirmed a hereditary link for this type of scoliosis.

What Are the Signs and Symptoms of Scoliosis?

Because scoliosis can develop very gradually, there may be no observed signs or symptoms in its early stages. Often, the curvature is first noticed in a teenager indirectly: one shoulder may become noticeably higher than the other, or a dress or jacket may not hang straight.

Early symptoms of scoliosis may include an unusually tired or achy feeling in the lower back after standing or sitting for a long time.

* **poliomyelitis** (po-lee-o-my-uh-LYE-tis) is a condition caused by the polio virus that involves damage of nerve cells. It may lead to weakness and deterioration of the muscles and sometimes paralysis.

* **ligament** (LIG-a-ment) is a fibrous band of tissue that connects bones or cartilages (CAR-ti-lij-ez), serving to support or strengthen joints.

* **sciatica** (sy-AT-i-ka) is pain along the course of either of the sciatic (sy-AT-ik) nerves, which run through the pelvis and down the backs of the thighs.

BACK BRACES, PAST, PRESENT, AND FUTURE

In the early 1900s, teenagers who had to wear back braces for scoliosis faced some very uncomfortable choices. As if being tortured, they were strapped to racks in an attempt to straighten their backs. Later on, metal jackets that weighed up to 30 pounds were worn to try to reduce the curvature. Lighter jackets, made of plaster of Paris, came next, but often they were hot and itchy.

In the early 2000s back braces are much improved. Many are made of lightweight materials and do not have to be worn all the time. There are several different types to choose from to suit the teenager's particular requirements. Some are worn only during sleep; others can be worn under clothing, so that they are not visible. Still others are of a low-profile type that comes up under the arms and are quite comfortable.

Wearing a back brace sometimes causes emotional problems. Some teenagers may resist the idea of wearing a back brace because they fear their friends or classmates may reject or ridicule them. Counseling or support groups often are helpful in sharing experiences and problems and should be considered as part of the treatment.

Future back braces undoubtedly will be even more adaptable, as medical engineers continue to design improvements in these devices.

For some, the curvature eventually may become more severe and easier to recognize. Severe scoliosis can cause chronic* back pain. If the curvature exceeds an angle of about 40 or 45 degrees, it can interfere with breathing and affect heart function.

How Do Doctors Diagnose and Treat Scoliosis?

Diagnosis Scoliosis is not always easy to diagnose, especially if it does not hurt or have visible signs. A physical examination of the spine, hips, and legs is the first step, followed by an x-ray if needed.

In the United States, public schools often do a simple test for scoliosis called the forward-bending test. The school nurse or another staff member has students bend over parallel to the floor with their shirts off to check for curvature. If scoliosis is suspected, the student is referred to a family doctor for further evaluation. The doctor might want to have an x-ray taken for a clearer view of the spine.

The severity of scoliosis is diagnosed by determining the extent of curvature of the spine. The curvature is the angle of slant of the spinal bones measured in degrees.

Treatment choices If the cause of scoliosis is known, such as an injury or unequal leg length, the treatment is designed to address the cause. For example, wearing a shoe with a raised heel can correct scoliosis caused by unequal leg length.

In idiopathic scoliosis, however, the choice of treatment depends largely on the severity of the condition. If the angle of curvature is slight (e.g., 10 to 15 degrees) nothing may need to be done other than having regular checkups to make sure the curvature does not worsen. Somewhat greater curvature can be treated by the person wearing any of several types of back braces. An angle of curvature of 40 degrees or more may mean that a corrective operation is needed.

Living with Scoliosis

Fortunately, much of the deformity of scoliosis can be prevented if the condition is detected early. In most instances, no lifestyle changes are needed, and people can carry on with their normal activities.

▶ *See also* **Genetic Diseases** • **Poliomyelitis**

Resources

Books and Articles

Silverstein, Alvin, Virginia Silverstein, and Laura Silverstein Nunn. *Scoliosis.* New York: Franklin Watts, 2002.

Organizations

National Institute of Arthritis and Musculoskeletal and Skin Diseases. 1 AMS Circle, Bethesda, MD, 20892-3675. Toll free: 877-226-4267. Web site: http://www.niams.nih.gov/Health_Info/Scoliosis/default.asp.

National Scoliosis Foundation. 5 Cabot Place, Stoughton, MA, 02072, Web site: http://www.scoliosis.org.

Southern California Orthopedic Institute. 6815 Noble Avenue, Van Nuys, CA, 91405. Telephone: 818-901-6600. Web site: http://www.scoi.com/scoilio.htm.

Scurvy

Scurvy is a disease that results when people do not get enough vitamin C (also called ascorbic acid) in the diet over a period of weeks or months. Some of the effects of scurvy are spongy gums, loose teeth, weakened blood vessels that cause bleeding under the skin, and damage to bones and cartilage, which results in arthritis-like pain.

What Is Scurvy?

Scurvy was one of the first recognized dietary deficiency diseases. During the sea voyages from the 15th through the 18th centuries, many sailors suffered from scurvy. For example, the Portuguese navigator Vasco da Gama (ca 1460–1524) lost half his crew to the disease during a voyage around the Cape of Good Hope, and the British admiral Sir Richard Hawkins (1532–1595) estimated that during his career, 10,000 sailors under his command died due to scurvy. One legend maintains that men sailing with Christopher Columbus developed scurvy and asked to be left on an island to die, but when Columbus returned, he found the men healthy. He named the island, which was rich in various kinds of fruit, Curacao, meaning cure in Portuguese.

To deal with dietary deficiencies, ships began to carry all manner of remedies, including sauerkraut, mustard, and dried vegetables for soup, but nothing seemed to work consistently to prevent scurvy. In 1747, the Scottish naval physician James Lind (1716–1794) conducted experiments to find out which foods or liquids were good treatments for scurvy. Sailors had long known the benefits of lime juice, but Lind's work was the first to confirm that citrus—and in particular lemons and oranges—was an effective treatment. Eventually, all ships embarking on long voyages carried a supply of citrus fruits or juice, and a British Navy mandated daily rations of lime juice.

Seventeenth-century Scottish physician James Lind supplied oranges and lemons to sailors with scurvy. ©*Bettmann/Corbis.*

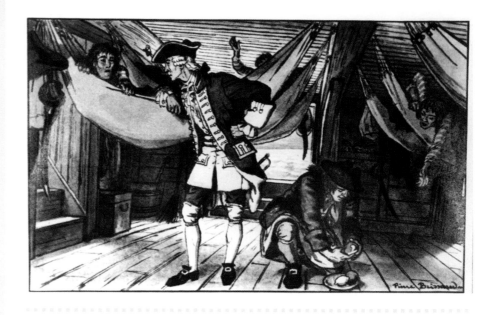

What Is the Role of Vitamin C in the Body?

Citrus fruits are rich sources of vitamin C, and vitamin C is necessary for strong blood vessels; healthy skin, gums, and connective tissue; formation of red blood cells; wound healing; and the absorption of iron from food. Scientists first learned about vitamin C in the late 1920s to early 1930s when an Hungarian research team and an American research team independently discovered the vitamin and identified it as ascorbic acid.

What Are the Symptoms of Scurvy?

The main symptom of scurvy is bleeding (hemorrhaging). Bleeding within the skin appears as spots or bruises. Bleeding can take place in the membranes covering the large bones and in the membranes of the heart and brain. Bleeding in or around vital organs can be fatal. Other symptoms include: slow and poor healing of wounds; swollen gums and gingivitis

---

HAVE YOU EVER HEARD OF A "LIMEY"?

In *Treatise of the Scurvy,* published in 1753, James Lind (1716–1794) wrote about the first example of a research experiment set up as a controlled clinical trial. To study the treatment of scurvy, Lind divided sailors who had it into several groups and then fed each group different liquids and foods. He discovered that the group fed lemons and oranges was able to recover from scurvy.

By the end of the 18th century, the British navy had its sailors drink a daily portion of lime or lemon juice to prevent scurvy. The American slang term for the English, "limeys," originated from that practice.

(jin-ji-VY-tis), which means inflammation of the gums; nausea; muscle and joint pain; loosening and sometimes outright loss of teeth; dry skin; and a general feeling of tiredness.

Scurvy develops slowly. In the beginning, a person usually feels tired, irritable, and depressed. In an individual in the advanced stages of scurvy, laboratory tests show a complete absence of vitamin C in the person's body.

Who Is at Risk for Scurvy?

Scurvy is less prevalent in modern times than it was in the time of Vasco da Gama and Richard Hawkins, but people who are on diets that lack a diversity of foods may develop scurvy or scurvy-like conditions. This statement applies to the following groups:

- infants who depend solely on processed cow's milk for nutrition and do not receive vitamin C supplements
- elderly people, whose diets often lack citrus fruits or vegetables that contain vitamin C
- people who follow diets that limit them to very few food choices.

How Is Scurvy Treated?

A simple blood test that checks for vitamin C levels can confirm whether a person has scurvy. If so, a medical professional will recommend vitamin C supplements (vitamin pills) and a diet that includes foods rich in vitamin C. In addition to citrus fruits such as oranges and grapefruits, good sources of vitamin C include broccoli, tomatoes, raw spinach, baked potatoes, red and green bell peppers, strawberries, cantaloupe, mangoes, and other fruits and vegetables.

▶ *See also* **Dietary Deficiencies • Gum Disease**

Resources

Books and Articles

Bown, Stephen R. *Scurvy: How a Surgeon, a Mariner, and a Gentleman Solved the Greatest Medical Mystery of the Age of Sail.* St. Martin's Griffin, 2005.

Organization

National Library of Medicine. 8600 Rockville Pike, Bethesda, MD, 20894, Web site: http://www.nlm.nih.gov/medlineplus/ency/article/000355.htm.

Seasickness *See Motion Sickness.*

* **neurotransmitter** (NUR-o-tranz-mit-er) is a brain chemical that lets brain cells communicate with each other and therefore allows the brain to function properly. In other words, a neurotransmitter transmits (carries) a chemical message from neuron to neuron.

* **serotonin** (ser-o-TO-nin) is a neurotransmitter, a substance that helps transmit information from one nerve cell to another in the brain. It is associated with feelings of well-being.

Seasonal Affective Disorder

Seasonal affective disorder (SAD) is a form of depression that occurs at the same time each year (usually with the onset of winter) and disappears at the same time each year (typically at the start of spring). SAD is linked to the availability of daylight and occurs most often in people who live in the Northern Hemisphere.

More than the Winter Blahs

Many people get the winter blahs or cabin fever as the days get shorter and colder, but for the approximately 10 million Americans with SAD, shorter days mean a slide into true depression. SAD is a seasonal pattern of depression. Women experience this form of depression four times more often than men, and it can also occur in children and teens. The farther individuals live from the equator, the higher the risk that they will experience SAD. One study has estimated the incidence of SAD in the general population as only 1.4 percent in Florida but 9.7 percent in New Hampshire. These numbers suggest that the condition strikes people who live in the northern state of New Hampshire about seven times more frequently than it does people who live in the southern state of Florida. The study also showed that SAD affected more people in other northern states: 4.7 percent in New York and 6.3 percent in Maryland.

What Causes Seasonal Affective Disorder?

As autumn arrives, the number of daylight hours declines. The effect is greater the farther north a person travels from the equator. Daylight also declines with increasing cloud cover in specific areas of the United States, such as the Great Lakes region and northwest coastal areas of Washington.

Researchers believe that for some people, the decrease in available daylight causes a decline in the neurotransmitter* serotonin*, in the brain. A decrease in serotonin in the brain has been linked to depression, because serotonin typically is associated with feelings of well-being. In the autumn, after a few weeks of reduced serotonin levels, a person can start to show signs of depression. If left untreated, the depression may continue throughout the winter and then disappear in the spring as the number of daylight hours increases.

Medical professionals diagnose SAD in people if they become depressed in the fall and winter for two or more consecutive years with periods of normal moods in the spring and summer and if they have no other problems that might account for seasonal depression. A rare form of SAD, called summer SAD, occurs in reverse of the normal pattern. People with summer SAD become depressed during the summer and feel better in the winter.

What Are the Symptoms of Seasonal Affective Disorder?

Not everyone who has SAD experiences all of the same symptoms. Common symptoms of SAD include fatigue and oversleeping; a craving for carbohydrates, such as breads and pasta; and a tendency to gain a little weight. In addition, a person may experience other common symptoms of depression such as the following:

- Depressed mood
- Feelings of helplessness, hopelessness, or guilt
- Pessimistic thoughts
- Loss of pleasure in previously enjoyable activities
- Difficulty concentrating or making decisions

How Is Seasonal Affective Disorder Treated?

Following a correct diagnosis, a medical professional may recommend that the patient begin light therapy to treat seasonal affective disorder. People with SAD sit in front of special bright light boxes or wear light visors for a period of 30 minutes to two hours every day, glancing occasionally at the light. To be effective, the light must enter the eyes and not just fall on the skin. Occasionally, people report eyestrain or headaches from the light devices, but they usually experience no other negative side effects. When natural daylight increases, people with SAD discontinue light treatment.

In addition to light therapy, some people with SAD benefit from antidepressant medications*. Some researchers have also advocated the use of melatonin, a light-sensitive hormone* that is believed to play a role in the normal sleep-wake cycle. They believe that SAD results when the body's normal cycle becomes skewed, and the timed administration of melatonin can help restore the normal pattern.

▶ *See also* **Depressive Disorders**

Resources

Books and Articles

Rosenthal, Norman E. *Winter Blues: Everything You Need to Know to Beat Seasonal Affective Disorder,* rev. ed. New York: Guilford Press, 2006.

Organizations

National Mental Health Association. 2000 N. Beauregard Street, 6th Floor, Alexandria, VA, 22311. Telephone: 703-684-7722. Web site: http://www1.nmha.org/infoctr/factsheets/27.cfm.

Seasonal Affective Disorder Association. P.O. Box 989, Steyning, England, BN44 3HG, Web site: http://www.sada.org.uk.

* **antidepressant medications** are used for the treatment and prevention of depression.

* **hormone** is a chemical substance that is produced by a gland and sent into the bloodstream carrying messages that have certain effects on other parts of the body.

* **Epilepsy** (EP-i-lep-see) is a condition of the nervous system characterized by recurrent seizures that temporarily affect a person's awareness, movements, or sensations. Seizures occur when powerful, rapid bursts of electrical energy interrupt the normal electrical patterns of the brain.

* **neurons** are nerve cells. Most neurons have extensions called axons and dendrites through which they send and receive signals from other neurons.

Seizures

Seizures (SEE-zhers) occur when the electrical patterns of the brain are interrupted by powerful, rapid bursts of electrical energy. A seizure may cause a person to lose consciousness, to fall down, to jerk or convulse, or simply to blank out for a few seconds. Infection, injury, or medical problems can cause a seizure. Epilepsy* is a disease of the nervous system characterized by recurring seizures.

Two Stories

Eric's story   As part of his sixth grade study of self-awareness, Eric was assigned to draw the frames of a film that would show the world as he saw it. Teachers were puzzled by what Eric drew. One frame showed him pouring milk, the next frame was completely black, and the next frame showed spilled milk. In another sequence, Eric drew a teacher calling on him to answer a math problem, followed by another black frame, and then a picture of the teacher complaining that Eric was not paying attention. The teachers realized that Eric's project did show the world as he saw it. The mysterious black frames were blackouts. Doctors determined that Eric had absence seizures, a type of seizure that causes a brief loss of consciousness. Medication successfully controlled Eric's seizures.

Carol's story   All the students in Carol's art class were preparing work for an art show when Carol stood up and began walking around the room. Looking like she was in a trance, Carol smacked her lips and tugged at the sleeve of her dress. About two minutes later, Carol became aware of her surroundings, only to discover that her classmates were laughing at her strange behavior. Embarrassed, she ran from the room. Carol had experienced a complex partial seizure.

What Is a Seizure?

Whether a person is sleeping or awake, millions of tiny electrical charges pass between neurons* in the brain and to all parts of body. These cells "fire," or transmit electrical impulses, in an orderly and controlled manner. Seizures occur when overactive nerve cells send out powerful, rapid electrical charges that disrupt the brain's normal function. The disruption can temporarily affect how a person behaves, moves, thinks, or feels.

Symptoms of a seizure can include combinations of the following:

- twitching and tingling in part of the body (for example, fingers and toes)
- muscle spasms spreading to arms and legs
- hallucinations

- intense feeling of fear or of familiarity (sometimes called déjà vu, which means "already seen" in French)
- a peculiar sensation, sometimes called an aura, immediately before the seizure (for example, seeing a flashing light or sensing strange odors)
- loss of consciousness.

How Do Seizures Differ?

There are two kinds of seizure disorders: an isolated seizure that occurs only once and epilepsy (EP-i-lep-see). Epileptic seizures occur more than once, and they occur over a period of time. In both epilepsy and isolated seizures, the seizure may have different symptoms or characteristics depending on where it begins in the brain and how the electrical discharge spreads across the brain. Seizures can be generalized or partial.

Generalized seizures   Generalized seizures affect nerve cells throughout the cerebral cortex* (the cauliflower-like outer portion of the brain), or all of the brain. Generalized seizures often are hereditary, which means they run in families. They may also be caused by imbalances in a person's kidney or liver function or in their blood sugar.

The most common generalized seizures are:

- **Generalized tonic-clonic seizure (formerly called grand mal seizure):** In the tonic phase of this seizure, people often lose consciousness, drop to the ground, and emit a loud cry as air is forced over their vocal cords. In the clonic phase, body muscles contract all at once or in a series of shorter rhythmic contractions, causing thrashing motions. Usually, this kind of seizure lasts for about one or two minutes and is followed by a period of relaxation, sleepiness, and possibly a headache.
- **Absence seizure (formerly called petit mal seizure):** Loss of consciousness in this seizure is often so brief (usually 10 to 30 seconds) that a person does not even change positions. The person may display a blank stare, rapid blinking, or chewing movements. Facial or eyelid muscles may jerk rhythmically. Absence seizures may be inherited and usually are seen for the first time in children between the ages of 6 and 12.
- **Infantile spasms:** This type of seizure occurs in children under the age of four and may cause a child to suddenly flex the arms, thrust the trunk forward, and extend the legs. The seizure lasts only a few seconds but can recur several times per day.
- **Atonic seizures:** Also seen primarily in children, these seizures cause a complete loss of muscle tone and consciousness, which means they pose a serious risk of injury due to falling.

* **cerebral cortex** (suh-REE-brul KOR-teks) is the part of the brain that controls functions such as conscious thought, listening, and speaking.

* **aura** is a warning sensation that precedes a seizure or other neurological event.

* **cerebrospinal fluid** (seh-ree-bro-SPY-nuhl) is the fluid that surrounds the brain and spinal cord.

Myoclonic seizures: These brief seizures are characterized by quick jerking movements of one limb or several limbs. The person experiencing the seizure does not lose consciousness.

Febrile seizures: These seizures occur in infancy or childhood and cause a child to lose consciousness and convulse. The seizures are accompanied by a high fever, and they are described as either simple or complex. Simple febrile seizures account for about 85 percent of febrile seizures. They occur once in 24 hours and last less than 15 minutes. Complex febrile seizures last more than 15 minutes or occur more than twice in 24 hours.

Partial seizures   Partial seizures affect nerve cells contained within one region of the cerebral cortex. Types of partial seizures include:

Simple partial: The seizure-related brain messages remain localized, and the individual is awake and alert. Symptoms vary depending on what area of the brain is involved. They may include jerking movements in one part of the body, emotional symptoms such as unexplained fear, an experience of peculiar smells, or nausea.

Complex partial: A person loses awareness of surroundings and is unresponsive or only partially responsive. There may be a blank stare, chewing movements, repeated swallowing, or other random activity. After the seizure, the person has no memory of the experience. In some cases, the person may become confused, begin to fumble, to wander, or to repeat inappropriate words or phrases.

What Causes A Seizure?

A seizure generally is easy to recognize, but finding the cause can be extremely difficult. Doctors begin with a thorough physical examination. They try to determine if the person has experienced other seizures or has a family history of seizures. Physicians also want to know if their patient has experienced an aura* because that can help establish the location in the brain of the seizure. They also will note the person's age and the nature of the movements the person made during the seizure.

An electroencephalogram (e-LEK-tro-en-SEF-a-lo-gram), commonly known as an EEG, records electric currents in the brain and can track abnormal electrical activity. Doctors may also look for structural brain abnormalities using other types of scans, including computerized tomography (CT) and magnetic resonance imaging (MRI). In some research centers, positron emission tomography (PET) is used to identify areas of the brain that are producing seizures.

A lumbar puncture, sometimes called a spinal tap, can detect infection. The procedure requires that a physician carefully insert a thin needle between two vertebrae (bones) in the patient's spine and draw out a small amount of cerebrospinal fluid* (CSF). The fluid is analyzed for the presence of bacterial or viral infections, tumors, or blood disorders that might provide a clue to the cause of the seizure.

Seizures are associated with the following diseases and conditions:

- Epilepsy, a disorder of the nervous system characterized by seizures that occur more than once and over a period of time
- Head trauma that damages the brain
- Loss of oxygen caused by birth trauma, carbon monoxide poisoning, or near drowning
- Brain infections, such as meningitis or encephalitis
- Brain tumor
- Stroke
- Toxic (poisonous) agents, including drug abuse or ingestion of poisons such as lead, alcohol, or strychnine
- Withdrawal from alcohol and drugs
- Metabolic imbalances such as hypoglycemia (very low blood sugar), uremia (kidney failure), or liver problems
- Eclampsia or toxemia, which may occur during pregnancy and is characterized by high blood pressure, protein in the urine, and fluid retention.

It is important to remain calm and not to panic when someone has a seizure. An adult usually asks if the person has epilepsy. If the person is unable to communicate, an adult checks for a medical identification bracelet or tag that carries information about the underlying cause of the seizure.

▶ *See also* **Brain Tumor • Diabetes • Encephalitis • Epilepsy • Fever • Hypoglycemia • Incontinence • Infection • Kidney Disease • Lead Poisoning • Lupus • Meningitis • Stroke • Substance Abuse**

Resources

Books and Articles

Kutscher, Martin L. *Children with Seizures: A Guide for Parents, Teachers, and Other Professionals.* Philadelphia, PA: Jessica Kingsley, 2006.

Wyllie, Elaine. *Epilepsy: Information for You and Those Who Care about You.* Cleveland, OH: Cleveland Clinic Press, 2008.

Organizations

Epilepsy Foundation. 8301 Professional Place, Landover, MD, 20785. Toll free: 800-332-1000. Web site: http://www.epilepsyfoundation.org.

National Library of Medicine. 8600 Rockville Pike, Bethesda, MD, 20894, Web site: http://www.nlm.nih.gov/medlineplus/seizures.html.

* **anxiety disorders** (ang-ZY-e-tee dis-OR-derz) are a group of conditions that cause people to feel extreme fear or worry that sometimes is accompanied by symptoms such as dizziness, chest pain, or difficulty sleeping or concentrating.

Selective Mutism

Selective mutism (se-LEK-tiv MU-ti-zum) is a condition in which children feel so inhibited and anxious that they do not speak in particular situations, most commonly in school. Children with selective mutism are capable of speaking and communicating normally and do so in other situations, for example, at home.

Brandon's Story

When Brandon first started kindergarten, his teacher just thought he was a very quiet boy and that he would come out of his shell in a week or two. As the weeks passed into months, though, Brandon still never spoke a word at school, even when the teacher called on him. Sometimes if he needed something, he would point or gesture, but he would not speak. His teacher was concerned, and when she called his parents, they told her that Brandon spoke easily at home and that he had always been a little shy around others. It was clear that Brandon's problem was more than normal shyness. Because it was interfering with his ability to participate in class and on the playground, his parents took Brandon to a mental health professional, who diagnosed his problem as selective mutism.

What Is Selective Mutism?

Selective mutism is a condition in which children feel anxious and inhibited and do not speak in certain situations. Children with selective mutism are capable of speaking normally and do so in other situations where they feel more comfortable. These children often talk normally at home, but they may completely stop talking around teachers, other children, or other adults. Their behavior gets in the way of their making friends and doing well in school.

Selective mutism, once thought to be quite rare, was beginning to be more widely recognized in the early 2000s. It used to be called elective mutism, because it was thought that children were purposely choosing not to talk. It was sometimes thought that a child's refusal to speak was a way to rebel against adults or a sign of anger. The problem affects at least 1 in 100 school-age children. It usually begins before the age of 5, but it may not cause problems until children start school. The condition may last for just a few months, but in some cases, if left untreated, selective mutism can last for years. Some experts believe that untreated selective mutism in children leads to social anxiety disorders* in their adult years. Experts concluded that selective mutism is an extreme form of social anxiety in a child. Social anxiety is an intense, lasting fear or extreme discomfort in social situations, and usually leads to avoidance of many social situations. With selective mutism, children seem to feel so self-conscious or anxious in certain situations that they avoid talking altogether.

What Causes Selective Mutism?

There is no single cause of selective mutism. As with other forms of anxiety, some children may be more likely to have this problem if anxiety or extreme shyness runs in the family, or if they are born with a shy nature. Beyond genetics, in some families in which adults are anxious, children may learn to feel socially anxious by watching the way adults react and behave. Upsetting or stressful events such as divorce, the death of a loved one, or frequent moves may trigger selective mutism in a child who is prone to anxiety.

What Are the Symptoms of Selective Mutism?

Many children are shy for a while when they first start kindergarten, but most eventually become comfortable in school, make friends, and talk to the teacher. Those with selective mutism remain silent and may not speak for a month or longer. Some children with selective mutism make gestures, nod, or write notes to communicate. Others use one-syllable words or whispers. Many children with selective mutism are very shy and fearful and may have nervous habits, such as biting their nails. They may cling to their parents and sulk around strangers but might throw temper tantrums and be stubborn and demanding at home. When pushed to speak, they may become stubborn in their refusal. It is sometimes hard for adults to understand that fear, not stubbornness, is at the root of selective mutism and that children with this condition experience speaking as risky, scary, or dangerous. Understood in this way, people can understand that a child's stubborn refusal to speak as a strong, but misguided, attempt at self-protection.

How Is Selective Mutism Diagnosed?

Some children with selective mutism will speak to a mental health professional, but others will not. Even if children are silent, though, a skilled professional therapist still can learn a lot by watching how they behave. The therapist can also talk to parents and teachers to find out more about the problem and possible factors that contribute to it. In addition, a number of tests may be used to exclude other possible causes for failing to speak. These include special medical tests to rule out brain damage, intelligence and academic tests to rule out learning problems, speech and language tests to rule out communication disorders*, and hearing tests to rule out hearing loss.

How Is Selective Mutism Treated?

Most children who have selective mutism want to feel comfortable talking. Although they resist efforts to help them talk at first, therapy can be effective in treating this problem. The most common treatment for selective mutism is behavioral (bee-HAY-vyor-al) therapy, which helps people gradually change specific, unwanted types of behavior. For example, after the therapist helps the child to feel comfortable, the child might be rewarded for speaking softly and clearly into a tape recorder. Once they have succeeded in this or at other times, they can move

* communication disorders affect a person's ability to use or understand speech and language.

* **systemic** (sis-TEM-ik) a problem affecting the whole system or whole body, as opposed to a localized problem that affects only one place on the body.

on to being rewarded for speaking to one child at school. Children who are selectively mute may speak to specific children. They then might be invited to participate in a group with the children to whom the selectively mute child speaks.

Often family therapy is added, which helps identify and change behavior patterns within the family that may play a role in maintaining mutism. When a child has selective mutism, it is common for the family members to speak for the child. While they begin to do this out of love and concern and the desire to be helpful, these patterns must be discontinued to help motivate reluctant children to begin to speak for themselves. Play therapy and drawing are often used to help these children to express their feelings and worries. In addition, some children with selective mutism are prescribed medications used for treating anxiety. These medications help lessen the anxiety that plays an important role in the selectively mute child's behavior, allowing the child to take the risks involved in talking.

▶ *See also* **Anxiety and Anxiety Disorders • School Avoidance • Social Phobia (Social Anxiety Disorder)**

Resources

Books and Articles

McHolm, Angela E., Charles E. Cunningham, and Melanie K. Vanier. *Helping Your Child with Selective Mutism: Practical Steps to Overcome a Fear of Speaking.* Oakland, CA: New Harbinger Publications, 2005.

Organizations

Selective Mutism Foundation. P.O. Box 13133, Sissonville, WV, 25360, Web site: http://www.selectivemutismfoundation.org.

Selective Mutism Group. 30 South J Street, 3A, Lake Worth, FL, 33460, Web site: http://www.selectivemutism.org.

Senile Dementia *See Alzheimer's Disease.*

Sepsis

Sepsis is a serious systemic* infection caused by bacteria in the bloodstream.

What Is Sepsis?

Sepsis is caused most commonly by bacteria in the bloodstream, a condition known as bacteremia (bak-tuh-REE-me-uh). These bacteria produce toxins* that provoke a response by the body's immune system. The effect of the toxins combined with the response of the immune system brings about the disease. Bacteremia may resolve by itself, or it can lead to sepsis if the bacteria are not removed by the immune system. Although bacteremia and sepsis frequently coexist, each can be present without the other. The bacteria may come from a local infection, such as pneumonia* or a urinary tract* infection, or they may come from the nose, skin, or intestines*, where bacteria live without causing problems unless they enter the bloodstream. The most common sources of infection that lead to sepsis are the lungs, skin, intestine, urinary tract, and gall bladder*.

Sepsis is most dangerous to people with weak immune systems, such as infants, the elderly, people with HIV/AIDS or cancer, or those who have undergone organ transplantation. In infants younger than three months, any fever may be a sign of sepsis or another serious infection. Doctors advise immediate evaluation of these infants and prompt treatment with antibiotics if sepsis is suspected. Group B streptococcus (strep-tuh-KAH-kus) bacteria passed from mother to baby during birth are a major cause of sepsis in infants. *Streptococcus pneumoniae* (strep-tuh-KAH-kus nu-MO-nye) and *Neisseria meningitidis* (nye-SEER-e-uh mehnin-JIH-tih-dis) bacteria are associated with sepsis in older children and in adults. Sepsis in adults most often is seen after surgery or some other medical procedure in the hospital, but it may occur outside the hospital, particularly associated with urinary tract infection.

How Common Is Sepsis?

Sepsis is not very common. According to the National Library of Medicine, sepsis develops in about 2 of every 10,000 people in the general population. In infants, sepsis occurs in fewer than 1 to 2 per 1,000 live births. Sepsis is a complication in about two of every 100 hospitalizations, where related intravenous (IV) lines, surgical wounds or drains, and bedsores* can be entry points for bacteria.

Is Sepsis Contagious?

Sepsis itself is not contagious, but the infectious agents that can cause sepsis can be transmitted from person to person. For example, in newborns, group B streptococcus organisms can spread from mother to baby during delivery.

What Are the Signs and Symptoms of Sepsis?

Early symptoms of sepsis may include fever, shaking chills, rapid breathing and heartbeat, confusion, delirium*, and rash. As the infection spreads, a person's blood pressure drops, leading to a condition known as shock*. Body organs that have important functions including the liver, lungs, and

* **toxins** are substances that cause harm to the body.

* **pneumonia** (nu-MO-nyah) is inflammation of the lungs.

* **urinary tract** (YOOR-ih-nair-e TRAKT) is the system of organs and channels that makes urine and removes it from the body. It consists of the urethra, bladder, ureters, and kidneys.

* **intestines** are the muscular tubes that food passes through during digestion after it exits the stomach.

* **gall bladder** is a small pear-shaped organ on the right side of the abdomen that stores bile, a liquid that helps the body digest fat.

* **bedsores** also called pressure sores, are skin sores caused by prolonged pressure on the skin and typically are seen in people who are confined by illness or paralysis to beds or wheelchairs.

* **delirium** (dih-LEER-e-um) is a condition in which a person is confused, is unable to think clearly, and has a reduced level of consciousness.

* **shock** is a serious condition in which blood pressure is very low and not enough blood flows to the body's organs and tissues. Untreated, shock may result in death.

* **clotting** is the body's way of thickening blood to stop bleeding.

* **platelets** (PLATE-lets) are tiny disk-shaped particles within the blood that play an important role in clotting.

* **dialysis** (dye-AL-uh-sis) is a process that removes waste, toxins (poisons), and extra fluid from the blood. Usually dialysis is done when a person's kidneys are unable to perform these functions normally.

* **respiratory failure** is a condition in which breathing and oxygen delivery to the body are dangerously altered. This may result from infection, nerve or muscle damage, poisoning, or other causes.

* **septic shock** is shock due to overwhelming infection and is characterized by decreased blood pressure, internal bleeding, heart failure, and, in some cases, death.

* **catheters** (KAH-thuh-ters) are small plastic tubes placed through a body opening into an organ (such as the bladder) or through the skin directly into a blood vessel. They are used to give fluids to or drain fluids from a person.

* **vaccination** (vak-sih-NAY-shun), also called immunization, is giving, usually by an injection, a preparation of killed or weakened germs, or a part of a germ or product it produces, to prevent or lessen the severity of the disease caused by that germ.

* **vagina** (vah-JY-nah) is the canal, or passageway, in a woman that leads from the uterus to the outside of the body.

kidneys, may begin to shut down. The blood-clotting* system may also be affected. Sepsis in young children may be more difficult to diagnose at first because it has fewer obvious symptoms. Children may have a fever or changing temperature, a change in heart rate, or difficulty breathing. They might also be irritable or sluggish, and they may lose interest in eating.

How Do Doctors Make the Diagnosis?

A diagnosis of sepsis is made based on a person's symptoms. Blood tests are performed to identify the bacteria and to look for a low platelet* count (an indicator of the blood-clotting problems seen with sepsis) and an abnormally low or high white blood cell count (both can occur with sepsis). Other tests can help show damage to vital organs, such as the kidneys.

Can Sepsis Be Treated?

As soon as a diagnosis of sepsis is suspected, treatment with intravenous antibiotics begins. Patients with sepsis are hospitalized in an intensive care unit, where they may be given oxygen, intravenous fluids, and medication to stabilize blood pressure, treat other symptoms, and kill the bacteria responsible for the condition. Dialysis* may be necessary if the patient's kidneys fail. If respiratory failure* occurs, patients usually are placed on a respirator, a machine that aids their breathing until they can breathe again on their own. If the patient survives, recovery from sepsis can take weeks.

What Are the Complications of Sepsis?

Septic shock* may occur in patients with sepsis. Disseminated intravascular coagulation is a complication associated with sepsis in which the body's blood-clotting system is out of control, a problem that can lead to serious internal bleeding. This complication usually improves when the cause of sepsis is treated. Sepsis can be fatal, depending on the infectious agent and on the age and overall health of the patient. Quick diagnosis and treatment can improve outcomes and save lives.

How Is Sepsis Prevented?

Sepsis may not be preventable in many cases, but an early response to symptoms may stop a bacterial infection from progressing to sepsis. Early treatment is particularly important with regard to people with weak immune systems. Among hospitalized patients, efforts are made to limit the use of intravenous and urinary catheters*, which are both common entry points for sepsis-causing bacteria. Following a recommended vaccination* schedule for children can lessen their risk of contracting certain infections that might lead to sepsis. Immunization against *Streptococcus pneumoniae* is recommended for infants and for adults and children at high risk due to age or medical problems. This vaccine is highly effective in preventing pneumonia and sepsis caused by this organism.

Pregnant women typically are tested to determine whether they are carrying group B streptococcus bacteria in their vagina*. Treating these women with antibiotics during pregnancy may reduce the risk of passing the bacterium from mother to child. People with medical conditions, such as sickle-cell disease*, that put them at greater risk for developing serious bacterial infections are prescribed antibiotics to decrease the chance that sepsis can develop.

▶ *See also* **Pneumonia • Skin and Soft Tissue Infections • Streptococcal Infections • Urinary Tract Infections**

Resources

Organizations

Mayo Clinic. 200 First Street SW, Rochester, MN, 55905, Web site: http://www.mayoclinic.com/health/sepsis/DS01004.

National Library of Medicine. 8600 Rockville Pike, Bethesda, MD, 20894, Web site: http://www.nlm.nih.gov/medlineplus/sepsis.html.

Severe Acute Respiratory Syndrome (SARS)

Severe acute respiratory* syndrome* (SARS) is a highly contagious*, potentially life-threatening respiratory illness caused by a coronavirus, which is a member of a family of viruses that includes the causative agents of numerous animal and human diseases, including SARS and the common cold.

What Is Severe Acute Respiratory Syndrome?

SARS, caused by the SARS-associated coronavirus (SARS-CoV), was the first newly emerging disease of the 21st century. It appeared in southeastern China in November 2002 and spread with lightning speed to every continent before it was contained just a few months later. It raised alarms among health officials and the general public because it underscored how rapidly a new infectious disease could spread around the world, potentially causing a pandemic*. Although SARS subsequently disappeared, it left a legacy of fear and severe economic consequences.

Coronaviruses are a group of viruses* so-named because they appear to be surrounded by a halo or corona when viewed under an electron microscope. They are large viruses carrying single-stranded RNA* as their genetic* material. In animals coronaviruses can cause serious respiratory, gastrointestinal*, liver*, and neurological* disease. However, in humans coronaviruses normally cause only mild to moderate upper respiratory

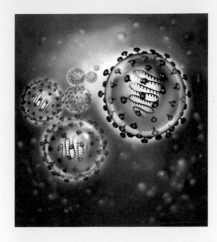

Illustration of the SARS virus. The membrane and protein envelope (violet) surround a genome of single stranded RNA. The entire virus is surrounded by glycoproteins (orange) that suggest a corona or crown. *Jim Dowdalls/Photo Researchers, Inc.*

* **sickle-cell disease** is a hereditary condition in which the red blood cells, which are usually round, take on an abnormal crescent shape and have a decreased ability to carry oxygen throughout the body.

* **respiratory** (RES-pi-ra-tor-ee) refers to the breathing passages and lungs.

* **syndrome** is a group or pattern of symptoms or signs that occur together.

* **contagious** (kon-TAY-jus) means transmittable from one person to another, usually referring to an infection.

* **pandemic** (pan-DEH-mik) is a worldwide outbreak of disease, especially infectious disease, in which the number of cases suddenly becomes far greater than usual.

* **viruses** (VY-rus-sez) are tiny infectious agents that can cause infectious diseases. A virus can only reproduce within the cells it infects.

* **RNA** or ribonucleic acid (ry-bo-nyoo-KLAY-ik AH-sid), is the chemical substance through which DNA sends genetic information to build new cells.

* **genetic** (juh-NEH-tik) refers to heredity and the ways in which genes control the development and maintenance of organisms.

* **gastrointestinal** (gas-tro-in-TES-tih-nuhl) means having to do with the organs of the digestive system, the system that processes food. It includes the mouth, esophagus, stomach, intestines, colon, and rectum and other organs involved in digestion, including the liver and pancreas.

* **liver** is a large organ located beneath the ribs on the right side of the body. The liver performs numerous digestive and chemical functions essential for health.

* **neurological** (nur-a-LAH-je-kal) refers to the nervous system, which includes the brain, spinal cord, and the nerves that control the senses, movement, and organ functions throughout the body.

* **mammals** are warm-blooded animals with backbones, who usually have fur or hair. Female mammals secrete milk from mammary glands to feed their young. Humans are mammals.

* **epidemic** (eh-pih-DEH-mik) is an outbreak of disease, especially infectious disease, in which the number of cases suddenly becomes far greater than usual. Usually epidemics are outbreaks of diseases in specific regions, whereas widespread epidemics are called pandemics.

* **respiratory failure** is a condition in which breathing and oxygen delivery to the body are dangerously altered. This may result from infection, nerve or muscle damage, poisoning, or other causes.

WHERE DID SEVERE ACUTE RESPIRATORY SYNDROME COME FROM?

Within weeks of the first recognized SARS cases, scientists had identified a coronavirus as the causative agent and immediately guessed that it was an animal virus that had crossed over to infect humans. Palm civets—small Asian weasel-like mammals*—were the suspected culprit. Civets are considered a delicacy in southern China and are commonly sold in live-food markets and restaurants. Early SARS victims included a waitress at a restaurant in Guangzhou, China, that served palm civet and a customer seated close to the restaurant's animal cages. SARS-CoV was subsequently found in other animals, including domestic cats, and bats were identified as a natural reservoir for SARS-like coronaviruses. Researchers eventually came to believe that the epidemic* SARS strain evolved through a series of transmission events between humans and palm civets in Chinese markets.

tract infections such as the common cold. Therefore, health officials were taken by surprise when the death toll from the first wave of SARS approached 15 percent and exceeded 50 percent in patients over age 65. Respiratory failure* is the most common cause of death from SARS; however, heart failure* or liver failure are also potential complications.

How Common Is Severe Acute Respiratory Syndrome?

According to the World Health Organization (WHO), 8,098 people became ill with SARS during the 2003 outbreak and 774 of them died. However, scientists believe that some of the cases originally diagnosed as SARS may actually have been avian influenza* or bird flu, a potentially far more deadly disease. Most of the early victims were healthcare workers or family members of SARS patients.

In the United States, only eight people were diagnosed with confirmed SARS, all of whom had traveled to regions of the world where SARS was being transmitted. There were no SARS-related deaths in the United States.

A second outbreak of a milder strain of SARS-CoV, which occurred in December 2003 and January 2004, resulted in only four diagnosed cases. Nine cases in March and May 2004 were traced to laboratory accidents in China, Hong Kong, and Singapore. By late 2004, SARS had seemingly disappeared, almost as quickly as it had emerged.

How Is Severe Acute Respiratory Syndrome Spread?

Like most other respiratory infections, SARS is spread primarily by close person-to-person contact, in the droplets produced when an infected person talks, coughs, or sneezes. Droplets can be propelled up to about three

How Did Severe Acute Respiratory Syndrome Move around the World?

In November 2002 a farmer in the Pearl Delta region of Guangdong province in southeastern China died of an undiagnosed illness. On November 27, 2002, Canada's Global Public Health Intelligence Network picked up Internet reports of a flu outbreak in China and forwarded the reports to WHO. However, the Chinese government restricted media coverage and did not inform WHO of the outbreak until February 2003.

On February 21, 2003, a Chinese doctor who had been treating patients in a Guangdong hospital checked into the Metropole Hotel in Hong Kong. On February 26, Johnny Chen, an American businessman living in Shanghai, stayed at the Metropole before catching a flight to Singapore. When he became ill on the airplane, the flight was diverted to Hanoi, Vietnam. There Carlo Urbani, an Italian WHO physician, identified Chen's illness as a new disease. Chen died of SARS after transmitting the virus to hospital workers in Hanoi. Urbani died of SARS on March 29, at the age of 46. About 80 percent of SARS cases in Hong Kong were eventually traced back to the Chinese doctor. Within a few weeks travelers who had stayed at the Metropole in February unwittingly spread the virus to Singapore, Taiwan, Europe, Africa, and North and South America.

Outside Asia, Toronto, Canada, was the city most affected by SARS. A Canadian woman died of SARS shortly after returning to Toronto from Hong Kong. Her son entered a Toronto hospital with an illness that was later identified as SARS. While waiting 16 hours in the crowded emergency room, he infected two other people. WHO advised travelers to avoid Toronto, but on May 17, 2003, the outbreak was declared over. Then on May 23, a second larger SARS outbreak was traced to another hospital. Healthcare workers accounted for 45 percent of the 375 SARS cases eventually diagnosed in the province.

* **heart failure** is a medical term used to describe a condition in which a damaged heart cannot pump enough blood to meet the oxygen and nutrient demands of the body. People with heart failure may find if hard to exercise due to the insufficient blood flow, but many people live a long time with heart failure.

* **influenza** (in-floo-EN-zuh), also known as the flu, is a contagious viral infection that attacks the respiratory tract, including the nose, throat, and lungs.

* **mucous membranes** (MU-kus) are the moist linings of the mouth, nose, eyes, and throat, as well as the respiratory, intestinal, and genital tracts.

* **susceptibility** (su-sep-ti-BIL-i-tee) means having less resistance to and higher risk for infection or disease.

* **immune system** (im-YOON SIS-tem) is the system of the body composed of specialized cells and the substances they produce that helps protect the body against disease-causing germs.

feet, encountering the mucous membranes* of another person's mouth, nose, or eyes. Droplet spread also occurs when someone touches a surface contaminated with an infected droplet and then touches their mouth, nose, or eyes. The virus is believed to survive in droplets for up to six hours. It can survive up to three hours after the droplets have dried. SARS-CoV can live in stool for up to four days and may survive for months or longer in temperatures below freezing. It is possible that SARS-CoV can also be spread through airborne particles, which travel further and remain in the air longer than droplets.

SARS is thought to be contagious only while symptoms of the illness are present. It is most contagious during the second week of illness. Susceptibility* to SARS increases with age, with children least likely to become ill.

Scientists have identified a variation in an immune system* gene that may make people much more susceptible to SARS. This variation is common in people of Southeast Asian descent, but rare in other populations.

* **quarantine** is the enforced isolation (for a fixed period) of apparently well people or animals who may have been exposed to infectious disease.

* **diarrhea** (di-ah-RE-a) refers to frequent, watery stools (bowel movements).

* **nausea** (NAW-zha) refers to a feeling of being sick to one's stomach or needing to vomit.

* **pneumonia** (nu-MO-nyah) is inflammation of the lungs.

* **hypoxia** (hip-AK-see-ah) is when insufficient oxygen reaches the tissues of the body.

* **oxygen** (OK-si-jen) is an odorless, colorless gas essential for the human body. It is taken in through the lungs and delivered to the body by the bloodstream.

HOW DID THE WORLD RESPOND TO SEVERE ACUTE RESPIRATORY SYNDROME?

On March 12, 2003, WHO issued a global SARS alert and travel advisories were issued. Fearing a pandemic, WHO tracked and reported the disease daily until June 7, 2003. Schools were closed throughout Hong Kong and Singapore and national economies were disrupted. International cooperation and quarantine* resulted in rapid containment of the virus.

However, China was sharply criticized for its initial response to SARS. In a letter circulated in the international news media, Jiang Yanyong, a surgeon in China's People's Liberation Army, reported that at least 100 people were being treated for SARS in Beijing hospitals. At that time Chinese authorities were asserting that there were only a handful of cases in all of China. China's leaders were forced to admit that they had given WHO false information. Jiang was hailed as a hero both in China and abroad. However, Jiang used his newfound fame to demand that Chinese leaders admit their mistakes in shooting down unarmed civilians in the 1989 Tiananmen Square pro-democracy protests. Jiang was arrested. In 2007 the New York Academy of Sciences awarded him the Heinz R. Pagels Human Rights of Scientists Award. However, Chinese authorities denied Jiang permission to travel to the United States to accept the award.

How Do People Know They Have Severe Acute Respiratory Syndrome?

SARS causes flu-like symptoms, usually within two to seven days of becoming infected, although it can take up to ten days for symptoms to appear. The first symptom is usually a fever of at least 100.4 degrees F (38.0 degrees C). Headache, muscle pain, body aches, and chills sometimes appear 12 to 24 hours before the fever.

Other initial symptoms may include:

- Overall discomfort
- Fatigue
- Decreased appetite
- Diarrhea* and/or nausea* in 10 to 20 percent of people
- Occasionally, early mild respiratory symptoms such as a sore throat A dry nonproductive cough develops between two and seven days after the first symptoms.

Most people with SARS develop pneumonia*. This may be accompanied by hypoxia*, in which oxygen* levels in the blood are low, leading to shortness of breath.

How Do Doctors Diagnose and Treat Severe Acute Respiratory Syndrome?

Diagnosis The symptoms of SARS are very similar to those of other acute* severe respiratory infections, such as influenza. SARS is only suspected in a patient with a fever who has recently traveled to a region where SARS has been reported or who has been in close contact with someone with SARS. A probable SARS case is one that meets the above criteria and has chest x-rays or computerized tomography* CT scans indicating atypical pneumonia or acute respiratory distress syndrome. Tests may be performed to rule out infection with other respiratory viruses or bacteria* that can cause pneumonia.

There are three laboratory tests that can confirm SARS:

- Reverse transcription polymerase chain reaction can detect the SARS-CoV genetic material in a patient's blood, stool, or nasal secretions.
- Serologic testing can detect antibodies* against SARS-CoV in a patient's blood.
- SARS-CoV can be cultured* from body tissue or fluid.

Other diagnostic tests may include:

- Pulse oximetry to measure the amount of oxygen in the blood
- Blood clotting*
- Blood chemistries to measure lactate dehydrogenase, creatine kinase, and C-reactive protein, all of which are sometimes elevated with SARS
- A complete blood count, because white blood cells and platelets* are often elevated with SARS

Treatment SARS requires immediate medical attention and hospitalization under isolation. There is no specific treatment. SARS is managed similarly to other community-acquired atypical pneumonias, with intensive, supportive medical care. About 10 to 20 percent of SARS patients require supplemental oxygen or mechanical ventilation with a respirator* due to breathing difficulties. Clinical studies have suggested that a combination of antiretroviral drugs used to treat AIDS* may prevent the most serious complications of SARS.

Can Severe Acute Respiratory Syndrome Be Prevented?

As with other infectious diseases, the best way to prevent SARS is frequent and effective hand washing with soap and water or a hand rub containing at least 60 percent alcohol. Unwashed hands should never touch the eyes, nose, or mouth.

The Centers for Disease Control (CDC) recommends that people traveling to parts of the world where SARS has been reported take the following precautions:

* **acute** describes an infection or other illness that comes on suddenly and usually does not last very long.

* **computerized tomography** (kom-PYOO-ter-ized toe-MAH-gruh-fee) or CT, also called computerized axial tomography (CAT), is a technique in which a machine takes many x-rays of the body to create a three-dimensional picture.

* **bacteria** (bak-TEER-ee-a) are single-celled microorganisms, which typically reproduce by cell division. Some, but not all, types of bacteria can cause disease in humans. Many types can live in the body without causing harm.

* **antibodies** (AN-tih-bah-deez) are protein molecules produced by the body's immune system to help fight specific infections caused by microorganisms, such as bacteria and viruses.

* **cultured** (KUL-churd) means subjected to a test in which a sample of fluid or tissue from the body is placed in a dish containing material that supports the growth of certain organisms. Typically, within days the organisms will grow and can be identified.

* **clotting** is a process in which blood changes into a jellylike mass that stops the flow of blood.

* **platelets** (PLATE-lets) are tiny disk-shaped particles within the blood that play an important role in clotting.

* **respirator** is a machine that helps people breathe when they are unable to breathe adequately on their own.

* **AIDS** or acquired immunodeficiency (ih-myoo-no-dih-FIH-shen-see) syndrome, is an infection that severely weakens the immune system; it is caused by the human immunodeficiency virus (HIV).

- Be informed about SARS
- Pack a kit with first-aid and medical supplies, including an alcohol-based hand rub
- Identify healthcare resources in the region to be visited
- Have health insurance that covers medical evacuation
- Turn off the air vents located above the seats on airplanes and carry disposable towelettes to clean hands during flights
- Avoid areas such as healthcare facilities where SARS is more likely to be transmitted
- Avoid live-food markets and direct contact with wildlife in China
- Monitor one's health for 10 days after returning
- If symptoms develop within the 10-day period, a healthcare provider should be alerted of the symptoms and regions visited before the medical appointment, so that precautions can be taken

The CDC recommends that a person suspected of having SARS should take the following precautions for 10 days after the fever and respiratory symptoms disappear:

- Cover the mouth and nose with a tissue before coughing or sneezing
- Limit activities outside the home and avoid public places and public transportation
- Wash hands frequently and effectively, especially after blowing one's nose
- Wear a surgical mask around other people or have household members wear masks
- Minimize contact with other household members
- Avoid sharing utensils, towels, bedding, clothing, or other items until they have been washed with soap and hot water
- Avoid sharing food or drink with others
- Clean all household surfaces with a disinfectant while wearing disposable gloves

▶ *See also* **Influenza • Travel-related Infections**

Resources

Books and Articles

Abraham, Thomas. *Twenty-first Century Plague: The Story of SARS.* Baltimore, MD: Johns Hopkins University Press, 2005.

Greenfeld, Karl Taro. *China Syndrome: The True Story of the 21st Century's First Great Epidemic.* New York: HarperCollins, 2006.

Pan, Philip P. "The Last Hero of Tiananmen." *The New Republic* 238, no. 12 (July 9, 2008): 16.

Organizations

Centers for Disease Control and Prevention. 1600 Clifton Road, Atlanta, GA, 30333. Toll free: 800-311-3435. Web site: http://www.cdc.gov/ncidod/sars/index.htm.

World Health Organization. Avenue Appia 20, CH - 1211 Geneva 27, Switzerland. Telephone: +41 22 791 2111. Web site: http://www.who.int/csr/sars/en.

Sexual Development *See Puberty and Sexual Development.*

Sexual Disorders

The term "sexual disorders" refers to any problem with sexual performance or the function of sexual organs. Many of these problems have psychological or psychosomatic origins. Those with a physical or medical origin represent only a small percentage of all cases, but a substantial number. These cases occur more often than previously thought, probably due to underreporting.

A Story of Gender Identity

Bruce Reimer was born a healthy boy with an identical twin* brother (Brian) in 1965. When they were about eight months old, it was discovered that each brother had a small penis deformity that doctors assured their parents could be solved through a circumcision*. Although Brian's circumcision turned out all right, the doctor made a serious mistake with Bruce's circumcision and his penis was horribly disfigured. After several agonizing months, Reimer's parents saw a television program profiling John Money (1921–2006) of Johns Hopkins University in Baltimore, a psychologist and sexologist who posited that boys could successfully be raised as girls if the process was started early enough in life. The family went to see Money and Bruce was deemed a perfect candidate for this process. At the age of 21 months, doctors removed Bruce's testicles* and on discharge from the hospital, Bruce was renamed Brenda and raised as a girl. In the following years, Money wrote papers and gave talks, claiming that Bruce had adapted well to being female and was living a happy life.

In reality, Brenda had not adjusted and was not living a happy life. For many years, Bruce, living as Brenda, knew that there was something wrong, and he suffered with depression*. He had a terrible childhood, full of emotional trauma, not being able to keep up with the boys in sports yet embarrassed by not being like feminine girls. His relationships were marred by the lack of identity, he was in no way a typical girl in social

* **identical twins** are twins produced when a single egg from the mother is fertilized and divides to form two separate embryos of the same sex with nearly identical DNA.

* **circumcision** is a surgical procedure in which the fold of skin covering the end of the penis is removed.

* **testicles** (TES-tih-kulz) are the paired male reproductive glands that produce sperm.

* **depression** (de-PRESH-un) is a mental state characterized by feelings of sadness, despair, and discouragement.

* **estrogen** (ES-tro-jen) a steroid
  hormone that stimulates
  the development of female
  sexual characteristics and
  maintenance of the female
  reproductive system.

* **chromosomes** (KRO-mo-somz)
  are threadlike chemical
  structures inside cells on
  which the genes are located.
  There are 46 (23 pairs) of
  chromosomes in normal human
  cells. Genes on the X and Y
  chromosomes (known as the sex
  chromosomes) help determine
  whether a person is male or
  female. Females have two X
  chromosomes; males have one
  X and one Y chromosome.

skills. He suffered in his psychosocial development, because he could not explain his core identity, his gender identity. Finally, at age 14, after threatening to commit suicide rather than return to see Dr. Money, he learned the truth from his father.

After hearing about the operation that turned him into Brenda, Bruce decided to live his life as a man. He stopped the estrogen* injections, which gave him female characteristics, and began testosterone injections to develop male sexual characteristics, and he changed his name to David. He worked from that point to regain his identity and his life. David later married but remained unhappy and he committed suicide at the age of 39.

At the twins' birth, Reimer's parents did not receive the counseling they needed, and it is probable that his medical care was incompetent, to say the least. This case, along with others, sensitized medical professionals to both the physical and psychological complications of surgically treating ambiguous genitalia.

What Are Pathophysiological Sexual Disorders?

Pathophysiological (physiological disruption of normal function) sexual disorder includes any sexual disorder that results from physical problems. The disorder can be as serious as structural deformities in the male or female sex organs. Further classification involves whether the disorder is congenital (existing from birth) or if it was acquired (shaped by a traumatic incident). Pathophysiological sexual disorders have similar symptoms to sexual dysfunction except the causes are different: Sexual dysfunction is often brought on by psychological or psychophysical (the influence of psychological factors on physical function) influences. Only 10 percent of sexual disorders are truly pathophysiological with a clear physical or medical origin. They include intersex (discrepancies between external genitals and internal sex organs) conditions, male pathophysiological sexual dysfunction, and female pathophysiological sexual dysfunction.

Intersex conditions   The term "hermaphrodite" was historically used to describe individuals who had both male and female sexual characteristics. In Greek mythology, Hermes and Aphrodite mated and Hermaphrodite was born of that union, an individual who had both male and female sexual identity. The term continues in the 21st century to be used to describe certain plants and animals that have both male and female sexual organs. Regarding humans, however, in the 20th century, the term "intersex" began to be used to describe individuals who in various ways incorporate both female and male physical sexual traits.

Intersex conditions take many forms. Four basic ways these conditions can be categorized are as follows:

- a child with male sex chromosomes* who has what appears to be female genitalia
- a child with female chromosomes who has what appears to be male genitalia

■ a child with partial genital characteristics of both sexes

■ a child with a mosaic chromosomal scheme (presence of two genotypes in one individual from one egg) without a clear chromosomal gender

Although these four categories as such are discussed in medical literature, the cases within any one of these categories can be further classified according to the circumstances influencing their cause.

One of the common causes of intersex conditions in both males and females is congenital adrenal hyperplasia, a serious medical imbalance in which the adrenal glands either do not produce enough vital hormones or else produce too much of one. This imbalance interferes with normal development and growth in all parts of the body, including the sex organs. In males, an intersex condition can be caused if the adrenal glands* do not produce enough testosterone; in females, an intersex condition can be caused if the adrenal glands produce too much testosterone.

A fetus* with male chromosomes may appear to be female at birth if the hormonal deficiency is experienced in the first twelve weeks of gestation. If the deficiency is experienced later in the pregnancy, it may lead to the baby having an extremely small penis, a condition known as microphallus. Masculine features are influenced after birth by the testosterone produced in the testes. If the testes are missing or weak due to prenatal hormonal deficiencies, then they cannot produce enough testosterone for full functioning of the male sex characteristics. Another problem is if the male baby does not have a testosterone deficiency but is missing the capacity to produce an enzyme that enables testosterone to effectively influence sex development. Many individuals with this condition have been unknowingly raised as females until puberty* increased the level of effective testosterone. The adolescent then surprisingly takes on more masculine features.

A genetically female fetus may be exposed to male sex hormones from a variety of sources other than congenital adrenal hyperplasia. The mother may have been prescribed progesterone as a means of preventing a miscarriage*. This artificial hormone sometimes crosses the placenta and acts as testosterone on the developing fetus. Another source of exposure to male hormones is the lack of an enzyme that converts the sex hormones to estrogen, which develops the female sex organs and other gender-related characteristics. Another source of male hormones is a tumor* in the glands. On rare occasions, the tumor may produce the male sex hormones in a young female.

Male pathophysiological sexual dysfunction
The most common sexual disorder in males is erectile dysfunction of the penis. This condition is most often caused by psychological problems or stress. However, there are several physical causes of the disorder, most of which are associated with aging. Although erectile dysfunction can happen to men of all ages for physical or medical reasons, about one-half of men over age 65 and three fourths of men over age 80 report erectile dysfunction. Three

* **adrenal glands** (a-DREEN-al glands) are the pair of endocrine organs located near the kidneys.

* **fetus** (FEE-tus) is the term for an unborn human after it is an embryo, from 9 weeks after fertilization until childbirth.

* **puberty** (PU-ber-tee) is the period during which sexual maturity is attained.

* **miscarriage** (MIS-kare-ij) is the end of a pregnancy through the death of the embryo or fetus before birth.

* **tumor** (TOO-mor) is an abnormal growth of body tissue that has no known cause or physiologic purpose. A tumor may or may not be cancerous.

* **diabetes** (dye-uh-BEE-teez) is a condition in which the body's pancreas does not produce enough insulin or the body cannot use the insulin it makes effectively, resulting in increased levels of sugar in the blood. This can lead to increased urination, dehydration, weight loss, weakness, and a number of other symptoms and complications related to chemical imbalances within the body.

* **clot** is the process by which the body forms a thickened mass of blood cells and protein to stop bleeding.

* **pituitary** (pih-TOO-ih-tare-e) is a small oval-shaped gland at the base of the skull that produces several hormones—substances that affect various body functions, including growth.

* **vulva** (VUL-vuh) refers to the organs of the female genitals that are located on the outside of the body.

* **vagina** (vah-JY-nah) is the canal, or passageway, in a woman that leads from the uterus to the outside of the body.

* **Bartholin glands** (BAR-tha-lin) are two very small glands, inside the vagina, that are important for vaginal lubrication during sexual intercourse.

* **cervix** (SIR-viks) is the lower, narrow end of the uterus that opens into the vagina.

* **fallopian tubes** (fa-LO-pee-an tubes) are the two slender tubes that connect the ovaries and the uterus in females. They carry the ova, or eggs, from the ovaries to the uterus.

main causes are: problems with the blood flow, problems with the nerves in the penile area, and problems with hormones.

The blood flow problems are of two types: not enough blood flows into the penis or the blood in the penis flows out too quickly. To sustain an erection, blood needs to engorge the penis. If the incoming blood vessels are too constricted, then not enough blood can flow into the penis to enlarge and stiffen the penis. However, if the outgoing blood vessels are not constricted enough, then blood cannot stay in the penis long enough to maintain an erection. These problems are caused by abnormalities in the blood vessels caused by previous surgery, diabetes*, blood clots*, or arteriosclerosis (hardening of the arteries).

Nerve damage in the penile area can interfere with the neurological communication that stimulates an erection in the penis. The nerve damage might be with the nerves sending the message from the brain to stimulate the functions that result in an erection. Alternatively, the damage may be in the nerves sending sensation to the brain diminishing the effects of sexual stimulation. This problem can be caused by spinal cord injuries from infection, external impact, or structural change. Other causes of penile nerve damage include diabetes, previous surgery, and nerve system irregularities.

Problems with hormones are related to failure of the testes to produce testosterone. The two hormones important for a balance leading to normal sexual functioning are testosterone and gonadotropin. Testosterone is responsible for all male sexual characteristics. Gonadotropin is produced by the pituitary* gland to stimulate production of testosterone. The presence of above average gonadotropin indicates that the testes are not producing enough testosterone. Too little testosterone and too much gonadotropin can lead to erectile dysfunction.

Female pathophysiological sexual dysfunction Dysparunia is the condition in which sexual intercourse is painful for women. As the pain is greater than any pleasure derived from sexual intercourse, a woman experiencing dysparunia is likely to avoid sexual relationships. The causes of this condition are varied, but they can be grouped according to whether the pain is felt during or after intercourse.

If the pain is felt during intercourse, it may be caused by infection to the vulva*, the vagina*, or the Bartholin glands*. Other causes include the after-effects of surgery from childbirth and congenital irregularities in the hymen (the membrane that covers the opening to the vagina) or the vaginal walls.

If the pain is felt after intercourse, its cause may be an infection of the cervix*, uterus, or fallopian tubes*. Most often these are the results of pelvic inflammatory disease caused by the sexually transmitted bacteria, chlamydia and gonorrhea. Other causes can be a pelvic tumor or internal scar tissue that forms after surgery or an infection.

Many women suffer pelvic pain and infertility due to endometriosis, a condition in which tissue cells similar to the ones lining the uterus are found outside the uterus in the abdominal cavity or in other organs.

When these cells line the ovaries or the fallopian tubes they can interfere with the normal functioning of these organs leading to infertility. Endometriosis can also be the cause of other sexual disorders.

Vaginismus, the involuntary contractions of vaginal muscles, is a symptom associated with many sexual dysfunctions. When this symptom occurs, the sexual act is interrupted as penetration becomes difficult or painful for the woman. It can be caused by current infections or by previous painful vaginal experience such as surgery or difficult childbirth. It is a natural reaction to anticipated pain of intercourse.

Vaginitis and vaginal atrophy are conditions resulting in irritation in the vagina. Vaginitis is usually the result of an infection. Vaginal atrophy is usually caused by the lack of lubrication associated with age.

Consistent irritation in the vulva area is referred to as vulvodynia. This condition occurs without warning and continues without relief. It is usually caused by damage to the nerves in that area. It usually occurs with (or is instigated by) a number of other conditions, including yeast infection, skin disorders, and diabetes. Vulvodynia can only be diagnosed by ruling out any other disorder as the cause.

Sexual arousal disorder is the condition in which a woman cannot be fully aroused to have sexual relations. It is often found to be caused by psychological conditions, such as fear of intimacy or loathing the current sex partner. However, there are several physical conditions that can lead to lack of sexual arousal. These include vaginitis, endometriosis, diabetes, or aging. If a woman knows that she has no psychological reason to reject sexual relations, she should have a health exam to determine if any medical problem could be the cause of her sexual arousal disorder.

How Common Is Pathophysiologic Sexual Dysfunction?

Most estimates of sexual dysfunction report that 43 percent of women and 31 percent of men experience some form of sexual dysfunction. However, less than 10 percent involve a physical cause. A survey of gynecologists found that when the doctor asked the patient about sexual problems, 12 percent reported a problem, presumably of a gynecological origin. Diabetes contributes to sexual dysfunction: 50 percent of men and 35 percent of women with Type 2 diabetes report trouble with sexual relations. One-half to two-thirds of patients with heart disease also experience sexual disorders. The occurrence of any intersex condition, regardless of how mild or severe, is estimated at 1 percent of all births.

How Do People Know They Have Pathophysiologic Sexual Dysfunction?

Many people live with a below average sexual drive and live relatively happy lives despite that fact. As many of the conditions of sexual disorders are not life-threatening, these people can lead normal lives without treatment. However, when individuals participating in a sexual relationship or anticipating a sexual relationship cannot function as they want, then

* **ultrasound** also called a sonogram, is a diagnostic test in which sound waves passing through the body create images on a computer screen.

treatment may be required. Similarly, some people are comfortable in an intersex state and content to remain the way they were born. However, if it is interfering with adapting to life, these individuals may seek medical advice and consider or undergo a gender reassignment operation.

If adults with diabetes or heart disease experience a decrease in sexual desire, they may have a sexual disorder related to the medical condition. Adolescents who do not develop sexually at the same rate as their peers may suspect a sexual disorder and seek medical advice and examination.

How Do Doctors Diagnose and Treat Pathophysiologic Sexual Disorders?

The diagnosis of any sexual disorder begins with taking a medical history and performing a physical exam. The common causes of sexual disorders are tested, such as diabetes, heart disease, or gland disorders. Blood and urine tests are used to analyze the presence of hormones and to determine the chromosomal gender. Any irregularities in hormonal or chromosomal balance would indicate a disorder. The effort would be made to identify and treat any underlying medical conditions. Many times the sexual disorder disappears when treatment for the underlying condition is effective. Hormonal imbalances indicate the need for diagnosis and treatment of any disorders in the glands producing the hormone.

Diagnosis The beginning of the search for a diagnosis is a complete history and a physical exam. A hormonal imbalance in men would be recognized by feminine characteristics such as a high-pitched voice, and legs and arms might be unusually large for the patient's age. Other symptoms include physical size below average for age in muscles and sexual organs. For women, a hormonal imbalance would be recognized by a large clitoris resembling a penis and a missing or malformed vagina.

For someone suspected of having an intersex condition because the sexual organs are not clearly male or female, a series of tests should be conducted. Blood tests would reveal the chromosomal gender. Sexual organs that are not in the genital area, such as testes that have not descended, can be detected by x-rays or ultrasound* imaging of the pelvic area. Amniocentesis, which is the analysis of fluids drawn from the uterus of a pregnant woman, can indicate developmental abnormalities of the fetus and the irregular presence of sex hormones.

The diagnosis for sexual dysfunction in men and women begins with a medical history and a physical exam for general physical health. Any problems with blood flow can be identified through testing the blood pressure in the legs. Any problems with the nerves in the penile area can be detected through rectal exams, which would indicate if the nerves in that area are healthy and fully functional. Problems with hormonal imbalance can be indicated through blood tests. The nature of female sexual disorders needs to be diagnosed by focusing on the specific cause. Endometriosis is identified through a series of tests. An ultrasound of the area can present visual evidence of the effects of endometriosis. A blood test analyzes the presence of a blood protein common in women with endometriosis. For men and women the doctor should do blood tests for specific diseases associated with sexual dysfunction.

Treatment Treatment focuses on resolving the specific complaint of patients with pathophysiological sexual disorder. Two well-known treatments are hormonal replacement therapy and sex reassignment surgery. Hormone replacement therapy involves prescribing synthetic hormones to imitate the effects of the normal hormonal levels. For men the synthetic hormone replaces testosterone; for women, the synthetic hormone replaces estrogen. For men and women, this treatment is fairly effective, but not without complications. Testosterone replacement in men is associated with liver disorders. Estrogen replacement in women contributes to higher risks of breast cancer.

Through much of the 20th century, doctors recommended sex reassignment operations at an early age, based on the assumption that young children can adapt to the reassigned sex and experience little trauma and discontinuity in development. Advocates also felt that early reassignment increased the effectiveness of parent/child bonding as the parents would know to treat the child as a member of the reassigned sex. The child would grow up knowing to accept the gender role of the reassigned sex. For this to be effective, the parents had to be strong in their decision from the start and had to continue with that decision through consistent behavior for the rest of the child's life.

Arguing for the contrary point of view is the case of David Reimer. David lived a traumatic childhood, partly because he thought he was a girl but did not feel like a girl. Once David found out that he was born male, he changed his life to live as a man, but he was unhappy and died early as a suicide. The Reimer case led to more criticism of early surgical sex reassignment for ambiguous genitalia and other physiological conditions of intersex. Critics point out that structural changes made surgically do not affect genetic composition.

Many serious studies of sex reassignment have found that most of the affected people do not adjust well. As much as possible, these individuals should be recognized by their chromosomal gender. If the chromosomal gender is clearly identified, minor operations may be done to reduce genital abnormalities. Also, if the sexual disorder is influenced by hormonal deficiencies, the doctor may recommend hormone treatments. If gender clarification surgery is necessary later in life, it should be at a time when affected individuals can have a voice in the decision making.

Complications Pathophysiological problems need a medical response. However, no matter what the cause, there are always psychological implications. The usual brain-to-body communication is interrupted through the physical disorder. The need to reestablish the connection may require psychotherapy. However, whereas most sexual disorders have a psychological component, without identifying and treating the physical cause, psychotherapy alone would not be effective.

* **cervix** (SIR-viks) is the lower, narrow end of the uterus that opens into the vagina.

* **uterus** (YOO-teh-rus) is the muscular, pear-shaped internal organ in a woman where a baby develops until birth.

* **fallopian tubes** (fa-LO-pee-an tubes) are the two slender tubes that connect the ovaries and the uterus in females. They carry the ova, or eggs, from the ovaries to the uterus.

* **epididymitis** (eh-pih-dih-duh-MY-tis) is a painful inflammation of the epididymitis, a structure attached to the testicles.

* **prostate** (PRAH-state) is a male reproductive gland located near where the bladder joins the urethra. The prostate produces the fluid part of semen.

Resources

Books and Articles

Colapinto, John. *As Nature Made Him: The Boy Who Was Raised as a Girl.* New York: HarperCollins, 2000.

Fagan, Peter J. *Sexual Disorders: Perspectives on Diagnosis and Treatment.* Baltimore, MD: Johns Hopkins University Press, 2004.

Goldstein, Andrew, Caroline Pukall, Irwin Goldstein. *Female Sexual Pain Disorders: Evaluation and Management.* Hoboken, NJ: Wiley, 2009.

Kandeel, Fouad R. *Male Sexual Dysfunction: Pathophysiology and Treatment.* New York: Informa Healthcare, 2007.

Van der Wijngaard, Marianne. *Reinventing the Sexes: Biomedical Construction of Femininity and Masculinity.* Indianapolis: Indiana University Press, 1997.

Organization

Intersex Society of North America. 979 Golf Course Drive, No. 282, Rohnert Park, CA, 94928, Web site: http://www.isna.org.

Sexually Transmitted Diseases (STDs)

Sexually transmitted diseases (STDs) are infections that pass from one person to another through sexual contact, which includes oral, genital, or anal intercourse.

What Are Sexually Transmitted Diseases?

STDs can be caused by bacteria, viruses, or parasites. Although the symptoms of a particular STD depend on the specific infection, many STDs cause vaginitis (vah-jih-NYE-tis), an inflammation of the vagina often accompanied by an abnormal discharge (fluid released from the body), and urethritis (yoo-ree-THRY-tis), an inflammation of the urethra (the tube through which urine passes from the bladder to the outside of the body), which can make urination painful. Several STDs can produce blisters or sores on the penis, vagina, rectum, or buttocks. In women, some STDs may spread to the cervix*, a condition called cervicitis (sir-vih-SYE-tis), or to the uterus* and fallopian tubes*, a condition known as pelvic inflammatory disease (PID). In men, STDs may spread to the testicle (causing epididymitis*) or prostate* (causing prostatitis, which is inflammation of the prostate). Sometimes, several STDs may occur in the

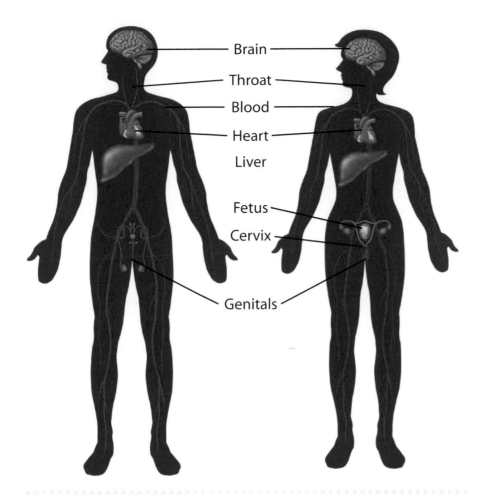

Brain

Throat

Blood

Heart

Liver

Fetus

Cervix

Genitals

Sexually transmitted diseases affect many parts of the body. *Illustration by Frank Forney. Reproduced by permission of Gale, a part of Cengage Learning.*

same person, and the presence of an STD can increase the risk of contracting infection with human immunodeficiency (ih-myoo-no-dih-FIH-shen-see) virus (HIV*), the virus that causes acquired immunodeficiency syndrome (AIDS), from an infected partner.

How Common Are Sexually Transmitted Diseases?

STDs are common in the United States, and medical professionals diagnose between 13 million and 15 million new cases every year. Although considerable information is available about preventing these infections and limiting their spread, the number of people infected is growing. About two-thirds of all reported cases occur in people who are younger than 25 years of age.

Are STDs Contagious?

STDs are contagious and are transmitted through sexual contact that involves vaginal, anal, or oral sex. The diseases can spread between people of the opposite sex or people of the same sex. The germs that cause many STDs move from person to person through semen (the sperm-containing whitish fluid produced by the male reproductive tract), vaginal (VAH-jih-nul) fluids, or blood. Other STDs such as herpes and genital warts

* **HIV** or human immunodeficiency virus (HYOO-mun ih-myoo-no-dih-FIH-shen-see), is the virus that causes AIDS (acquired immunodeficiency syndrome).

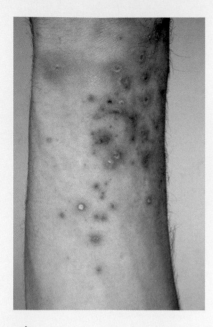

▲

Skin abscesses caused by gonococcal infection. *Biophoto Associates/Photo Researchers, Inc.*

* **lymph nodes** (LIMF) are small, bean-shaped masses of tissue containing immune system cells that fight harmful microorganisms. Lymph nodes may swell during infections.

* **paralysis** (pah-RAH-luh-sis) is the loss or impairment of the ability to move some part of the body.

* **dementia** (dih-MEN-sha) is a loss of mental abilities, including memory, understanding, and judgment.

can spread by intimate skin-to-skin contact, often with the sores that the disease causes. A mother can transmit certain STDs to her baby during pregnancy or childbirth. STDs do not pass from one person to another by simply hugging, shaking hands, or sharing utensils.

What Are Some Common Sexually Transmitted Diseases?

Gonorrhea   The bacterium *Neisseria gonorrhoeae* (nye-SEER-e-uh gah-no-REE-eye) causes gonorrhea (gah-nuh-REE-uh). Women who are infected may not have any symptoms. When they do, symptoms include vaginal discharge and pain during urination. Lower belly pain usually occurs when the infection has spread past the cervix and caused PID. Most men with gonorrhea have a discharge from the penis and pain during urination. Doctors prescribe antibiotics to patients with gonorrhea; the antibiotics kill the bacteria. Not infrequently, individuals with gonorrhea are also infected with Chlamydia.

Syphilis   The bacterium *Treponema pallidum* (treh-puh-NEE-muh PAL-ih-dum) causes syphilis (SIH-fih-lis). Unlike many other STDs, this illness has distinct stages. In the first stage, a small, hard sore called a chancre (SHANG-ker) appears where the bacteria entered the body. In the next stage, a red or brown rash develops, sometimes on the palms of the hands and soles of the feet. In some cases, patients also may have a fever, swollen lymph nodes*, muscle aches, and headaches. If the disease goes untreated, it can progress to the third and most serious stage, when it may damage the bones, organs, and nervous system. At this point, it can result in blindness, paralysis*, dementia*, heart problems, and sometimes even death. As they do with gonorrhea, doctors can treat syphilis with antibiotics. Medical professionals reported more than 36,000 cases of syphilis in the United States in 2006, which indicates a marked increase since the beginning of the new millennium.

Herpes simplex virus   Herpes simplex (HER-peez SIM-plex) virus causes herpes. Herpes comes in two types, one of which—type 2—usually spreads through sexual contact and causes genital herpes. In a person with genital herpes, small, painful blisters develop on the vagina, cervix, penis, buttocks, or thighs. Once infection occurs, the herpes virus remains in the body and can recur throughout a person's life. Antiviral medications may shorten outbreaks of symptoms and make them less severe, but they do not kill the virus. In the United States, an estimated 45 million people over the age of 12 have genital herpes infection.

Chlamydia   Chlamydia (kla-MIH-dee-uh) results from infection with the bacterium *Chlamydia trachomatis* (kla-MIH-dee-uh truh-KO-mah-tis). In many infected people, it produces no symptoms. The most common symptoms in both men and women are discharge and pain during urination. Because infection with *Chlamydia* often goes unnoticed, it can spread and produce other symptoms, including epididymitis in men and PID in women. The Centers for Disease Control and Prevention estimates that *Chlamydia* bacteria infect 2.8 million people in the United States each year. Medical professionals use antibiotics to treat the infection effectively.

HIV   Infection with HIV damages immune system cells in the body that normally fight infections, leaving the body unable to defend itself against a variety of illnesses. A person can be infected with HIV and not have AIDS, although most people with untreated HIV infection eventually develop AIDS. The first symptoms of HIV infection are fever, muscle aches, sore throat, and, in some cases, a rash that looks somewhat like that of measles*. Other symptoms usually take much longer to appear—perhaps years—and may include rapid weight loss, recurring fever, a dry cough, night sweats, pneumonia*, white spots on the tongue or throat, long-lasting diarrhea, and skin rashes and yeast infections. A person with AIDS* may also have memory loss, depression, and extreme tiredness.

Despite significant advances in treatment, HIV infection continued in the early 2000s to be an epidemic of global proportions. The CDC estimated as of 2008 that more than one million Americans may be infected with HIV, but 25 percent of them are unaware of their infection. In the United States, estimates indicate that more than 56,000 new HIV infections occur every year. Between the early 1980s when the disease was first identified in the United States and 2008, more than 540,000 people in the United States died due to complications of AIDS. No cure for AIDS exists, but a combination of medications can help an infected person live longer and have a better quality of life.

Human papillomavirus   Genital and anal warts are caused by human papillomavirus (pah-pih-LO-mah-vy-rus), or HPV, a very common virus. The warts are soft and skin-colored, and they can grow alone or in bunches on the genitals; on the skin around the genitals, rectum, or buttocks; or in the vagina or cervix. Like herpes, genital warts can reappear many times, because once this type of virus enters the body, it remains there for life. Doctors can remove genital warts by freezing, burning, or cutting them off or by coating them with medication that destroys the warts. In women, infection with HPV can affect the cells of the cervix, which may lead to cervical cancer.

Trichomoniasis   A parasite causes trichomoniasis (trih-ko-mo-NYE-uh-sis), which is a very common STD. Most women with trichomoniasis have a frothy, yellow, foul-smelling vaginal discharge, along with itching and irritation in the vagina and discomfort during sex and urination. Men with this STD typically do not have symptoms; those who do have symptoms may feel irritation in the penis or a burning sensation after they urinate or ejaculate*. Medical professionals diagnose more than 2 million cases each year in the United States. Doctors use antibiotics to treat trichomoniasis.

* **measles** (ME-zuls) is a viral respiratory infection that is best known for the rash of large, flat, red blotches that appear on the arms, face, neck, and body.

* **pneumonia** (nu-MO-nyah) is inflammation of the lungs.

* **AIDS** or acquired immunodeficiency (ih-myoo-no-dih-FIH-shen-see) syndrome, is an infection that severely weakens the immune system; it is caused by the human immunodeficiency virus (HIV).

* **ejaculate** (e-JAH-kyoo-late) means to discharge semen from the penis.

preparations of killed or
weakened germs, or a part of
a germ or product it produces,
given to prevent or lessen the
severity of the disease that can
result if a person is exposed to
the germ itself. Use of vaccines
for this purpose is called
immunization.

Can Sexually Transmitted Diseases Be Prevented?

The only sure way to prevent STDs is to refrain from having sexual contact with anyone. In most cases, it is impossible or very difficult to tell whether another person has an STD. People may not always tell the truth about their sexual past, or they may have an STD and not know it. For people who do have sex, the safest choices are to limit the number of sexual partners and to use latex condoms. Latex condoms lower the risk of contracting many STDs, including becoming infected with HIV. Certain STDs such as genital warts and herpes may present additional problems, because the warts or herpes blisters can be on the skin around the genitals, and condoms only protect against infection from the warts and blisters they cover. Avoiding skin-to-skin contact is the best option for preventing these kinds of STDs.

In addition, vaccines* are available against some STDs, such as hepatitis B and specific HPVs. These vaccines are most effective at the time in a person's life before he or she has engaged in any sexual contact.

▶ See also **AIDS and HIV Infection • Bacterial Infections • Chlamydial Infections • Fungal Infections • Genital Warts • Gonorrhea • Herpes Simplex Virus Infections • Human Papilloma Virus (HPV) • Nonspecific Urethritis • Rape • Syphilis • Trichomoniasis • Urinary Tract Infections • Viral Infections**

Resources

Books and Articles

Hunter, Miranda, and William Hunter. *Staying Safe: A Teen's Guide to Sexually Transmitted Diseases.* Philadelphia, PA: Mason Crest, 2005.

Marr, Lisa. *Sexually Transmitted Diseases: A Physician Tells You What You Need to Know,* 2nd ed. Baltimore, MD: Johns Hopkins University Press, 2007.

Radziszewicz, Tina. *Ready or Not? A Girl's Guide to Making Her Own Decisions about Dating, Love, and Sex.* New York: Walker, 2006.

Silverstein, Alvin, Virginia Silverstein, and Laura Silverstein Nunn. *The STDs Update.* Berkeley Heights, NJ: Enslow Elementary, 2006.

Organizations

Centers for Disease Control and Prevention. 1600 Clifton Road, Atlanta, GA, 30333. Toll free: 800-232-4636. Web site: http://www.cdc.gov/std.

Food and Drug Administration. 5600 Fishers Lane, Rockville, MD, 20857. Toll free: 888-INFO-FDA. Web site: http://www.fda.gov/oashi/aids/condom.html.

National Institute of Allergy and Infectious Diseases. Office of Communications and Public Liaison, 6610 Rockledge Drive, MSC 6612, Bethesda, MD, 20892-6612. Toll free: 866-284-4107. Web site: http://www3.niaid.nih.gov/topics/sti.

* **aortic aneurysm** (ay-OR-tik AN-yoo-rizm) is a weak spot in the aorta, the body's largest blood vessel. The weak spot can rupture or break, causing massive internal bleeding.

Shin Splints *See Strains and Sprains.*

Shingles *See Varicella (Chicken Pox) and Herpes Zoster (Shingles).*

Shock

Shock is a dangerous physical condition in which the flow of blood throughout the body is drastically reduced, causing weakness, confusion, or loss of consciousness. It can result from many kinds of serious injuries and illnesses. If shock is not treated quickly, a person can suffer permanent organ damage and die.

What Is Shock?

"I studied for days, but I failed the test. I'm in shock," says one teenager to another.

In everyday speech, the use of the word "shock" is common and sometimes even enjoyable. People line up to see horror movies because they want to be shocked. They want to feel an emotional jolt from seeing something sudden, surprising, and scary. Their hearts may beat a little faster for a moment, but when the movie ends, they are as healthy as before.

This kind of emotional shock has nothing to do with the medical condition called shock. Shock in the medical sense can also be sudden, surprising, and scary, but it is a specific physical condition that is extremely serious.

Shock occurs when the amount of blood reaching the brain and other parts of the body drops sharply. In other words, it occurs when the blood pressure falls very low. Because the blood carries oxygen needed by every cell in the body, the drop in blood flow deprives the cells of oxygen. The brain, the biggest user of oxygen, is affected, and the person becomes confused or dazed or may lose consciousness. As cells struggle to function without enough oxygen, many chemical processes in the body are disrupted. Organs, including the lungs, kidneys, liver, and heart, start to fail. Unless the blood flow is restored quickly, the damage may be fatal.

What Causes Shock?

Shock has underlying causes. Often, a case of shock involves two or all three of these types of underlying problems. They are as follows:

- The bloodstream does not contain enough fluid. This kind of shock is called hypovolemic (hy-po-vo-LEEM-ik) shock. Its causes include heavy bleeding from an injury, such as a gunshot wound or wounds suffered in a car crash, or from severe bleeding due to a medical condition, such as an aortic aneurysm* or bleeding stomach ulcers.

Electrical Shock

An electric current that passes through the body is called a shock. Although such a shock is often dangerous (electrical accidents kill about 1,000 people per year in the United States), electrical shock is different from the medical shock discussed in this entry.

Medical shock is a reduction in blood flow. Electrical shock, by contrast, primarily causes internal burns and disruption of heart rhythms. In some cases, an electrical shock can cause medical shock. This situation occurs if the burns lead to rapid loss of fluid and the heart problems prevent adequate pumping of blood.

* **blood clot** is a thickening of the blood into a jelly-like substance that helps stop bleeding. Clotting of the blood within a blood vessel can lead to blockage of blood flow.

* **leukemia** (loo-KEE-me-uh) is a form of cancer characterized by the body's uncontrolled production of abnormal white blood cells.

* **blood transfusion** is the process of giving blood (or certain cells or chemicals found in the blood) to a person who needs it due to illness or blood loss.

It can also result if a person loses large amounts of fluids other than blood. This situation can occur, for instance, if a person has severe vomiting and diarrhea or has experienced bad burns over a large part of the body.

- The blood vessels dilate (expand) too much, which causes the blood pressure (the pressure within the blood vessels) to become so low that it cannot push along enough blood to reach vital tissues. The most common example of this kind of shock is septic (SEP-tik) shock, which results from a severe bacterial infection.

- The heart fails to pump the blood strongly enough, which is called cardiogenic (kar-dee-o-GEN-ik) shock. It can result from many heart problems, including a heart attack, an abnormal heart rhythm, a blood clot* in the heart, or a buildup of fluid around the heart that presses on the organ. Severe damage to a heart valve can also cause cardiogenic shock.

What Is Septic Shock?

Septic shock occurs when a person becomes infected with bacteria that get into the bloodstream and produce a dangerous level of toxins (poisons). Even when treated, it is sometimes fatal.

It is most common among hospitalized people who have recently had surgery or who have had drainage tubes, breathing tubes, or other devices inserted into their body. Such devices increase the chances that bacteria will get into the bloodstream.

Other people at risk for septic shock are those with weakened immune systems, including those who have diabetes, cirrhosis, leukemia*, or AIDS. Newborns and pregnant women are also at risk.

Toxic shock syndrome is a form of septic shock that experts originally linked to the use of certain tampons.

What Is Anaphylactic Shock?

Anaphylactic (an-a-fi-LAK-tik) shock is a severe allergic reaction. Depending on the individual, the trigger may be a certain medication, a blood transfusion*, a bee sting, or particular foods, such as peanuts. During anaphylactic shock, fluid leaks out from the blood vessels and the blood vessels dilate. This type of shock is sometimes fatal.

What Are the Symptoms of Shock?

Whatever its cause, people with shock have rapid and shallow breathing, cold and clammy skin, a weak but rapid pulse, low blood pressure, and weakness all over the body. They are dizzy, confused, and may become unconscious.

How Is Shock Treated?

People in shock require immediate transport by ambulance to a hospital. Until the ambulance arrives, a friend, family member, or other onlooker should take on the role of caregiver and have the person lie down on the back with the feet raised about a foot higher than the head. This position helps get the blood flowing to the brain and heart. The caregiver should also cover the person with a coat or blankets to keep the individual warm.

Medical workers will try to raise the blood pressure by giving fluids intravenously (through a needle into a vein). If the shock was caused by blood loss, they may also start a blood transfusion. If the blood pressure still remains dangerously low, they may use drugs known as pressors to raise the blood pressure. For anaphylactic shock, medical professionals give the drug epinephrine (ep-i-NEF-rin), also called adrenaline*, to constrict (narrow) the blood vessels. For septic shock, doctors may give a drug called drotrecogin alpha, and in some cases they may prescribe corticosteroids but only at low dosage. Several studies of high-dosage corticosteroid therapy have shown it is not beneficial and may even be damaging.

Another common treatment for shock is oxygen. Medical professionals routinely administer oxygen, and in some cases they may put the patient on a ventilator (a breathing machine) to increase the amount of oxygen getting to the cells. If septic shock is suspected, they may also give intravenous antibiotics.

Once the person is out of immediate danger, doctors can try to treat the underlying cause of the shock.

How Can Shock Be Prevented?

Individuals can reduce their chances of experiencing shock by following safety rules to prevent fires and serious accidents, including car crashes. To avert bacterial infections that can cause septic shock, hospitals have rules about sterilizing equipment and washing hands. To prevent anaphylactic shock, people with allergies must take care to avoid the foods or other substances that trigger them.

▶ *See also* **Burns • Heart Disease • Toxic Shock Syndrome**

Resources

Organization

National Library of Medicine. 8600 Rockville Pike, Bethesda, MD, 20894, Web site: http://www.nlm.nih.gov/medlineplus/ency/article/000039.html.

Shyness *See Social Phobia (Social Anxiety Disorder).*

Siamese Twins *See Conjoined Twins*

---

* **adrenaline** (a-DREN-a-lin), also called epinephrine, (ep-e-NEF-rin), is a hormone, or chemical messenger, that is released in response to fear, anger, panic, and other emotions. It readies the body to respond to threat by increasing heart rate, breathing rate, and blood flow to the arms and legs. These and other effects prepare the body to run away or fight.

* **hemoglobin** (HE-muh-glo-bin) is the oxygen-carrying pigment of the red blood cells.

* **inflammation** (in-fla-MAY-shun) is the body's reaction to irritation, infection, or injury that often involves swelling, pain, redness, and warmth.

* **anemia** (uh-NEE-me-uh) is a blood condition in which there is a decreased hemoglobin in the blood and, usually, fewer than normal numbers of red blood cells.

* **genes** (JEENS) are chemical structures composed of deoxyribonucleic acid (DNA) that help determine a person's body structure and physical characteristics. Inherited from a person's parents, genes are contained in the chromosomes found in the body's cells.

Sickle-Cell Anemia

Sickle-cell anemia, also called sickle-cell disease, is a hereditary disorder in which abnormal hemoglobin* within the red blood cells (RBCs) causes the cells to take on abnormal sickle (crescent) shapes. This shape decreases the ability of the hemoglobin to transport oxygen throughout the body. The sickled cells tend to bunch up and clog the blood vessels, and they tend to break apart more easily than normal RBCs, which may cause inflammation*, pain, tissue damage, and anemia*.

What Are the Sickle-Cell Trait and Sickle-Cell Disease?

Normally, red blood cells (RBCs) are round and flat, like a saucer. They pass easily through the tiniest blood vessels. Red blood cells sickle or take on the crescent shape when they carry an abnormal form of hemoglobin called hemoglobin S. The abnormality in hemoglobin S occurs due to the presence of a faulty gene*.

People inherit one set of genes from each parent. They can inherit either two normal hemoglobin genes (HbA), one normal hemoglobin gene and one gene for the abnormal hemoglobin gene (HbS), or two abnormal HbS genes, depending on the composition of their parents' genes.

When a person carries one HbS and one HbA gene, the presence of the normal gene is sufficient to override the effects of the HbS gene so the symptoms of sickle-cell disease do not develop. These people, however,

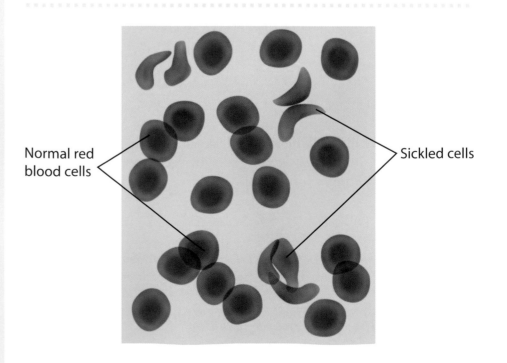

Normal red blood cells

Sickled cells

The shape of sickled red blood cells compared to normal red blood cells. *Illustration by Frank Forney. Reproduced by permission of Gale, a part of Cengage Learning.*

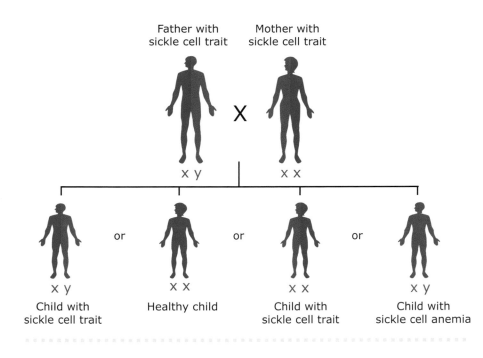

Father with
sickle cell trait

Mother with
sickle cell trait

X

x y   x x

x y   x x   x x   x y

Child with
sickle cell trait

Healthy child

Child with
sickle cell trait

Child with
sickle cell anemia

The inheritance pattern for the sickle-cell gene HbS. *Illustration by Frank Forney. Reproduced by permission of Gale, a part of Cengage Learning.*

are said to have the sickle-cell trait or to be carriers of the sickle-cell trait, and they may pass it on to their children. Prospective parents who are likely to carry the HbS gene may wish to be tested for its presence and receive genetic counseling before having children.

When people inherit two abnormal HbS genes, one from each parent, they have sickle-cell disease, and they show symptoms of that disease. They have only abnormal HbS genes to pass on to their children.

Sickle-cell disease is a genetic* disorder, and its frequency varies in different populations worldwide. It is found most frequently in Africa, where in some locations up to 40 percent of the population has at least one HbS gene. The gene is also found in people in Mediterranean and Middle Eastern countries, such as Italy, Greece, and Saudi Arabia. There are groups of people in India, Latin America, the Caribbean, and the United States in which the HbS gene is also found.

Among people of African ancestry in the United States, about 8 in every 100 individuals carries at least one HbS gene (has the sickle-cell trait) and about 40,000 people carry two copies of the HbS gene and have sickle-cell disease.

What Are the Effects of Sickle-Cell Disease?

People who have sickle-cell disease get infections more frequently than other people. In 1987 the National Institutes of Health recommended that all babies, regardless of ethnic or racial background, be tested at birth for the presence of the HbS. Babies with sickle-cell disease are often given antibiotics* to prevent infections. Before this screening became common, many babies born with sickle-cell disease died in infancy. Later the use of preventive antibiotics significantly reduced the number of babies who died.

* **genetic** (juh-NEH-tik) refers to heredity and the ways in which genes control the development and maintenance of organisms.

* **antibiotics** (an-tie-by-AH-tiks) are drugs that kill or slow the growth of bacteria.

* **central nervous system** (SEN-trul NER-vus SIS-tem) is the part of the nervous system that includes the brain and spinal cord.

Infants, older children, and adults with sickle-cell disease periodically experience bouts of critical illness called crises. They also suffer from complications of anemia.

Because sickle-cell disease is hereditary, people are born with it and will have it all their lives. There is no way one person can catch sickle-cell disease or sickle-cell trait from another person, and there is no way the disease can be cured.

Crises Sickle-shaped red blood cells clump more easily than normal RBCs. Sickle-cell crises start suddenly when clumping of sickled RBCs in the blood vessels obstructs the normal flow of blood, depriving various tissues and organs of oxygen. The first crises usually appear in early childhood.

Crises may be brought on by respiratory infection, by a loss of body fluids from vomiting or diarrhea, by situations in which the body's need for oxygen is increased, or they may occur for no obvious reason. They may last for several days and cause fever and sharp, intense pain in the back, abdomen, chest, arms, and legs. In infants, the hands and feet may become swollen and painful.

Crises may damage nearly any part of the body, but especially the bones, kidneys, intestines, lungs, liver, spleen, and the central nervous system*, including the brain. There may also be eye damage, stroke,

---

IN THE FOREFRONT OF MEDICAL SCIENCE

In 1949, Linus Pauling (1901–1994) and associates published an article in *Science* magazine ("Sickle-Cell Anemia, a Molecular Disease"). This paper explains how protein electrophoresis was used to show how sickle-cell hemoglobin differed in structure from normal hemoglobin. Hemoglobin S (sickle-cell) differs from normal adult hemoglobin (called hemoglobin A) only by a single amino acid substitution (a valine replacing a glutamine in the 6th position of the beta chain of globin).

This breakthrough concept marked the birth of molecular biology as a field of study. Medical science entered the era of molecular biology, a time in which the focus is to try to understand health and disease in terms of the structure of molecules.

In the 1970s the understanding began to grow that sickle trait conveys a survival advantage to people in malarial areas, which represented a breakthrough concept in the field of human genetics. It explained that clustering and concentration of hemoglobin S genes in certain areas of the world and constituted an example of human evolution in action.

In the 21st century, with the development of genetic engineering, it became possible to remove the gene for sickle hemoglobin from the genome of families with sickle-cell anemia so that their children will not carry the disease.

convulsions*, or paralysis. The damage is caused because the clumping of RBCs in a blood vessel deprives tissues of oxygen.

Many people with sickle-cell disease go for long periods during which they may feel relatively well and engage in most normal activities and are free of crises (in remission). Others may experience pain on a daily basis, and some need to be hospitalized as a result of crises several times per year.

Anemia Sickle cells are more easily broken down and destroyed than normal RBCs. Sickle cells have a lifespan of 10 to 20 days compared to 90 to 120 days for a normal RBC. People with sickle-cell anemia thus cannot keep up a normal level of oxygen-carrying hemoglobin in their blood. This situation exists despite the fact that they make red blood cells faster than people without the disease. The result is that they are anemic.

The anemia may become so severe that a person will need to have a blood transfusion*. The long-term effect of anemia is that the heart has to work harder to pump more blood through the body. Over time the heart enlarges, increasing the risk of heart attack and heart failure.

Other complications of sickle-cell disease People who have sickle-cell disease are more susceptible to all kinds of bacterial and fungal infections. They are more likely to have strokes* and to experience kidney failure. In some people, the liver enlarges, and by age 30, 70 percent of people with sickle-cell disease have developed gallstones.

Modern medicine has increased the survival of people with sickle-cell disease. About half the people with sickle-cell disease live beyond 50 years of age. Still, living with the pain and complications of this condition can cause emotional stress on both the person with the disease and the family.

How Is Sickle-Cell Disease Diagnosed?

Sickle-cell disease and sickle-cell trait can be diagnosed by a blood test, which detects the presence of HbS and other abnormal hemoglobins. A complete blood count (CBC) counts the number of RBCs and checks for abnormal shapes.

How Is Sickle-Cell Disease Treated?

There is no cure for sickle-cell anemia. Much treatment is preventive and directed toward symptoms. Antibiotics may be given to prevent infections. Fluid intake is important to prevent dehydration*, a major cause of sickling. Folic acid may be given daily to lessen the anemia by helping to make new red cells. Children are given a complete set of immunizations. Lifestyle habits that can help sickle-cell patients stay healthy and have fewer crises include drinking plenty of water, avoiding extremes of heat and cold, avoiding stress and overexertion, getting enough sleep, and having regular medical check-ups.

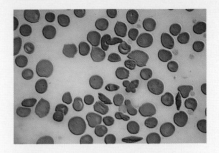

Both normal red blood cells and deformed cells can be seen in this sample of blood taken from a person with sickle cell anemia. *Dr. David M. Phillips/Visuals Unlimited/Getty Images.*

A Possible Benefit of the Sickle-Cell Trait

Sickle-cell disease is especially prevalent among people of African or African American descent. No one knows for sure why this is so. However, it is believed that the gene that causes sickle-cell disease also provides natural resistance to malaria, an often-fatal disease. The parts of Africa where malaria is most prevalent, such as Ghana and Nigeria, are also the areas where the incidence of sickle-cell anemia and sickle-cell trait is greatest. It is believed that the gene that causes the sickle-cell trait gives these people some advantage in surviving malaria, which allows them to live and reproduce, thereby passing the gene along to later generations. However, people with sickle-cell disease (two copies of the HbS sickle-cell gene) do not have this advantage and are more likely to die of malaria.

* **convulsions** (kon-VUL-shuns), also called seizures, are involuntary muscle contractions caused by electrical discharges within the brain and are usually accompanied by changes in consciousness.

* **blood transfusion** is the process of giving blood (or certain cells or chemicals found in the blood) to a person who needs it due to illness or blood loss.

* **strokes** are events that occur when a blood vessel bringing oxygen and nutrients to the brain bursts or becomes clogged by a blood clot or other particle. As a result, nerve cells in the affected area of the brain cannot function properly.

* **dehydration** (dee-hi-DRAY-shun) is a condition in which the body is depleted of water, usually caused by excessive and unreplaced loss of body fluids, such as through sweating, vomiting, or diarrhea.

* **bone marrow** is the soft tissue inside bones where blood cells are made.

Treatment in a sickle-cell crisis may require oxygen therapy, pain relieving medications, antibiotics, and intravenous fluids to offset dehydration. Blood transfusions may also have to be performed. Treatment of pain is a major concern. The benefits of different pain relievers and their unwanted side effects must be balanced for each patient.

Research is ongoing to find better ways to treat people with sickle-cell disease. Some of these research efforts are directed at stimulating the production of fetal hemoglobin, a form of hemoglobin found in infants, even those with sickle-cell disease. Other research is directed toward the development of drugs that block dehydration in cells. Gene therapy and the transplantation of healthy bone marrow* that makes normal red blood cells are also under investigation.

▶ *See also* **Anemia, Bleeding, and Clotting • Genetic Diseases**

Resources

Books and Articles

Jones, Phill. *Sickle Cell Disease.* New York: Chelsea House, 2008.

Peak, Lizabeth. *Sickle Cell Disease.* Detroit, MI: Lucent Books, 2008.

Peterson, Judy Monroe. *Sickle Cell Anemia.* New York: Rosen, 2009.

Silverstein, Alvin, Virginia Silverstein, and Laura Silverstein Nunn. *The Sickle Cell Anemia Update.* Berkeley Heights, NJ: Enslow, 2006.

Organizations

National Heart, Lung, and Blood Institute. P.O. Box 30105, Bethesda, MD, 20824-0105. Telephone: 301-592-8573. Web site: http://www.nhlbi.nih.gov/health/dci/Diseases/Sca/SCA_WhatIs.html.

Sickle-Cell Disease Association of America. 200 Corporate Pointe, Suite 495, Culver City, CA, 90230-7633. Toll free: 800-421-8453. Web site: http://www.sicklecelldisease.org.

Sickle Cell Information Center. Grady Memorial Hospital, P.O. Box 109, Atlanta, GA, 30303, Web site: http://www.scinfo.org.

SIDS *See Sudden Infant Death Syndrome.*

Silicosis *See Pneumoconiosis.*

Sinusitis

Sinusitis (sy-nyoo-SY-tis) is an inflammation of the sinuses (SY-nuh-ses), the hollow chambers or cavities located in the bones of the face that surround the nose.

What Causes Sinusitis?

People have four pairs of paranasal sinuses (the sinuses surrounding the nose):

- Frontal sinuses, located in the forehead and over the eyebrows
- Ethmoid (ETH-moyd) sinuses, located between the eyes at the bridge of the nose
- Sphenoid (SFEE-noyd) sinuses, located behind the ethmoid sinuses
- Maxillary (MAX-ih-lary) sinuses, located in the cheekbones

The sinuses and the narrow tube-like structures that link them to the nasal passages are lined with the same mucous membranes* that line the nose. Colds, allergies*, and exposure to some chemicals can cause swelling and inflammation in the lining of the sinus passages and block sinus drainage. Bacteria* (such as *Streptococcus pneumoniae,* strep-tuh-KAH-kus nu-MO-nye), viruses*, and fungi* that live in the body may become trapped, multiply, and invade the inflamed sinuses.

People with allergies, asthma*, and cystic fibrosis* are more likely to have sinus infections. Other candidates for sinusitis are people with a weakened immune system, such as those who have AIDS* or cancer; people with narrow sinus passages or with growths or blockages in the nasal area, such as tumors* or polyps*; and people with previously broken or deformed nasal bones. The risk of sinusitis also is higher when people swim or dive, due to the pressure this activity puts on the sinus cavities.

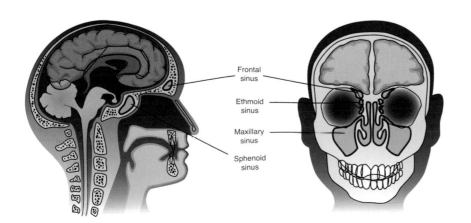

Frontal sinus

Ethmoid sinus

Maxillary sinus

Sphenoid sinus

* **mucous membranes** are the thin layers of tissue found inside the nose, ears, cervix (SER-viks) and uterus, stomach, colon and rectum, on the vocal cords, and in other parts of the body.

* **allergies** (AL-uhr-jeez) are immune system-related sensitivities to certain substances, for example, cat dander or the pollen of certain plants, that cause various reactions, such as sneezing, runny nose, wheezing, or swollen, itchy patches on the skin, called hives.

* **bacteria** (bak-TEER-ee-a) are single-celled microorganisms, which typically reproduce by cell division. Some, but not all, types of bacteria can cause disease in humans. Many types can live in the body without causing harm.

* **viruses** (VY-rus-sez) are tiny infectious agents that can cause infectious diseases. A virus can only reproduce within the cells it infects.

* **fungi** (FUNG-eye) are micro-organisms that can grow in or on the body, causing infections of internal organs or of the skin, hair, and nails.

* **asthma** (AZ-mah) is a condition in which the airways of the lungs repeatedly become narrowed and inflamed, causing breathing difficulty.

* **cystic fibrosis** (SIS-tik fy-BRO-sis) is a disease that causes the body to produce thick mucus that clogs passages in many of the body's organs, including the lungs.

The four pairs of paranasal sinuses in the human skull. *Illustration by Frank Forney. Reproduced by permission of Gale, a part of Cengage Learning.*

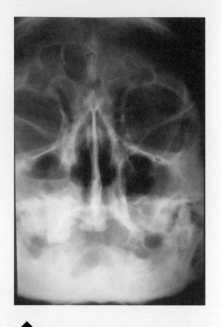

On the right side of this x-ray is an example of the inflammation associated with sinusitis. If the patient's sinusitis is severe, the doctor may recommend surgery to help drain the sinus cavities. *Custom Medical Stock Photo, Inc. Reproduced by permission.*

* **AIDS** or acquired immunodeficiency (ih-myoo-no-dih-FIH-shen-see) syndrome, is an infection that severely weakens the immune system; it is caused by the human immunodeficiency virus (HIV).

* **tumors** (TOO-morz) are abnormal growths of body tissue that have no known cause or physiologic purpose. Tumors may or may not be cancerous.

* **polyps** (PAH-lips) are bumps or growths usually on the lining or surface of a body part (such as the nose or intestine). Their size can range from tiny to large enough to cause pain or obstruction. They may be harmless, but they also may be cancerous.

* **acute** describes an infection or other illness that comes on suddenly and usually does not last very long.

What Are Different Types of Sinusitis?

Physicians classify sinusitis in three ways:

- Acute* sinusitis often develops after a person has had a cold, with symptoms lasting less than three weeks.
- Chronic* sinusitis can last three to eight weeks or longer. It often occurs in people who have allergies or asthma.
- Recurrent sinusitis consists of several acute episodes of sinusitis in one year.

How Common Is Sinusitis?

The National Institute of Allergy and Infectious Diseases estimates that every year 37 million people in the United States have sinusitis.

Is Sinusitis Contagious?

No one can catch a sinus infection from another person, but the viruses and bacteria that cause colds and other respiratory tract* infections that can trigger sinusitis may spread from person to person in drops of fluid from the nose or mouth. When people who have sinusitis cough, sneeze, laugh, or talk, they can transmit germs to their hands, to the surfaces around them, and into the air. Others can then breathe in the germs or touch contaminated surfaces with their hands and spread the germs to their noses and mouths. Such infections sometimes develop into sinusitis.

What Are the Symptoms of Sinusitis?

Symptoms of a cold (runny nose and low fever) often give way to pain and pressure in the sinuses, which are usually the first signs of sinusitis. Other symptoms of sinusitis include pain or puffiness around the eyes; a bad-smelling, yellow-green discharge from the nose; bad breath; a headache in the morning; aching in the upper jaw and the back teeth; weakness or extreme tiredness; and coughing, especially at night. People with sinusitis occasionally develop earaches, neck pain, or a sore throat caused by mucus* draining into the throat.

Some other conditions have similar symptoms to sinusitis, but they are not the same condition. Many people confuse nasal congestion with sinusitis. In addition, considerable confusion exists about people call "sinus headaches," and some studies have indicated that up to 90 percent of these headaches are actually not related to the sinuses.

How Is Sinusitis Diagnosed?

To diagnose sinusitis, doctors look for the signs and symptoms of the condition in the patient. They suspect sinusitis if a patient has cold symptoms that last for more than 10 days, or if the patient has other sinusitis symptoms. A doctor may, for example, tap the patient's face to determine if sinuses are tender. If a patient has complicated or repeated cases of sinusitis, a doctor may order x-rays or a computerized tomography* (CT) scan to determine whether the sinuses are inflamed.

How Is Sinusitis Treated?

Bacterial sinusitis usually clears up after treatment with antibiotics. Most cases of acute sinusitis, however, result from viruses. Because antibiotics have no effect on viruses, the initial treatment of acute sinusitis generally does not involve antibiotics. Rather, it includes decongestants and pain medications. However, some patients still demand antibiotics. Such overuse of antibiotics is ill-advised because it can contribute significantly to antibiotic resistance*. Medical professionals typically only consider antibiotic use in treating acute sinusitis if the patient has no improvement in 48 hours after using decongestants and pain medications.

Beyond these treatments, individuals can try to relieve the symptoms of sinusitis in several ways. They can take acetaminophen* to help ease the pain and use nonprescription decongestants (dee-kon-JES-tents), taken by mouth or in sprays, to lessen stuffiness. Using a decongestant nasal spray for more than a few days, however, may itself cause swelling of the sinuses and slow recovery. Saline or salt sprays may also reduce swelling in the sinuses. Some patients find relief by placing a warm compress over the infected sinuses, using a steam vaporizer*, or sitting in a warm, steamy bathroom. Doctors may prescribe special nasal sprays or oral (by mouth) medications for people with chronic sinusitis who have allergies that contribute to the infection. Chronic sinusitis sufferers often benefit from sinus irrigation or flushing, and many different devices are available for this purpose. For chronic or recurrent sinusitis, doctors may refer the patient to an ear, nose, and throat specialist.

In some cases, people with severe chronic sinusitis may undergo surgery to enlarge their sinus passages, to remove a polyp, or to fix a deviated septum* that might be blocking sinus drainage.

Does Sinusitis Have Complications?

Complications of sinusitis are rare, but they do occur. Sinusitis can cause osteomyelitis* when the infection from the sinus spreads into the bones of the face or skull. Sinusitis can also lead to an infection of brain tissue or meningitis (inflammation of the meninges*). In addition, a sinus infection can spread to invade the tissues surrounding the eyes.

Can Sinusitis Be Prevented?

Because no practical way exists to prevent all colds or to eliminate all allergies, sinusitis is not entirely preventable. People can limit their exposure to the viruses and bacteria that cause the infections by washing their hands thoroughly and frequently, and by only using their own, rather than sharing, eating or drinking utensils. Individuals should also avoid smoking as well as exposure to tobacco smoke to help limit the risk of sinusitis. People with allergies should avoid whatever triggers their allergy symptoms and control their allergies with the treatment recommended by their doctors. Drinking plenty of fluids and keeping the air in the house moist by using a vaporizer can help thin mucus and prevent its buildup in

* **chronic** (KRAH-nik) lasting a long time or recurring frequently.

* **respiratory tract** includes the nose, mouth, throat, and lungs. It is the pathway through which air and gases are transported down into the lungs and back out of the body.

* **mucus** (MYOO-kus) is a thick, slippery substance that lines the insides of many body parts.

* **computerized tomography** (kom-PYOO-ter-ized toe-MAH-gruh-fee) or CT, also called computerized axial tomography (CAT), is a technique in which a machine takes many x-rays of the body to create a three-dimensional picture.

* **antibiotic resistance** occurs when bacteria evolve to withstand attack by antibiotics.

* **acetaminophen** (uh-see-teh-MIH-noh-fen) is a medication commonly used to reduce fever and relieve pain.

* **vaporizer** is a device that converts water (or a liquid medication) into a vapor, a suspension of tiny droplets that hang in the air and can be inhaled.

* **deviated septum** is a condition in which the wall of tissue between the nasal passages, the septum, divides the passageways unevenly, sometimes causing breathing difficulties and blockage of sinus drainage.

* **osteomyelitis** (ah-stee-o-my-uh-LYE-tis) is a bone infection that is usually caused by bacteria. It can involve any bone in the body, but it most commonly affects the long bones in the arms and legs.

* **meninges** (meh-NIN-jeez) are the membranes that enclose and protect the brain and the spinal cord.

* **congenital** (kon-JEH-nih-tul) means present at birth.

the sinuses. Limiting alcohol consumption also may help, because alcohol can cause nasal membranes to swell. In addition, air travel and underwater diving can cause significant discomfort in individuals with acute or chronic sinusitis, so they may consider using decongestants prior to these activities.

▶ *See also* **Antibiotic Resistance • Common Cold • Fever • Headache • Infection • Influenza • Osteomyelitis**

Resources

Books and Articles

Bruce, Debra Fulghum, and Murray Grossan. *The Sinus Cure: Seven Simple Steps to Relieve Sinusitis and Other Ear, Nose, and Throat Conditions,* rev. updated ed. New York: Ballantine Books, 2007.

Hirsch, Alan R. *What Your Doctor May Not Tell You about Sinusitis: Relieve Your Symptoms and Identify the Real Source of Your Pain.* New York: Warner Books, 2004.

Wynn, Rhoda, and Winston C. Vaughan. *100 Questions & Answers about Sinusitis and Other Sinus Diseases.* Sudbury, MA: Jones and Bartlett, 2008.

Organizations

American Academy of Otolaryngology, Head and Neck Surgery. 1650 Diagonal Road, Alexandria, VA, 22314-2857. Telephone: 703-836-4444. Web site: http://www.entnet.org.

American Rhinologic Society. P.O. Box 495, Warwick, NY, 10990-0495. Telephone: 845-988-1631. Web site: http://www.american-rhinologic.org/patientinfo.phtml.

Medical College of Wisconsin. 8701 Watertown Plank Road, Milwaukee, WI, 53226, Web site: http://healthlink.mcw.edu/article/924452495.html.

National Institute of Allergy and Infectious Diseases. Office of Communications and Public Liaison, 6610 Rockledge Drive, MSC, 6612, Bethesda, MD, 20892-66123. Toll free: 866-284-4107. Web site: http://www3.niaid.nih.gov/topics/sinusitis.

Situs Inversus

Situs inversus (SI-tus in-VER-sus) is a congenital* condition in which major organs in the body are in reversed or mirrored position.

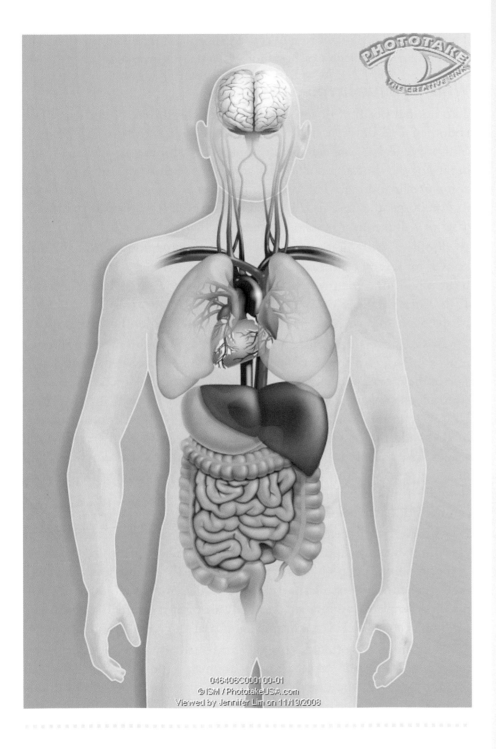

PHOTOTAKE
THE CREATIVE LINK

A total visceral inversion (situs inversus) where the visceral organs are reversed— the heart is on the right, the liver is on the left, etc. ©*ISM/Phototake. Reproduced by permission.*

◄

046406C000100-01
© ISM / PhototakeUSA.com
Viewed by Jennifer Lim on 11/19/2008

Marlowe's Story

Marlowe was a normal, happy girl of 18. Suddenly, she started to experience diffuse pain under and around her belly button (navel or umbilicus). Over the next few hours, the pain became worse and started to move to the left side of Marlowe's abdomen. When the pain continued to worsen, she called her family doctor to ask for advice. The doctor was initially stumped but then remembered a comment from his anatomy class in medical school.

* **dextrocardia** mirror image rotation that is confined to the heart.

* **CT scans** or CAT scans are the shortened name for computerized axial tomography (to-MOG-ra-fee), which uses computers to view structures inside the body.

* **MRI** which is short for magnetic resonance imaging, produces computerized images of internal body tissues based on the magnetic properties of atoms within the body.

* **ultrasound** also called a sonogram, is a diagnostic test in which sound waves passing through the body create images on a computer screen.

* **appendicitis** (ah-pen-dih-SY-tis) is an inflammation of the appendix, the narrow, finger-shaped organ that branches off the part of the large intestine in the lower right side of the abdomen.

* **appendix** (ah-PEN-diks) is the narrow, finger-shaped organ that branches off the part of the large intestine in the lower right side of the abdomen. Although the organ is not known to have any vital function, the tissue of the appendix is populated by cells of the immune system.

The doctor told Marlowe to report to the hospital for an examination. The doctor made two diagnoses: appendicitis and situs inversus.

What Is Situs Inversus?

The normal position of internal organs of the thorax (THOR-ax) and abdomen (AB-do-men) is known as situs solitus (SI-tus so-LEE-tus). Situs inversus is a congenital condition in which some or all of the major organs of the thorax and abdomen are in reversed or mirrored positions compared to normal. The prevalence of situs inversus is less than one in 10,000 people. It is usually an autosomal recessive disorder, although cases of X-linked transmission have been described.

Problems with rotation or mirrored position of body organs have been known for several centuries. A variant of situs inversus dextrocardia* (the heart is positioned on the right side of the thorax) was first described in the 17th century. Full or complete situs inversus (totalis) was first described by the Scottish physician Matthew Baillie at the end of the 18th century.

In situs inversus totalis, all major organs are positioned as the exact mirror opposite to the usual location. The heart is located on the right side of the thorax, the liver is on the left side of the abdomen, whereas the stomach and spleen are on the right side. In situs inversus the right lung has two lobes, and the left lung has three lobes (the exact opposite of normal). In addition, all of the blood vessels, intestines, nerves, and lymph vessels are transposed. If all these organs are transposed as described, and in the absence of any congenital heart defects, no functional problems should be present in affected individuals. Individuals with situs inversus can live normal lives.

However, when there is dextrocardia without situs inversus, or situs inversus with levocardia (mirror image rotation of the heart in which the direction of rotation is opposite that of normal cardiac development), there is a much higher rate of significant congenital cardiac abnormalities. Many people with complete situs inversus are not aware of their unusual anatomy. The condition is often discovered during an unrelated medical examination.

Situs inversus is often discovered accidentally by a radiologist evaluating an x-ray, CT scan*, MRI* image or an image produced by ultrasound*. It is also discovered by a physician making a diagnosis in which the bodily position of the problem does not match with the doctor's expectation. Marlowe had appendicitis*. Normally, the appendix* is in the right lower portion of a person's abdomen. The normal pattern of pain associated with appendicitis is to become localized in the appendix. Marlowe's history was consistent with appendicitis. The explanation for the incorrect position is that Marlowe also has situs inversus.

On an x-ray of the large intestine, the cecum (initial portion of the large intestine) is on the left side instead of the right. The ascending colon is also on the left, the descending colon is on the right, and the sigmoid colon (the final portion of the large intestine) curves to the right as it connects with the rectum.

Correct labeling of x-ray images is important. Situs inversus may be overlooked if labels are incorrectly applied by an x-ray technician. Such errors occur but they are uncommon.

Is Situs Inversus Serious?

Generally, situs inversus is not serious. As noted, situs inversus with levocardia is associated with a much higher rate of significant congenital cardiac abnormalities. People with known situs inversus should inform physicians and other medical personnel about their condition, as this will expedite medical care and prevent unnecessary confusion.

What Causes Situs Inversus?

Situs inversus results when events of twisting and folding embryonic development occur in a direction that is opposite to normal. Although the affected organs are mirror images of usual, they function in a normal manner.

Living with Situs Inversus

People with situs inversus have a normal life expectancy. When situs inversus is accompanied by anomalies involving the heart, life expectancy is reduced. The degree of reduced life expectancy depends on the severity of the defect. Not recognizing situs inversus may lead to problems during surgical procedures.

Males and females experience situs inversus in about the same proportion. It occurs with the same frequency in people of all races throughout the world.

Resources

Organizations

American Academy of Family Physicians. P.O. Box 11210, Shawnee Mission, KS, 66207-1210. Toll free: 800-274-2237. Web site: http://www.aafp.org.

American Academy of Pediatrics. 141 Northwest Point Boulevard, Elk Grove Village, IL, 60007-1098. Telephone: 847-434-4000. Web site: http://www.aap.org/default.htm.

American College of Physicians. 190 N. Independence Mall West, Philadelphia, PA, 19106. Toll free: 800-523-1546. Web site: http://www.acponline.org.

Skin and Soft Tissue Infections

Skin and soft tissue infection is an infection involving the layers of the skin and the soft tissues directly beneath it.

Donny Osmond and Situs Inversus

Donny Osmond was not aware of his situs inversus until he had appendicitis. His doctor initially missed the diagnosis because Donny had pain on the left side of his abdomen and the appendix is normally on the right side. Like Marlowe, people with situs inversus are usually unaware of their condition until a medical problem develops but is not in its expected location.

* **viruses** (VY-rus-sez) are tiny infectious agents that can cause infectious diseases. A virus can only reproduce within the cells it infects.

* **bacteria** (bak-TEER-ee-a) are single-celled microorganisms, which typically reproduce by cell division. Some, but not all, types of bacteria can cause disease in humans. Many types can live in the body without causing harm.

* **fungi** (FUNG-eye) are microorganisms that can grow in or on the body, causing infections of internal organs or of the skin, hair, and nails.

* **antifungal drugs** (an-ty-FUNG-al drugs) are medications that kill fungi.

* **pus** is a thick, creamy fluid, usually yellow or ivory in color, that forms at the site of an infection. Pus contains infection-fighting white cells and other substances.

What Causes Skin and Soft Tissue Infections?

Viruses*, bacteria*, and fungi* generally cause skin and soft tissue infections by entering the body at a spot where a cut, scrape, bite, or other wound has broken the skin; some infections are even the result of bacteria that normally live on the body. These infections can affect the layers of the skin or deeper tissues, such as muscle and connective tissue (the interlacing framework of tissue that forms ligaments, tendons, and other supporting structures of the body), and they may bring about symptoms in other parts of the body.

Many infections such as varicella (chicken pox) and measles (rubeola) affect the skin, but these infections involve the whole body and do not primarily arise within the skin or soft tissues.

What Are Some Types of Skin and Soft Tissue Infections?

Dermatophyte infections Dermatophytes (dur-MAH-toh-fites) are fungi that live on the dead outer layer of skin. Sometimes they can produce symptoms of infection. Tinea (TIH-nee-uh) infections, commonly called ringworm (although they have nothing to do with worms), usually are caused by the *Trichophyton* group of these organisms. They include tinea pedis (PEE-dis), or athlete's foot; tinea cruris (KRU-ris), or jock itch; tinea capitis (KAH-pih-tis), or ringworm of the scalp; tinea unguium (UN-gwee-um), or ringworm of the nails; and tinea corporis (KOR-poor-us), or ringworm of the body. Damaged skin is more vulnerable to infection, as is skin in warm, moist areas of the body. When the fungus takes hold, it typically causes a ring-like rash of red, flaking skin. The border of the rash may be raised, as if a worm were under the skin. The rash's shape and this raised edge led people to call the infection ringworm. When the nails are infected, they usually become yellow, thickened, and brittle.

Tinea versicolor, or pityriasis (pih-tih-RYE-uh-sis) versicolor, is caused by the fungus *Malassezia furfur*. Symptoms include scaly patches of skin, ranging in color from light to dark. The patches occur on the chest, neck, back, underarms, and upper arms. Hot, humid weather encourages the growth of tinea versicolor. These fungal skin infections typically are treated with antifungal creams or ointments. In severe cases or when the infections do not improve with this therapy, several antifungal* medications are available that may be given by mouth.

Impetigo Impetigo (im-pih-TEE-go) is a skin infection in which red blister-like bumps develop that contain a yellowish fluid or pus*. After the blisters break open, they crust over. Impetigo is most common on the face, especially around the nose and mouth. Usually, either streptococcus (strep-tuh-KAH-kus) or staphylococcus (stah-fih-lo-KAH-kus) bacteria are the cause of the infection. Impetigo can spread easily, especially among children, who may scratch the lesions and then touch other areas of their skin or another person. People also can contract impetigo from handling clothing or blankets that have been in contact with infected skin.

Doctors prescribe antibiotics to treat impetigo. The infection generally clears without leaving permanent skin damage.

Skin abscesses

Skin abscesses (AB-seh-sez) may occur in areas of the skin where the body has been fighting a bacterial infection. To isolate the infection, the body forms a wall of tissue around the collection of pus, and this area is the abscess. Abscesses are usually round, raised, and red, and they may feel warm and tender. A furuncle (FYOOR-ung-kul), or boil, is an abscess that forms at the base of a hair follicle*. A carbuncle (KAR-bung-kul) forms when the infection spreads to include several follicles and the surrounding skin and deeper tissues. Like furuncles, carbuncles are red, raised, and painful to the touch.

Most skin abscesses eventually burst to allow the pus to drain out, but treatment with antibiotics may be needed to clear up the infection in some cases. When a skin abscess does not improve on its own, it likely needs to be lanced (punctured and drained) by a doctor.

Cellulitis

Cellulitis (sel-yoo-LYE-tis) is an inflammation of the skin and/or the tissues beneath it. The culprits behind the infection are almost always group A streptococcus or *Staphylococcus aureus* (stah-fih-lo-KAH-kus ARE-ree-us) bacteria. Cellulitis may occur in people with diabetes* or those who have immune system problems even if they do not have a skin injury. The infection can occur anywhere on the body, but it is found most frequently on the face and lower legs. It appears as tender, red, swollen areas of skin. The skin in the infected area may feel stretched and warm. A few days after the first symptoms, patients may experience fever, chills, and muscle aches. Red streaks also may appear on the skin, signaling the spread of the infection into the lymphatic vessels. Some people call these streaks "blood poisoning," but they do not really involve the blood.

Antibiotics are used to treat cellulitis. Even after the infection is gone, the skin may look different for several weeks. Complications are rare, but they can include sepsis*, gangrene*, and lymphangitis*. Cellulitis may involve infection of deeper tissue called the fascia (FAY-she-uh). Infection in this layer can be very serious or even life threatening and often requires surgery to remove the infected tissue.

Bites

Any type of bite that breaks the skin (cat, dog, human) puts an individual at very high risk of skin and soft tissue infection. Dog bites tend to be particularly damaging to the skin and underlying tissues and muscle, but cat bites and human bites have a higher rate of infection, usually occurring several days after the actual biting incident. Signs of infection include redness, swelling, warmth of the skin overlying and surrounding the wound, pain, and pus oozing from the wound. These signs can develop within several hours following a cat bite, much quicker than the usual one or two days. Rodent bites and the bites of wild animals (especially raccoons,

* **hair follicle** (FAH-lih-kul) is the skin structure from which hair develops and grows.

* **diabetes** (dye-uh-BEE-teez) is a condition in which the body's pancreas does not produce enough insulin or the body cannot use the insulin it makes effectively, resulting in increased levels of sugar in the blood. This can lead to increased urination, dehydration, weight loss, weakness, and a number of other symptoms and complications related to chemical imbalances within the body.

* **sepsis** is a potentially serious spreading of infection, usually bacterial, through the bloodstream and body.

* **gangrene** (GANG-green) is the decay or death of living tissue caused by a lack of oxygen supply to the tissue and/or bacterial infection of the tissue.

* **lymphangitis** (lim-fan-JIE-tis) is inflammation of the lymphatic system, the system that carries lymph through the body. Lymph is a clear fluid that contains white blood cells.

* **rabies** (RAY-beez) is a viral infection of the central nervous system that usually is transmitted to humans by the bite of an infected animal.

* **HIV** or human immunodeficiency virus (HYOO-mun ih-myoo-no-dih-FIH-shen-see), is the virus that causes AIDS (acquired immunodeficiency syndrome).

* **hepatitis** (heh-puh-TIE-tis) is an inflammation of the liver. Hepatitis can be caused by viruses, bacteria, and a number of other noninfectious medical conditions.

skunks, bats, and foxes) or domestic animals of unknown rabies* vaccine status put the bite victim at high risk of contracting the potentially fatal viral infection called rabies. In most instances, when rabies status of the biting animal cannot be confirmed, the individual is given a series of six shots to prevent the development of this life-threatening infection. A tetanus booster shot is also given to people who suffer an animal or human bite, and who have not had a tetanus booster within the previous five years. Additionally, human bites put the recipient at risk of contracting other infections, such as HIV* or hepatitis*.

Methicillin-resistant staphylococcus aureus

While the staphylococcus bacterium has long been implicated in skin and soft tissues infections, a later strain that is resistant to methicillin and other antibiotics exists. Whereas in the past this type of infection tended to affect only already-ill, hospitalized patients, a later form, called community-associated methicillin-resistant staphylococcus aureus (MRSA), is of particular concern because it may be more contagious via contact between previously healthy individuals than other forms of staph infections. People who have close physical contact are vulnerable to this type of infection, which includes children in daycare or other close school settings, people participating in contact sports, prisoners, military personnel, homeless people, homosexual men, and illegal intravenous (IV) drug users. Because of the unusual destructiveness and virulence of MRSA, it is important to maintain a high level of suspicion when an infection does not respond immediately to treatment or when an infection spreads unusually rapidly. Infections caused by this type of bacteria will not respond to the usual types of antibiotics, although there are some oral antibiotics that can be effective. More severe infections require IV antibiotics. In some severe cases, a wide-excision of all infected tissue is required in order to rid the body of the organism and lower the risk for systemic spread of this virulent organism.

Necrotizing fasciitis

Necrotizing fasciitis (NEH-kro-tie-zing fash-e-EYE-tis), also called flesh-eating disease, is a rare but potentially fatal disease, which can be caused by group A streptococcus bacteria infection. It affects the deeper layers of skin and tissues beneath the skin. Necrotizing fasciitis starts with sudden painful swelling and discoloration (red, purple, or bronze) of the skin. Often, the appearance of the affected skin does not reflect how far the infection has spread into the deeper layers of tissue. The disease can spread rapidly, with the infected area growing larger and darker. The ability to feel in the infected area disappears as the skin tissue dies. As the infection quickly progresses, the patient can become very ill. Early treatment with antibiotics and surgery to remove the damaged tissue is extremely important. Recovery may take several months.

Molluscum contagiosum

Molluscum contagiosum (moh-LUS-kum kon-tay-jee-O-sum), caused by a virus, produces small, solid, dome-shaped bumps on the surface of the skin. They are flesh-colored and pearly with a dimple in the center. The growths are similar to warts. Viruses cause both conditions: poxvirus in the case of molluscum contagiosum and human papillomavirus in the case of warts. Growths can be single, but they most often appear in groups on the trunk, arms, legs, and genitals*, and occasionally on the face.

The disease usually clears up by itself over several months, although new growths may arise on the skin if the virus spreads through contact with infected areas. Doctors may recommend home treatment with over-the-counter medications or removal of the growths by freezing, surgery, laser therapy, or acid treatments.

Herpes simplex virus   There are two types of the herpes simplex virus (HSV): HSV-1 and HSV-2. Both can show up as skin infections. HSV-1 can cause small, clear blisters (also known as cold sores, fever blisters, or oral herpes) around the lips on the face, and HSV-2 can cause similar looking blisters in the genital area. These blisters can break and form ulcers and then crust over. When the crust falls off red spots of healing skin are seen.

There is no cure for either HSV-1 or HSV-2. As of 2009, antiviral medications could help control outbreaks of herpes virus and were used to treat genital herpes or sometimes recurrent cold sores from HSV-1.

Warts   Warts are caused by human papillomavirus (pah-pih-LO-mah-vy-rus), or HPV. They can be skin-colored, pink, tan, or white, and they may appear anywhere on the body. Common warts usually are seen on the hands (especially around the nails), feet, and face, because the virus spreads most easily to those areas. Common warts are rough and raised, but plantar warts, found on the soles of the feet, are flat. Unlike other warts, plantar warts can be painful.

Many warts disappear by themselves after months or even years. Treatments are available for those that do not, including over-the-counter medications or professional treatment by freezing, surgery, laser therapy, or acid treatments.

Are Skin and Soft Tissue Infections Contagious?

Necrotizing fasciitis, cellulitis, and abscesses are not contagious from person to person, but the bacteria that can cause these infections can spread between people. Dermatophytes, warts, and molluscum contagiosum spread fairly easily through skin-to-skin contact.

How Are Skin and Soft Tissue Infections Diagnosed?

A doctor examines the size, shape, and color of the affected area and checks it for tenderness and warmth. The doctor may order blood tests for cellulitis to assess the extent of the infection; tests of skin scrapings for suspected fungal infections or molluscum contagiosum; or tests on a tissue sample for necrotizing fasciitis. Doctors can use a special type of filtered ultraviolet*

* **genitals** (JEH-nih-tuls) are the external sexual organs.

* **ultraviolet** light is a wavelength of light beyond visible light; on the spectrum of light, it falls between the violet end of visible light and x-rays.

light to check for tinea capitis because the fungi that cause it glow a characteristic color when the light is shined on the infected area.

Can Skin and Soft Tissue Infections Be Prevented?

The best way to prevent skin and soft tissue infections is to avoid getting cuts, scrapes, bites, or any kind of open wound. Frequent hand washing can curb the spread of bacteria. Doctors also advise keeping any opening in the skin clean and dry. It is wise to consult a doctor if the area around the wound becomes red, hot, or painful or if the infected person develops a fever. Dermatophyte infection is best avoided by keeping the skin dry, such as in areas where sweating occurs.

▶ *See also* **Abscesses • Fungal Infections • Gangrene • Impetigo • Ringworm • Sepsis • Skin Parasites • Staphylococcal Infections • Streptococcal Infections • Warts**

Resources

Organization

American Academy of Dermatology. P.O. Box 4014, Schaumburg, IL, 60168-4014. Toll free: 866-503-SKIN. Web site: http://www.aad.org.

Skin Cancer

Skin cancer is a disease in which rapidly multiplying, abnormal cells (cancer cells) are found in the outer layers of the skin.

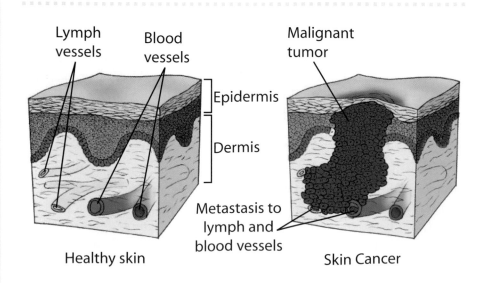

Lymph vessels · Blood vessels · Malignant tumor · Epidermis · Dermis · Metastasis to lymph and blood vessels · Healthy skin · Skin Cancer

Healthy skin cells protect the body (left), but cancer cells grow and divide uncontrollably (right), crowding out the healthy cells nearby. Melanoma is particularly dangerous because it can spread throughout the body. *Illustration by Frank Forney. Reproduced by permission of Gale, a part of Cengage Learning.*

What Is Skin Cancer?

In 1985, former president Ronald Reagan had a growth called a basal (BAY-zuhl) cell carcinoma removed from the side of his nose. The president had often been described as looking tanned and healthy, and when the news broke, it raised public awareness of skin cancer and the dangers of overexposure to the sun. Each year, about one million Americans are diagnosed with skin cancer.

The skin is the largest organ of the body. It protects people by keeping water and other fluids inside the body, by helping to regulate body temperature, by manufacturing vitamin D, and by performing a range of other complex functions. The skin also is a critically important barrier between people and such foreign invaders as bacteria. The skin is a basic part of physical appearance; it is the surface of the body that people present to the world.

Skin cancer is the most common of all cancers. It accounts for 50 percent of all cases of cancer. Cancers of the skin are divided into two general types: melanoma (mel-a-NO-ma) and nonmelanoma. Nonmelanoma are the most common cancers of the skin. They are also the most curable. Melanoma is much less common, but it is far more aggressive and causes 75 percent of all skin cancer deaths.

What Are the Types of Skin Cancer and Their Development?

Melanoma   The outer layer of the skin, the epidermis (ep-i-DER-mis), consists of layers of flat, scaly cells called squamous (SQUAY-muss) cells, under which are round cells called basal cells. The deepest part of the epidermis consists of melanocytes (MEL-a-no-sites), which are the cells that give skin its color. Melanoma begins in the melanocytes.

Nonmelanoma   The two main types of nonmelanoma are basal cell carcinoma and squamous cell carcinoma. These cancers develop in different layers of the skin, but they both appear more commonly on sun-exposed areas of the body. Squamous cell carcinomas grow more quickly than basal cell carcinomas.

How skin cancer develops   Skin cancer begins with damage to the DNA* of the cells in skin. DNA is information people inherit from their parents that tells the cells of the body how to perform all the activities needed for life. DNA is contained in genes*, and each cell has an identical set of genes. Some of these genes carefully control when cells grow, divide, and die. If a gene is damaged, the cell receives the wrong instructions or no instructions at all. When that happens, the cell can begin to grow and divide uncontrollably, forming an unruly cluster that crowds out its neighbors and forms a cancerous growth, or tumor. Melanoma is potentially serious because it has the ability to spread to other places in the body. Nonmelanoma, however, tends to stay put and is less likely to spread.

ABCDs of Melanoma Screening

The American Academy of Dermatology recommends checking the skin on a regular basis for changes in moles, freckles, and beauty marks. Their ABCD system for recognizing changes is as follows:

A: asymmetrical shape

B: border with ragged, blurred, or irregular shape

C: color variations

D: diameter greater than 6 millimeters (size of a pencil eraser)

Moles that match any of the ABCDs should be seen by a doctor.

---

* **DNA** or deoxyribonucleic acid (dee-OX-see-ry-bo-nyoo-klay-ik AH-sid), is the specialized chemical substance that contains the genetic code necessary to build and maintain the structures and functions of living organisms.

* **genes** (JEENS) are chemical structures composed of deoxyribonucleic acid (DNA) that help determine a person's body structure and physical characteristics. Inherited from a person's parents, genes are contained in the chromosomes found in the body's cells.

* **ultraviolet** light is a wavelength of light beyond visible light; on the spectrum of light, it falls between the violet end of visible light and x-rays.

What Causes Skin Cancer?

Certain kinds of risk factors suggest who might be likely to develop cancer. A risk factor is anything that increases a person's chances of getting a disease.

Melanoma   One risk factor is having certain types of moles. Another risk factor is having fair skin. The risk of melanoma is about 20 times higher for light-skinned people than it is for dark-skinned people. But dark-skinned people can still get melanoma. A person's chances of getting melanoma are greater if one or more close relatives have gotten it. People who have been treated with medicines that suppress the immune system (the body's defenses against infection) have an increased risk of developing melanoma. Exposure to ultraviolet* radiation—for example, sunlight, tanning lamps, and tanning booths—also is a risk factor for melanoma. Studies have shown no protective benefit of sunscreens in preventing melanoma.

Nonmelanoma   Most cases of nonmelanoma are caused by unprotected exposure of the area that has the cancer to ultraviolet radiation. Most of this radiation comes from sunlight, but it may also come from artificial sources. Although children and young adults usually do not get skin cancer, they may get a lot of exposure to the sun that could result in cancer later on. Other risk factors for nonmelanoma include having fair skin and having a weakened immune system as a result of medical treatment for other conditions. In addition, exposure to certain kinds of chemicals increases a person's risk of getting nonmelanoma.

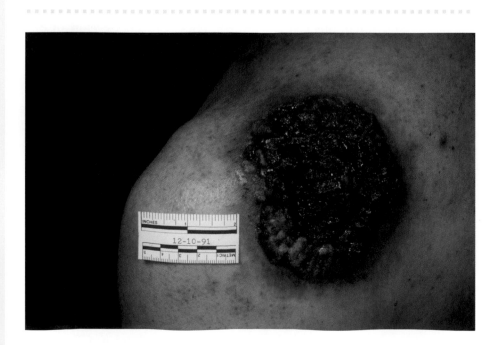

Large red, blistery irregular-shaped growth of basal cell carcinoma. *M. Abbey/Photo Researchers, Inc.*

SUNSHINE AND SKIN CANCER

Cumulative Effects of Tanning

Long-term exposure to the ultraviolet (UV) rays of the sun damages the body's skin cells and can lead to cancer. For example, repeated sunburn and tanning cause the skin to wrinkle and to lose its ability to hold its shape. Dark patches called lentigos (len-TEE-goes) (age spots or liver spots) may appear, along with scaly precancerous growths and actual skin cancers. The sun's UV radiation also increases a person's risk of developing eye problems, including cataracts, which can cause blindness.

Burning and Peeling

Burning and peeling are signs that a person's skin has been damaged. The sun can also damage the DNA of cells, and if a person is exposed to the sun (or other forms of UV light) over many years, skin cancer may result.

Sunglasses

Sunglasses are an effective way of preventing sun damage to the eyes. But not just any sunglasses will do. The right sunglasses are wraparound UV-absorbent sunglasses, which block 99 to 100 percent of ultraviolet radiation. If the label on the glasses reads, "UV absorption up to 400 nm," or "special purpose," or "meets ANSI UV requirements," then the glasses block at least 99 percent of UV rays. Whether the glasses are dark or light does not matter. The protection comes from an invisible chemical that is applied to the lenses. Any type of eyewear can be treated to make it UV-absorbent.

How Is Skin Cancer Diagnosed?

Melanoma may show up as a change in the size, color, texture, or shape of a mole or other darkly pigmented area. Bleeding from a mole that is not the result of a scratch or other injury may also be a warning sign of cancer. Nonmelanoma can be hard to tell from normal skin. The most important warning signs are a new growth, a spot or bump that seems to be growing larger (over a few months or a year or two), or a sore that does not heal within three months.

When either melanoma or nonmelanoma is suspected, the doctor will take a sample (biopsy) of the abnormal tissue for examination under the microscope.

How Is Skin Cancer Treated?

The first step in treating skin cancer is to stage it, that is, to determine whether and how far it might have spread. Staging a cancer is an important step in choosing the best treatment. It also helps to determine the patient's prognosis (outlook for survival). The most common system for describing skin cancer, assigns five stages: 0, I, II, III, and IV. So, for example, stage 0 means the cancer has not spread beyond the tissue beneath the skin; stage IV means that the cancer has spread to other organs such as the lung, liver, or brain, and is less likely to be curable.

Fortunately, most nonmelanoma can be completely cured by a variety of types of surgery depending on the size of the cancer and where it is. If a squamous cell cancer appears to have a high risk of spreading, surgery may sometimes be followed by radiation, which uses high-energy rays to kill cancer cells, or chemotherapy (kee-mo-THER-a-pee), which uses anticancer drugs that can be injected into a vein in the arm or taken as tablets. For some precancerous conditions, chemotherapy may simply be placed directly on the skin as a cream.

Treatment for melanoma includes surgery and chemotherapy. Radiation therapy is not usually used to treat the original melanoma that developed on the skin.

How Is Skin Cancer Prevented?

A popular anti-skin cancer slogan in Australia states: "Slip on a shirt. Slap on a hat. Slop on some sunscreen. Seek shade." The most important way of lowering the risk of nonmelanoma is to stay out of the sun. Sunscreen does not seem to prevent melanoma. This is especially important in the middle of the day, when sunlight is most intense. Because no one wants to stay indoors all day, children and adults can protect their skin by covering it with clothing and by using a sunscreen. The sunscreen should protect users from both UVA and UVB radiation. It should have a skin protection factor (SPF) of at lease 50 on areas of the skin that are exposed to the sun. Wide-brimmed hats and wrap-around sunglasses with 99 to 100 percent ultraviolet absorption help to protect the eyes. Tanning booths should be avoided.

What Skin Cancer Research Has Been Conducted?

Scientists have made enormous progress in understanding how ultraviolet light damages DNA and how DNA changes cause normal skin cells to become cancerous. In addition, researchers have explored ways of treating skin cancers by enlisting the patient's immune system (the body's defenses against tumors and infection) to fight cancer cells.

One possible treatment involves the immune system. The goal of this approach is to recognize and then attack cancerous cells. Other immunotherapies were anticipated to treat melanoma. As of 2009, much more work remained before therapies could be used by the general public. In June 2008, researchers in Israel announced they had developed a new vaccine that decreases recurrence of melanoma in prior sufferers and increases survival among the current ones. Plans were in place for further tests on this treatment.

Living with Skin Cancer

The most important fact to remember about skin cancer is that most of it is preventable. It is never too late for people to begin to protect their skin. Because a person who has had one skin cancer is at risk for another one, monthly self-examinations should become part of a routine. Cancer is most likely to recur (that is, to come back) in the first five years after treatment. Individuals who love being in the sun must take steps to protect their skin from more exposure. But except for staying out of the sun, almost everyone with skin cancer can go back to the life they had before they got cancer.

▶ *See also* **Cancer: Overview • Skin Conditions • Tumor**

Resources

Books and Articles

Kaufman, Howard L. *The Melanoma Book: A Complete Guide to Prevention and Treatment.* New York: Gotham Books, 2005.

McClay, Edward F., Mary-Eileen T. McClay, and Jodie Smith. *100 Questions & Answers about Melanoma and Other Skin Cancers.* Boston, MA: Jones and Bartlett, 2004.

Poole, Catherine M. *Melanoma: Prevention, Detection, and Treatment,* 2nd ed. New Haven, CT: Yale University Press, 2005.

So Po-Lin. *Skin Cancer.* New York: Chelsea House, 2008.

Organizations

Abramson Cancer Center of the University of Pennsylvania. 3400 Spruce Street, Philadelphia, PA, 19104. Web site: http://www.oncolink.upenn.edu.

American Academy of Dermatology. P.O. Box 4014, Schaumburg, IL, 60168-4014. Toll free: 866-503-SKIN. Web site: http://www.aad.org.

American Cancer Society. 1599 Clifton Road NE, Atlanta, GA, 30329-4251. Toll free: 800-227-2345. Web site: http://www.cancer.org.

National Cancer Institute. Public Inquiries Office, 6116 Executive Boulevard, Room 3036A, Bethesda, MD, 20892. Toll free: 800-4-CANCER. Web site: http://cancernet.nci.nih.gov/cancertopics.

Skin Cancer Foundation. 149 Madison Avenue, Suite 901, New York, NY, 10016. Telephone: 212-725-5176. Web site: http://www.skincancer.org.

Did You Know?

- The average adult body has two square yards of skin, which make up about 15 percent of the body's total weight.

- A one-inch square of skin contains millions of cells as well as many special nerve endings for sensing heat, cold, and pain.

- The average thickness of skin is one-tenth of an inch, but it ranges from very thin on the eyelids to thick on the soles of the feet.

* **allergens** are substances that provoke a response by the body's immune system or cause a hypersensitive reaction.

Skin Conditions

Skin conditions include various rashes, diseases, infections, injuries, growths, and cancers that affect the skin.

Leaves of Three, Let Them Be

Alison loved to take long walks in the woods in the summer, but one day she developed a streaky rash two days after she had gone on a hike. At first, her skin was red and swollen in spots. Soon, however, little blisters formed and began to itch intensely. Alison had developed contact dermatitis (der-ma-TY-tis), an allergic response to touching the oily resin urushiol (u-ROO-she-ol), an allergen* in poison ivy. Cool showers and a soothing lotion helped relieve the intense itchiness. Within a few days, the blisters began to scab over. It took about 10 days for the rash to heal completely. Afterward, Alison was careful to wear long-sleeved shirts and long pants when walking in the woods and to stay away from poison ivy, identifiable by its clusters of three, deep-veined leaves, with the center leaf on a short stalk.

What Does the Skin Do?

The skin is the largest and most visible organ of the body. It also is one of the most complex, because it has so much to do. The main job of the skin is to protect a person's inside parts from harmful factors in the outside

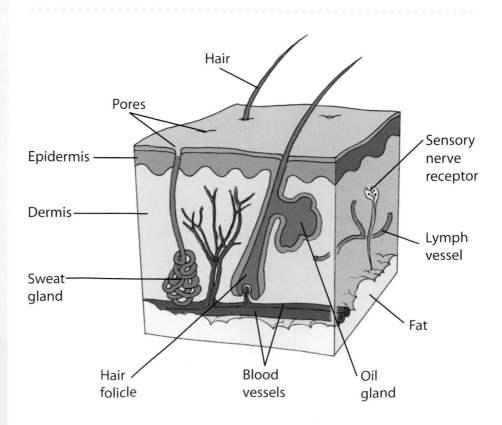

Anatomy of the skin. *Illustration by Frank Forney. Reproduced by permission of Gale, a part of Cengage Learning.*

world. It acts as a shield against sun, wind, heat, cold, dryness, pollution, and fluids. All of these can injure the skin over time. In addition, the skin comes into contact with and helps protect the body from germs; allergens, which are substances that can cause allergic reactions; and irritants, which are harsh chemicals that can hurt the skin. In addition, special nerve endings in the skin alert the brain to heat, cold, and pain.

What Can Go Wrong?

It is not surprising that many things can go wrong with an organ so big and complicated. Allergens and irritants can make the skin break out in a rash. Dermatitis is a general term for red, inflamed skin from a variety of causes.

There can also be problems in the way the skin functions. For example, it can make too much oil, leading to acne*. If the skin makes too many new cells, the result can be psoriasis (so-RY-a-sis). If the skin makes too little or too much coloring matter, called pigment, the result can be patches of abnormally light skin (hypopigmentation) or dark skin (hyperpigmentation).

The skin can also be injured, as in sunburn, and by viral infections, such as cold sores. Other kinds of skin infections are caused by bacteria and fungi. In addition, the skin can be affected by both non-cancerous growths, such as birthmarks, and skin cancers.

What Are Some Common Skin Problems?

The following are some of the most common skin problems seen by dermatologists (der-ma-TOL-o-jists), doctors who specialize in treating skin problems:

- **Acne:** a rash of pimples, blackheads, whiteheads, and deeper lumps, mostly on the face. Almost all teenagers have at least a little acne, and some adults have the problem as well. Acne develops when the skin makes too much oil and sheds dead cells too fast. Bacteria also play a role.

- **Athlete's foot:** a fungal infection that may cause the skin on the foot and between the toes to look red and peel, crack, flake, or even blister. Sweaty feet and tight shoes provide the perfect setting for a fungus to grow. Athlete's foot is most common among people who engage in sports and wear socks that are moist with sweat or who walk on pool decks and locker-room floors that are contaminated with the fungus.

- **Atopic (ay-TOP-ik) dermatitis, also called eczema (EK-zem-ah):** a red, itchy rash that often runs in families and accompanies allergies. In babies, it typically leads to itching, oozing patches with scabs, mainly on the face. In older children, the patches tend to be dry, and the affected skin may flake and thicken. In teenagers, the patches usually occur on the inside of the arm at the elbow bend, on the backs of legs at the knees, ankles, wrists, face, neck, and upper chest.

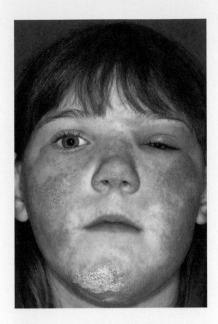

▲

Girl with a poison ivy rash on her face, which she is treating with calamine lotion. *Scott Camazine/Alamy.*

Names for Certain Skin Abnormalities

The following are medical terms for some common skin spots and bumps:

- **Comedo** (KOM-ee-do): a blackhead, whitehead, or pimple. Example: acne.

- **Macule** (MAK-yool): a small, flat, colored spot. Example: freckles.

- **Papule** (PAP-yool): a small solid elevation of the skin that usually occurs in clusters and often accompanies rashes.

- **Plaque** (PLAK): a large, raised patch of skin. Example: psoriasis.

- **Pustule** (PUS-tyool): a pimple filled with pus. Example: acne.

- **Wheal** (WEEL): a short-lasting, swollen bump. Example: hives.

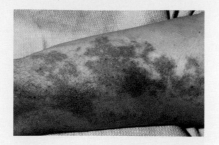

▲
A "port wine stain" birthmark. *Custom Medical Stock Photo, Inc. Reproduced by permission.*

* **acne** (AK-nee) is a condition in which pimples, blackheads, whiteheads, and sometimes deeper lumps occur on the skin.

* **benign** (be-NINE) refers to a condition that is not cancerous or serious and will probably improve, go away, or not get worse.

* **virus** (VY-rus) is a tiny infectious agent that can cause infectious diseases. A virus can only reproduce within the cells it infects.

* **histamine** (HIS-tuh-meen) is a substance released by the body during inflammation. It causes blood vessels to expand and makes it easier for fluid and other substances to pass through vessel walls.

* **immune system** (im-YOON SIS-tem) is the system of the body composed of specialized cells and the substances they produce that helps protect the body against disease-causing germs.

Birthmarks: a skin mark that develops before or shortly after birth. Several kinds of common birthmarks are caused by overgrowth of blood vessels. Such marks are painless and benign*.

Cold sores: an infection caused by the herpes (HER-peez) simplex virus* that leads to sores, usually around the mouth and nose. Some sores are barely noticeable, but others hurt. Cold sores are common among children and are easily spread from person to person by kissing or sharing dishes or towels.

Contact dermatitis: a red, itchy rash that occurs when the skin comes into contact with an allergen or something else to which the skin is sensitive. Examples include poison ivy and sensitivities to nickel, rubber, and skin care products.

Dandruff: flaking of the skin on the scalp. Some flaking is part of the normal process by which the outer layer of skin cells is regularly shed. If the flaking becomes obvious on a person's hair and clothes, it is called dandruff. If the scalp is red or if there are large flakes along with flaking elsewhere, the problem may be something else.

Hives: pale red, swollen bumps that occur in groups on the skin. Hives are usually itchy, but they may also burn or sting. They are caused when the body releases a chemical called histamine* as part of a reaction to substances such as foods, medications, and insect stings.

Irritant dermatitis: a red, itchy rash that occurs when the skin comes into contact with a harsh chemical. Examples of irritants include strong soaps or detergents and industrial chemicals.

Moles: growths that can appear anywhere on the skin, alone or in groups. They are usually brown and can have various shapes and sizes. Everyone has at least a few moles, and some people have forty or more. Most moles are not cancerous, but some may turn into a serious form of skin cancer called malignant melanoma (mel-a-NO-ma).

Poison ivy: a common type of contact dermatitis that occurs when a sensitive person comes into contact with the oily resin in the sap of poison ivy plants. Poison oak and poison sumac (SOO-mak) plants can have the same effect. The result is a streaky rash with redness and swelling, followed by blisters and itching. About 85 percent of all people have this kind of allergic reaction to poison ivy.

Psoriasis: a long-lasting skin disease caused when too many new cells are made, resulting in patches of red, thickened skin covered with silvery flakes. Four to 5 million Americans have psoriasis. It may result from a problem with the immune system*, which normally fights germs and other foreign substances in the body.

Ringworm: a skin infection caused by a fungus (not a worm). Ringworm is marked by red, itchy, ring-shaped patches that may flake or blister. It commonly affects the feet, scalp, trunk, nails, and groin.

- **Rosacea (ro-ZAY-she-a):** a skin disease that causes redness and swelling on the face that may gradually spreads on the cheeks and chin. Small blood vessels and tiny pimples may appear on or around the red area. Fair-skinned adults, especially women, are most likely to get rosacea.

- **Seborrheic (seb-o-REE-ik) dermatitis:** a common condition that causes red skin and greasy-looking flakes, mainly on the scalp, on the sides of the nose, between the eyebrows, on the eyelids, behind the ears, or on the chest. In babies, this condition is called cradle cap. In adults, it often occurs in people with oily skin and hair, and it may occur in those with acne or psoriasis.

- **Shingles:** a skin eruption caused by the same virus that causes chickenpox. It starts with pain or tingling on one side of the body or face, followed by a red rash with small blisters. After a person has chickenpox, the virus may live on in the nerve cells and come out years later as shingles. An episode of shingles may last weeks.

- **Skin cancer:** the most common of all types of cancer, including various kinds of growths on the skin. About 700,000 Americans get skin cancer each year. The main cause is the sun's harmful rays.

- **Sunburn:** the immediate result of getting too much sun. The skin is injured, just as if it had been burned by heat, and becomes red and painful. If the sunburn is severe, blisters may form. The long-term effects of sun damage include wrinkles, certain skin bumps and spots, and skin cancer.

- **Vitiligo (vit-i-LY-go):** a condition that causes white patches of skin due to a loss of pigment in the cells and tissues. It affects one or two out of every 100 people. Although vitiligo strikes people of all races, it is particularly noticeable in individuals with dark skin.

- **Warts:** small, hard bumps on the skin or inner linings of the body that are caused by a virus. Most are skin-colored, raised, and rough, but some are dark, flat, or smooth. Warts are common on the fingers, hands, arms, and feet. Some warts occur on the genitals and can be spread during sex.

- **Wrinkles:** a common sign of skin aging. The main cause of wrinkles is getting too much sun over a lifetime. Cigarette smoking also plays a major role.

How Are Skin Conditions Diagnosed?

Nearly everyone has a skin problem at some time. Such problems can affect anyone, from newborns to older adults. A doctor can identify many skin problems just by looking closely at the skin. The doctor may also ask about the person's current symptoms, past illnesses, and family history.

In some cases, the doctor may need to do a biopsy*. This procedure involves removing a small bit of tissue so that it can be looked at under a microscope. If an infection caused by a fungus is suspected, the doctor

Botox and Wrinkle Relief

One of the drugs in the fight against wrinkles is Botox. The name is short for botulism toxin type A, a byproduct produced by the bacterium *Clostridium botulinum*. In food, the bacterium causes a potentially fatal type of food poisoning known as botulism. To remove wrinkles, a small amount of Botox is injected into the muscles under the wrinkled skin. The Botox temporarily paralyzes the muscles. The result, after three to five days, is that the wrinkles temporarily disappear. This treatment is controversial.

* **biopsy** (BI-op-see) is a test in which a small sample of skin or other body tissue is removed and examined for signs of disease.

* **ultraviolet** light is a wavelength of light beyond visible light; on the spectrum of light, it falls between the violet end of visible light and x-rays.

may scrape off some skin flakes, which can be checked at a lab for signs of fungus. Another way to check for an infection caused by bacteria or a fungus is with a culture, which involves taking a sample from the site of possible infection and placing it in a nourishing substance called a medium to see what kind of bacteria or fungi grow.

If contact or allergic dermatitis is suspected, the doctor may do patch testing to find out what allergens are to blame. Doing so involves putting tiny amounts of different substances on the skin under a patch. The skin is checked two days later to see which substances, if any, caused a reaction.

How Are Skin Conditions Treated?

Following are various ways to treat skin conditions:

- **Medicines:** Many medicines used to treat mild skin conditions are sold without a prescription in creams, lotions, gels, pads, and shampoos. Stronger medicines that are put on the skin, taken by mouth, or given in a shot are available only from a doctor or with a doctor's prescription.

- **Surgery:** Doctors use several kinds of surgery to remove or destroy abnormal skin tissue. Excision involves removing a skin growth by cutting. Cryosurgery involves destroying a skin growth by freezing it with an extremely cold liquid such as liquid nitrogen. Electrosurgery involves destroying a skin growth by burning it with electricity. Laser surgery involves destroying skin tissue with a laser, a tool that produces a very narrow and intense beam of light. Surgery is used for such problems as warts, skin cancer, moles, and birthmarks.

- **Light therapy:** Doctors treat certain skin problems with lamps that give off ultraviolet* rays. In some cases, the person also takes a drug that makes the skin more sensitive to ultraviolet light. This therapy is used for such problems as psoriasis and vitiligo.

Skin Care Suggestions

These tips can help keep a person's skin feeling healthy and looking its best:

- Protect the skin from the sun's harmful rays. Avoid the midday sun, cover up with clothing, and use a sunscreen with an sun protection factor (SPF) of around 45.

- Wash the face gently with lukewarm water, a mild soap, and a washcloth or sponge to remove dead cells.

- Reduce dry skin by keeping baths short and using warm water. Use moisturizing soap for dry or sensitive skin.

- Use a light moisturizer after bathing or showering if prone to dry skin.

- Dry off the skin after bathing by brushing it lightly with the hands or patting it with a towel.

▶ *See also* **Acne** • **Athlete's Foot** • **Herpes Simplex Virus Infections** • **Hives** • **Psoriasis** • **Ringworm** • **Skin Cancer** • **Vitiligo** • **Warts**

Resources

Books and Articles

Kunin, Audrey, with Bill Gottlieb. *The Dermadoctor Skinstruction Manual: The Smart Guide to Healthy Beautiful Skin and Looking Good at Any Age.* New York: Simon & Schuster, 2005.

Spilsbury, Louise. *Why Should I Wash My Hair? and Other Questions about Healthy Skin and Hair.* Chicago: Heinemann Library, 2003.

Organizations

American Academy of Dermatology. P.O. Box 4014, Schaumburg, IL, 60168-4014. Toll free: 866-503-SKIN. Web site: http://www.aad.org.

American Society for Dermatologic Surgery. 930 N. Meacham Road, Schaumburg, IL, 60173. Toll free: 800-441-2737. Web site: http://www.asds-net.org.

National Institute of Arthritis and Musculoskeletal and Skin Diseases. 1 AMS Circle, Bethesda, MD, 20892-3675. Toll free: 877-226-4267. Web site: http://www.niams.nih.gov.

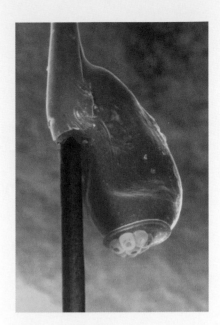

▲

Magnification of an egg laid by head lice. These eggs, called "nits," are visible to the naked eye. The term "nit-pick," which means to be concerned with insignificant details, derives from the process of taking the tiny eggs out of the hair by hand, a method used for centuries before more effective treatment became widely available. *Custom Medical Stock Photo, Inc. Reproduced by permission.*

Skin Parasites

Skin parasites (PAIR-uh-sites) are tiny organisms that invade the skin, often causing irritation and itching.

What Are Skin Parasites?

Parasites live off other living beings (including people), often feeding and reproducing on them. Some parasites thrive on human blood and cannot live long without it. Parasites may lay their eggs on people's skin. Before long, that person could become the host (an organism that provides another organism, such as a parasite or virus, with a place to live and grow) for hundreds or more of the parasites.

Skin parasites are found worldwide and infest large numbers of people. For example, as many as 6 to 12 million people worldwide contract head lice every year, according to the Centers for Disease Control and Prevention. Head lice most often affect children in school and daycare settings.

* **hair follicles** (FAH-lih-kulz) are the skin structures from hair develops and grows.

* **hives** are swollen, itchy patches on the skin.

What Are Some Common Skin Parasites?

There are many parasites that infest human skin, but lice, scabies (SKAY-beez), and chiggers are among the most common.

Head lice   Also known as *Pediculus humanus capitis* (peh-DIH-kyoo-lus HYOO-mah-nus KAH-pih-tis), head lice are six-legged parasites with tiny claws that cling to hairs. They are found on the scalp, neck, and behind the ears. Lice lay visible, whitish eggs called nits. In about seven days, the nits hatch into young called nymphs (NIMFS). Nymphs grow up fast, and in just one week they have matured into adult lice that must feed on blood to stay alive. Head lice may not cause any symptoms immediately, but as with other insect bites, the body reacts to the invaders, leading to itching and sores from scratching.

Pubic lice   Pubic lice, or *Phthirus pubis* (THEER-us PYOO-bus), invade the pubic hair and sometimes other body hair such as beards, eyebrows, eyelashes, and armpit hair. They often are called "crabs" because of their crab-like appearance. Pubic lice cause intense itching, especially at night, when they feed by burying their heads into hair follicles*. The nits or adult lice can be seen on pubic hairs or surrounding skin.

Scabies   Microscopic *Sarcoptes scabiei* (sar-KOP-teez SKAY-be-eye) mites cause an infestation called scabies. The mites work their way under the top layer of skin and lay their eggs. Most people are not even aware of the intruders until intense itching begins two to six weeks later. Red, pimple-like bumps appear on the skin, and there may be wavy lines on the skin tracing the mites' paths, especially in the webbing between the fingers and in the skin folds at the back of the knees and the inside of the elbows.

Chiggers   Chiggers are mites that tend to live in weeds, tall grass, or wooded areas. The chigger larvae (LAR-vee, immature mites) feed on a variety of animals, including humans. The larvae crawl onto the skin of passersby and can use their tiny claws to grab onto human hair. They then attach to the skin, usually at the ankles or waist or in skin folds, with hooked mouthparts and feed on skin cells. Unlike lice and scabies, chiggers only feed on their host for a couple of days, then let go and fall off. Chigger bites can cause a red bump that continues to grow in size, a skin rash, hives*, and severe itchiness. Sometimes the larvae are visible in the center of the bump.

How Are Skin Parasites Spread?

Despite what many believe, people do not get skin parasites because of poor hygiene. Instead, skin parasites tend to spread in situations where they can walk or fall from one person to another (or in the case of chiggers, from vegetation to human skin). The parasites often require relatively prolonged and close contact to move between people, and they spread most easily in crowded conditions, from sharing personal items, and from skin-to-skin contact.

Head lice in particular fall easily onto their next victims in close quarters. They also can infest hairbrushes, barrettes, hats, and sometimes clothes or bed linens. Other people become infested by using these items. Pubic lice spread mostly through sexual contact, but people also can get them from bed linens and clothes.

Scabies spread quickly in crowded living conditions or in places with lots of skin-to-skin contact (such as daycare centers and nursing homes). Like lice, scabies can be passed through sexual contact and by sharing clothes, towels, and bed linens.

How Are Skin Parasites Diagnosed and Treated?
Doctors often diagnose skin parasite infestations just by spotting the parasites, their eggs, larvae, or characteristic red bumps on the skin. With scabies, a skin scraping might be taken to check for mites, eggs, and mite feces (FEE-seez, or bowel movements). However, this test is not always accurate because the mites may have moved from the spot that was scraped.

Over-the-counter and prescription lotions and shampoos (known as pediculicides, peh-DIH-kyoo-lih-sides) can be used to kill head lice. In some cases, treatment may need to be repeated or replaced with stronger medications because lice are becoming resistant to some treatments. Other people living in the same house with the infested person may be treated at the same time.

Pubic lice also are treated with a pediculicide, similar to the treatment of head lice. If the infestation includes the eyelashes, petroleum jelly is applied several times a day to the eyelids for a week or more.

Patients with scabies are given medicated lotions to apply over the entire body, and the lotion must stay on for 8 to 12 hours. Chigger bites do not require any special treatment to heal, but antihistamines* may ease itching.

Infestation with lice and scabies can persist until they are treated properly. Once treatment begins, patients usually are no longer contagious after a day or two, but sores and itching may continue for several weeks. Chigger bites heal quickly.

Can Skin Parasites Cause Medical Complications?

Complications of skin parasites are rare. Frequent or rough scratching of bites or sores can lead to bacterial infections, such as impetigo*. If lice spread to eyebrows or eyelashes, the eyelids may become infected. Norwegian or crusted scabies is a form of scabies that can be severe in people with weak immune systems*, such as those with a chronic* illness and elderly people.

How Infestation with Skin Parasites Be Prevented?

To avoid skin parasites, experts recommend that people take the following precautions:

- shower daily, wash hands frequently, and wear clean clothes
- avoid anyone who has lice or scabies until that person is treated

* **antihistamines** (an-tie-HIS-tuh-meens) are drugs used to combat allergic reactions and relieve itching.

* **impetigo** (im-pih-TEE-go) is a bacterial skin infection that usually occurs around the nose and mouth and causes itching and fluid-filled blisters that often burst and form yellowish crusts.

* **immune system** (im-YOON SIS-tem) is the system of the body composed of specialized cells and the substances they produce that helps protect the body against disease-causing germs.

* **chronic** (KRAH-nik) lasting a long time or recurring frequently.

■ never share brushes, hats, bed linens, or clothes

■ practice abstinence (not having sex); birth control does not prevent pubic lice or scabies

■ avoid chigger-infested areas and wear socks, long pants, and long sleeves in wooded or grassy areas

To prevent the spread of parasites in a home when a family member has been diagnosed with an infestation, it is wise to do the following:

■ wash bed linens, towels, and clothes in hot water, then dry them on high heat

■ vacuum the entire house, then throw the vacuum cleaner bag away

■ disinfect combs and hair items

■ seal items that cannot be cleaned in airtight plastic bags for two weeks; at the end of that time, any parasites on those items will have died

In addition, children who have skin parasites should stay home from school or daycare until a day or two after they begin their treatment.

▶ See also **Lice** • **Scabies**

Resources

Organizations

Bohart Museum of Entomology, University of California. 1124 Academic Surge, Davis, CA, 95616, Web site: http://delusion. ucdavis.edu.

Centers for Disease Control and Prevention. 1600 Clifton Road, Atlanta, GA, 30333. Toll free: 800-311-3435. Web site: http://www. cdc.gov.

Slapped Cheek Syndrome *See Fifth Disease.*

Sleep Apnea

Sleep apnea (AP-nee-a) is a disorder in which a person temporarily stops breathing while sleeping.

Will He Snooze or Snore?

James loved his grandfather, but he was dreading this year's visit. Sharing his room with Grandpa last year, James had not slept all week. Sometimes his grandfather's snoring would stop, but then James had to hop out of bed to make sure his grandfather was breathing. Each time, Grandpa started breathing again after about 10 seconds, but he would choke and gasp for air before starting to snore again. In the morning, Grandpa had no memory of the night's noisy events.

When Grandpa arrived, he announced he would be a better room-mate this year. His snoring had been caused by sleep apnea, and his doc-tor had given him a device to wear in his nose at night to make it easier for him to breathe.

What Is Sleep Apnea?

While sleeping, a person with sleep apnea stops breathing briefly, usually for about 10 seconds at a time. This interruption in breathing can happen hundreds of times a night. The result is that the body does not get enough oxygen* or a restful night's sleep. People with sleep apnea often are very tired during the day, have trouble concentrating, and may feel anxious at night and have difficulty falling asleep. Sometimes, they wake up in a panic because they think they are choking, and many wake up with head-aches and are depressed and moody during the day.

Obstructive sleep apnea (OSA) is the most common type of sleep apnea; it affects an estimated 12 million Americans. It occurs when some-thing in the throat, such as the tongue or tonsils*, blocks the airway. Central sleep apnea is another type of sleep apnea that occurs when the brain temporarily "forgets" to tell the body to breathe. Mixed apnea is a combination of OSA and central sleep apnea.

Sleep apnea can affect people of all ages, but it is most common in older individuals. OSA occurs most often in men who are 50 or older, and many people with OSA are overweight. People with sleep apnea often do not know that they have it. Family members, however, are well aware of the problem because the most common symptom is loud snoring.

Living with Sleep Apnea

In some people, sleep apnea is just an annoying problem; in others, it can lead to heart problems and stroke*. Many people with OSA also have hypertension, which can also be dangerous. To determine if someone has sleep apnea, doctors may check how long it takes for the person to fall asleep, and they may monitor different body functions while the individ-ual sleeps. Sometimes, these tests occur at sleep clinics, which are special places where researchers can measure such factors as brain waves, heart rate, eye movement, body muscle tone, breathing, snoring, and blood oxygen levels during sleep.

Because sleep apnea can be dangerous, individuals who suspect they have sleep apnea should visit a doctor to learn more about their particular condition. In general, people with sleep apnea should not drink alcohol or take sleeping pills before bed, and they should try to lose weight if they are overweight. For many people, sleeping on their sides eliminates, or at least lessens, snoring. Various prescription drugs relieve apnea in some

Snoring

One of the symptoms of sleep apnea is snoring, but snoring can have other causes, including alcohol consumption, sedative medication use, chronic nasal congestion, or obstruction caused by enlarged adenoids and tonsils.

In most cases, medical professionals do not know what causes snoring: Some people just snore. Sometimes, how-ever, they can find a cause. If a patient' snoring is punctuated by extended quiet periods before snoring resumes, a doctor may identify the snoring as a symptom of sleep apnea and then suggest treatment options.

* **oxygen** (OK-si-jen) is an odorless, colorless gas essential for the human body. It is taken in through the lungs and delivered to the body by the bloodstream.

* **tonsils** are paired clusters of lymphatic tissue in the throat that help protect the body from bacteria and viruses that enter through a person's nose or mouth.

* **stroke** is a brain-damaging event usually caused by interference with blood flow to the brain. A stroke may occur when a blood vessel supplying the brain becomes clogged or bursts, depriving brain tissue of oxygen. As a result, nerve cells in the affected area of the brain, and the specific body parts they control, do not properly function.

people. Special devices worn in the nose or mouth can keep the airways clear as well. In some cases, doctors may recommend surgery to remove tissues, such as tonsils and adenoids, that block the airway.

▶ *See also* **Insomnia • Obesity • Sleep Disorders**

Resources

Books and Articles

Chokroverty, Sudhansu. *Questions and Answers about Sleep Apnea.* Sudbury, MA: Jones and Bartlett, 2009.

Pascualy, Ralph A. *Snoring and Sleep Apnea: Sleep Well, Feel Better,* 4th ed. New York: Demos Health, 2008.

Organization

American Sleep Apnea Association. 6856 Eastern Avenue, NW, Suite 203, Washington, DC, 20012. Telephone: 202-293-3650. Web site: http://www.sleepapnea.org.

Sleep Disorders

A sleep disorder is just what its name implies: something abnormal about the way individuals sleep. It might be that these people cannot get enough sleep, as is the case in insomnia (in-SOM-nee-a). In hypersomnia (HY-per-SOM-nee-a), individuals sleeps too much. In still other kinds of sleep disorders, events such as night terrors or restless leg syndrome may interfere with sleep.

Why Are Sleep Disorders Important?

When people do not get a normal refreshing sleep, they are not at their best. They may be impatient or careless, or they may show poor judgment in their actions. They may also be irritable with family and friends. Sleeplessness can cause serious accidents, as when someone "nods off" while driving a car or operating machinery.

An estimated 30 million to 40 million Americans have serious sleep problems that can be damaging to their health. In the case of insomnia alone, estimates of the cost in terms of lost productivity reach many billions of dollars.

In order to understand sleep disorders, it is necessary to understand something about sleep itself and the wide range of normal variations in the way people sleep.

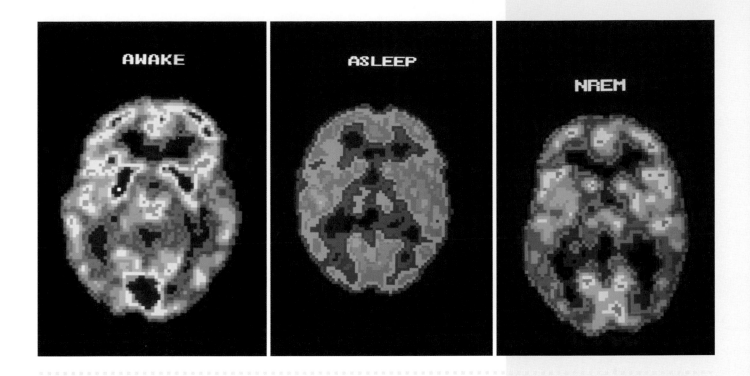

What Is Normal Sleep?

On average, about one-third of a person's life is spent sleeping. However, the amount and timing of sleep vary considerably in different people, based on their age and lifestyle. Newborn infants may sleep up to 20 hours per day. Young and middle-aged adults sleep about eight hours on average. Elderly people tend to get less sleep at night but may take naps during the day.

The timing of sleep often is determined by such factors as work schedules, but it is affected by lifestyle as well. Some individuals seem to be morning people, or "early birds," by nature, whereas others are "night owls," preferring to stay up late.

What Are the Types and the Stages of Sleep?

Scientists at sleep laboratories have discovered that there are two distinct types of sleep. One is called rapid eye movement, or REM, sleep, because the eyes can be seen moving rapidly beneath the closed eyelids. Dreaming takes place during REM sleep, and the brain waves of someone in REM sleep look much like those of someone who is awake when the waves are measured on an electroencephalogram (EEG)*.

The other type, non-REM sleep, consists of four stages in which the brain waves progressively become deeper and slower but then speed up again until the REM stage occurs. This cycle normally is repeated with some variation at approximately 90-minute intervals, with REM sleep usually taking up about 25 percent of the total.

Studies conducted at sleep laboratories have contributed greatly to the diagnosis and treatment of sleep problems. The following are some of the more common sleep disorders.

▲

Researchers use electroencephalograms (EEGs) and positron emission tomography (PET scans) to study sleep disorders. These PET scans show various stages of sleep and wakefulness. When awake (left), the brain shows active areas in red and yellow, with inactive areas in blue. During normal sleep (center), the brain is less active, and most areas show as blue. During deep sleep and non-REM sleep (right), the brain is active but not as active as during REM sleep (not shown) or wakefulness. *Hank Morgan/ Photo Researchers, Inc.*

* **electroencephalogram** instrument that records the electrical activity of the brain.

Researchers believe that the body's daily "clock," also called its circadian rhythm, is linked to the pineal gland and to the suprachiasmatic nucleus region of the hypothalamus. These structures within the brain receive information from the eye's retina about daylight and darkness, and send signals about regulating body responses to the spinal cord and elsewhere in the nervous system. *Illustration by Frank Forney. Reproduced by permission of Gale, a part of Cengage Learning.*

▶

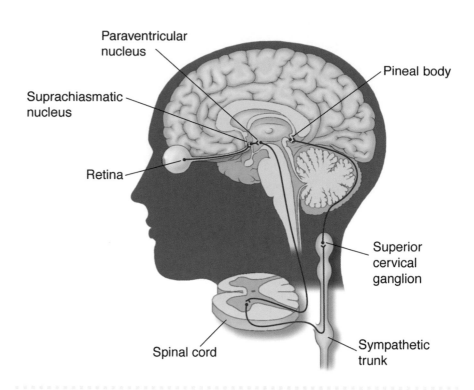

* **stroke** is a brain-damaging event usually caused by interference with blood flow to the brain. A stroke may occur when a blood vessel supplying the brain becomes clogged or bursts, depriving brain tissue of oxygen. As a result, nerve cells in the affected area of the brain, and the specific body parts they control, do not properly function.

* **hallucinations** (ha-LOO-sin-AY-shuns) occur when a person sees or hears things that are not really there. Hallucinations can result from nervous system abnormalities, mental disorders, or the use of certain drugs.

* **paralysis** (pah-RAH-luh-sis) is the loss or impairment of the ability to move some part of the body.

Sleep Disorder Conditions

Sleep disorder conditions include insomnia, sleep apnea, narcolepsy, hypersomnia, restless leg syndrome, and situational sleep loss.

Insomnia is a general term for trouble sleeping ("somnia" comes from the Latin *somnus,* which means sleep). People with insomnia may have difficulty falling asleep, or they may wake up too early in the morning. Some wake up frequently during the night and then find it hard to go back to sleep.

A person with sleep apnea (AP-nee-a) stops breathing intermittently while asleep, for periods of about 10 seconds or more. The most common and severe type is obstructive sleep apnea. In this disorder, the muscles at the back of the throat relax and sag during sleep until they obstruct the airway. The pressure to breathe builds up until the sleeper gasps for air. These episodes may occur hundreds of times a night and are accompanied by awakenings so brief that they usually are not remembered. People with sleep apnea typically complain of being very tired during the day. Severe sleep apnea can induce high blood pressure and increase the risk of stroke*, heart attack, and even heart failure.

Narcolepsy (NAR-ko-lep-see), like sleep apnea, involves excessive daytime sleepiness. In narcolepsy, however, the person cannot resist falling asleep. Some people with narcolepsy also experience frightening hallucinations* or sleep paralysis*, an inability to move or speak, while falling asleep or waking up. Research has shown that during a sleep attack, the REM stage of sleep intrudes suddenly into the waking state. It is a lifelong condition of unknown cause. Narcolepsy runs in families.

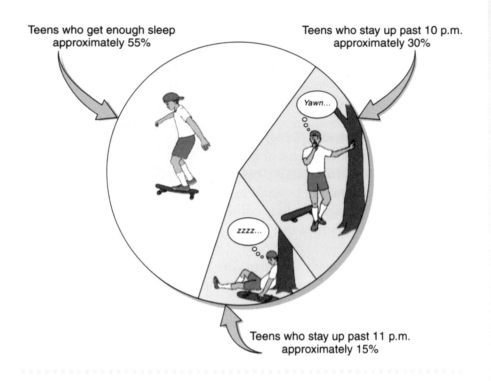

Teens who get enough sleep approximately 55%

Teens who stay up past 10 p.m. approximately 30%

Yawn...

zzzz...

Teens who stay up past 11 p.m. approximately 15%

Research shows that the brain makes proteins essential for neuron function at a faster rate during sleep than during waking hours. But close to half of all teens do not get as much sleep as they need, leading to feelings of "burn out," possibly because the brain is burning through proteins faster than it can replace them. *Illustration by Frank Forney. Reproduced by permission of Gale, a part of Cengage Learning.*

Sometimes socially embarrassing or inconvenient, this disorder can also be severely disabling and cause injury.

People with hypersomnia may sleep excessively during the day or longer than normal at night. Drowsiness or sleep periods last longer than with narcolepsy. Psychological depression* is often the main cause.

Restless leg syndrome is characterized by frequent leg movements due to discomfort inside the legs such as aching or prickling sensations that prevent individuals from falling asleep. In some individuals, sleep is then disrupted by involuntary leg jerking, which in some women is more troublesome during pregnancy.

Situational sleep loss (also known as situational insomnia) occurs as a result of a stressful event such as a family, work, or financial issue. When the worries surrounding the specific event are resolved the insomnia usually dissipates as well. Patients with situational sleep loss may benefit from relaxation techniques and/or pharmacologic treatment options from their physician, counselor, or therapist.

Nightmares, night terrors, and sleepwalking

Almost everyone has nightmares occasionally. These unpleasant, vivid dreams occur during REM sleep, usually in the middle or late hours of the night. Upon awakening, the dreamer often remembers the nightmare clearly and may feel anxious. Nightmares are especially common in young children. In adults, they may be a side effect of certain drugs or of traumatic events, such as accidents.

A night terror is quite different from a nightmare. It occurs in children during deep non-REM sleep, usually an hour or two after going to bed. During an episode, they may sit up in bed shrieking and thrashing about with their eyes wide open. Typically, the next day they remember nothing

Melatonin

Some over-the-counter sleep aids contain melatonin (mel-a-TO-nin). Melatonin is a hormone secreted during darkness by the pineal (PIN-e-al) gland, a small structure located over the brain stem (the part of the brain that connects to the spinal cord and controls the basic functions of life, such as breathing and blood pressure).

Melatonin appears to be part of the system that regulates sleep-wake cycles in humans. Some research studies have shown that a small dose of melatonin at night helps make falling asleep easier and that melatonin may be beneficial to travelers who have jet lag.

Melatonin is available for sale without a prescription, but the Food and Drug Administration does not regulate its production or sale. Studies continued on this product to determine whether melatonin is safe for use.

Did You Know?

■ People's eyes move when they dream much as they do when they are awake.

■ A person who lives to be 70 has spent about six years dreaming.

■ In one sleep disorder, apnea, people can stop breathing hundreds of times each night.

■ In another, narcolepsy, someone can fall asleep while having a conversation.

■ Night terrors are different from nightmares.

■ People who sleepwalk are not acting out their dreams.

* **depression** (de-PRESH-un) is a mental state characterized by feelings of sadness, despair, and discouragement.

* **psychotherapy** (sy-ko-THER-a-pea) is the treatment of mental and behavioral disorders by support and insight to encourage healthy behavior patterns and personality growth.

of the event. Night terrors occur chiefly in preschool children. Although frightening, they generally are harmless and are soon outgrown.

Sleepwalking also occurs during non-REM sleep. It was once believed to be the acting out of dreams, but such is not the case. It takes place most commonly in children. The sleepwalker wanders about aimlessly, appearing dazed and uncoordinated, and remembers nothing of the episode afterward.

How Do Doctors Diagnose and Treat Sleep Disorders?

Most sleep disorders can be treated successfully if diagnosed properly. Anyone who sleeps poorly for more than a month or has daytime sleepiness that interferes with normal activities may wish to consult a doctor or be referred to a specialist in sleep disorders.

At a sleep clinic, patients are first asked questions about their medical history and sleep history. A polysomnogram (pol-ee-SOM-no-gram) is sometimes used to measure brain waves, muscle activity, breathing, blood oxygen level, and other body functions during sleep.

Many sleep disorders, such as jet lag, short-term insomnia, and most nightmares, do not need treatment. Some others, such as night terrors, are outgrown.

Chronic insomnia often is treated successfully with behavior therapy, which involves various relaxation techniques and reconditioning to change poor sleeping habits. Sleeping pills may be used temporarily, but their long-term use is controversial due to unwanted side effects.

Obstructive sleep apnea is often treated with dental appliances or one of two devices: the CPAP (continuous positive airway pressure) or the BiPAP (bi-level positive airway pressure). These devices keep the airway open. Operations (to widen the area at the back of the throat or to provide a new opening into the windpipe below the Adam's apple) sometimes are performed to treat severe obstructive sleep apnea.

For restless leg syndrome, people can alter their routines, incorporating stretching, walking, and regular exercise into their daily patterns. Massage may also be helpful. If the problem requires medical treatment, physicians can prescribe various types of drugs, for example, a dopamine agonist such as ropinirole (Requip) or some kind of sedative, such as zolpidem (Ambien).

Hypersomnia due to depression is often helped by psychotherapy*.

There is no cure for narcolepsy and restless legs, but medications can help control or ease symptoms.

Guidelines for Prevention

Most sleep disorders can be prevented or minimized by making a few changes in one's lifestyle. The following are some simple guidelines:

■ Avoid excessive amounts of caffeine or alcoholic beverages, especially soon before bedtime. The same goes for smoking cigarettes.

■ Avoid frequently disrupted sleep-wake schedules.

- Avoid excessive napping in the afternoon or evening.
- Exercise regularly, but not just before retiring.

▶ *See also* **Depressive Disorders • Insomnia • Jet Lag • Narcolepsy • Sleep Apnea**

Resources

Books and Articles

Colligan, L. H. *Sleep Disorders.* New York: Marshall Cavendish Benchmark, 2009.

Epstein, Lawrence J., with Steven Mardon. *The Harvard Medical School Guide to a Good Night's Sleep.* New York: McGraw-Hill, 2007.

Marcovitz, Hal. *Sleep Disorders.* San Diego, CA: ReferencePoint Press, 2008.

Wilson, Sue, and David Nutt. *Sleep Disorders.* New York: Oxford University Press, 2008.

Organizations

Center for Narcolepsy, Sleep, and Health Research. College of Nursing, Suite 208, University of Illinois at Chicago. 845 South Damen Avenue (M/C 802), Chicago, IL 60612. Telephone: 312-996-5176. Web site: http://www.uic.edu/nursing/CNSHR/index.html.

National Heart, Lung, and Blood Institute. P.O. Box 30105, Bethesda, MD, 20824-0105. Telephone: 301-592-8573. Web site: http://www.nhlbi.nih.gov/health/dci/Browse/Sleep.html.

National Sleep Foundation. 1522 K Street NW, Suite 500, Washington, DC, 20005. Telephone: 202-347-3471. Web site: http://www.sleepfoundation.org.

Slipped (Herniated) Disk

Slipped disk is a condition in which a disk in the spinal column moves out of its correct position in the spine and presses on the spinal nerves, causing pain and sometimes muscle weakness.

What Is a Slipped Disk?

The spine is made up of bones called vertebrae (VUR-te-bray) that protect the delicate spinal cord. These vertebrae are separated from each other and cushioned by disks. The disks contain a soft inner layer and a tough outer layer. If the outer layer tears, the soft inner layer can push out and

Healthy disk between vertebrae (bottom) compared to slipped disk pressing on spinal nerve (middle). *Illustration by Frank Forney. Reproduced by permission of Gale, a part of Cengage Learning.*

▶

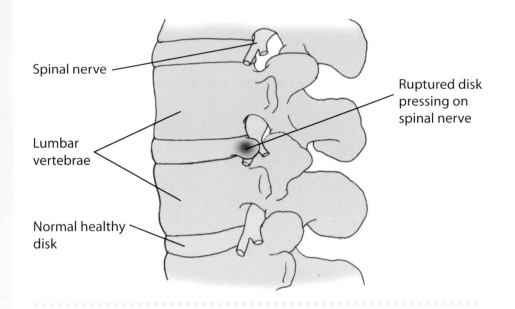

Spinal nerve

Lumbar vertebrae

Normal healthy disk

Ruptured disk pressing on spinal nerve

put pressure on the spinal nerves. This condition can cause severe pain as well as muscular weakness. Slipped disks are also described as "herniated," "protruded," and "bulging."

Most slipped disks occur in the lower back. However, slipped disks can occur in any part of the spine, including the neck.

What Causes Slipped Disks?

In most cases, the condition develops gradually over a number of years. A person may be totally unaware that anything is wrong, until the disk begins to cause pain. There are a small number of cases of slipped disk that occur to people who have made a sudden difficult movement, such as lifting a heavy object or making a sudden awkward movement. Slipped disks can also be the result of normal wear and tear on the disks due to aging.

The correct posture when carrying loads, lifting, or wearing a backpack can prevent back injuries. *Illustration by Frank Forney. Reproduced by permission of Gale, a part of Cengage Learning.*

▼

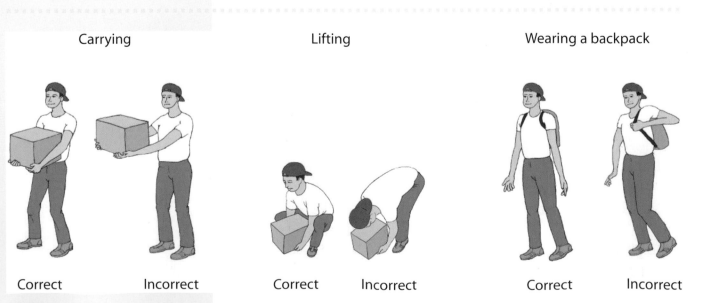

Carrying

Correct   Incorrect

Lifting

Correct   Incorrect

Wearing a backpack

Correct   Incorrect

How Common Is Slipped Disk?

Slipped disk is a fairly common. It happens mainly to people between the ages of 30 and 40. However, it can occur in younger people and even in children. After the age of 40, disks become more stable because extra tissue forms around them. Between the ages of 30 to 40, disks tend to lose fluid and become less resistant to pressures put on them. Slipped disk is more common in men than in women. People of either sex, however, who sit for long periods of time are more susceptible to the condition.

How Is Slipped Disk Diagnosed?

Individuals suffering from severe, sudden back pain should be evaluated by a physician to determine if they have a slipped disk, particularly if there is muscular weakness or pain and numbness in the legs or feet. The doctor administers nerve-reflex and muscle-strength tests after taking a personal history of the patient.

Among the tests used to locate and confirm a diagnosis, x-rays and other imaging tests may be performed. A test called an electromyogram (e-LEK-tro-MY-o-gram) can measure the amount of electrical activity in the muscles and help determine how much muscle or nerve damage the patient has.

What Is the Treatment for Slipped Disk?

Total bed rest used to be prescribed for two weeks. Doctors later came to believe that this much bed rest does not help, and patients may be told to stay in bed two to three days. Medications are given to help relax muscle spasms and to relieve pain. After their initial symptoms have improved, patients are given certain exercises to strengthen the muscles of the back and abdomen, and they are told to avoid twisting the spine. Lifting should be done by bending the knees first and keeping the spine upright. Most patients recover within three months.

However, if these treatments are not successful, surgery may be necessary. Disk surgery involves removing a part of the disk that has slipped against a nerve. Exercise, weight management, and lifestyle changes are recommended following surgery to avoid a recurrence of the injury.

▶ *See also* **Sciatica**

Resources

Organizations

Emory Orthopaedics, Spine Center & Sports Medicine Center. 59 Executive Park South, Atlanta, GA, 30329, Web site: http://www.emoryhealthcare.org/departments/spine/sub_menu/ herniated_disk_.html.

Spine-health.com. 790 Estate Drive, Deerfield, IL, 60015. Telephone: 312-224-4150. Web site: http://www.spine-health.com.

A Smallpox Death and Its Results

On September 11, 1978, Janet Parker, a medical photographer, died from smallpox. She is the last known person to do so. She contracted the virus from a research laboratory at the University of Birmingham Medical School in Birmingham, England.

After Parker's death, the World Health Organization (WHO) ordered all known stocks of smallpox to be destroyed or transferred to one of two WHO reference laboratories: the Centers for Disease Control and Prevention (CDC) in the United States and the State Research Center of Virology and Biotechnology VECTOR in Russia.

* **vaccine** (vak-SEEN) is a preparation of killed or weakened germs, or a part of a germ or product it produces, given to prevent or lessen the severity of the disease that can result if a person is exposed to the germ itself. Use of vaccines for this purpose is called immunization.

* **epidemic** (eh-pih-DEH-mik) is an outbreak of disease, especially infectious disease, in which the number of cases suddenly becomes far greater than usual. Usually epidemics are outbreaks of diseases in specific regions, whereas widespread epidemics are called pandemics.

* **lesions** (LEE-zhuns) is a general term referring to a sore or a damaged or irregular area of tissue.

Smallpox

Smallpox is a contagious and often fatal infection caused by the variola (ver-e-O-luh) virus.

What Is Smallpox?

What do Queen Mary II of England, King Louis XV of France, and Czar Peter II of Russia have in common? Other than being royalty, they all died from smallpox, one of the deadliest diseases in history. This devastating illness first surfaced thousands of years ago, and many believe smallpox killed more people than all other diseases combined before it was wiped out in the late 1970s. The variola (from the Latin word "svarus," meaning "spotted") virus causes two types of smallpox: variola major and variola minor. Variola major (the type discussed in this entry) is extremely serious and can be fatal in up to 30 percent of cases. The milder variola minor is fatal in less than 1 percent of patients.

How Common Is the Disease?

Thanks to the vaccine* developed by Edward Jenner in 1796 and the intensified immunization program begun in 1967 by the World Health Organization (WHO), smallpox is no longer found in the world; the last naturally occurring case was reported in Somalia in Africa in 1977. Before this successful eradication program, the illness affected millions of people of all ages every year. Those who survived the severe period of infection often were left scarred or blinded.

Is It Contagious?

Smallpox is so contagious that just one infected person can launch an epidemic*. As soon as the first symptoms of the disease appear, an infected person can spread the virus by coughing, sneezing, or even talking. These actions expel tiny virus-packed drops of moisture into the air. When a healthy person breathes in these drops, the virus finds a new home. Less often, touching patients' sores or even just their bed linens or clothes can spread the infection. Smallpox is typically most contagious during the first week of illness. Outbreaks of the disease in a community tended to occur at two- to three-week intervals.

What Are the Signs and Symptoms of Smallpox?

Once the virus enters the body, it quickly reproduces and takes over healthy cells. An infected person usually is not even aware of the viral intruders for at least a week. Then the first wave of smallpox symptoms appears, often resembling those of a cold or the flu: fever, extreme tiredness, headache, backache, and, occasionally, nausea (NAW-zee-uh) and vomiting. These symptoms can last up to a week. About two to three days after the onset of symptoms, a rash of red blisters or lesions* appears

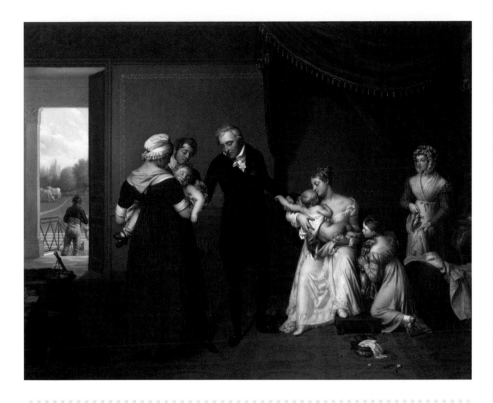

Dr. Alibert performs a smallpox vaccination on an infant in the year 1800. The doctor has scratched the skin with cowpox, which conferred immunity against smallpox (painting by Constant Desbordes). *Jean-Loup Charmet/Photo Researchers, Inc.*

suddenly on the face, arms, and palms. Within a few days, the lesions fill with fluid and pus* and spread to other parts of the body, including the inside of the nose and mouth. The sores can expand and break open, causing pain. Eventually, scabs form and later fall off. During its early stages, smallpox can be confused with chicken pox, which is caused by a different virus (varicella zoster, var-uh-SEH-luh ZOS-ter). Chicken pox produces a much milder rash that usually develops on the body and is less prominent on the face, arms, and hands.

How Do Doctors Make the Diagnosis?

Because smallpox was wiped out in the last quarter of the twentieth century, very few doctors practicing in the 21st century have ever seen a case. With the heightened awareness of the possibility that smallpox could be used as a weapon in biological warfare*, doctors are trained to recognize the disease. To make a diagnosis of smallpox, tests would be done on blood and fluid from a patient's lesions to identify the virus. To prevent a widespread outbreak, the patient would be isolated, and those in close contact with the person would be vaccinated. In the early 2000s, one diagnosed case of smallpox could cause a public health emergency.

What Is the Treatment for Smallpox?

There is no known cure for smallpox. Receiving the smallpox vaccine within four days of being exposed to someone who has the disease may prevent infection or lessen symptoms. Scientists are looking for new medicines as possible treatments for the disease. Public health agencies

* **pus** is a thick, creamy fluid, usually yellow or ivory in color, that forms at the site of an infection. Pus contains infection-fighting white cells and other substances.

* **biological warfare** is a method of waging war by using harmful microorganisms to purposely spread disease to many people.

* **immunology** (ih-myoo-NOL-uh-jee) is the science of the system of the body composed of specialized cells and the substances they produce that help protect the body against disease-causing germs.

* **malignant** (ma-LIG-nant) refers to a condition that is severe and progressively worsening.

* **pneumonia** (nu-MO-nyah) is inflammation of the lungs.

* **encephalitis** (en-seh-fuh-LYE-tis) is an inflammation of the brain, usually caused by a viral infection.

* **vaccination** (vak-sih-NAY-shun), also called immunization, is giving, usually by an injection, a preparation of killed or weakened germs, or a part of a germ or product it produces, to prevent or lessen the severity of the disease caused by that germ.

* **immunity** (ih-MYOON-uh-tee) is the condition of being protected against an infectious disease. Immunity often develops after a germ has entered the body. One type of immunity occurs when the body makes special protein molecules called antibodies to fight the disease-causing germ. The next time that germ enters the body, the antibodies quickly attack it, usually preventing the germ from causing disease.

BIRTH OF A VACCINE

Edward Jenner (1749–1823) often is called the father of modern immunology* because of his major contribution to ending small-pox. As an English country doctor, Jenner was fascinated that milkmaids exposed to cowpox (a disease that affects cows and is caused by a virus similar to variola) did not contract smallpox. He developed a vaccine containing live cowpox virus and injected it into an eight-year old boy. The boy did not contract smallpox, and vaccinations for the disease quickly became standard. Following Jenner's discovery, fatalities from smallpox dropped significantly. Jenner believed that his vaccine provided lifelong immunity to the disease. It is now thought, however, that the vaccine may not protect people for more that 10 years.

---

recommend that patients who have symptoms of smallpox be isolated immediately—either in a special unit of a hospital or at home—so that the infection does not spread to others. Healthcare workers are advised to take careful precautions when treating these patients. In the absence of a cure, treatment focuses on easing symptoms and preventing further infections. Patients may receive intravenous fluids (fluids injected directly into a vein), pain relievers, and antibiotics (to combat bacterial infections that can develop in the open sores) while the disease runs its course.

What Should an Infected Person Expect?

Smallpox infection can last from three to four weeks or until the last scabs fall off. The lesions often leave behind deep, pitted scars. When smallpox is fatal, patients usually die during the second week of illness. Smallpox can lead to serious complications, including the following:

- Hemorrhagic (heh-muh-RAH-jik) smallpox, which is associated with bleeding in the skin and body membranes
- Malignant* smallpox, in which the sores are flat and close together
- Blindness
- Bacterial infections
- Pneumonia*
- Encephalitis*

How Can Smallpox Be Prevented?

Widespread vaccination* in the United States for smallpox ended in 1972. In 1980 the WHO declared the disease eradicated. It is unknown how long vaccine-generated immunity* lasts. Many experts believe that it prevents infection for at least 10 years, but scientists think that few people in the world as of 2009 were still immune to smallpox.

DID YOU KNOW?

Before Jenner developed the cowpox vaccine, a technique called variolation achieved similar results. Medical practitioners in Asia would deliberately infect patients with a mild form of smallpox by blowing dried smallpox scabs into their noses. When they recovered, patients were immune to the disease. Thirty percent of the people who naturally contracted smallpox died, but only about 1 or 2 percent of people who had been variolated died.

By the 18th century, this dried-scab form of variolation was practiced in Africa, India, and much of the Ottoman Empire. Europeans practiced a form that involved puncturing the skin. Variolation was introduced into North America by African slaves. In Massachusetts, the Puritan clergyman Cotton Mather (1663–1728) learned about it from his slave Onesimus. Because of Mather's support of the technique, variolation was first tried during a smallpox epidemic in Boston in 1721.

Variolation was dangerous, however. Patients died from the procedure, and the mild form of the disease they contracted was still contagious and could spread to others, causing an epidemic. One son of King George III died after being variolated.

Two official facilities store samples of the virus: the CDC in Atlanta, Georgia, and the Russian State Research Center of Virology and Biotechnology in Koltsovo. In the unlikely event that bioterrrorists were to get access to any of these stored samples, it is possible that they might try to use the virus to launch a biological attack. If this were to happen, vaccines would be in high demand. To prepare for such a potential emergency, mass production of the vaccine was under way in the United States in the early 2000s.

Owing to possible side effects of the smallpox vaccine, the CDC suggests that it be given only to those at greatest risk of being exposed to the virus, including military personnel and first responders, for example, medical care providers, law enforcement personnel, and laboratory workers. About one in a million people who are vaccinated die from the effects of the vaccine, and a small percentage experience scarring or serious infections.

▶ *See also* **Bioterrorism • Encephalitis • Varicella (Chicken Pox) and Herpes Zoster (Shingles)**

Resources

Books and Articles

Finer, Kim R. *Smallpox.* Philadelphia, PA: Chelsea House, 2004.

Peters, Stephanie True. *Epidemic! Smallpox in the New World.* New York: Benchmark Books, 2005.

Underwood, Deborah. *Has a Cow Saved Your Life?* Chicago: Raintree, 2007.

Organizations

Centers for Disease Control and Prevention. 1600 Clifton Road, Atlanta, GA, 30333. Toll free: 800-311-3435. Web site: http://emergency.cdc.gov/agent/smallpox/index.asp.

World Health Organization. Avenue Appia 20, CH - 1211 Geneva 27, Switzerland. Telephone: +41 22 791 2111. Web site: http://www.who.int/csr/disease/smallpox/en.

Smoking *See Addiction; Lung Cancer; Pregnancy; Sudden Infant Death Syndrome; Tobacco-Related Diseases.*

Snail Fever *See Schistosomiasis.*

Snake Bites *See Animal Bites and Stings.*

Social Phobia (Social Anxiety Disorder)

Social phobia (FO-bee-a), also known as social anxiety (ang-ZY-e-tee) disorder, is an intense, long-lasting fear of social situations in which embarrassment may occur.

Angie's Story

Kim was shy. He did not like to raise his hand in class, but when the English teacher asked him a question, he answered in a soft voice. Angie, by contrast, was so afraid of being called on that she began skipping English class. Her problem went beyond ordinary shyness. She suffered from social phobia.

What Is Social Phobia?

Social phobia is an intense, long-lasting fear of embarrassment in social situations. It is different from shyness or stage fright, however. Social phobia involves extreme anxiety, an intense feeling of fear, worry, or nervousness. It may cause people to avoid social situations or to feel intensely self-conscious or uncomfortable and may lead to problems at home, work, or school.

Some people with social phobia are afraid of one particular type of social activity, such as giving a speech, talking in class, eating in a restaurant, or going to a party. Others have a broad form of the disorder, in which they fear and avoid almost any interaction with other people. In its most extreme form, the disorder can greatly limit people's lives. It makes it hard for them to go to school or work. It also makes it almost impossible for them to form relationships with others. Some children who have a particular and intense form of social phobia that causes them to be too anxious to speak in certain situations may have another type of disorder, known as selective mutism.

What Causes Social Phobia?

There are probably several causes for social phobia. People may learn their fear in part from watching how other people behave and what results from their behavior. Research also suggests that some people may inherit a tendency for anxiety. Research points to the possible role of the amygdala (a-MIG-da-la), a small structure inside the brain that is believed to be the seat of fear responses, whether learned or inherited. In addition, some studies have looked at the role of various hormones*, which have an effect on how the body responds to stress. Scientists have explored the theory that certain hormones may influence some people to overreact to criticism expressed by others.

What Are the Symptoms of Social Phobia?

Children with social phobia may cry, throw tantrums, freeze, shy away from others, or avoid or refuse to participate or perform in certain situations without really understanding what the problem is. Teenagers and adults, by contrast, realize the source of their fears. While they know their fears can be extreme, unreasonable, or out of proportion, they feel they cannot control them. Instead, they avoid the feared situation, or they face it with great distress. People with social phobia commonly fear situations that include the following:

- giving a speech
- performing on stage
- eating in a restaurant
- using a public restroom
- talking in class
- talking to a teacher
- going on dates
- going to parties
- meeting someone new
- talking on the phone

About 7 percent of adults in the United States show symptoms of social anxiety disorder in any given year. The problem typically starts in

---

Speaking Up

A common form of social phobia is fear of public speaking. Many people have a less extreme form of this fear. Toastmasters International is an organization with more than 11,700 clubs in 92 countries and more than 235,000 members worldwide. The aim of this group is to help people become more comfortable with and skilled at speaking in public. Some of the organization's tips for successful public speaking are:

- Know the material that you will present. Practice your speech, and change it if necessary.

- Imagine yourself giving the speech successfully. Imagine your voice as loud, clear, and confident.

- Realize that people do not want you to fail. They want you to be interesting and fun to listen to.

- Do not apologize for nervousness or problems. Doing so just calls attention to any problems you have.

- Think about what you are saying, not how you are saying it. Focus on getting your message across.

* **hormones** are chemical substances that are produced by various glands and sent into the bloodstream carrying messages that have certain effects on other parts of the body.

* **serotonin** (ser-o-TO-nin) is a neurotransmitter, a substance that helps transmit information from one nerve cell to another.

* **neurotransmitters** (nur-o-trans-MIH-terz) are chemical substances that transmit nerve impulses, or messages, throughout the brain and nervous system and are involved in the control of thought, movement, and other body functions.

the mid-teens although the person may have shown social inhibition or shyness since childhood. It can also begin in childhood. The problem occurs more often in women than men, but a higher percentage of men who have social phobia seek treatment for it.

How Are Teenagers Affected?

Most teenagers feel self-conscious at times, but those who are gripped by social phobia may be so overcome by self-doubt and worry that they find it hard to join in social activities. Instead, they may withdraw to the point where they have trouble making and keeping friends or participating in class. Their constant fear of being criticized or judged harshly may lead them to fret too much about their health and appearance. Some teenagers may try to escape the anxiety by drinking alcohol or using other drugs. Others may try to mask fear by acting like class clowns. Still others may stop going to school or taking part in after-school activities and may avoid opportunities to socialize with friends. As a result, their grades may fall, and their self-esteem may decline.

How Is Social Anxiety Disorder Treated?

Medications Four out of five people with social anxiety disorder feel better when treated with medications, psychotherapy, or both. Several kinds of medications have been shown to help people with the disorder. Although they cannot cure social anxiety, certain medications, called selective serotonin* reuptake inhibitors, can decrease the intensity of anxiety, allowing people to learn and practice new ways to feel comfortable in social situations. These medications work to correct imbalances in neurotransmitters* (such as serotonin), which play a part in mood conditions such as anxiety and depression. Other medications that are sometimes used are benzodiazepines (BEN-zo-dy-AZ-a-peenz), fast-acting agents that help people relax and decrease physical symptoms of anxiety such as sweating, trembling, and a pounding heart.

Psychotherapy In psychotherapy (sy-ko-THER-a-pee), people talk about their feelings with a mental health professional, who can help them change the thoughts, behaviors, or relationships that play a part in their problems. With social phobia, certain approaches to therapy can be especially helpful. Exposure (ex-PO-zhur) therapy is a technique in which people are gradually introduced, in a relaxed and supportive environment, to situations that frighten them, until they begin to feel more and more comfortable. Anxiety management training includes various techniques, such as deep breathing, that people can be taught to use to help control their distress. Cognitive techniques help people learn to identify beliefs they have that might not be reasonable (for example, "I will die if I have to give this talk") and replace them with more realistic ideas about the likelihood of danger in social situations (for example, "It might be uncomfortable, but I know the material, and I will be okay").

▶ *See also* **Anxiety and Anxiety Disorders • Selective Mutism**

Resources

Books and Articles

Hollander, Eric, and Nicholas Bakalar. *Coping with Social Anxiety: The Definitive Guide to Effective Treatment Options.* New York: Holt, 2005.

Organizations

Anxiety Disorders Association of America. 8730 Georgia Avenue, Suite 600, Silver Spring, MD, 20910. Telephone: 240-485-1001. Web site: http://www.adaa.org.

National Institute of Mental Health. Science Writing, Press, and Dissemination Branch, 6001 Executive Boulevard, Room 8184, MSC 9663, Bethesda, MD, 20892-9663. Toll free: 866-615-6464. Web site: http://www.nimh.nih.gov/health/topics/social-phobia/index.shtml.

Social Phobia/Social Anxiety Association. 2058 E. Topeka Drive, Phoenix, AZ, 85024, Web site: http://www.socialphobia.org.

Soft Tissue Infections *See Skin and Soft Tissue Infections.*

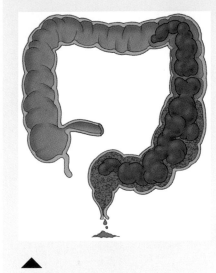

▲

Soiling results when solid body waste becomes hard and compacted in the large intestine, blocking it and causing it to stretch out of shape. If softer waste (liquid stool) seeps around the blockage, it can leak out of the anus, causing soiling. *Illustration by Frank Forney. Reproduced by permission of Gale, a part of Cengage Learning.*

Soiling (Encopresis)

Soiling, also called encopresis (en-ko-PREE-sis), is having uncontrolled bowel movements in one's underwear.

What Is Soiling?

Young children routinely have bowel movements in their diapers or underwear, but by about three years of age most children are able to maintain good bowel control and can be toilet-trained. When people who have established bowel control begin to have a bowel movement in their pants, the condition is called soiling, or encopresis. This soiling is often a leaking and not a full bowel movement. Most people who have a problem with soiling do not even realize that it is happening, because they do not feel as if they are having a bowel movement. In the majority of cases, encopresis is a medical problem. This medical problem can have serious psychological effects, ranging from embarrassment to family stress to teasing.

Why Does Soiling Happen?

Soiling is related to constipation (kon-sti-PAY-shun). Constipation is infrequent, hard, and painful bowel movements. When food goes through the digestive system, it is broken down into a thick, sludge-like liquid. The nutrients that the body needs, such as sugars, are absorbed from this liquid in the small intestine. The rest of the material passes into the large intestine, where water is reabsorbed. The remaining solids, called feces (FEE-seez), are then passed out of the body as a bowel movement.

When the bowels move infrequently, the large intestine reabsorbs so much water that the feces become hard and compacted. As a result, bowel movements are painful, causing many people to try to avoid having them. Doing so only makes the problem worse. Eventually, the mass of hard solids in the large intestine causes it to stretch out of shape. As it stretches, small amounts of liquid sludge from the small intestine seep around the hard mass of feces in the large intestine and then leak out of the body. This is the material that causes soiling.

Some adults think that children soil on purpose or that soiling is evidence of a psychological problem. In reality, soiling accidents are not intentional. Sometimes children who are teased or embarrassed about soiling can have emotional or behavior problems. Generally, once the soiling is treated and stops, these problems disappear.

How Is Soiling Treated?

There are three steps to treating soiling:

- Empty the large intestine
- Establish regular bowel movements
- Maintain regular bowel movements

An enema or a laxative medication often is used to empty the large intestine. With an enema, liquid is pushed into the large intestine to soften the hard mass of feces and create the urge to expel it. Sometimes strong laxatives are used instead to encourage the intestine to contract and push out the feces.

Once the large intestine is unblocked, it is important to establish regular bowel movements to keep it clear. A doctor may recommend laxatives taken by mouth, such as milk of magnesia, products that contain senna, or mineral oil. These laxatives keep waste material moving quickly through the large intestine so that it remains soft. Setting aside time each day to try to have a bowel movement (usually after breakfast or dinner) also helps establish a regular schedule.

Once a person is having regular daily bowel movements, laxatives are reduced and then gradually eliminated so that a regular schedule can be maintained without artificial assistance. Eating a high-fiber diet and drinking plenty of liquids also help maintain bowel regularity. Once feces move through the large intestine in a regular, painless way, the problem of soiling disappears. Unfortunately, it often takes time for soiling to be diagnosed correctly and properly treated. Sometimes consultation with a mental health professional, who works with a person's doctor, helps in developing a good behavioral treatment program that also minimizes emotional difficulties.

▶ *See also* **Bedwetting (Enuresis)**

Resources

Books and Articles

Galvin, Matthew. *Clouds and Clocks: A Story for Children Who Soil,* 2nd ed. Washington, DC: Magination Press, 2007.

Organizations

American Academy of Pediatrics. 141 Northwest Point Boulevard, Elk Grove Village, IL 60007-1098. Telephone: 847-434-4000. Web site: http://www.aap.org/publiced/BK5_Soiling.htm.

Somatoform Disorders

Somatoform (so-MAT-a-form) disorders are a group of conditions in which physical symptoms suggest a disease or medical condition, but no physical cause can be found. The term "somatoform" is derived from the Greek "soma," meaning "body." A "somatoform disorder" is one in which emotional problems are transformed into body symptoms. These disorders include hypochondria*, conversion disorder, and somatization (so-ma-ti-ZA-shun) disorder. Somatoform disorders do not include malingering or Munchausen syndrome, both of which involve pretending to be physically ill or intentionally producing the symptoms of an illness.

How Can Somatoform Disorders Be Told Apart?

Somatoform disorders are alike in that they involve physical symptoms without evidence of physical disease. The symptoms stem from an emotional cause. To understand how the disorders differ from each other, it may be helpful to consider the cases of three young people in a doctor's waiting room who were all having trouble with their voices. Tommy, a teenager, was only hoarse, but he feared this meant that he was getting throat cancer. Nine-year-old Mary had suddenly lost her voice completely and could not speak. Lillian, who was 25, was also hoarse and coughing, but she had many other symptoms, including dizziness and a stomachache.

As it turned out, Tommy was suffering not from cancer but from hypochondria. He had been much too worried about his hoarseness,

* **hypochondria** (hy-po-KON-dree-a) is a mental disorder in which people believe that they are sick, but their symptoms are not related to any physical illness.

which had come from cheering for his high school football team. The doctor could find nothing wrong with Mary's larynx, or voice box. Her mother said that Mary had been punished severely for "talking back," and the doctor suspected that she had lost her voice because of conversion disorder. None of Lillian's many symptoms, which had come and gone for years, could be traced to any physical disorder. The doctor thought that she must have somatization disorder. Tommy, Mary, and Lillian were referred to mental health professionals for treatment.

More Symptoms of Somatoform Disorders

Hypochondria   People with hypochondria have the fear or belief that they have a serious illness, such as heart disease or cancer, even though medical tests show no sign of disease. People with this condition may be excessively concerned with a wide range of common, usually minor, symptoms, such as coughing, nausea, dizzy spells, and various aches and pains. When their physician reassures them that these symptoms do not mean that they are seriously ill, they are not always convinced and may remain anxious, worried, and preoccupied with their symptoms. They may then go to various other doctors, seeking a "true" diagnosis of the same symptoms.

Conversion disorder   Conversion disorder, a much rarer somatoform disorder, might cause people to lose their voice, sight, or hearing or to become paralyzed in one or more of their limbs. They also may have trembling or lose feeling in various parts of their bodies. The condition is psychological, because medical examination can find no physical explanation for the symptoms. It typically begins suddenly after an extremely stressful event in a person's life. The symptom or affected body part is usually related in some way to the trauma or stress that triggered the conversion reaction. For example, a soldier who is extremely distressed after killing people during combat might develop "paralysis" in his weapon arm. Conversion disorder resulting from war experience has also been called shell shock or battle fatigue. Someone who has witnessed the murder of a loved one may develop "blindness" as a conversion symptom.

Somatization disorder   In somatization disorder, there are many different recurring symptoms in various parts of the body. These may include headache, backache, and pains in the abdomen, chest, and joints. There also may be digestive symptoms, such as nausea and abdominal bloating, or symptoms that involve the reproductive and nervous systems. As in other somatoform disorders, medical examinations and testing generally detect no clear physical cause for the symptoms.

Pain disorder and body dysmorphic disorder   Two other kinds of somatoform disorders are pain disorder and body dysmorphic (dis-MOR-fik) disorder. Pain disorder is similar to somatization disorder, except that pain is the main symptom. The pain may be in one or several areas of the body, but it does not fit a pattern of any particular medical illness or injury, and diagnostic tests fail to show the presence of any disease. In body dysmorphic disorder, a person becomes extremely concerned about some imagined or very slight body defect. Sometimes called "imagined ugliness," body dysmorphic disorder can cause great distress and cause a person to avoid being seen in public. In some cases, a person may seek unnecessary plastic surgery.

What Causes Somatoform Disorders?

The causes of somatoform disorders are not clearly understood. In hypochondria, a person may be overly sensitive to body sensations, or they may exaggerate the meaning of normal body sensations. A distressing memory of childhood illness may also play a part. It is believed that conversion disorder, somatization disorder, and pain disorder are all caused by the conversion, or shifting, of stressful emotional events or feelings of conflict into body symptoms to relieve anxiety*. Body dysmorphic disorder involves a distorted body image and may be influenced by cultures that emphasize the importance of physical appearance and early experiences which may have interfered with developing self-esteem.

How Are Somatoform Disorders Diagnosed and Treated?

Somatoform disorders are diagnosed by performing a medical evaluation and testing to determine whether there is a physical reason for a patient's symptoms and complaints. If there is not, a somatoform disorder may be diagnosed by looking closely at the particular signs and symptoms. A correct diagnosis is important, in order to avoid unnecessary surgery and other medical procedures and to begin proper treatment for the particular disorder.

Psychotherapy Psychotherapy* is the appropriate treatment for somatoform disorders. With the help of a mental health professional, a person tries to understand and resolve anxiety, trauma, or conflicts that are behind these conditions. Treatment may take varying lengths of time, depending on the severity of a disorder in a particular person.

▶ *See also* **Anxiety and Anxiety Disorders • Body Image • Conversion Disorder • Hypochondria • Malingering • Munchausen Syndrome • Stress and Stress-Related Illness**

Resources

Organizations

American Academy of Family Physicians. P.O. Box 11210, Shawnee Mission, KS, 66207-1210. Toll free: 800-274-2237. Web site: http://familydoctor.org/online/famdocen/home/common/pain/disorders/162.html.

* **anxiety** (ang-ZY-e-tee) can be experienced as a troubled feeling, a sense of dread, fear of the future, or distress over a possible threat to a person's physical or mental well-being.

* **psychotherapy** (sy-ko-THER-a-pea) is the treatment of mental and behavioral disorders by support and insight to encourage healthy behavior patterns and personality growth.

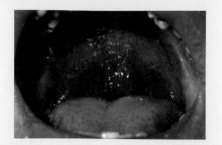

▲

A red and inflamed throat from pharyngitis, an infection caused by Streptococcus bacteria. *Dr. P. Marazzi/ Photo Researchers, Inc.*

* **bacteria** (bak-TEER-ee-a) are single-celled microorganisms, which typically reproduce by cell division. Some, but not all, types of bacteria can cause disease in humans. Many types can live in the body without causing harm.

* **influenza** (in-floo-EN-zuh), also known as the flu, is a contagious viral infection that attacks the respiratory tract, including the nose, throat, and lungs.

* **adenovirus** (ah-deh-no-VY-rus) is a type of virus that can produce a variety of symptoms, including upper respiratory disease, when it infects humans.

* **mononucleosis** (mah-no-nu-klee-O-sis) is an infectious illness caused by a virus with symptoms that typically include fever, sore throat, swollen glands, and tiredness.

* **immune system** (im-YOON SIS-tem) is the system of the body composed of specialized cells and the substances they produce that helps protect the body against disease-causing germs.

* **diarrhea** (di-ah-RE-a) refers to frequent, watery stools (bowel movements).

Children's Hospital Boston. 300 Longwood Avenue, Boston, MA 02115. Telephone: 617-355-6000. Web site: http://www. childrenshospital.org/views/august06/somatoform_disorders.html.

Sore Throat/Strep Throat

The pain and discomfort of a sore throat, also called pharyngitis (fair-un-JY-tis), are usually the result of inflammation due to infection or irritation.

Strep throat is caused by bacteria* in the Streptococcus (strep-to-KOK-us) family. Its main symptoms are sore throat and fever. The medical term for strep throat is streptococcal pharyngitis.

What Is a Sore Throat?

A sore throat can be a symptom of many infectious diseases. Viral infections such as the common cold, influenza*, adenovirus* infection, and infectious mononucleosis* cause most sore throats. Bacterial infections are less common, but the sore throats they produce usually are more severe. Group A beta hemolytic streptococci (he-muh-LIH-tik strep-tuh-KAH-kye) are the most common bacterial culprits, and they cause strep throat. Rarely, fungal infections can cause a sore throat, usually in people with a weakened immune system*. Non-infectious causes of sore throat include allergies, postnasal drip (the dripping of mucus from the back of the nose into the throat), and too much yelling or straining the voice. Smoking and other irritants can also cause a sore throat.

Are Sore Throats Common?

Sore throats are very common, especially in children. It is not unusual for children between the 5 and 10 years of age to develop several sore throat infections over the course of a year. Most of these illnesses are common viral respiratory infections. About 15 percent of all sore throats are caused by group A streptococci.

All of the infections that cause sore throats are contagious. They can spread through contact with drops of fluid from an infected person that can be coughed or sneezed into the air. The drops can be inhaled or transferred by the hand to the mouth or nose. The infections that cause sore throats also can spread through direct contact with an infected person, such as through kissing.

What Are the Signs and Symptoms of a Viral Sore Throat?

Sore throats are painful, sometimes swollen, and red. Many viral infections that cause sore throats are associated with other symptoms, including hoarseness, runny nose, cough, and diarrhea*.

Sore throat is a common symptom of infectious mononucleosis, a viral infection caused by the Epstein-Barr (EP-steen BAR) virus. The tonsils* become very swollen and may have white patches or an extensive coating. Swallowing is difficult, and in a few cases, the tonsils enlarge enough to cause difficulty breathing. Other signs and symptoms of mononucleosis include swollen lymph nodes* in the neck, fever, extreme tiredness, muscle aches, and an enlarged spleen.

What Are the Symptoms of Strep Throat?

People with strep throat feel generally weak and tired. The tonsils often are enlarged, there may be white specks and pus* on them, or they may be covered with a gray or white coating. Other symptoms of strep throat include high fever; headache; enlarged and tender lymph nodes in the neck; and abdominal* pain.

How Do Doctors Diagnose the Cause of a Sore Throat?

If a patient's sore throat and other symptoms match those of a common viral cold or respiratory infection, the doctor may base the diagnosis on the physical symptoms alone. Nasal and throat swabs can be tested to detect other causes of a sore throat, if necessary.

If the doctor suspects that a patient might have a strep throat infection, the doctor uses a cotton swab to take a sample from the throat and tonsils for a culture*. Often, the doctor will do a rapid strep test of the bacteria from the throat swab in the office. This quick test can give the doctor results in 10 to 15 minutes. A positive result indicates that strep bacteria are present; a negative result means that the strep bacteria may or may not be present and the more extensive culture should be done.

Infectious mononucleosis is diagnosed by examining blood samples for antibodies* to the virus.

How Is a Sore Throat Treated?

Treatment of a sore throat depends on the diagnosis. If it stems from a common cold caused by a virus, treatment is aimed at relieving symptoms until the illness disappears. Drinking plenty of fluids can help prevent dehydration* and clear out mucus* in the back of the throat. Water, ginger ale, warm tea with honey, and clear soups are good choices, but not acidic juices (such as lemonade or orange juice), because they can irritate the throat. Gargling with warm salt water can help soothe a sore throat, and over-the-counter pain relievers and throat drops can help ease symptoms as well. Antibiotics are not effective for treating viral infections such as colds. Most viral sore throats go away on their own without complications, and they generally clear up within a few days to a week.

The best treatment for infectious mononucleosis is rest. In addition, over-the-counter medications such as acetaminophen* can help relieve pain and fever. Studies have shown that one type of antiviral medication

* **tonsils** are paired clusters of lymphatic tissue in the throat that help protect the body from bacteria and viruses that enter through a person's nose or mouth.

* **lymph nodes** (LIMF) are small, bean-shaped masses of tissue containing immune system cells that fight harmful microorganisms. Lymph nodes may swell during infecti ons.

* **pus** is a thick, creamy fluid, usually yellow or ivory in color, that forms at the site of an infection. Pus contains infection-fighting white cells and other substances.

* **abdominal** (ab-DAH-mih-nul) refers to the area of the body below the ribs and above the hips that contains the stomach, intestines, and other organs.

* **culture** (KUL-chur) is a test in which a sample of fluid or tissue from the body is placed in a dish containing material that supports the growth of certain organisms. Typically, within days the organisms will grow and can be identified.

* **antibodies** (AN-tih-bah-deez) are protein molecules produced by the body's immune system to help fight specific infections caused by microorganisms, such as bacteria and viruses.

* **dehydration** (dee-hi-DRAY-shun) is a condition in which the body is depleted of water, usually caused by excessive and unreplaced loss of body fluids, such as through sweating, vomiting, or diarrhea.

* **mucus** (MYOO-kus) is a thick, slippery substance that lines the insides of many body parts.

* **acetaminophen** (uh-see-teh-MIH-noh-fen) is a medication commonly used to reduce fever and relieve pain.

* **corticosteroids** (kor-tih-ko-STIR-oyds) are chemical substances made by the adrenal glands that have several functions in the body, including maintaining blood pressure during stress and controlling inflammation. They can also be given to people as medication to treat certain illnesses.

* **antibiotics** (an-tie-by-AH-tiks) are drugs that kill or slow the growth of bacteria.

* **scarlet fever** is an infection that causes a sore throat and a rash.

* **rheumatic fever** (roo-MAH-tik) is a condition associated with fever, joint pain, and inflammation affecting many parts of the body, including the heart. It occurs following infection with certain types of strep bacteria.

* **kidney** is one of the pair of organs that filter blood and remove waste products and excess water from the body in the form of urine.

* **abscesses** (AB-seh-sez) are localized or walled off accumulations of pus caused by infection that can occur anywhere within the body.

(valacyclovir) may be useful in reducing the severity of symptoms. Severe cases of infectious mononucleosis may benefit from the administration of corticosteroids* to reduce swelling and inflammation. Infectious mononucleosis can take from one to two months to subside, and other symptoms from the illness, such as tiredness, can remain for months after.

How Is Strep Throat Treated?

When strep throat has been diagnosed, a course of antibiotic* is usually prescribed. A doctor may recommend a 10-day course of treatment or alternatively a one-time antibiotic shot, which can be an advantage if a patient experiences difficulty swallowing, nausea or vomiting. Regardless of type, any antibiotic should be taken as directed to prevent complications. Symptoms of strep throat usually improve within one to two days of starting the antibiotic.

What Are the Complications of a Strep Throat?

Strep throat can lead to scarlet fever*, rheumatic fever*, kidney* problems, including post-streptococcal glomerulonephritis, or throat abscesses*. Prompt treatment with antibiotics can prevent most of these complications.

Can Sore Throats Be Prevented?

Many respiratory infections both viral and bacterial are spread through contact with respiratory fluids from infected people. People who have respiratory infections and sneeze or cough in a classroom, on a playground, or in another crowded environment, can spread the infection to other people. Moisture droplets from their coughing or sneezing are passed into the air. Others inhale these germs, and then they too become infected.

Another way respiratory infections can be passed along is by hand-to-hand contact or by touching objects that an infected person has recently handled. That is why doctors tell people to wash their hands regularly. If someone has an infection or has been in close contact with someone who does, it is wise not to share utensils, food, and drinking glasses with that person.

▶ *See also* **Common Cold** • **Glomerulonephritis** • **Influenza** • **Laryngitis** • **Mononucleosis, Infectious** • **Rheumatic Fever** • **Scarlet Fever** • **Streptococcal Infections**

Resources

Books and Articles

Glaser, Jason. *Strep Throat.* Mankato, MN: Capstone Press, 2007.

Powell, Jillian. *Sore Throat.* North Mankato, MN: Cherrytree Books, 2007.

Organizations

American Academy of Family Physicians. P.O. Box 11210, Shawnee Mission, KS, 66207-1210. Toll free: 800-274-2237. Web sites: http://familydoctor.org/online/famdocen/home/common/infections/cold-flu/163.html; http://familydoctor.org/online/famdocen/home/common/infections/common/bacterial/670.html.

National Institute of Allergy and Infectious Diseases. Office of Communications and Public Liaison, 6610 Rockledge Drive, MSC 6612, Bethesda, MD, 20892-66123. Toll free: 866-284-4107. Web site: http://www3.niaid.nih.gov/topics/strepThroat/default.htm.

National Library of Medicine. 8600 Rockville Pike, Bethesda, MD, 20894, Web sites: http://www.nlm.nih.gov/medlineplus/streptococcalinfections.html; http://www.nlm.nih.gov/medlineplus/ency/article/003053.htm.

Spastic Colon *See Irritable Bowel Syndrome.*

Speech Disorders

A speech disorder is a condition that interferes with a person's ability to speak clearly and be understood. It may be caused by congenital problems, developmental delays, hearing problems, accidents, strokes, or defects in any of the organs or muscles involved in producing speech or in any of the areas of the brain that control speech.

How Does Speech Develop?

Speech and language develop most intensively during the first three years of life. When babies are born, they can make sounds by pushing air out of the lungs and through the vocal cords in the throat. The air vibrates these vocal cords, located in the larynx (LAR-inks) or voice box, creating sound.

Newborns learn that a cry will bring food, comfort, and companionship, and they begin to recognize certain sounds. As the jaw, lips, tongue, throat and brain develop over the first nine months of life, infants learn how to use the voice to mimic simple controlled sounds, such as "ba ba" or "da da." During this time, they learn to regulate the action of muscles in the face, mouth, neck, chest, and abdomen to produce speech-like sounds. At first, these sounds do not convey meaning as words do. Eventually, however, children begin to use words that others can understand. The responses they get encourage them to speak more and more. With practice, words become more understandable.

SIGN LANGUAGES

Spoken language is not the only way that people can communicate. Many people who are deaf and/or unable to speak learn to communicate through manual communication or signed language. In the early 2000s, three signed languages were used in the United States: American Sign Language (ASL), Signed Exact English, and Cued Speech.

In the mid-1700s, a French educator working with poor deaf children developed a system for spelling out French words with a manual alphabet, expressing whole concepts with one or two hand signs, and adding emphasis with standardized facial expressions. In 1816, Thomas Gallaudet (1787–1851) brought French Sign Language to the United States. French Sign Language was modified to incorporate English terms, while maintaining French sentence structure, to form what later was called American Sign Language (ASL). Gallaudet University in Washington, D.C., is named for Thomas Gallaudet.

Signed Exact English was developed by educators in California who worked with children with hearing loss and deafness. This language takes the same alphabet and hand signs as American Sign Language, but places them into English sentence structure.

Cued Speech, developed in 1966 by the American scientist R. Orin Cornett, uses hand signs to represent sounds, rather than letters or concepts. It is used in conjunction with mouthing of word cues, such as the most prominent vowel in each word.

During the preschool years, children increase their mastery of speech sounds, word and sentence formation, word and sentence understanding, the tone and rhythm of speech, and effective use of language.

What Can Go Wrong?

Speech disorders arise from many different conditions and have a wide range of causes. Two main parts of the brain are involved in producing and understanding speech: Broca's area and Wernicke's area. Broca's area coordinates the muscles of the lips, tongue, jaw, and vocal cords to produce understandable speech. Wernicke's area controls the comprehension, or understanding, of others' speech. Damage to these or other portions of the brain or to the nerve connections to the organs that make speech (tongue, mouth, chest, and so forth) can result in disordered speech.

Stroke, trauma, or infection may be the root cause of these disruptions. Severe mental retardation often has a negative impact on speech development. In some cases, anatomy plays a role in speech disorders, for example cleft palate, cleft lip, hearing problems, and damage to the larynx all can interfere with speech.

Speech disorders are fairly common in children. Many children show delays in developing speech, a condition that is frequently outgrown. Often the cause of a child's speech disorder is never known.

When adults develop a speech disorder after years of speaking normally, it usually is easier to locate the cause. For instance, a stroke, head injury, brain tumor, or dementia* may involve damage to the areas of the brain that affect speech or speech understanding. In other cases, an accident, a surgical procedure, or a viral infection can cause damage to the nerves that control the functions of the larynx.

Phonological (Articulatory) Disorders

Phonological (articulatory) (ar-TIK-yoo-la-tor-ee) disorders interfere with the process whereby the muscles of the mouth, tongue, jaw, throat, and diaphragm work together to produce clear, understandable sounds. These problems typically begin in childhood and can persist into adulthood. They also may be called fluency disorders.

It is normal for children to have problems with articulation as they are learning to speak. For instance, many children between the ages of two and three are unable to pronounce the sound "th." Other children in this age group stutter, which means that they repeat sounds occasionally or hesitate between words. Most children outgrow such problems rather quickly. If problems persist, however, they are considered speech disorders.

Lisp   A lisp is a relatively common speech disorder in which a person has trouble pronouncing the sounds of the letters *s* and *z*. One of the most well-known lispers is the cat, Sylvester, featured in the Tweety Bird cartoons, whose favorite exclamation is "thuffering thuccotash!" (suffering succotash)

Lisping can happen for a variety of reasons: an abnormal number or position of teeth; unconscious imitation of other lispers; defects in the structure of the mouth, such as a cleft palate; or hearing loss. Usually lisps can be corrected by working with a speech-language therapist who coaches the person with the lisp on how to make the sound correctly.

Stuttering   Stuttering often begins in early childhood and may persist into adulthood. People who stutter repeat certain speech sounds, or prolong certain sounds, or hesitate before and during speaking. Stuttering often is referred to as a fluency disorder because it disrupts the smooth flow of speech. More than million Americans stutter, and most began stuttering between the ages of two and seven.

Stuttering can have social and emotional consequences. People who stutter may be self-conscious about their speech. Some show signs of tension, such as twitching, unusual facial expressions, or eye blinks, when trying to get words out. Experts are not sure what causes stuttering, although some studies show that stuttering has a tendency to run in families, suggesting that it may have a genetic component.

Other cases of stuttering may be neurogenic (noor-o-JEN-ik), meaning that that they are caused by signal problems between the brain and the nerves or muscles that control speech. Stuttering also may result from emotional trauma, stress, or other psychological causes.

* **dementia** (dih-MEN-sha) is a loss of mental abilities, including memory, understanding, and judgment.

SUCCESSFUL SPEAKERS

What do singers Carly Simon and Mel Tillis, television journalist John Stossel, and actors James Earl Jones, Marilyn Monroe, and Bruce Willis have in common? All had the problem of stuttering. Their public successes point to one of the unique features of stuttering: although it is a problem in everyday conversation, it often disappears when someone is singing or delivering memorized lines. Further, people who stutter often can learn strategies for overcoming the problem as they grow older.

James Earl Jones

In his autobiography, actor James Earl Jones describes how he overcame his stuttering problem by reading Shakespeare aloud to himself and then reading to audiences, debating, and acting. Jones provided the voices for Darth Vader in *Star Wars* and King Mufasa in the animated *Lion King*; he has also acted on stage and in numerous films.

John Stossel

As a reporter for the television news magazine *20/20*, John Stossel depends on his voice to make a living. He stuttered as a child and worked hard to hide the condition. Stossel started his career in news as a researcher, but eventually he was asked to go on the air. He considered quitting when he found himself stumbling over certain words, but he got help overcoming his stuttering through speech therapy at the Hollins College speech clinic in Roanoke, Virginia. Stossel later became a spokesman for the National Stuttering Association.

Researchers have found that stuttering affects males about three times more often than females. Certain situations, such as speaking before a group of people or talking on the telephone, may make stuttering more severe for some, whereas singing or speaking alone often improve fluency.

Most young children outgrow their stuttering, and it is estimated that less than 1 percent of American adults stutter. However, children who do not outgrow stuttering by the time they enter elementary school may need speech therapy. Many people have overcome stuttering and gone on to achieve success in careers that require public speaking, acting, and singing.

Brain Disorders

Speech disorders in adults usually are the result of damage to the portions of the brain that control language. Damage may be caused by head injury, brain tumor, or stroke. Adults who have aphasia (a-FAY-zha) have trouble speaking and difficulty understanding what others are saying. Dysphasia (dis-FAY-zha) is a condition that causes similar, but less severe, challenges in speaking and understanding. The symptoms of aphasia and dysphasia depend on which area of the brain is affected: Broca's area or Wernicke's area.

Broca's aphasia   Broca's aphasia results from damage to the area that coordinates the muscles of the lips, tongue, jaw, and vocal cords that produce understandable speech. People with damage to Broca's area frequently speak in short, meaningful phrases that are produced with great effort, omitting small words such as "is," "and," and "the." People with Broca's aphasia often are aware of their speech difficulties and may become frustrated by their speech problems.

Wernicke's aphasia   Wernicke's aphasia results from damage to the area of the brain responsible for understanding speech. People afflicted with this form of aphasia have trouble understanding others and often are unaware of their own problems. They may speak in long rambling sentences that have no meaning, often adding unnecessary words. They may even create nonsense words.

Global aphasia   Global aphasia results from damage to large portions of the language areas of the brain. Individuals with global aphasia have severe communication difficulties and may be extremely limited in their ability to speak or to comprehend language.

How Are Speech Disorders Diagnosed and Treated?

Diagnosis   Many adults recognize when they develop a speech difficulty and seek help from doctors and trained speech-language therapists. Parents of children with speech disorders often are the first to call the condition to the attention of healthcare providers.

Speech-language therapists often make an initial evaluation to help determine what problems exist and the best way to treat them. Because talking and hearing are closely related, children with speech disorders often undergo a hearing evaluation done by an audiologist (aw-dee-OL-o-jist), who is educated in the study of the hearing process and hearing loss. The audiologist can determine if a person has a hearing loss, identify the type of loss, and recommend how the person can make the best use of any remaining hearing. When the speech disorder is caused by damage to the nerves or brain, a neurologist* may also be involved in the evaluation process.

Treatment   People with aphasia often benefit from speech-language therapy, which focuses on helping people make the most of their remaining abilities and learning other methods of communicating. Supplemental methods of communication that assist an individual in speaking are called Augmentative Communication Devices (ACDs). Available ACDs include portable communication computers, personalized language boards, and picture exchange programs. As technology continues to improve and become more portable, communication possibilities for aphasic and dysphasic adults continue to expand.

▶ *See also* **Alzheimer's Disease • Brain Tumor • Cleft Palate • Deafness and Hearing Loss • Infection • Intellectual Disability • Laryngitis • Stroke • Trauma • Viral Infections**

* **neurologist** (new-RHAL-eh-jist) a physician who specializes in diagnosing and treating diseases of the nervous system.

Resources

Books and Articles

Bryant, John E. *Taking Speech Disorders to School.* Plainview, NY: JayJo Books, 2004.

Feit, Debbie, with Heidi M. Feldman. *The Parent's Guide to Speech and Language Problems.* New York: McGraw-Hill, 2007.

Hulit, Lloyd M. *Straight Talk on Stuttering: Information, Encouragement, and Counsel for Stutterers, Caregivers, and Speech-language Clinicians,* 2nd ed. Springfield, IL: Charles C. Thomas, 2004.

Jones, James Earl, and Penelope Niven. *Voices and Silences: With a New Epilogue.* New York: Limelight Editions, 2002.

Libal, Joyce. *Finding My Voice: Youth with Speech Impairment.* Broomall, PA: Mason Crest Publishers, 2004.

O'Connor, Frances. *Frequently Asked Questions about Stuttering.* New York: Rosen, 2008.

Organizations

American Speech-Language-Hearing Association. 2200 Research Boulevard, Rockville, MD, 20850-3289. Toll free: 800-638-8255. Web site: http://www.asha.org/public/speech/disorders.

National Aphasia Association. 350 Seventh Avenue, Suite 902, New York, NY, 10001. Toll free: 800-922-4622. Web site: http://www.aphasia.org.

National Institute on Deafness and Other Communication Disorders, National Institutes of Health. 31 Center Drive, MSC 2320, Bethesda, MD, 20892-2320. Toll free: 800-241-1044. Web site: http://www.nidcd.nih.gov.

National Stuttering Association. 119 W. Fortieth Street, 14th Floor, New York, NY, 10018. Toll free: 800-937-8888. Web site: http://www.nsastutter.org.

Stuttering Foundation of America. P.O. Box 11749, 3100 Walnut Grove Road, Suite 603, Memphis, TN, 38111-0749. Toll free: 800-992-9392. Web site: http://www.stutteringhelp.org.

Spina Bifida

Spina bifida (SPY-na BI-fi-da) is a birth defect in which the spinal column does not form properly, leaving a gap or opening in the spine.

Brian Teaches Class

As part of a sixth-grade science project, Brian chose to report on a condition called spina bifida. He showed a picture of the ring-shaped bones, or vertebrae, of the spine and demonstrated how the vertebrae protect the spinal cord and anchor muscles. He explained that in people with spina bifida, some of the bony plates that should cover the spine do not close, leaving an unprotected opening at the back of the spine.

No one in Brian's class had ever heard of spina bifida, and they all were surprised to learn that Brian had been born with it. He had a mild form of the condition, but he underwent a surgical procedure that corrected it when he was an infant. He ended his presentation by showing the small scar on his lower back.

What Is Spina Bifida?

Spina bifida is a Latin term meaning "split spine" or "open spine." It is the most common of several birth defects called neural tube defects. The neural tube contains the cells that ultimately make the spinal cord, spine, and brain, and it develops during the first three to four weeks of pregnancy (often before a woman even knows that she is pregnant).

Spina bifida results when the sides of the neural tube fail to join together properly, leaving an open area. Often the gap occurs in the lower back at the base of the spine. The spinal cord is part of the central nervous system, which allows individuals to move and sense the world around them. Because spina bifida involves the central nervous system, it can cause a range of physical and mental problems.

Prenatal Testing for Spina Bifida

Sometimes parents can find out whether their baby has spina bifida before birth. Several commonly used tests can help to provide this information.

Maternal-Serum Alfa-Fetoprotein (AFP) Test This test is performed between the sixteenth and eighteenth weeks of pregnancy. Alfa-fetoprotein is a substance made by the developing fetus. Because the mother and fetus are connected via their circulatory systems, AFP from the fetus gets into the mother's bloodstream. By measuring the amount of AFP in the mother's blood, doctors get an indication of the likelihood that the fetus has certain birth defects. This test does not give a definite answer, and high levels of AFP only suggest that the fetus *might* have spina bifida. If AFP levels are high, doctors repeat the test. If the results are again high, doctors order other tests to confirm that the fetus has spina bifida. Many times, high AFP readings are false alarms and the baby is just fine.

Ultrasound Medical professionals can use ultrasound to confirm or rule out spina bifida. An ultrasound works by bouncing sound waves off of internal structures. A computer converts the returning sound waves into an image of the fetus inside the uterus. Sometimes the defect in the developing spine is visible on the ultrasound image.

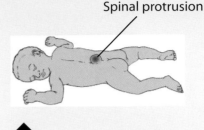

Spinal protrusion

▲

Babies born with spina bifida often have an unprotected opening at the back of the spine. *Illustration by Frank Forney. Reproduced by permission of Gale, a part of Cengage Learning.*

Amniocentesis is a procedure medical professionals can perform between the sixteenth and eighteenth week of pregnancy. In this procedure, a needle passes through the mother's belly into her uterus to collect some of the fluid that surrounds the fetus. This fluid, called amniotic fluid, contains cells and chemicals from the fetus. In this fluid, medical professionals can measure the levels of AFP to help them determine whether the fetus may have spina bifida. Like the AFP test of the maternal blood, though, the test of the amniotic fluid does not give a definite answer.

Is Spina Bifida Always Serious?

Spina bifida is a common birth defect, but it does not always cause serious problems. At birth, the gap may be so slight that it is invisible and harmless. However, sometimes the spinal cord bulges out through the malformed vertebrae and serious neurological (nerve) problems result.

Spina bifida occulta Brian was born with spina bifida occulta, the mildest form of spina bifida. "Occulta" means hidden, and in many cases, the gap in the spine is never detected. Often an opening in one or two of the vertebrae occurs, but the spinal cord is not affected. A dimple, a birthmark, or a patch of hair may be visible on the skin overlying the site of the gap.

Scientists estimate that up to 40 percent of all Americans have this form of spina bifida, but few ever know they have it. Most people with spina bifida occulta never need treatment. Brian was an exception. He needed surgery because as he grew, the lower end of his spinal cord got caught against his vertebrae, causing him to have problems controlling his bladder. The doctors "unhooked" the spinal cord and closed the gap surgically.

Spina bifida manifesta Spina bifida manifesta includes two forms of spina bifida that together represent one of the most common disabling birth defects. On average, 1 out of 1,000 babies in the United States is born with one of these forms, either meningocele (me-NING-go-seel) or myelomeningocele (MY-e-lo-me-NING-go-seel).

Meningocele Of babies born with spina bifida manifesta, about 4 percent have the meningocele form. The meninges (me-NIN-jez) consist of three layers of tough membranes that cover and protect the brain and spinal cord. The brain and spinal cord are also bathed in a fluid called cerebrospinal fluid (CSF). A meningocele is a CSF-filled sac formed when the meninges balloon through the gap in the vertebrae. It looks like a large blister covered by a thin layer of skin. The sac can range in size from as small as a grape to as large as a grapefruit.

A meningocele is harmless if the sac contains only CSF. However, if nerves are caught in the sac, the affected baby can have problems controlling muscles and the bladder. Babies with this form of spina bifida usually have surgery during infancy to put the meninges back inside the vertebrae and to close the gap in the vertebrae.

Myelomeningocele When many people think of spina bifida, they think of the myelomeningocele form. Approximately 96 percent of babies born with spina bifida manifesta have myelomeningocele, and it is the most serious type of spina bifida. As in meningocele, the meninges bulge through the gap in the spine, but in myelomeningocele, part of the spinal cord bulges out as well. The sac may be covered with skin or the nerves may actually be exposed.

People with myelomeningocele have a variety of physical and mental problems, the severity of which depends on the location of the defect in the spine. A gap high on the spinal column creates more problems than a gap at the lower back. People often experience loss of movement and feeling (paralysis) below the abnormal vertebrae. The most severely impaired children cannot walk or control their bowel or bladder. Most babies born with myelomeningocele also have hydrocephalus, which means that they have too much fluid inside and surrounding their brain. If hydrocephalus is left untreated, the excess pressure in the skull can cause blindness and permanent brain damage.

Myelomeningocele requires surgery within 24 to 48 hours of birth. Surgeons must close the gap in the vertebrae to protect the spinal cord and prevent infection. They also must treat hydrocephalus, if it is present. They do this by placing a device called a shunt into the brain to drain excess fluid and relieve pressure on the brain.

What Causes Spina Bifida?

Spina bifida sometimes runs in families, which suggests that genes may play a role in some cases. In 90 to 95 percent of cases, however, babies are born to families that have never before had a child with the condition. Mothers who have diabetes, a high fever during pregnancy, or who have taken a drug called valproic acid to treat epilepsy* seem to have a greater chance of having a baby with spina bifida than other mothers. In addition, scientists have linked a deficiency of folic acid (a B vitamin) in the mother's diet to a higher risk of having a baby with spina bifida. Adding folic acid to the diet significantly reduces the chance that a woman will give birth to a baby with spina bifida.

Living with Spina Bifida

Most children with spina bifida occulta, and many with meningocele, live normal lives without any impairment. Children born with myelomeningocele, however, often have multiple problems resulting from damage to their spinal cord. Surgery to repair the gap in the vertebrae and to place a shunt in the brain can prevent further damage to the nervous system. It cannot, however, reverse the nerve problems that are already present at birth.

The severity of symptoms caused by myelomeningocele varies from child to child. A common problem is the inability to control the bowel and bladder. Catheters*, diapers, and attentive caregivers can all play a role in helping to control this problem and/or in alleviating associated embarrassment.

Preventing Spina Bifida: The Role of Folic Acid

Scientists have linked spina bifida to a deficiency of folic acid during the first weeks of pregnancy. One of the B vitamins, folic acid is essential for proper functioning of the human body. During pregnancy and during fetal development, the mother's body and the fetus's body need more folic acid than usual.

Scientists estimate that the incidence of spina bifida can be decreased by about 70 percent if all women of child-bearing age consume 0.4 mg of folic acid each day.

Good sources of folic acid include dark-green, leafy vegetables (such as spinach and broccoli); eggs; and orange juice. In addition, the U.S. Food and Drug Administration mandates that breads, enriched grains, and cereals have folic acid added to them. Even with folic acid supplements added to common foods, the average American diet does not contain 0.4 mg of folic acid per day. Most multivitamins, however, contain the recommended dose of folic acid.

* **epilepsy** (EP-i-lep-see) is a condition of the nervous system characterized by recurrent seizures that temporarily affect a person's awareness, movements, or sensations. Seizures occur when powerful, rapid bursts of electrical energy interrupt the normal electrical patterns of the brain.

* **catheters** (KAH-thuh-ters) are small plastic tubes placed through a body opening into an organ (such as the bladder) or through the skin directly into a blood vessel. They are used to give fluids to or drain fluids from a person.

* **catheter** (KAH-thuh-ter) is a small plastic tube placed through a body opening into an organ (such as the bladder) or through the skin directly into a blood vessel. It is used to give fluids to or drain fluids from a person.

Many affected children cannot walk without crutches or leg braces, and many need a wheelchair. In addition, some children have learning difficulties, particularly with reading and math. Special education classes can help them in their academic work.

Children with spina bifida often develop sensitivity or an allergy to latex (natural rubber), which is used in such healthcare products as gloves and catheter* tubes. The allergy probably develops because they come into contact with latex so often and at such a young age as a result of their medical care.

Even with the disabilities caused by spina bifida, children who have the condition often live well into adulthood. With the help of early and continuing medical, psychological, and educational treatment, children with spina bifida can lead full and productive lives.

▶ *See also* **Birth Defects and Brain Development** • **Hydrocephalus** • **Incontinence** • **Paralysis**

Resources

Books and Articles

Lutkenhoff, Marlene. *Children with Spina Bifida: A Parents' Guide,* 2nd ed. Bethesda, MD: Woodbine House, 2007.

Sandler, Adrian. *Living with Spina Bifida: A Guide for Families and Professionals.* Chapel Hill: University of North Carolina Press, 2003.

Organizations

March of Dimes. 1275 Mamaroneck Avenue, White Plains, NY, 10605. Telephone: 914-997-4488. Web site: http://www.marchofdimes.com/pnhec/4439_1224.asp.

Spina Bifida Association. 4590 MacArthur Boulevard, NW, Washington, DC, 20007. Toll free: 800-621-3141. Web site: http://www.sbaa.org.

Spinocerebellar Ataxia

A spinocerebellar ataxia (SCA) is one of a group of inherited disorders in which individuals experience degeneration of the cerebellum leading to uncoordinated and clumsy movements that get worse over time. The word "ataxia" literally means "without order" and refers to the symptom of uncoordinated (or unordered) movement.

What Is Spinocerebellar Ataxia?

When it comes to movement, a vital part of the body is the cerebellum (sare-uh-BELL-um), a portion of the brain located at the back of the head. It helps the body make smooth and coordinated movements. A group of 28 different types of disorders, together called spinocerebellar ataxias or spinal cerebellar ataxias (SCA), interfere with that control and lead to uncoordinated movement, which is known as "ataxia." The 28 types of SCA are distinguished by the age of onset, the genes* involved, the symptoms in addition to ataxia, the degree of severity of symptoms, the progression of the disease, and the prognosis. The types of SCA are classified either by the chronological order of gene discovery or by the names of families in which they were first discovered (such as Machado-Joseph disease), or by the chronological order of gene discovery (such as SCA 3).

How Common Is Spinocerebellar Ataxia?

The SCAs are rare diseases and accurate estimates of their incidence were unavailable as of 2009. Type 3 is the most common (23% of all SCAs). Other more common SCAs are Type 1 (16%), 2 (18%), 6 (17%), and 7 (2–5%). Some types occur more often in certain ethnic groups, such as SCA 3 in Portuguese and German persons, SCA 10 in Mexicans, SCA 13 in French individuals, and SCA 14 in Japanese people.

People who experience ataxias usually begin having symptoms when they are between 30 and 50 years of age, and the symptoms worsen over 10 to 20 years. The onset exceptions are SCA 2 and SCA 7, which start in childhood.

Is Spinocerebellar Ataxia Inherited?

Spinocerebellar ataxias are inherited disorders. They arise because of a mutation* that disrupts the construction of DNA*, which in turn affects the production of proteins that are essential to properly running bodily functions. The problem in SCAs begins in the building blocks of DNA.

How Does DNA Make Proteins? DNA has the shape of a twisted ladder, but unlike an actual ladder, DNA can peel apart like a zipper into two halves, which are called strands. When DNA unzips, its "rungs" are split in two with half a rung going to each strand. Each "half-rung" of the DNA is a chemical compound called a base. DNA has only four different bases. The four bases are cytosine (C), guanine (G), adenine (A), and thymine (T). These bases line up in a particular order on the strand. Part of a DNA strand, for instance, may have the following order: CAGGTCAATCGCCAAA. Each of the four bases has a certain shape that fits nicely with one—and only one—other base: C and G fit together, and A and T fit together. As a result, the strand on the other side of the DNA "zipper" has the exact opposite order. Scientists call this opposite order "complementary." In this example, the order would be GTCCAGTTAGCGGTTT.

To make a protein, the DNA unzips, leaving its bases exposed, and an enzyme (called RNA polymerase) starts making a new complementary strand. The new complementary strand is called messenger RNA, or mRNA. From there, another structure, called a ribosome, latches onto and runs along the newly formed mRNA. The ribosome is a matchmaker

* **genes** (JEENS) are chemical structures composed of deoxyribonucleic acid (DNA) that help determine a person's body structure and physical characteristics. Inherited from a person's parents, genes are contained in the chromosomes found in the body's cells.

* **mutation** (myoo-TAY-shun) is a change in an organism's gene or genes.

* **DNA** or deoxyribonucleic acid (dee-OX-see-ry-bo-nyoo-klay-ik AH-sid), is the specialized chemical substance that contains the genetic code necessary to build and maintain the structures and functions of living organisms.

* **nervous system** is a network of specialized tissue made of nerve cells, or neurons, that processes messages to and from different parts of the human body.

* **brain stem** is the part of the brain that connects to the spinal cord. The brain stem controls the basic functions of life, such as breathing and blood pressure.

* **autonomic nervous system** is a branch of the peripheral nervous system that controls various involuntary body activities, such as body temperature, metabolism, heart rate, blood pressure, breathing, and digestion. The autonomic nervous system has two parts—the sympathetic and parasympathetic branches.

of sorts. It reads the bases on the mRNA three at a time and then matches that three-base set, which is called a codon (COE-don), with a particular amino acid, which is another type of chemical compound that serves as a building block of proteins. All of the proteins in the human body are made of 20 amino acids, and these different amino acids correspond to specific codons. By reading one codon after another on the mRNA, the ribosome can link together an exact chain of amino acids, which becomes a particular type of protein that has an explicit job to do in the body.

A person with an inherited spinocerebellar ataxia has a mutation that can throw off the entire DNA-RNA-amino acid-protein pathway. The mutation causes numerous repeated three-base sequences. These repeats, called trinucleotide repeats, result in the production of an abnormal protein (such as ataxin in SCA 1) that may lead to dysfunction or degeneration of parts of the nervous system* and other organs. Even healthy people have a certain number of trinucleotide repeats, and this normal condition does not cause SCA. When too many repeats exist, however, an individual can develop SCA. With a moderate number of repeats, a person has the disease but may or may not manifest the symptoms.

Individuals with a moderate or large number of repeats will transmit SCA by autosomal dominant inheritance, which means that a child need only inherit an abnormal gene from one parent to get the disease. In other words, every child born to an affected parent has a 50 percent chance of inheriting SCA. The number of repeats increases with each generation (which is called "anticipation"), and symptoms start earlier with an increasing number of repeats. Thus, a child may develop symptoms at an earlier age than his or her parents or even the grandparents. In some individuals, SCA is not inherited. Instead, a mutation occurs for the first time in the egg or sperm and causes SCA. Such a first-time mutation is called a "de novo" mutation.

What Are the Symptoms and Signs of Spinocerebellar Ataxia?

All SCAs have some common symptoms even though different genetic mutations cause them. Symptoms include a drunken or wide-based gait with falls and dysarthric (slurred) or staccato (clipped) speech. Swallowing becomes difficult, and patients may inadvertently inhale some food and choke. Eye movements become slowed and nystagmus (jerky). When reaching for an object, patients' hands may start to shake, and they may overshoot the item they are attempting to grasp. Individuals with SCA1 may have jerky or otherwise abnormal muscle movements that result from dysfunction (improper function) of the motor pathways (the muscle-controlling nerve pathways) in the brain stem* and spinal cord. Dysfunction of the nerves leads to muscle wasting, cramps and twitching, decreased muscle stretch reflexes (a muscle contraction that follows a stretch), and loss of feeling in the feet or legs in SCA 1, 2, 3 and 4. Dysfunction of the autonomic nervous system*, which are the nerves that control automatic functions such as heart rate and digestion, causes dizziness on standing in SCA 3. Other eye abnormalities include slowed eye movements in SCA 2 and 3, an inability to close the eyes and a "staring" look in SCA 3, and vision loss due to retinal* degeneration in SCA 7. Types of SCA that start in infancy (e.g., SCA 2 and SCA 7) lead to poor muscle tone and developmental delay. Abnormal writhing or jerky limb movements can occur in SCA 3. Problems with memory and spatial difficulty (problems judging distances, causing the patient to bump into barriers or knock over items) occur in SCA 3, 12, and 13. A unique feature of SCA 6 is positional vertigo*, which causes a disconcerting spinning sensation. Convulsions* occur in SCA 7 and 10. Heart involvement occurs in SCA 7.

How Is Spinocerebellar Ataxia Diagnosed?

A neurologist* or a movement disorders specialist usually makes the diagnosis after taking a thorough medical and family history and conducting a physical exam. Frequently, the medical professional will also order blood tests to rule out other conditions, such as vitamin or thyroid gland* deficiency, and may order magnetic resonance imaging* (MRI) of the brain. The MRI will show whether the patient has a shrunken cerebellum and will also exclude other causes of ataxia such as multiple sclerosis *, ischemic strokes* or tumors*.

Genetic testing   The only way to differentiate the specific type of SCA a patient has is to look for genetic mutations in DNA, which is usually obtained from blood. As of 2009, such tests were commercially available for SCA 1, 2, 3, 5, 6, 7, 8, 10, 13, 14, and 17. Medical professionals can also run tests on adults (not children) who do not have SCA but have a strong family history of SCA. Doing so determines the likelihood that these individuals will develop symptoms later in life. Such tests are only conducted after individuals have undergone genetic and psychological counseling so they can understand the personal, professional, and health implications of a positive test. Testing cannot, however, pinpoint when symptoms will start if they have no symptoms.

Prenatal (prior to birth) tests, such as chorionic villus sampling* and amniocentesis*, can determine if the fetus has inherited SCA. Based on the results, a couple can decide if they want to continue with the pregnancy or proceed to abortion on medical grounds. Such genetic testing can also look for SCA in artificially implanted embryos.

How Is Spinocerebellar Ataxia Treated?

As of 2009, no treatment was available for SCA. Over time, patients may need walkers or wheelchairs. Some patients may also require speech therapy. Therapists can help with impaired swallowing, and nutritionists can instruct patients about what types of foods they can eat. Physical and occupational therapists* can help patients learn how to modify their home and work environment to make life as easy as possible.

* **retina** (RET-i-na) is the tissue that forms the inner surface of the back of the eyeballs; it receives the light that enters the eye and transmits it through the optic nerves to the brain to produce visual images.

* **vertigo** (VER-ti-go) is the feeling that either the environment or one's own body is revolving or spinning, even though they are not.

* **convulsions** (kon-VUL-shuns), also called seizures, are involuntary muscle contractions caused by electrical discharges within the brain and are usually accompanied by changes in consciousness.

* **neurologist** (new-RHAL-eh-jist) a physician who specializes in diagnosing and treating diseases of the nervous system.

* **thyroid gland** (THY-roid GLAND) is located in the lower part of the front of the neck. The thyroid produces hormones that regulate the body's metabolism (me-TAB-o-LIZ-um), the processes the body uses to produce energy, to grow, and to maintain body tissues.

* **magnetic resonance imaging** or MRI, uses magnetic waves, instead of x-rays, to scan the body and produce detailed pictures of the body's structures.

* **multiple sclerosis** (skluh-RO-sis), or MS, is an inflammatory disease of the nervous system that disrupts communication between the brain and other parts of the body. MS can result in paralysis, loss of vision, and other symptoms.

* **ischemic strokes** are events that occur when a blood vessel bringing oxygen and nutrients to the brain becomes clogged by a blood clot or other particle. As a result, nerve cells in the affected area of the brain cannot function properly.

* **tumors** (TOO-morz) are abnormal growths of body tissue that have no known cause or physiologic purpose. Tumors may or may not be cancerous.

* **chorionic villus sampling** (KOR-ee-on-ik VIL-lus sampling) is a test in which a small tube is inserted through the cervix and a small piece of the placenta supporting the fetus is removed for genetic testing.

* **amniocentesis** (am-nee-o-sen-TEE-sis) is a test in which a long, thin needle is inserted in the mother's uterus to obtain a sample of the amniotic fluid from the sac that surrounds the fetus. The fetal cells in the fluid are then examined for genetic defects.

* **physical and occupational therapists** are professionals who are trained to treat injured people by means of activities designed to help them recover or relearn specific functions or movements and restore their abilities to perform the tasks of daily living.

* **pneumonia** (nu-MO-nyah) is inflammation of the lungs.

What Is the Prognosis for Spinocerebellar Ataxia?

Patients with milder forms can anticipate a normal life expectancy, whereas SCAs that start in infancy lead to severe disability and death in adulthood. Most people die from respiratory failure or lung complications such as pneumonia*.

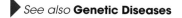 *See also* **Genetic Diseases**

Resources

Books and Articles

Icon Health Publications. *Ataxia: A Medical Dictionary, Bibliography, and Annotated Research Guide to Internet References.* San Diego, CA: Author, 2004.

Rangamani, G. N. *Managing Speech and Swallowing Problems: A Guidebook for People with Ataxia,* 2nd ed. Minneapolis, MN: National Ataxia Foundation, 2006.

Organizations

National Ataxia Foundation. 2600 Fernbrook Lane, Suite 119, Minneapolis, MN, 55447. Toll free: 762-553-0167. Web site: http://ataxia.org.

WE MOVE. 204 West Eighty-fourth Street, New York, NY, 10024. Toll free: 800-437-MOV2. Web site: http://www.wemove.org.

Sports Injuries

Sports injuries include the physical, musculoskeletal injuries that result from taking part in a sport.

The Chris Benoit Story

Odell and his friend Jason were huge fans of pro wrestling. They never missed a weekly broadcast, and the highlight of their year was when Odell's dad took the boys to a live match. But one day in 2007, Jason called with bad news. "Did you hear? The Rabid Wolverine! He's dead!"

Odell turned on the news. It was true: One of his favorite wrestlers, Chris Benoit, a.k.a. "The Rabid Wolverine," had been found dead at his home. But the news got worse: Benoit's son and wife were dead, too. Police believed that Benoit killed them and then himself.

As he watched the report, Odell thought, "How could this have happened? He was in great shape."

* **ethics** is a guiding set of principles for conduct, a system of moral values.

Just because an athlete looks great doesn't mean he or she is not suffering from a sports-related injury.

What Are Sports Injuries?

The general term "sports injuries" includes the physical, musculoskeletal injuries that result from taking part in a sport. The most common musculoskeletal sports injuries are ankle sprains; muscle strains such as of the hamstring and groin; knee injuries, including rupture or tear of the anterior cruciate ligament (ACL); and injuries to the elbow. Generally speaking, these injuries get better with home care, which includes icing and elevating the affected area, rest, and the use of analgesics, particularly nonsteroidal anti-inflammatory drugs (NSAIDs). Approximately 4 million emergency-room visits in the United States each year involve injuries sustained while people engage in sports.

However, possible sports injuries go beyond sprains and strains, particularly among professional or hyper-fit athletes of both sexes.

What Pressures do Athletes Face?

Professional sports is a multi-billion dollar industry. In the National Football League, the value of the 31 teams averaged $531 million as of 2002; in Major League Baseball team values averaged $295 million. Clearly, a great deal of money is riding on the performance on professional sports teams, and that does not take into consideration the value of endorsements, products, and other income sources, or other professional sports and sports entertainment, such as bicycling and pro wrestling, or amateur athletics, including college and high-school sports.

When so much money is at stake, ethics* and personal welfare can easily take a back seat to winning.

What are Perfomance Enhancing Drugs?

The human body has natural limits. Training and practice hone the athlete's skills to push the edge of those limits and produce astonishing performances. But there is always the desire to be better, stronger, or faster, whether it comes from wanting personal glory or the cash rewards that follow winning. Once the natural limits are reached, some athletes turn to performance-enhancing drugs.

Anabolic steroids Anabolic steroids can be synthetic or naturally produced by the body. The male hormone testosterone is an anabolic steroid; it promotes the development of muscle and influences male traits, such as a deep voice and body hair. Men and women who take anabolic steroids develop more muscle in a relatively short amount of time. However, anabolic steroids have side effects. Men may develop shrunken testicles, prominent breasts, baldness, and a higher voice. Women may find themselves with more body hair, a deeper voice, an enlarged clitoris, and an increased appetite. Both sexes can experience baldness, increased levels of cholesterol, elevated blood pressure, and acne.

Detroit Lions linebacker Reggie Brown works with weights during a rehabilitation session at a rehabilitation institute in Houston, TX, January 12, 1998. Brown was recovering from a severe neck injury sustained in a game against the New York Jets where he collided with another player dislocated his top two neck vertebrae, bruising his spinal cord and leaving him unable to breathe and with no feeling below the neck. *AP Images.*

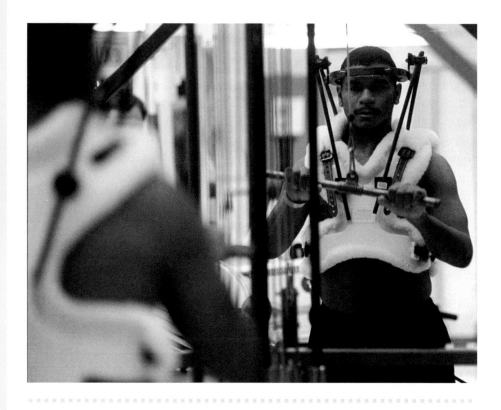

More worrisome, however, is the psychological condition commonly called "roid rage." High levels of steroids have been linked to increased aggression, which can range from a mild person simply becoming more assertive to someone overreacting violently. The drugs may also uncover an underlying psychological disorder.

It is estimated that between 500,000 and 1 million young athletes have tried anabolic steroids.

Human growth hormone The ready availability of human growth hormone (HGH) and the fact that it is undetectable in standard drug tests have led some athletes to inject themselves with it. However, a 1993 study conducted by the University of Vienna with serious athletes and a study on non-athletes that appeared in the *American Journal of Physiology* found that a course of HGH injections had no effect on body weight, body fat, or the strength of the biceps or quadriceps. The researchers concluded that while HGH may help people who lack the hormone, it apparently does not change the strength or body composition of those who do not lack the hormone.

Stimulants Athletes may also turn to stimulants or diuretics to enhance their performance. Stimulants are drugs that act on the nervous system to increase heart rate and metabolism and reduce fatigue. They also sharpen focus and aggressiveness.

This group of drugs includes caffeine, amphetamines, ephedrine, cocaine, and methamphetamine. It is easy to become addicted to stimulants, which can also cause heart problems, hypertension, weight loss, convulsions*, and brain hemorrhages.

Diuretics   Diuretics remove water from the body, and athletes use them to lose weight quickly. However, as a diuretic removes fluids, it also washes out the electrolytes they carry. Electrolyte imbalances can cause muscle cramps and heart arrhythmia, and overuse of diuretics can also lead to dehydration*.

What Other Injuries Can Athletes Face?

Head and Brain Injuries   Head injuries can occur in any field in sports. More than 64,000 cyclists went to emergency rooms for head injuries in 2007, far exceeding the number of football players (36,412), baseball/softball players (25,079), and basketball players (24,701).

Between 15 and 40 percent of former boxers show symptoms of chronic brain injuries, ranging from speech problems to needing institutional care. One study showed that most professional boxers have some brain damage, a result of being hit with the equivalent of a 13-pound bowling ball traveling at 20 miles an hour every time a punch is landed.

Former professional football players also have been found to suffer brain injuries. In 2007, doctors studied the brain of Justin Strzelczyk, a former Pittsburgh Steelers lineman who had died, in a car accident. They found that Stezelczyk, who was 36 when he died, had a condition more often found in people in their 80s: chronic traumatic encephalopathy. Between 1995 and 2004, 44 football players died from head injuries; during the same time period, high school and college players suffered 48 head injuries. The NFL estimates that 160 concussions occur among pro players each year. Regarding the double murder-suicide of Chris Benoit, the conclusion suggested by an autopsy* on Benoit's brain was that Benoit suffered brain damage from years of blows to the head and that this damage caused dementia*, which seemed to explain his erratic behavior and may have contributed to his violent acts.

Amenorrhea   Male and female athletes, especially runners and gymnasts, have very little body fat. Female athletes can experience a decrease in or a halt to their menstrual cycle*, a condition called amenorrhea. Because female athletes may experience considerable stress during competition, have low body weight, and expend a great deal of energy, their bodies may cease to menstruate.

This condition is not permanent, and it can be corrected. A physician may prescribe birth control pills to an amenorrheic female athlete in order to restore a normal cycle.

MRSA Infections   An unexpected side effect of the collegial atmosphere surrounding team sports is the spread of bacteria, including MRSA. MRSA, or methicillin-resistant Staphylococcus aureus, is a

* **convulsions** (kon-VUL-shuns), also called seizures, are involuntary muscle contractions caused by electrical discharges within the brain and are usually accompanied by changes in consciousness.

* **dehydration** (dee-hi-DRAY-shun) is a condition in which the body is depleted of water, usually caused by excessive and unreplaced loss of body fluids, such as through sweating, vomiting, or diarrhea.

* **autopsy** (AW-top-see) is an examination of a body after death to look for the cause of death or the effects of a disease.

* **dementia** (dih-MEN-sha) is a loss of mental abilities, including memory, understanding, and judgment.

* **menstrual cycle** (MEN-stroo-al SYkul) culminates in menstruation (men-stroo-AY-shun), the discharging through the vagina of blood, secretions, and tissue debris from the uterus that recurs at approximately monthly intervals in females of reproductive age.

A Brief History of Performance-Enhancing Drugs

The use of drugs to enhance athletic performance was first suspected in 1886, when the 24-year-old Welshman Arthur Linton died during a race in France; he likely took the stimulant trimethyl.

1935: German scientists develop anabolic steroids.

1954: The doctor of the Soviet Olympic power-lifting team admits to injecting the Soviet lifters with testosterone.

1958: Ciba Pharmaceuticals releases the anabolic steroid methandrostenolone.

1960: A major article in *Sports Illustrated* discloses the use of tranquilizers, amphetamines, and other drugs among athletes.

1973: East German women win 10 of 14 gold medals at the world swimming championships.

1975: The Olympics bans anabolic steroids.

1983: Four weightlifters are stripped of their medals for using steroids at the Pan Am Games; a total of 23 medals, including 11 gold medals, are forfeited.

1988: Canadian sprinter Ben Johnson loses both his gold medal and his world record after testing positive for anabolic steroids.

1990: Federal law makes illegal the possession of steroids without a prescription.

1992: Former NFL player Lyle Alzado dies of brain cancer, that he attributed to more than 20 years of using steroids and human growth hormone. He was 43.

1998: A team is ejected from the Tour de France bicycling competition after the director admits to giving his team performance enhancing drugs, including erythropoietin.

2001: Retired baseball player Ken Caminiti admits to using steroids and estimates that half of the players in major league baseball also use them. Two years later, he suffers a heart attack and dies at age 41.

2004: A *New York Times* article estimates that between 500 and 2,000 of East German athletes who were involved in using performance-enhancing drugs face serious health problems ranging from infertility to liver tumors to heart disease.

2007: Pro wrestler Chris Benoit is found dead in his home, along with his wife and son. Police rule it a murder-suicide. Autopsy results suggest Benoit had brain damage from repeated concussions, which caused his erratic and violent behavior.

2007: Olympic runner Marion Jones is stripped of her five medals from the Sydney Olympics after admitting to using steroids.

2008: The Committee on Oversight and Government Reform in the U.S. House of Representatives begins investigations of steroid and HGH use in professional baseball and wrestling.

form of bacterial infection that can be spread by sharing equipment, uniforms, and even towels, or by the cuts and scrapes associated with team play.

The antibiotics used to treat regular staph infections cannot kill this type of bacterial infection, and so it is important for the athlete to have an infected wound tested before antibiotics are used.

To guard against MRSA infections, athletes should not share equipment, towels, or razors with teammates and should be sure to shower with soap and water after practice or a game.

What to Do If You Are Injured

The choice of treatment depends on the severity of the injury. When an injury occurs athletes should stop playing or exercising and not try to "play through the pain."

When to call the doctor The doctor should be called when the following situations occur:

- The injury causes severe pain, swelling, or numbness
- The athlete cannot put weight on the area
- An old injury aches, hurts, or swells
- A joint does not feel normal or feels unstable
- If the pain or other symptoms increase after home treatment

When and how to treat the injury yourself If the injury does not have the above criteria, the athlete can treat the injury at home using the R-I-C-E method for 48 hours after the injury occurs to reduce pain and swelling and promote healing.

- **Rest.** Reduce regular activities and take the weight off an injured foot, ankle, or knee.
- **Ice.** Place ice on the injured area using a cold pack or ice bag for 20 minutes four to eight times a day. To avoid cold injury do not leave the ice on the injury longer than 20 minutes.
- **Compression.** Put even pressure such as an elastic wrap bandage, boot, air cast, or splint on the injured area to help reduce swelling.
- **Elevation.** Keep the injured area above the heart by elevating it on a pillow.

How Can Sports Injuries Be Prevented?

There are a number of actions a person can take to prevent injury while exercising or engaging in athletic activity. These include the following:

- Always do a proper warm up routine of exercises and stretches.
- Always do a proper cool down after exercising.
- Wear the proper shoes and equipment for the activity.
- Make sure one's body is mature enough and properly trained to do the activity (i.e., it is suggested youth leagues limit the number of times participants pitch per week to avoid injuries).
- Don't play if injured.

▶ *See also* **Brain Injuries • Broken Bones (Fractures) • Concussion • Substance Abuse**

Resources

Books and Articles

Deyssig, R., H. Frisch, W. F. Blum, et al. "Effect of Growth Hormone Treatment on Hormonal Parameters, Body Composition, and Strength in Athletes." *Acta Endocrinology* (Copenhagen) 128, no. 4 (April 1993):313–318.

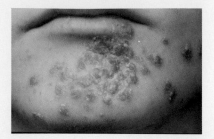

▲

The staph infection impetigo most often involves the face. Impetigo is more common among young children. In young adults, it may be a complication of other skin problems. *Custom Medical Stock Photo, Inc. Reproduced by permission.*

* **bacteria** (bak-TEER-ee-a) are single-celled microorganisms, which typically reproduce by cell division. Some, but not all, types of bacteria can cause disease in humans. Many types can live in the body without causing harm.

Furgang, Kathy. *Frequently Asked Questions about Sports Injuries.* New York: Rosen, 2008.

Kita, Joe, ed. *Sports Injuries Handbook.* Emmaus, PA: Rodale, 2005.

Lennard-Brown, Sarah. *Sports Injuries.* Chicago: Raintree, 2005.

McCallum, Jack. "Steroids in America." *Sports Illustrated,* March 11, 2008.

Pfeiffer, Ronald P., Alton Thygerson, Nicholas F. Palmieri, and American Academy of Orthopaedic Surgeons. *Sports First Aid and Injury Prevention.* Sudbury, MA: Jones and Bartlett, 2008.

Schwarz, Alan. "Lineman, Dead at 36, Exposes Brain Injuries." *New York Times,* June 15, 2007. http://www.nytimes.com/2007/06/15/sports/football/15brain.html?_r=1.

Organizations

American Association of Neurological Surgeons. 5550 Meadowbrook Drive, Rolling Meadows, IL, 60008, Web site: http://www.neurosurgerytoday.org.

National Institute of Arthritis and Musculoskeletal and Skin Diseases. 1 AMS Circle, Bethesda, MD, 20892-3675. Toll free: 877-226-4267. Web site: http://www.niams.nih.gov/Health_Info/Sports_Injuries/sports_injuries_ff.asp.

National Library of Medicine. 8600 Rockville Pike, Bethesda, MD, 20894. Toll free: 888-346-3656. Web site: http://www.nlm.nih.gov/medlineplus/sportsinjuries.html.

Sprains *See Strains and Sprains.*

Staphylococcal Infections

Staphylococcal (stah-fih-lo-KAH-kul) infections are infections caused by the organism Staphylococcus aureus (stah-fih-lo-KAH-kus ARE-ree-us) and related species of bacteria, over thirty species in all.

What Are Staphylococcal Infections?

They cannot be seen with the naked eye, but bacteria* cover the skin's surface. *Staphylococcus aureus* (*S. aureus*) bacteria, also called staph (pronounced "staff") bacteria, often live on people's skin, particularly around openings such as the nose, mouth, genitals*, and anus*, and sometimes inside the nose and mouth, without causing disease. But when a person's skin is broken or cut, the bacteria can enter the wound and cause an infection. Staph infections range from minor skin infections to joint, bone, or lung infections to widespread or systemic infections that can be life threatening. Some strains* of staph produce a toxin (or poison) that causes illness.

Newborns, elderly people, and people with immune systems* weakened by diseases such as cancer and AIDS* are at greater risk of serious staph infections. Some serious infections, often resistant to many antibiotics, can be acquired in a hospital when a patient is being treated for another condition. In fact, in the United States, staph infections are considered the leading cause of primary infections that result from being medically treated within hospitals and healthcare centers; or, what are called nosocomial (nas-eh-KO-meh-el) infections.

How Common Are Staphylococcal Infections?

Some species of staph bacteria are present on people's skin all the time. The more dangerous *Staphylococcus aureus* may come and go regularly from people's noses and skin. Skin infections caused by staph, such as boils, are quite common. Many staph infections are minor and do not require treatment; serious staph infections are less common. Overall, studies have shown that staph bacteria exist on the skin or inside the nose of about 20 to 30 percent of all healthy people in the United States. They can remain there indefinitely without any medical problems. They exist less frequently in the mouth; mammary glands; and intestinal, upper respiratory, and urinary tracts. However, if a break in the skin occurs or the bacteria is able to invade the body by other means, then serious health problems can result when the body's immune system cannot effectively counter them. The immune system is especially vulnerable to such outbreaks in newborn infants, breastfeeding women, and people with compromised immune systems, surgical incisions, and serious diseases or illnesses.

Overall, the incidence of staph infections steadily increased during the late 1990s and early 2000s in the United States and other developed countries. Globally, if left untreated such infections, as a group, potentially kill the majority of people afflicted. People more prone to staph infections and serious symptoms are more apt to die from such infections.

Are Staphylococcal Infections Contagious?

Sometimes staph infections of the skin are contagious. In such circumstances, they are called communicable (contagious) diseases because bacteria can be transmitted between humans. Infrequently, staph bacteria are spread through the air. However, they are usually transmitted from human-to-human contact. If a person touches another person who has a staph infection of the skin, with either open sores or bodily fluids, and then touches his or her own mouth, nose, or an area of broken skin, the staph infection can spread. A person also can spread the bacteria from one

* **genitals** (JEH-nih-tuls) are the external sexual organs.
* **anus** (A-nus) is the opening at the end of the digestive system, through which waste leaves the body.
* **strains** are various subtypes of organisms, such as viruses or bacteria.
* **immune system** (im-YOON SIS-tem) is the system of the body composed of specialized cells and the substances they produce that helps protect the body against disease-causing germs.
* **AIDS** or acquired immunodeficiency (ih-myoo-no-dih-FIH-shen-see) syndrome, is an infection that severely weakens the immune system; it is caused by the human immunodeficiency virus (HIV).

part of the body to another through touch. Staph can also be transmitted via contaminated surfaces and food.

What Are Some Types of Staphylococcal Infections?

Impetigo (im-pih-TEE-go) is a skin infection that usually occurs around the nose and mouth. In impetigo, fluid-filled blisters appear and often burst and form yellowish crusts of skin. Impetigo is a contagious infection that can spread if a person scratches the blisters and then scratches or touches another area of the body.

THE EVOLUTION OF ANTIBIOTIC-RESISTANT STAPH

Antibiotics are used widely to treat infections such as those caused by staph. Over time, staph bacteria may become stronger so that the antibiotics may not be as effective against the germ; this change is known as antibiotic resistance. When Scottish biologist Alexander Fleming (1881–1955) discovered penicillin in 1928, staph bacteria were highly sensitive to it. By the early 2000s, few staph bacteria were killed by penicillin. These bacteria often are resistant to many antibiotics.

The more important strains of antibiotic-resistant staph are known as methicillin-resistant staphylococcus aureus (MRSA). MRSA is resistant to commonplace antibiotics, but it is still susceptible to the last-resort, more powerful medications. A more serious strain of staph infection, vancomycin intermediate S. aureus (VISA), can resist vancomycin, one of the most powerful (and last-resort) antibiotics available. Although all strains of the bacteria found so far have been treatable with some type of antibiotic, VISA potentially could defy all medication available in the early 2000s to treat it. Fortunately, VRSA was quite rare.

In the past, MRSA and VISA infections usually developed only in a hospital or healthcare facility where prolonged treatment of patients with several antibiotics is common. As of 2008, however, community-acquired MRSA (those infections within a local community but outside a health facility) was widespread, even in previously healthy individuals without a history of recent antibiotic treatments. In fact, the Centers for Disease Control and Prevention (CDC) states that approximately 12 percent of MRSA infections (throughout the United States) were as of 2008 community-associated, although the percentages varied widely depending on region. The spread of community-acquired MRSA alters its treatment especially concerning the initial choices of antibiotics. As of 2009, the progression of MRSA was a great health concern, emerging as a serious public health problem. Of utmost importance for anyone who may have MRSA is the need to get prompt medical attention for any and all skin and soft tissue infections.

Overall, the prudent use of antibiotics remained especially important as more bacterial strains become more resistant to antibiotics.

Carbuncles (KAR-bung-kulz) and furuncles (FYOOR-ung-kulz), also known as boils, are staph infections that produce a red, swollen bump filled with pus* in the skin surrounding a hair follicle*. With boils pus forms in a single hair follicle, whereas carbuncles form from grouped furuncles and have several small chambers, like a series of connected boils.

Cellulitis (sel-yoo-LYE-tis) is an infection of the deeper layers of the skin and the connective tissues below the skin's surface. People with cellulitis usually have an area of red, swollen, tender, warm skin. They also may have fever, swollen lymph nodes*, and a general feeling of being ill. Cellulitis is most common on the face and lower legs.

In women who are breastfeeding their infants an inflammation of the breast can develop. Called mastitis, the infection can cause bacteria to be released in the mother's milk, which can harm the child.

Scalded skin syndrome (formally called staphylococcal scalded skin syndrome, and also known as Ritter disease) is a staph infection that typically occurs in infants and children less than five years of age (but can occur in people of all ages) and causes large portions of skin to be shed from the body. In this condition, the staph bacteria produce a toxin that damages skin. Fluid collects beneath the skin and loosens it so that large portions slip off when rubbed. Where the skin slips off, raw areas remain that eventually crust over. When the area under the skin is exposed, the child is at risk of excessive fluid loss and additional bacterial infections. Other symptoms include fever and skin redness and tenderness. Babies with this condition may become extremely ill.

Toxic shock syndrome (TSS) is a severe infection that, like scalded skin syndrome, is caused by a toxin produced by staph bacteria. With initial symptoms of severe headache, high fever reaching 105° Fahrenheit (40.5° Celsius), sore throat, and sunburn-looking rash, it can develop into a life-threatening condition when such symptoms as dehydration* and diarrhea* occur, followed by peeling skin over much of the body. Muscle, kidney, and liver damage can lead quickly to loss of life. TSS was first recognized in the late 1970s and early 1980s, mostly among women who were using certain types of very absorbent tampons, but it can occur in people of both sexes and in both children and adults. After this type of absorbent tampon was no longer available, TSS usually developed after surgery or in wounds that, in most cases, did not look infected but contained the toxin-producing staph. Skin abscesses* or other staphylococcal infections may also lead to TSS. Symptoms of TSS include sudden fever, low blood pressure, very red rash, vomiting, diarrhea, and muscle pain.

Staph bacteria can produce other types of toxins that cause food poisoning if a person eats contaminated food (usually meats, poultry, eggs, and dairy products) that has not been heated or refrigerated at the proper temperature. Symptoms include belly pain, nausea (NAW-zee-uh), and vomiting. If the food poisoning is severe, a person may experience headaches, muscle aches, and blood pressure changes.

Some staph infections affect internal organs. Staph is a common cause of the bone infection osteomyelitis (ah-stee-o-my-uh-LYE-tis). Staph infections

* **pus** is a thick, creamy fluid, usually yellow or ivory in color, that forms at the site of an infection. Pus contains infection-fighting white cells and other substances.

* **hair follicle** (FAH-lih-kul) is the skin structure from which hair develops and grows.

* **lymph nodes** (LIMF) are small, bean-shaped masses of tissue containing immune system cells that fight harmful microorganisms. Lymph nodes may swell during infections.

* **dehydration** (dee-hi-DRAY-shun) is a condition in which the body is depleted of water, usually caused by excessive and unreplaced loss of body fluids, such as through sweating, vomiting, or diarrhea.

* **diarrhea** (di-ah-RE-a) refers to frequent, watery stools (bowel movements).

* **abscesses** (AB-seh-sez) are localized or walled off accumulations of pus caused by infection that can occur anywhere within the body.

* **catheter** (KAH-thuh-ter) is a small plastic tube placed through a body opening into an organ (such as the bladder) or through the skin directly into a blood vessel. It is used to give fluids to or drain fluids from a person.

* **colonized** means that a group of organisms, particularly bacteria, are living on or inside the body without causing symptoms of infection.

* **culture** (KUL-chur) is a test in which a sample of fluid or tissue from the body is placed in a dish containing material that supports the growth of certain organisms. Typically, within days the organisms will grow and can be identified.

* **susceptibility** (su-sep-ti-BIL-i-tee) means having less resistance to and higher risk for infection or disease.

* **intravenous** (in-tra-VEE-nus) or IV, means within or through a vein. For example, medications, fluid, or other substances can be given through a needle or soft tube inserted through the skin's surface directly into a vein.

also may cause pneumonia (nu-MO-nyah), an inflammation of the lungs; blood infection (sepsis); and, more rarely, meningitis (meh-nin-JY-tis), an inflammation of the membranes that surround the brain and the spinal cord (the meninges, meh-NIN-jeez). The bacteria may spread from an infection elsewhere in the body, or they can come from a medical device, such as a catheter*, that has been colonized* by staph bacteria. *Staphylococcus aureus* also may infect the heart valves, where it causes inflammation and gives rise to a condition called endocarditis (endo-kar-DYE-tis).

How Is a Staphylococcal Infection Diagnosed?

A doctor may diagnose and treat a staph infection based on its appearance, but a definite diagnosis is made by identifying the organism under a microscope or by culture* with the use of a laboratory. Samples are taken from the site of the infection, which may be the skin, the blood, or an abscess. Imaging scans such as x-rays can help with diagnoses in identifying locations of the infection. Staph food poisoning generally is diagnosed based on symptoms, dietary history, and sometimes illness in other people who have eaten the same food or eaten at the same place. Minor superficial infections are usually diagnosed without the need of blood samples and cultures. However, serious infections rely on the laboratory, especially when the infection lies within the bloodstream, heart, or lungs. In such cases, samples and cultures of blood and affected fluids are taken and analyzed by skilled laboratory personnel to verify the proper course of medical treatment.

What Is the Treatment for Staphylococcal Infections?

Minor skin infections caused by staph bacteria often can be treated with an over-the-counter antibiotic ointment, or they can heal on their own. The choice of the antibiotic often depends on the severity of the infection, its location, and the susceptibility* of the particular staph strain. If a person has an abscess that stems from a staph infection, surgery to drain the pus may be necessary in addition to antibiotics, to allow the infection to heal.

More serious staph infections, such as endocarditis, osteomyelitis, TSS, and scalded skin syndrome, usually require hospitalization and supportive care, such as antibiotics, intravenous* fluids to prevent dehydration, and other medications. Endocarditis caused by staph may require surgery in which the infected, damaged heart valve is removed and an artificial valve is inserted. Scalded skin syndrome is treated with intravenous antibiotics so that the skin can be protected from becoming dehydrated and, consequently, from peeling off.

Because antibiotics are used widely to treat both minor and serious infections caused by staph and other bacteria, some strains of bacteria have become resistant to common antibiotics. Discovery of new medications and forms of treatment are important, and scientists continue to work in the early 2000s on developing a *Staphylococcus aureus* vaccine that might help people with weakened immune systems resist staph infections.

How Long Does a Staphylococcal Infection Last?

Minor skin infections caused by staph bacteria usually clear up within a week, whereas more serious widespread illnesses may take several weeks to more than a month to resolve.

What Are the Complications of Staphylococcal Infections?

Minor staph skin infections rarely result in complications, but some can produce more widespread infection, such as sepsis, a serious systemic infection caused by bacteria invading the bloodstream. TSS can lead to shock*, organ failure, and death. Scalded skin syndrome can give rise to other infections, dehydration, and sepsis. Osteomyelitis can cause permanent bone damage and may require surgical treatment. Under normal circumstances, healthy patients fully recover from staph infections within a short period. However, even healthy people can develop repeat infections, which can eventually become more serious.

Can Staphylococcal Infections Be Prevented?

There are several ways to help prevent the spread of staph infections:

- Washing hands with warm water and antibacterial soap before eating and after using the toilet or touching the nose
- Washing any cuts, scrapes, or open sores
- Showering, rather than bathing, in order to reduce the risk of spreading the infection to other parts of the body
- Using separate towels, washcloths, bed linens, and other related materials from other members of a household, and laundering them daily in hot water and bleach
- Not sharing brushes, combs, clothing, and other personal items
- Keeping wounds covered with a clean bandage after applying an antiseptic

Food poisoning can be prevented by washing hands before food preparation, storing food properly before cooking, cooking food to the appropriate temperatures, using clean utensils and dishes, and refrigerating or freezing food as soon as possible after cooking. To lessen the risk of TSS, women are advised to use less-absorbent tampons, to change them frequently, and not to use only tampons during a menstrual period, or to avoid tampons altogether.

▶ *See also* **Antibiotic Resistance**

** **shock** is a serious condition in which blood pressure is very low and not enough blood flows to the body's organs and tissues. Untreated, shock may result in death.*

Resources

Books and Articles

Tilden, Thomasine E. Lewis. *Help! What's Eating My Flesh? Runaway Staph and Strep Infections!* New York: Franklin Watts, 2008.

Organizations

Centers for Disease Control and Prevention. 1600 Clifton Road, Atlanta, GA, 30333. Toll free: 800-311-3435. Web site: http://www.cdc.gov.

National Institute of Allergy and Infectious Diseases. Office of Communications and Public Liaison, 6610 Rockledge Drive, MSC, 6612, Bethesda, MD, 20892. Toll free: 866-284-4107. Web site: http://www3.niaid.nih.gov.

STDs	*See Sexually Transmitted Diseases (STDs).*

Stealing	*See Conduct Disorder.*

Stings	*See Animal Bites and Stings.*

Stomach Cancer

Stomach cancer, also called gastric cancer, is a disease in which the cells in the stomach divide without control or order and take on an abnormal appearance. These cancerous cells often spread to nearby organs and to other parts of the body.

How Does Stomach Cancer Develop?

The stomach is the sac-like organ located in the upper abdomen, under the ribs, which plays a role in the digestion of food. It connects the esophagus (e-SOF-a-gus), the tube that carries swallowed food, with the small intestine, which absorbs the nutrients needed by the body. When food enters the stomach, the muscles in its wall create a rippling motion that mixes and mashes it. The glands in the lining of the stomach release juices that help to digest the mixture. After a few hours, the food becomes a liquid and moves into the small intestine, which makes it easier for the intestine to continue the process of digestion and absorb the substances that the body needs for energy.

Stomach cancer begins when some of its cells take on an abnormal appearance and begin to divide without control or order. If left untreated, these cancer cells can grow through the stomach wall, and they can spread to nearby organs or to nearby lymph nodes*. Through the lymphatic system, the cancer cells can spread to distant areas of the body, including the lungs and the ovaries.

About 95 percent of all stomach cancers are adenocarcinomas, which start in the glandular cells of the stomach. Other types of stomach cancer include malignant* transformation of the immune* tissue of the stomach wall, which causes lymphoma of the stomach wall; cancer affecting the hormone-producing cells in the stomach that causes a condition called carcinoid tumor; and gastrointestinal stromal tumors, a rare form of stomach cancer that affects nervous system tissue within the stomach.

Who Gets Stomach Cancer and Why?

Each year, about 24,000 people in the United States learn that they have cancer of the stomach. Like most other forms of cancer, stomach cancer occurs most frequently in older people, usually 55 years of age or older. Fortunately, for reasons that scientists cannot fully explain, the number of people who get this disease dropped steadily between the 1940s and the early 2000s.

Stomach cancer is much more common in other countries, especially Japan, Chile, and Iceland. Researchers think the reason may be that people in these countries eat many foods that are preserved by drying, smoking, salting, or pickling. Eating foods preserved in this way may raise someone's risk for developing stomach cancer. People who smoke cigarettes may also be at higher risk of developing stomach cancer.

What Happens When People Have Stomach Cancer?

Symptoms   At first, stomach cancer does not cause any symptoms. And when it eventually causes symptoms, they often are mistaken for less serious stomach problems, such as indigestion, heartburn, or a virus. Therefore, it is hard to find stomach cancer early, which makes it more difficult to treat. Possible symptoms include:

   Discomfort or pain in the abdomen

   Nausea and vomiting after meals

   Bloating of the stomach after meals

   Anemia

   Weakness, fatigue, or weight loss

   Vomiting blood or passing black, tar-like stools

* **lymph nodes** (LIMF) are small, bean-shaped masses of tissue containing immune system cells that fight harmful microorganisms. Lymph nodes may swell during infections.

* **malignant** (ma-LIG-nant) refers to a condition that is severe and progressively worsening.

* **immune** (ih-MYOON) means resistant to or not susceptible to a disease.

* **feces** (FEE-seez) is the excreted waste from the gastrointestinal tract.

* **CT scans** or CAT scans are the shortened name for computerized axial tomography (to-MOG-ra-fee), which uses computers to view structures inside the body.

* **ultrasound** also called a sonogram, is a diagnostic test in which sound waves passing through the body create images on a computer screen.

* **chemotherapy** (KEE-mo-THER-a-pee) is the treatment of cancer with powerful drugs that kill cancer cells.

Diagnosis When people report these symptoms to their family doctor, they may be referred to a gastroenterologist (gas-tro-en-ter-OL-o-jist), a doctor who specializes in diagnosing and treating digestive problems. The gastroenterologist may order additional diagnostic tests to figure out what is wrong.

One of the most common procedures is called endoscopy (en-DOS-ko-pee), which involves passing a very thin, lighted tube down the esophagus and into the stomach. This tube allows doctors to look directly at the inside of the stomach. If an abnormal area is seen, doctors can remove some tissue from it through the tube and have the tissue examined under a microscope. This process, called a biopsy (BY-op-see), determines whether cancer cells are present.

A person might also have an upper GI series, which is a series of x-rays of the upper gastrointestinal (gas-tro-in-TES-ti-nal) tract, including the esophagus and stomach. These pictures are taken after the person drinks a thick chalky liquid called barium (BA-ree-um). The barium outlines the stomach on the x-rays, helping doctors locate tumors or other abnormal areas.

Doctor might also want to test for blood in the feces*, the solid waste that people produce when they go to the bathroom. This test involves placing a small amount of feces (stool) on a slide and having it tested in the laboratory. Sometimes, blood in the stool is a sign of stomach cancer or other cancers of the digestive tract.

If cancer is diagnosed, then doctors need to find out whether it has spread to other parts of the body. They often use imaging tests such as CT scans* or ultrasound* to check for this possibility.

How Is Stomach Cancer Treated?

Because the symptoms associated with stomach cancer seem so minor at first, people rarely report them right away. Therefore, the cancer usually has spread into the stomach wall or even beyond the stomach when it is found, which makes it difficult to cure.

The most common treatment is an operation called gastrectomy (gas-TREK-to-mee), during which surgeons remove part or all of the stomach and some of the surrounding tissue. If all of the stomach needs to be removed, then surgeons connect the esophagus directly to the small intestine. The nearby lymph nodes usually are removed, too.

People with stomach cancer may also be treated with radiation therapy or chemotherapy*, either in an attempt to destroy some of the cancer cells or to ease some of their symptoms, such as pain. Radiation therapy focuses high-energy rays on the body to destroy cancer cells and to stop or slow their growth. During chemotherapy, anti-cancer drugs are given by mouth or by injection into a muscle or blood vessel.

Because stomach cancer is so difficult to cure, researchers have looked at other ways to treat this disease. Studies called clinical trials have been conducted to evaluate some new treatments in cancer patients. One example is biological therapy, which triggers the body's own immune system to attack and destroy cancer cells.

Living with Stomach Cancer

Because people with stomach cancer often have part or all of the stomach removed, they need time to readjust to eating after the surgery. At first, patients are fed intravenously (in-tra-VEE-nus-lee), through a vein in the hand or arm. Within several days, they usually can start taking in liquids, then soft foods, and then more solid foods. Often they need to follow a special diet until they can adjust to having a smaller stomach or none at all. People with stomach cancer need to work with dietitians and nutritionists to make sure that they are getting the nutrients their body needs.

▶ *See also* **Cancer: Overview • Tumor**

Resources

Books and Articles

Shah, Manish A., Natasha Pinheiro, and Brinda M. Shah. *100 Questions & Answers about Gastric Cancer.* Sudbury, MA: Jones and Bartlett, 2008.

Organizations

American Cancer Society. 1599 Clifton Road NE, Atlanta, GA, 30329-4251. Toll free: 800-ACS-2345. Web site: http://www3. cancer.org/cancerinfo.

Cedars-Sinai Medical Center. 8700 Beverly Boulevard, Los Angeles, CA, 90048. Telephone: 310-4-CEDARS. Web site: http://www. csmc.edu/5548.html.

Memorial Sloan-Kettering Cancer Center. 1275 York Avenue, New York, NY, 10065. Telephone: 212-639-2000. Web site: http://www. mskcc.org/mskcc/html/1467.cfm.

National Cancer Institute. Public Inquiries Office, 6116 Executive Boulevard, Room 3036A, Bethesda, MD, 20892-8322. Toll free: 800-4-CANCER. Web site: http://cancernet.nci.nih.gov/wyntk_ pubs/stomach.htm.

United Ostomy Associations of America. P.O. Box 66, Fairview, TN, 37062-0066. Toll free: 800-826-0826. Web site: http://www.uoaa.org.

Stomach Ulcer *See Helicobactor Pylori Infection.*

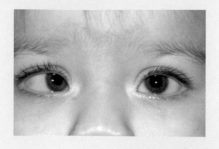

▲

An uncorrected case of strabismus can create the appearance of crossed eyes. *Biophoto Associates/Photo Researchers, Inc.*

* **Down syndrome** is a genetic disorder that can cause mental retardation, shortness, and distinctive facial characteristics, as well as many other features.

* **cerebral palsy** (se-RE-bral PAL-zee) is a group of conditions, all of which affect a person's ability to move. They are usually caused by injury to the brain before or soon after birth.

* **hydrocephalus** (HY-droe-SEF-uh-lus) is a condition, sometimes present at birth, in which there is an abnormal buildup of fluid within the skull, leading to enlargement of the skull and pressure on the brain.

* **tumor** (TOO-mor) usually refers to an abnormal growth of body tissue that has no known cause or physiologic purpose and is not an inflammation.

* **cataracts** (KAH-tuh-rakts) are areas of cloudiness of the lens of the eye that can interfere with vision.

* **stroke** is a brain-damaging event usually caused by interference with blood flow to the brain. A stroke may occur when a blood vessel supplying the brain becomes clogged or bursts, depriving brain tissue of oxygen. As a result, nerve cells in the affected area of the brain, and the specific body parts they control, do not properly function.

Strabismus

Strabismus is a condition in which the eyes cross or do not work together normally, which may lead to permanent loss of vision in one eye.

What Is Strabismus?

When people cross their eyes, the world suddenly doubles. Images, like the words on this page, become blurred, and it appears as if there are two of each. When the eyes function correctly, they work together to focus images and to allow the brain to develop a three-dimensional view of the world. But when the eyes cannot work together, as when people cross their eyes, the brain sees double. The result is double vision.

Fortunately, both eyes work together for most people. But some people have an eye disorder that causes the eyes to fail to line up properly, resulting in blurred or double vision. This condition is called strabismus (stra-BIZ-mus), which comes from a Greek word that means squinting. Often in strabismus, one eye may remain straight and the other eye may turn in, which may look to others as if the person is crossing one eye.

Why Do People Have Strabismus?

Strabismus usually develops during infancy or early childhood. In most cases, there is no known cause, although sometimes several members of the same family have the disorder, which may mean that in some cases strabismus is inherited, like eye color is. Other possible causes include the following:

- Farsightedness, causing focus difficulties
- Damage to one eye or to the part of the brain that controls the muscles involved in eye movement
- Other disorders that affect the brain, including Down syndrome*, cerebral palsy*, and hydrocephalus*
- Less commonly, vision is blocked by a tumor* or cataracts* that causes cloudiness in the normally clear lens of the eye. Strabismus affects about 3 to 5 percent of children in the United States. It occurs in boys and girls equally. Fortunately, if it is diagnosed and treated early, there is a good chance of saving or improving vision in the affected eye.

Some adults have strabismus, perhaps because they were not treated for it as a child or because the treatment was not effective. Other adults may develop strabismus when a disorder such as stroke* causes the eyes to cross or not work together normally.

How Do Six Muscles in Each Eye Work as One?

The eyes and the nerves that connect them to the brain work like the two lenses of binoculars. They merge the image seen by each eye into one image. Six muscles are attached to each eye, and they control how the eyeball moves left and right or up and down. To make it possible for the brain to develop a single three-dimensional image, the muscles must work together to focus, just as the two lenses of binoculars must be aligned to focus together.

People with strabismus have trouble with one or more of the muscles in an eye. Instead of working together, one eye is out of alignment. Sometimes strabismus seems to come and go, depending on how tired the eyes are, and sometimes the eyes remain out of correct position. There are different forms of strabismus:

- When one eye points inward toward the nose, which makes the person look cross-eyed, the condition is esotropia (es-o-TRO-pe-a).

- When one eye points away from the nose, as if looking to the outside, the condition is exotropia (ek-so-TRO-pe-a) or walleye.

- When the brain turns off the vision in the turned eye in favor of the vision in the straight eye, the condition is called strabismic amblyopia (stra-BIZ-mik am-blee-O-pee-a) or lazy eye. Amblyopia does not mean that the eye is lazy. Instead, the brain turns off the image coming from the optic nerve in that eye so the person sees only one clear image of the world instead of having blurred or double vision.

A Little Pirate

Mrs. Apple noticed that the eyes of her baby Chloe often did not work together. She had read in a book how babies sometimes appear cross-eyed or how it seems one eye is looking off in another direction from the other, which can be normal for a very young baby. But when Chloe was about four months old, Mrs. Apple became worried. Chloe's left eye seemed to be looking at her nose when Mrs. Apple moved her face close, and the right eye seemed to be looking straight ahead. Mrs. Apple took the baby to an ophthalmologist* for an eye exam and was told that Chloe likely had strabismus.

It is usually a parent who first notices the signs of strabismus when children are infants or preschoolers. The children are too young to complain about double or poor vision. If Mrs. Apple had not taken action because of her worries, the strabismus might have developed into amblyopia, leaving Chloe without vision in the crossed eye. Without treatment, amblyopia may become permanent.

The ophthalmologist recommended that Chloe wear an eye patch over her normal eye. The doctor explained that this could force the weaker eye to develop vision more properly.

How Do Doctors Diagnose Strabismus and Amblyopia?

Diagnosis Doctors use a variety of methods to diagnose strabismus and amblyopia. Most involve observation of how the child looks at objects, because most children are too young to recognize the letters on a standard eye chart. The doctor will cover one eye and then the other, holding and moving

Will Crossed Eyes Become Stuck?

Many people have received the following warning: "If you keep crossing your eyes like that, they could stay that way forever!"

Although the warning may be intended to stop a silly behavior, it is not medically true. Voluntarily crossing the eyes will not harm them or put them at risk of strabismus.

* **ophthalmologist** (off-thal-MOLL-o-jist) is a medical doctor who specializes in treating diseases of the eye.

objects and watching to see if the child squints or tries to cover or close one eye in favor of the other. The doctor also will check the alignment of the eyes by shining a light in both eyes to see if the reflection falls in the same place in the pupils (the black spot in the center of the eye) of both eyes.

Many children do not like to have their eyes covered during these exams. Some are frightened of the equipment that may be held close to their faces. Some techniques under development in the early 2000s used computers to track eye movements from a distance, sometimes while the child is watching a cartoon.

Treatment   The most common treatment of strabismus involves wearing a patch like Chloe's over the stronger eye. The brain now starts to try to send and receive signals from the weaker eye, and the muscles that control it try to bring the eye back to a normal focus. The same result often is achieved with eye drops that blur the vision in the normal eye to make the other eye work harder. Doctors may also prescribe special eyeglasses for some children with strabismus. Some of these eyeglasses use prisms that change how the image is sent into the eye.

Some techniques involve disabling or weakening one or more of the muscles in the eye. This strategy is designed to force the other muscles to work harder to bring the affected eye into focus with the normal eye. Surgery can reposition the eye muscles of one or both eyes. The operation can leave the eyes straight and vision normal, although sometimes the eyes appear straight but people still need eyeglasses to achieve good vision. Sometimes, injections are used to disable one or more eye muscles for a period of time, which may achieve similar results to surgery.

Treatment is most effective when children are young, which is why vision testing and early diagnosis are important. Strabismus and amblyopia do not simply go away, as some people believe. With treatment, children like Chloe can have almost normal vision and no restrictions on activities as they grow up.

▶ *See also* **Cataracts • Farsightedness • Marfan Syndrome**

Resources

Books and Articles

Sutton, Amy L., ed. *Eye Care Sourcebook,* 3rd ed. Detroit, MI: Omnigraphics, 2008.

Organizations

American Association for Pediatric Ophthalmology and Strabismus. P.O. Box 193832, San Francisco, CA, 94119-3832. Telephone: 415-561-8505. Web site: http://www.aapos.org/index.cfm.

American Optometric Association. 243 N. Lindbergh Boulevard, St. Louis, MO, 63141, Web site: http://www.aoa.org/strabismus.xml.

* **inflammation** (in-fla-MAY-shun) is the body's reaction to irritation, infection, or injury that often involves swelling, pain, redness, and warmth.

Optometrists Network. 93 Bedford Street, Suite 5D, New York, NY, 10014, Web sites: http://www.strabismus.org/all_about_strabismus. html; http://www.strabismus.org/references.html.

Strains and Sprains

Strains and sprains are injuries to the body's soft tissues. Strains are injuries to muscles and/or tendons, which are the cords that connect muscles and bones. Sprains are injuries to ligaments, which are bands of strong connective tissue that support the joints (areas in the body where two bones meet) and connect the bones to each other. Strains and sprains may result from sudden injury or from long-term overuse.

What Are Strains and Sprains?

Strains and sprains are injuries to the body's soft tissues—its muscles, tendons, and ligaments. They are everyday occurrences for athletes but can happen to anyone as the result of a fall, a twist, or any other sudden blow to the body.

Strains are injuries to muscles or to tendons, which support the bones and connect them to the muscles. Sprains are injuries to ligaments, which are bands of connective tissue that support the joints and connect the bones to each other.

Strains occur most often in the muscles and tendons of the legs and back: Hamstring pulls, groin pulls, and sore back muscles are common forms of strain. Sprains most often affect the joints, such as the ankles, knees, and wrists. Both strains and sprains cause pain, swelling, and inflammation*. The injured area may also be discolored if it has been bruised and blood pools underneath the skin.

Most people recover from strains and sprains if they see their doctor promptly and follow the doctor's instructions, which often involve what is known as a R.I.C.E. protocol: rest, ice, compression, and elevation.

What Are the Different Types of Strains and Sprains?

Doctors usually classify strains and sprains by the degree of damage done to the muscles or ligaments.

First degree A first-degree strain or sprain is the least serious of the three degrees and causes the least amount of damage or stretching of ligaments or muscle fibers. No tears occur in the tissue fibers, pain and swelling are minimal, and range of motion (movement up and down, or sideways) usually is not affected to any significant degree. People who have a first-degree strain or sprain may experience some slight disability

Strains and sprains are injuries to the muscles, tendons, and ligaments. *Illustration by Frank Forney. Reproduced by permission of Gale, a part of Cengage Learning.*

▶

Sprained (partially torn) ligament

Muscle strain

Torn tendon

* **edema** (e-DEE-ma) means swelling in the body's tissues caused by excess fluids.

in using the affected joint, but on the whole, they can resume normal activities after a short recovery period.

Second degree   In a second-degree strain or sprain, up to 80 percent of the tissue fibers are ruptured. The individual experiences more pain, edema*, and reduced range of motion. Unlike first-degree injuries, two to three weeks may pass before the pain and swelling begin to show real improvement. Athletes who resume their sports activity too soon risk the real possibility that the second-degree injury will turn into a third-degree injury, which requires a longer recovery time.

Third degree   In third-degree injury, a 100 percent rupture occurs in all the tissues that surround the joint capsule: muscles, tendons, and ligaments. A person with a third-degree sprain or strain can no longer use the injured part of the body and will experience pain and visible bruising. X-rays may show that even though bones have not been broken, they may have been chipped. Doctors call such bone chips avulsion (a-VUL-shun) fractures. Medical professionals usually tell patients to protect the injured area for 8 to 10 weeks and may order surgery to repair damaged joints.

What Is the Treatment for Strains and Sprains?

Doctors who treat strains and sprains use the expression "RICE DIETS" to describe the steps required for healing. The "RICE" part of the term refers more to first-aid practices, whereas "DIETS" refers to more definitive therapies performed by or under doctor's supervision.

- **R: Rest.** The amount of rest depends on the degree of injury.
- **I: Ice.** Ice causes blood vessels to constrict (get small) which helps reduce inflammation.
- **C: Compression.** Bandages and wraps play a role in reducing pain and swelling, and in helping ruptured small blood vessels to heal more quickly.
- **E: Elevation.** Lifting the injured area above level of the heart helps keep swelling down and blood from pooling in the area of damage.
- **D: Drugs.** Doctors may recommend the use of aspirin, ibuprofen*, or other anti-inflammatory medications during the first few days after the injury.
- **I: Incision, drainage, and injection.** Third-degree sprains sometimes require these procedures.
- **E: Exercise.** Patients may be taught how to do certain leg exercises that will help them after their injuries.
- **T: Therapy.** Patients may benefit greatly from physical therapy to get the injured part of the body back in use without hurting it again.
- **S: Surgery.** A bad strain or sprain may need surgery to repair damaged tissue or fractured (broken) bones.

Can Strains or Sprains Be Prevented?

Many strains and sprains can be avoided. Precautions at home include the following:

- Clearing ice away from porches, steps, and sidewalks
- Wearing shoes and boots with nonskid soles
- Holding hand rails on stairways
- Using rubber mats in tubs and shower stalls
- Choosing rugs with nonskid backing
- Making sure night-time entrances have adequate lighting
- Keeping a night light or wall light on between the bedroom and the bathroom
- Keeping tools, toys, and other items away from places where people can trip over them
- Ensuring that ladders are steady when they are used

Sports Medicine

Athletes and those who exercise for physical fitness are at risk for strains and sprains. The branch of medicine that specializes in treating these injuries is called sports medicine.

Doctors who specialize in sports medicine can help athletes improve performance without injuring the body. They can also test athletes for drug use, treat injuries that result from exercise or sports, advise about proper clothing and protective gear, and supervise diet and fluid intake during training and travel, especially abroad.

* **ibuprofen** (eye-bew-PRO-fin) is a nonsteroidal anti-inflammatory drug (NISAD) used to reduce fever and relieve pain or inflammation.

* **strains** are various subtypes of organisms, such as viruses or bacteria.

Rules for athletes include starting slowly, stretching frequently, and always remembering to warm up and cool down before and after strenuous exercise.

▶ *See also* **Carpal Tunnel Syndrome • Repetitive Stress Syndrome • Trauma**

Resources

Books and Articles

Silverstein, Alvin, Virginia Silverstein, and Laura Silverstein Nunn. *Pains and Strains.* New York: Franklin Watts, 2003.

Organizations

American Academy of Orthopaedic Surgeons. 6300 North River Road, Rosemont, IL, 60018-4262. Telephone: 847-823-7186. Web site: http://orthoinfo.aaos.org/topic.cfm?topic=A00111. Web site: http://orthoinfo.aaos.org/topic.cfm?topic=A00410. Web site: http://orthoinfo.aaos.org/topic.cfm?topic=A00065.

American Physical Therapy Association. 1111 North Fairfax Street, Alexandria, VA, 22314-1488. Telephone: 703-684-2782. Web site: http://www.apta.org/consumer.

National Institute of Arthritis and Musculoskeletal and Skin Diseases. 1 AMS Circle, Bethesda, MD, 20892-3675. Telephone: 301-495-4484. Web site: http://www.niams.nih.gov/Health_Info/ Sprains_Strains/default.asp.

Strep Throat *See Sore Throat/Strep Throat.*

Streptococcal Infections

Streptococcal (strep-tuh-KAH-kul) infections are caused by various strains* of Streptococcus *(strep-tuh-KAH-kus) bacteria.*

What Are Streptococcal Infections?

Streptococci (strep-tuh-KAH-kye) are common bacteria that live in the human body, including the nose, skin, and genital tract. These bacteria can destroy red blood cells, damage them, or cause no damage at all. The amount of damage they do is used to classify streptococcus strains. The ones that destroy red blood cells are known as beta-hemolytic (he-muh-LIH-tik), and these strains are categorized as groups A through T.

Groups A and B streptococci are most often associated with disease. Group A strep (GAS) infections range from superficial skin infections and strep throat to serious and life-threatening illnesses such as toxic shock syndrome and necrotizing fasciitis (NEH-kro-tie-zing fash-e-EYE-tis). Group B strep (GBS) is the leading cause of life-threatening infections in newborns. In pregnant women, GBS can lead to bladder infections, infections of the womb, and death of the fetus*.

Alpha-hemolytic streptococci are strains that damage red blood cells but do not destroy them. Two important strains are *S. viridans* (VEER-ih-dans), which is found in the mouth and is involved in tooth decay and endocarditis* and *S. pneumoniae* (nu-MO-nye), which can cause pneumonia*, middle ear infection, and meningitis*.

Group A Streptococcus (GAS) Infections

How common are they? According to the National Institute of Allergy and Infectious Diseases (NIAID), more than 10 million cases of mild GAS infections, such as skin and throat infections, are diagnosed each year. Between 9,000 and 10,000 cases of more serious infections, including toxic shock syndrome and necrotizing fasciitis, occur annually. People with immune systems weakened by diseases such as diabetes or cancer, are at a greater risk for developing serious GAS infections.

Are they contagious? GAS bacteria are contagious and spread through contact with fluid from the mouth or nose of an infected person or contact with infected skin lesions*.

Examples of GAS infections

■ Strep throat, or streptococcal pharyngitis (fair-un-JY-tis), is a painful inflammation of the throat. Symptoms include a sore throat with white patches on the tonsils*, swollen lymph nodes* in the neck, fever, and headache.

■ Scarlet fever, which often occurs along with strep throat or other strep infections, is caused by strains of group A strep that produce a toxin (or poison) that results in a very red rash and a bright red tongue, along with a high fever.

■ Impetigo (im-pih-TEE-go) is a superficial skin infection common in young children. Symptoms include fluid-filled blisters (one or more) surrounded by red skin. The blisters eventually break and form a honey-colored crust.

■ Cellulitis (sel-yoo-LYE-tis) is an inflammation of the skin and/or its underlying soft tissues. Symptoms include skin that is red, tender, and painful to the touch; fever; and chills.

* **fetus** (FEE-tus) is the term for an unborn human after it is an embryo, from 9 weeks after fertilization until childbirth.

* **endocarditis** (en-do-kar-DYE-tis) is an inflammation of the valves and internal lining of the heart, known as the endocardium (en-doh-KAR-dee-um), usually caused by an infection.

* **pneumonia** (nu-MO-nyah) is inflammation of the lungs.

* **meningitis** (meh-nin-JY-tis) is an inflammation of the meninges, the membranes that surround the brain and the spinal cord. Meningitis is most often caused by infection with a virus or a bacterium.

* **lesions** (LEE-zhuns) is a general term referring to a sore or a damaged or irregular area of tissue.

* **tonsils** are paired clusters of lymphatic tissue in the throat that help protect the body from bacteria and viruses that enter through a person's nose or mouth.

* **lymph nodes** (LIMF) are small, bean-shaped masses of tissue containing immune system cells that fight harmful microorganisms. Lymph nodes may swell during infections.

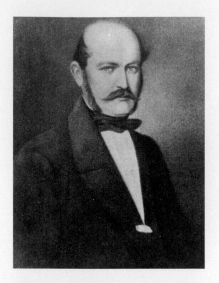

After Hungarian physician Ignaz Semmelweis (1818–1865) had the physicians at a Vienna, Austria, hospital wash their hands regularly with an antiseptic, the hospital's mortality rate fell dramatically. *The Library of Congress.*

* **shock** is a serious condition in which blood pressure is very low and not enough blood flows to the body's organs and tissues. Untreated, shock may result in death.

* **arthritis** (ar-THRY-tis) refers to any of several disorders characterized by inflammation of the joints.

* **culture** (KUL-chur) is a test in which a sample of fluid or tissue from the body is placed in a dish containing material that supports the growth of certain organisms. Typically, within days the organisms will grow and can be identified.

* **intravenous** (in-tra-VEE-nus) or IV, means within or through a vein. For example, medications, fluid, or other substances can be given through a needle or soft tube inserted through the skin's surface directly into a vein.

■ Bacteremia (bak-tuh-REE-me-uh) is the presence of bacteria in the bloodstream, which can spread infection to other organs. Bacteremia that causes symptoms, which is known as sepsis, is associated with fever, rapid heart rate, and low blood pressure that may lead to shock*.

■ Toxin-producing strains of GAS can cause a rare but serious illness called streptococcal toxic shock syndrome. The infection may occur anywhere in the body, and the toxin is released into the bloodstream, causing low blood pressure and shock.

■ Necrotizing fasciitis (or flesh-eating disease) is a rare, rapidly progressing infection of the deeper layers of skin, muscle, and other tissues. Symptoms usually start at the site of an injury, where the skin becomes painful, swollen, discolored (e.g., red, purple, or bronze), and hot to the touch. The skin gradually becomes darker and blisters can form while the tissues beneath the skin are being damaged. Fever, shock, and multiple organ damage may accompany this serious infection.

■ Rheumatic (roo-MAH-tik) fever, a syndrome involving arthritis* and inflammation of the heart, is actually a complication of untreated strep throat. Rashes and neurological problems may also occur, and people with rheumatic fever may have permanent damage to one or more heart valves.

Making the diagnosis   With skin infections, a doctor may take a sample from the affected area to culture*. For other types of suspected infections, blood samples are drawn and swabs of fluid from the patient's nose and throat are cultured for bacteria. A rapid strep test on a sample taken with a throat swab can also be done in a doctor's office.

Treatment   Superficial skin infections often are treated with topical (on the skin) antibiotic ointments. Other GAS infections are treated with oral (by mouth), intramuscular (IM), or intravenous* (IV) antibiotics. Serious GAS infections require hospitalization, during which patients receive IV fluids and antibiotics. In some cases, such as with necrotizing fasciitis, surgical removal of damaged tissue is necessary. Treatment of rheumatic fever depends on the severity of the disease but includes using antibiotics to treat strep infections, anti-inflammatory medicines such as high-dose aspirin, and medications to treat heart complications.

What to expect   Symptoms of strep throat usually improve within one to two days after starting antibiotics. Skin infections often clear up within a week, but more serious infections can take weeks or even months to heal. Complications from serious bacterial infections include sepsis, shock, organ damage and failure, and death.

Prevention   Maintaining good health and hygiene can help reduce the risk of bacterial infection. Not sharing food or eating utensils, washing hands frequently, and cleaning and bandaging cuts and scrapes can help prevent the spread of bacteria.

Group B Streptococcus (GBS) Infections

How common are they?   According to the Centers for Disease Control and Prevention, GBS is the most frequent cause of life-threatening infections in newborns. Early screening of pregnant women for GBS and treatment have reduced infection rates by approximately 70 percent. In the early 2000s, 17,000 cases of GBS infection occurred annually in the United States.

Are they contagious?   GBS infections are contagious and can pass from mother to child before or during birth. At least 25 percent of women are carriers of GBS at some point in their lives but do not become ill from it. The bacteria can be found in the bowel, vagina*, bladder, and throat.

Examples of GBS Infections

■ Newborns can develop sepsis, pneumonia, and meningitis due to infection with GBS. Symptoms of GBS infection in newborns include fever, irritability, extreme sleepiness, breathing difficulties, and poor feeding.

■ GBS bacteria in pregnant women can cause urinary tract infections* as well as chorioamnionitis (kor-e-o-am-nee-on-EYE-tis, infection of the womb and membranes surrounding the fetus) and stillbirth (a fetus that is dead at birth). Symptoms of urinary tract infection include fever, pain, and a burning sensation during urination. Women with chorioamnionitis often do not show symptoms of infection until after childbirth. Symptoms include fever, belly pain, and rapid pulse.

■ The most common GBS infections in other people are urinary tract infections, sepsis, tissue infections, and pneumonia. GBS infections, including pneumonia and sepsis, are more likely to be found in people with weakened immune systems or chronic diseases, such as diabetes.

Making the diagnosis   GBS infections are diagnosed by performing cultures of blood, urine, or cerebrospinal fluid* to identify the bacteria.

Treatment   GBS infections are treated with antibiotics, often intravenously, and they usually require a hospital stay, particularly for newborns. Pregnant women with urinary tract infections usually are treated with antibiotics as well.

What to expect   Recovery can take several weeks. Complications in infants, particularly those with meningitis, include hearing and vision loss and brain damage. Approximately 5 percent of cases of GBS disease in newborns are fatal.

Shaking Hands with Semmelweis

Ignaz Philipp Semmelweis (1818–1865) was a Hungarian physician working at the Vienna (Austria) General Hospital in 1847, who suspected that doctors could spread disease by not washing their hands thoroughly after working with cadavers before delivering babies. At the time, up to 30 percent of women who gave birth in hospitals died of puerperal (pyoo-ER-puh-rul) fever, a group A strep bacterial infection that occurred after childbirth. Semmelweis noticed that women who delivered their babies with midwives were less likely to become ill. He had his student doctors wash their hands with an antiseptic, which is a solution that prevents the growth of bacteria. Because the idea that germs could cause disease had not yet been introduced, Semmelweis' ideas about hand washing were not well received until many years later.

* **vagina** (vah-JY-nah) is the canal, or passageway, in a woman that leads from the uterus to the outside of the body.

* **urinary** (YOOR-ih-nair-e) **tract infection** or UTI, is an infection that occurs in any part of the urinary tract. The urinary tract is made up of the urethra, bladder, ureters, and kidneys.

* **cerebrospinal fluid** (seh-ree-bro-SPY-nuhl) is the fluid that surrounds the brain and spinal cord.

* **rectum** is the final portion of the large intestine, connecting the colon to the outside opening of the anus.

* **vaccines** (vak-SEENS) are preparations of killed or weakened germs, or a part of a germ or product it produces, given to prevent or lessen the severity of the disease that can result if a person is exposed to the germ itself. Use of vaccines for this purpose is called immunization.

* **sinuses** (SY-nuh-ses) are hollow, air-filled cavities in the facial bones.

* **sputum** (SPYOO-tum) is a substance that contains mucus and other matter coughed out from the lungs, bronchi, and trachea.

Prevention   Most newborn cases can be prevented by testing women in the 35th to 37th week of pregnancy for the bacteria. A culture swabbed from the vagina and rectum* can determine whether a woman has GBS. If she does, giving IV antibiotics during labor reduces the risk of passing GBS to the baby. Vaccines* to prevent GBS infections during pregnancy were being developed in the early 2000s.

Alpha-Hemolytic Streptococcus Infections

How common are they?   Infections with alpha-hemolytic strep bacteria are common; many strains live naturally in humans.

Examples of alpha-hemolytic strep infections

S. PNEUMONIAE (NU-MON-YI) INFECTIONS

◻ Bacterial pneumonia is an inflammation of the lungs that often occurs after or along with an upper respiratory infection. Symptoms may develop quickly and can include fever, chills, cough, rapid breathing, chest pain, belly pain, and vomiting. Before antibiotics were developed, bacterial pneumonia was the most common cause of death in adults.

◻ Otitis (o-TIE-tis) media is an inflammation of the middle ear. The infection usually is associated with ear pain and sometimes with fever.

◻ Sinusitis (sy-nyoo-SY-tis) is an inflammation of the sinuses*, usually due to infection. Symptoms include a stuffy nose, colored discharge (green, yellow, or tinged with blood) from the nose, tenderness around the eyes, and headache or a feeling of pressure in the head.

◻ Meningitis is an inflammation of the membranes covering the brain and the spinal cord. Symptoms include fever, weakness, vomiting, irritability, and stiff neck.

S. VIRIDANS (VEER-IH-DANZ) INFECTION

◻ Endocarditis is an infection of the inner surface of the heart or heart valves that can be caused by *S. viridans* and other bacteria. Bacteria can enter the bloodstream (during a dental procedure, for example) and attach to already damaged heart tissue or an abnormal heart valve, causing more damage. Symptoms include extreme tiredness, weakness, fever, chills, night sweats, and weight loss. The infection can progress, resulting in problems with heart function in some cases.

Making the diagnosis   Depending on the type of infection, a diagnosis is made by testing blood, sputum*, or cerebrospinal fluid samples for signs of the bacteria.

Treatment   Oral or IV antibiotics are used, depending on the severity of the infection. A hospital stay may be needed, particularly in cases of pneumonia or meningitis. Long courses of antibiotics, lasting several weeks or more, may be required to treat endocarditis.

Prevention   Vaccines against *S. pneumoniae* are given routinely to infants and the elderly, as well as to children and adults with weakened immune systems or certain medical conditions. People with abnormal or damaged heart valves are given courses of antibiotics when they have some types of surgical procedures, including dental work, to help prevent endocarditis from developing from the shedding of bacteria into the bloodstream that occurs with these procedures.

▶ *See also* **Impetigo • Meningitis • Otitis (Ear Infections) • Scarlet Fever • Sepsis • Sore Throat/Strep Throat • Toxic Shock Syndrome**

Resources

Books and Articles

Glaser, Jason. *Strep Throat.* Mankato, MN: Capstone Press, 2007.

Lewis Tilden, Thomasine E. *Help! What's Eating My Flesh? Runaway Staph and Strep Infections!* New York: Franklin Watts, 2008.

Organizations

Centers for Disease Control and Prevention. 1600 Clifton Road, Atlanta, GA, 30333. Toll free: 800-311-3435. Web site: http://www.cdc.gov/ncidod/dbmd/diseaseinfo/groupastreptococcal_g.htm. Web site: http://www.cdc.gov/groupBstrep.

National Library of Medicine. 8600 Rockville Pike, Bethesda, MD, 20894, Web site: http://www.nlm.nih.gov/medlineplus/streptococcalinfections.html.

Stress and Stress-Related Illness

Stress is a physical and/or emotional response to a difficult, painful, or challenging experience and may affect children, teenagers, and adults. The body's stress response system can cause a rapid heartbeat, a rise in blood pressure, and other physical changes. Stress-related illnesses are physical or mental maladies that may be brought on or made worse by stress. They can include headaches, stomachaches, sleeplessness, depression, anxiety, and other conditions. Relaxation and stress management techniques often help people deal with stress.

The body's stress hormone response. When the brain perceives stress, the hypothalamus releases corticotropin-releasing factor (1), which triggers the release of adrenocorticotropin (ACTH) (2) from the pituitary gland. ACTH (2) travels through the bloodstream and (along with signals from the brain sent through the autonomic nervous system) stimulates the adrenal glands to release cortisol and epinephrine into the bloodstream (3). Cortisol and epinephrine (3) help provide energy, oxygen, and stimulation to the heart, the brain, and other muscles and organs (4) to support the body's response to stress. When the brain perceives that the stress has ended, it allows hormone levels to return to their baseline values. *Illustration by Frank Forney. Reproduced by permission of Gale, a part of Cengage Learning.*

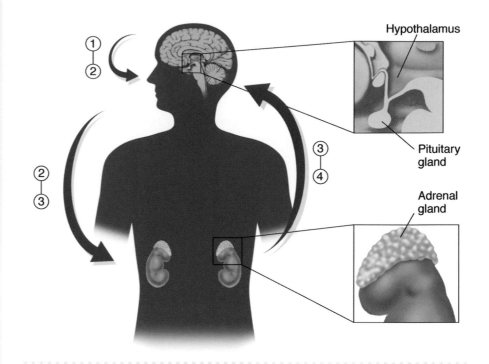

Good Stress and Bad Stress

Everyone experiences stress, which is the body's general response to any event, real or imagined, that requires an adaptation or extra effort. In most cases, an event or situation is not stressful by itself. Rather, it is how people view the event and what they believe about their own ability to respond to it that create stress. About 10 percent of modern stress can be linked to actual physical threats to life or safety, such as being threatened with a weapon or needing to slam on the brakes to avoid an accident. The other 90 percent of stress seems to result from people's perceptions of life events, such as arguments with friends or family, concerns about school or work, or problems individuals do not know how to solve. The causes for a majority of doctor visits are believed to be stress-related.

Stressors Stressors are the triggers for the body's stress response. These triggers are unique to each person. An event that one person finds relaxing may create tension in another. Stressors fall into several different categories:

- Physical stressors affect a person's body. These biological stressors may include exercise, illness, or disabilities.

- Environmental stressors include noise, overcrowding, poverty, natural disasters, or even technology that causes too much change in too short a period of time.

- Life situations create both good and bad stressors. These may include moving to a new home, changing schools or jobs, or experiencing changes in the family structure, such as marriage, divorce, the birth or adoption of a new child, or the death of a friend or family member.

- Behaviors can also be stressors. These may include smoking cigarettes, taking drugs, not sleeping enough, eating too little or too much, or exercising too little or too much.

- Certain patterns of thinking (cognitive actions) can be stressors, too. These may include fearing change, interpreting minor losses as catastrophes, or recalling difficult life events.

Stress, anxiety, and excitement Stress is often associated with negative thoughts or events that people find unpleasant, frightening, or anxiety-producing. It may come about as a result of being bullied or teased by peers, being anxious about a test, feeling disappointed about not achieving a goal, or from efforts to bundle too many activities into too little time. Sometimes life events that cause stress initially result in anxiety that turns instead into positive excitement. An audition, a game point, or a date to the prom are positive stressors. Stress is the body's natural response to the difficult demands or exciting new challenges it encounters everyday.

Trauma and stress Some events are so stressful that they overwhelm people, and no amount of deep breathing or positive thinking may seem to help. Accidents, injuries, abuse, violence, war, serious threats to physical safety, or the sudden death of a loved one are examples of traumas that cause a stress response within the body.

Which Illnesses Are Stress-Related?

It is difficult for researchers to establish a definite cause-and-effect relationship between stress and specific physical symptoms or illnesses. Not only do people's minds and bodies react differently to stress, but there are other factors at work when someone gets sick. The following conditions are known or believed to be stress-related (as opposed to stress-caused):

- Pain caused by muscular problems, such as tension headaches, back pain, jaw pain, and repetitive stress syndrome. Pain of many kinds seems to be caused or made worse by stress.

- Gastrointestinal (gas-tro-in-TES-ti-nal) problems, such as heartburn, stomach pain, and diarrhea.

- Insomnia, or difficulty sleeping.

- Substance abuse, including smoking, drug addiction, and heavy drinking of alcohol. Substance abuse, in turn, can lead to other illnesses, including heart disease and cancer.

- Asthma attacks in people who already have the condition or who are susceptible to it.

- Post-traumatic stress disorder, a mental disorder in which people relive a terrifying experience in dreams and memories long after the event has passed, and acute stress disorder, in which they have similar symptoms immediately after the event.

Coping with Stress

Tips for coping with stress include the following:

■ Be realistic.

■ Don't try to be perfect.

■ Don't expect others to be perfect.

■ Take one thing at a time.

■ Be flexible.

■ Share feelings.

■ Maintain a healthy lifestyle.

■ Meditate.

■ Ask for help when necessary.

■ Have fun.

Tips for helping others cope with stress include the following:

■ Pay attention.

■ Take them seriously.

■ Be patient.

■ Offer help when necessary.

---

* **eating disorders** are conditions in which a person's eating behaviors and food habits are so unbalanced that they cause physical and emotional problems.

* **schizophrenia** (skit-so-FREE-nee-ah) is a serious mental disorder that causes people to experience hallucinations, delusions, and other confusing thoughts and behaviors, which distort their view of reality.

■ Other mental disorders, including eating disorders*, anxiety, depression, and possibly schizophrenia*.

■ Cardiovascular (car-dee-o-VAS-kyu-lar) problems, such as irregular heartbeat, hardening of the arteries, and heart attack. Stress makes the heart beat more quickly and increases blood pressure temporarily. Although long-term effects have not been proven, many scientists suspect that they exist.

What Is the Stress Response?

Stressors both good and bad set off a series of events within the body's neuroendocrine system. Often called the "fight or flight" response, these events are triggered by the brain, which alerts the body's autonomic nervous system* to prepare all systems to react to an emergency. The autonomic nervous system sends a message in a split second through nerve fibers, which signal all the other body systems.

During this alarm period, various hormones are activated with many dramatic effects on other body systems. The heart beats faster, blood pressure is raised, and blood vessels dilate (open wider) to increase blood flow to the muscles. The pupils dilate to aid vision. The digestive system slows down so that the body's resources and energy can be used wherever else they are needed, and the production of saliva decreases. The bronchi dilate to aid breathing. The skin sweats to cool the body, and the liver releases its stores of glucose, the major fuel of the body, to increase the person's energy level. The body stays in this states until the brain tells it that the emergency has ended.

What Happens with Too Much Stress?

Researchers have found that chronic stress and post-trauma stress can suppress the immune system*, interfering with the body's natural ability to defend itself against infection. Chronic stress may also contribute to many other problems of mind and body, including:

■ Headaches or stomachaches

■ Allergic responses, such as skin rashes or asthma

■ Irritability, aggression, or conduct disorders

■ Bruxism (grinding the teeth)

■ Sleep disorders

■ Eating disorders

■ Alcoholism or substance abuse

■ Anxiety

■ Phobias

■ Depression

Long-term stress (chronic stress), frequently recurring stress, or extreme stress from a life-threatening event can keep the body's stress response system activated for a long time. Long-term stress may lead to

HANS SELYE AND STRESS RESEARCH

Hans Selye (1907–1982) is considered the founder of modern stress research. He authored 39 books, wrote more than 1,700 scholarly papers, and was cited as a source in more than 362,000 scientific papers and countless articles in magazines and newspapers around the world. He also established the International Institute on Stress at the University of Montreal. The body's "general adaptation syndrome" is often called "Selye syndrome."

Selye defined stress as "the nonspecific response of the body to any demand," which means the body's reaction to any change in its environment. Selye linked physical illnesses not just to bacterial and viral infections but also to hormones within the body that become activated whenever the body responds to external stressors, such as temperature extremes, pain, and threats to safety. Selye determined that many of the body's hormonal responses to stress were helpful and adaptive (positive change in response to environment), but others were maladaptive (unhelpful change) and placed physical demands on the body that could result in disease.

Still, Selye described stress as the spice of life; it might make one person sick while invigorating another. In one of his bestselling books, *The Stress of Life,* Selye offered this rhymed advice: "Fight for your highest attainable aim/But never put up resistance in vain." When people choose wisely about when to invest effort and emotional energy, they reduce the damaging side effects of stress, keep distress to a minimum, and increase our enjoyment of life.

* **autonomic nervous system** is a branch of the peripheral nervous system that controls various involuntary body activities, such as body temperature, metabolism, heart rate, blood pressure, breathing, and digestion. The autonomic nervous system has two parts—the sympathetic and parasympathetic branches.

* **immune system** (im-YOON SIS-tem) is the system of the body composed of specialized cells and the substances they produce that helps protect the body against disease-causing germs.

* **chronic** (KRAH-nik) lasting a long time or recurring frequently.

emotional or behavioral problems, post-traumatic stress disorder, or the development of stress-related illnesses. Chronic* stress is believed to be a factor in many cases of abuse, violence, and suicide. Over the long term, chronic stress may contribute to the development of cardiovascular problems, such as high blood pressure, heart disease, and stroke. People who experience chronic stress can benefit from working with a doctor or therapist to learn stress management techniques.

What Is the Antidote for Too Much Stress?

The antidote for stress is relaxation, creating a state of ease, rest, and repose within the body. Taking a deep breath almost always is the first step toward relaxation, allowing individuals to determine that the emergency that triggered the body's stress response has ended.

Relaxation response At the end of a stress response cycle, the body begins a relaxation response: Breathing slows down, hearts stop racing, muscles stretch out, minds become peaceful, and levels of stress hormones return to their baseline values. There are various techniques for achieving a relaxation response. Some people listen to music or sing, go for a long walk

* **paralysis** (pah-RAH-luh-sis) is the loss or impairment of the ability to move some part of the body.

or a run in the park, or practice meditation. Other techniques that promote a relaxation response include yoga, abdominal breathing, progressive muscle relaxation, biofeedback, guided imagery or visualization, hypnosis, prayer, belonging to support groups, or spending time with pets or loved ones. Because stress is an inevitable part of living, the long-term antidote for stress is learning coping strategies that allow people to live with it successfully.

Resilience Resilient people who experience high levels of stress but recover quickly and show low levels of illness are stress-resistant personalities. According to researchers, such resilient people seem to have several characteristics in common:

- They view change as a challenging and normal part of life, rather than as a threat.
- They have a sense of control over their lives, they believe that setbacks are temporary, and they believe that they will succeed if they work toward their goals.
- They have commitments to work, family, friends, support networks, and regular activities that promote relaxation, including hobbies, vacations, sports, yoga, and meditation.

Some people seem to be born with resilient personalities and good stress management skills. They know instinctively how to manage and how to find the help they need from others. However, at times when a little help is not enough and only extra-strength help will do, or when a person needs some coaching to improve coping skills, it may be useful to turn to a doctor, counselor, or therapist.

Resources

Books and Articles

Donovan, Sandy. *Keep Your Cool! What You Should Know about Stress.* Minneapolis, MN: Lerner, 2009.

Greenberg, Jerrold S. *Comprehensive Stress Management.* New York: McGraw-Hill, 2008.

Organization

American Institute of Stress. 124 Park Avenue, Yonkers, NY, 10703. Telephone: 914-963-1200. Web site: http://www.stress.org.

Stroke

A stroke is the sudden destruction of brain cells when blood flow to the brain is disrupted, usually by a blockage in a blood vessel. It can cause weakness, speech problems, paralysis*, and death, although most people survive.

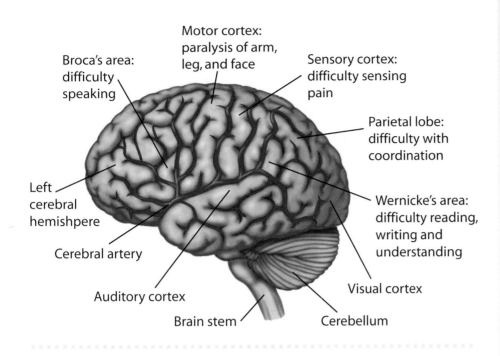

Broca's area: difficulty speaking

Motor cortex: paralysis of arm, leg, and face

Sensory cortex: difficulty sensing pain

Parietal lobe: difficulty with coordination

Left cerebral hemishpere

Cerebral artery

Auditory cortex

Brain stem

Cerebellum

Visual cortex

Wernicke's area: difficulty reading, writing and understanding

Strokes can affect many different parts of the brain. Illustration by Frank Forney. Reproduced by permission of Gale, a part of Cengage Learning.

Carmen's Story

While eating lunch with her grandfather on a sunny afternoon, 14 year-old Carmen was in the midst of describing her summer camp plans when suddenly one side of her grandfather's face went slack. He tried to speak, but he was slurring his words. Without warning, he clutched the picnic table, and the drinking glass he held smashed to the ground.

"Grandma," Carmen called. As her grandmother rushed to dial for emergency aid, Carmen held her grandfather's trembling hand.

In a few minutes, the ambulance arrived to carry him to the hospital, where a brain scan showed that Carmen's grandfather had undergone an ischemic (is-KEE-mik) stroke. Because Carmen and her grandmother acted quickly, the diagnosis was made in the Emergency Department less than three hours after his symptoms started, and the doctors were able to give him t-PA, a powerful drug that dissolved a blood clot that was blocking the flow of blood to his brain. Special guidelines specify that t-PA may be given only within *three hours* from the onset of stroke symptoms, so it was especially important that Carmen took prompt action. In a few days, her grandfather was ready to return home. Over several months, with the help of physical, occupational, and speech therapies, Carmen's grandfather was able to make a full recovery.

What Is a Stroke?

A stroke occurs when the blood supply to part of the brain is suddenly interrupted, or when a blood vessel in the brain bursts, spilling blood into the spaces surrounding neurons (nerve cells). Like other cells, brain cells die when they no longer receive oxygen and nutrients from the bloodstream or when they are damaged by sudden bleeding into or around the brain.

There are two major types of strokes. Ischemic strokes involve a reduced blood flow to the brain. Hemorrhagic (hem-o-RAJ-ik) strokes involve bleeding in the brain. "Ischemia" (is-KEY-me-a) is the term used to describe the loss of oxygen and nutrients when there is inadequate blood flow. If ischemia is left untreated, it can lead to infarction (in-FARK-shun), or cell death and tissue death in the surrounding area.

Ischemic Strokes

Ischemic strokes occur when a blood vessel to the brain becomes blocked, suddenly decreasing or stopping blood flow and ultimately causing an infarction. Ischemic strokes account for approximately 80 percent of all strokes. A blood clot (also called a thrombus) is the most common cause of vessel blockage and brain infarction.

Blood clots   Blood clotting is necessary in the body to stop bleeding and to allow repair of damaged areas, but when blood clots develop in the wrong place within an artery, they can cause injury by stopping the normal flow of blood. Problems with clots develop more frequently as people age.

An embolus is a clot that has formed in a blood vessel somewhere in the body, often in the heart. It can break away from the wall of the vessel where it was formed, travel through the circulatory system, and become wedged in the brain, causing an embolic stroke. Ischemic strokes also can be caused by the formation of a blood clot in one of the cerebral arteries (arteries supplying blood to the brain). If the clot grows large enough, it will block blood flow.

Stenosis   Stenosis, or a narrowing of the arteries, also can cause ischemia. Occurring in large arteries or small arteries, stenosis is called blood vessel disease or small vessel disease. The most common blood vessel

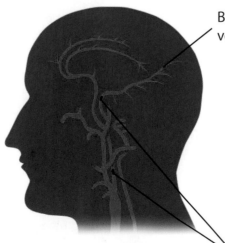

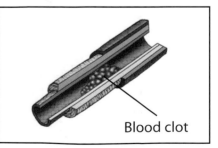

Blood clot blocks small vessels within the brain.

Blood clot

Blood clots create blockages in cerebral arteries.

A blockage in an artery that supplies blood to the brain can cause an ischemic stroke. *Illustration by Frank Forney. Reproduced by permission of Gale, a part of Cengage Learning.*

disease that causes stenosis is atherosclerosis. Deposits of plaque (a mixture of cholesterol and other fatty substances) build up along the inner walls of larger and medium sized arteries causing thickening, hardening, and loss of elasticity of the artery walls.

Transient ischemic attacks Some people get a warning that they may be headed for a future stroke. A transient ischemic attack (TIA) is a very small stroke caused by a temporarily blocked blood vessel. Unlike a full stroke, a TIA leaves no permanent damage. Symptoms are similar to those of a full stroke, but they usually last 24 hours or less. It is impossible to know whether the symptoms are caused by a stroke or by a TIA, so any symptoms should receive immediate medical attention. Having a TIA increases the risk of having a full stroke in the future, and medical attention can sometimes prevent or lessen the severity of the stroke.

Hemorrhagic Strokes

Hemorrhagic strokes are caused by burst blood vessels. In a healthy brain, the neurons do not come into direct contact with blood. Oxygen and nutrients move across a membrane from the blood vessel to the brain cells. Neuroglial (noo-ro-GLEE-al) cells help control which fluids and nutrients reach the neurons of the brain. When an artery in the brain bursts, blood spills out into the surrounding tissue, overriding the control of neuroglial cells and disrupting the delicate chemical balance of the brain.

Hemorrhagic strokes may occur in several ways. Aneurysms, or weak spots on artery walls, can stretch or "balloon" until eventually they break and spill blood into surrounding brain cells. Hemorrhages can also happen when plaque-encrusted arteries lose their elasticity and become brittle and thin enough to crack. Hypertension (high blood pressure) increases the risk that a brittle artery wall will give way and release blood into surrounding brain tissue.

Individuals who have an arteriovenous (ar-ter-ee-o-VEN-us) malformation (a tangle of defective blood vessels and capillaries within the brain that can rupture) can also be at increased risk for hemorrhagic stroke. Although hemorrhagic strokes are less common than ischemic strokes, they have a much higher fatality rate, because more brain tissue can be damaged more quickly.

How Do People Know They Are Having a Stroke?

Symptoms of stroke, such as those experienced by Carmen's grandfather, appear suddenly. They may include:

- Numbness or weakness of the face, arm, or leg, particularly on one side
- Confusion, trouble talking, and trouble understanding speech
- Difficulty seeing in one or both eyes
- Dizziness, difficulty walking, loss of balance, or loss of coordination
- Severe headache with no known cause

The United States and the World

- Stroke is the third leading cause of death in the United States, killing more than 160,000 people each year. About 75 percent of all strokes occur in people over the age of 65.

- Stroke is a significant cause of long-term disability.

- Strokes can occur at any age; however, the risk for stroke more than doubles each decade after the age of 55.

- Stroke may strike individuals of any race, but death due to stroke is higher for African Americans than for whites.

- In 2005, costs associated with stroke totaled about $57 billion.

- The southeastern region of the United States has the highest stroke mortality rates in the country, but it is not yet clear why this is the case.

- Approximately 700,000 strokes occur each year, and of these, about 500,000 are first strokes, whereas 200,000 occur in people who have had at least one previous stroke.

- The World Health Organization (WHO) estimates that strokes killed approximately 5.5 million people worldwide in 1999.

---

* **electrocardiogram** (e-lek-tro-KAR-dee-o-gram), also known as an EKG, is a test that records and displays the electrical activity of the heart.

* **CT scans** or CAT scans are the shortened name for computerized axial tomography (to-MOG-ra-fee), which uses computers to view structures inside the body.

Strokes are medical emergencies and require immediate medical attention.

How Is Stroke Diagnosed?

Doctors have diagnostic techniques and imaging tools to help diagnose strokes quickly and accurately. When a person with signs and symptoms of stroke arrives at the hospital, the first diagnostic step is a physical examination and a medical history. Often, an electrocardiogram* and a CT scans* will be done to check for signs of heart disease, evidence of prior TIAs, and heart rhythm disturbances. The patient may be asked to answer questions and to perform several physical and mental tests to evaluate the possibility or severity of brain damage.

Imaging tests also help healthcare professionals to evaluate stroke. The CT scan may rule out a hemorrhage or may show evidence of early infarction. If the stroke is caused by a hemorrhage, a CT scan can reveal any bleeding into the brain. MRIs* may be taken to detect subtler changes in brain tissue or areas of dead tissue soon after a stroke.

How Is Stroke Treated?

Stroke treatment most often involves medication and rehabilitation. Acute stroke therapy uses medication to stop a stroke while it is happening by quickly dissolving the blood clot that is causing the stroke or by stopping the bleeding of a hemorrhagic stroke. Surgery is almost never used for acute stroke treatment. Very rarely, and only in hemorrhagic stroke, a neurosurgeon may consider placing an intraventricular drain to remove some blood from a ventricle and relieve pressure on the brain. Carotid endarterecomy (surgery to remove plaque buildup in carotid arteries) may be indicated to prevent an ischemic stroke from happening, although it is rarely performed as an emergency procedure.

Medication and surgery   Various medications can be used to treat stroke:

- Antithrombotics work to counteract the chemicals in the body that cause blood to clot.

- Antiplatelet drugs prevent clotting by decreasing the activity of cells that contribute to the clotting properties of blood. They can reduce the risk of ischemic stroke.

- Anticoagulants reduce the stroke risk by thinning the blood and reducing its clotting properties.

- Thrombolytic agents can sometimes be used to treat an ongoing stroke. These drugs work by dissolving the blood clot that is blocking the blood vessel supplying the brain.

- Tissue plasminogen activator (t-PA) can be effective if given intravenously within three hours of the onset of stroke symptoms when a CT scan confirms that a person has suffered an ischemic stroke. However, t-PA increases the risk of major bleeding, so it can be used only when a patient fully meets the established guidelines, including the onset of symptoms less than three hours in duration. As of 2009, the majority of patients with ischemic stroke turned out to be ineligible for the t-PA treatment.

Surgery is not used to treat an ischemic stroke, but it is sometimes used to treat a hemorrhagic stroke. An attempt to surgically remove accumulated blood and intracranial pressure caused by a hemorrhagic stroke is a delicate procedure, as the surgery itself may generate additional bleeding, thus causing more harm. The surgeon may insert a tube called a shunt, to allow drainage and relieve pressure around the brain. In addition, surgery is sometimes used to repair vascular malformations in and around the brain.

Rehabilitation Post-stroke rehabilitation helps people overcome the disabilities that result from stroke damage. For some people, like Carmen's grandfather, acute stroke treatment and post-stroke therapy lead to a full recovery. For others, recovery is only partial.

Although strokes occur in the brain, they may affect the entire body and all activities of daily living. Some of the disabilities that may result from a stroke include paralysis, or partial paralysis, of different parts of the body, difficulties with memory and concentration, speech problems, and emotional distress as people cope with their changed circumstances. Rehabilitation may involve several different forms of therapy:

- Physical therapy helps people to regain movement, balance, and coordination and to reestablish skills such as sitting, walking, and moving from one activity to another.

- Occupational therapy helps people who have had strokes readapt to everyday life by relearning practical skills needed at home, such as dressing, eating, bathing, reading, and writing.

- Speech therapy addresses the speech and language problems that arise when a stroke causes brain damage in the language parts of the brain. Speech therapy helps people who have no deficits in cognition or thinking but have problems understanding written words, or problems forming speech. One common problem for people who have suffered stroke is aphasia (a-FAY-zha), a condition in which comprehension or expression of words is impaired. Speech therapists help stroke patients by working to improve language skills, develop alternative ways of communicating, and develop coping skills to deal with the frustration of not being able to communicate easily.

- Psychotherapy often is useful following a stroke, because depression, anxiety, frustration, and anger are common post-stroke symptoms.

Preventing Stroke

The most important risk factors* for stroke are hypertension (high blood pressure), heart disease, diabetes, and smoking. Others factors that increase the risk of having a stroke are heavy alcohol consumption, high

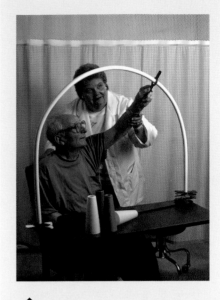

Physical therapy helps people who have had strokes regain movement, balance, and muscular coordination. *©Dwight Cendrowski/Alamy.*

* **MRI** which is short for magnetic resonance imaging, produces computerized images of internal body tissues based on the magnetic properties of atoms within the body.

* **risk factors** are any factors that increase the chance of developing a disease.

Dwight D. Eisenhower

Dwight D. Eisenhower (1890–1969) was a U.S. Army general and the thirty-fourth president of the United States. "Ike," as he was known, had a meteoric rise as a military commander during World War II. In 1953, he was elected to his first term in the White House. Despite having a heart attack in 1955 and a stroke in 1957, he was elected to a second term. Eisenhower completed his presidency in 1961, when John F. Kennedy was sworn in as thirty-fifth president.

* **atrial fibrillation** (AY-tree-al fib-ri-LAY-shun) is the arrhythmic or irregular beating of the left upper chamber of the heart. This leads to an irregular flow of blood and to the formation of blood clots that can leave the heart and travel to the brain, causing a stroke.

cholesterol levels, and genetic or congenital conditions, such as vascular (blood vessel) abnormalities.

Hypertension People with hypertension (high blood pressure) have a risk for stroke that is four to six times greater than those without hypertension. One-third of adults in the United States have high blood pressure. Antihypertensive drugs and attention to diet can decrease a person's risk for stroke.

Heart disease After hypertension, the second most powerful risk factor for stroke is heart disease, particularly the condition known as atrial fibrillation*. This condition is more prevalent in older people. Other forms of heart disease that can increase the chances of having stroke include malformations of heart muscle and some heart valve diseases. Cardiac surgery to correct heart malformation or the effects of heart disease can also cause stroke. Strokes occurring during surgery often are the result of dislodged plaques.

Diabetes People with diabetes have three times the risk of stroke as those without diabetes. The relative risk is highest in the fifth and sixth decades of life and decreases after that. People with diabetes who control their blood sugar level well, who avoid smoking, and who avoid or control hypertension, are less likely to have strokes.

Cigarette smoking Smokers have a 40 to 60 percent greater chance of having a stroke than nonsmokers. Smoking increases a person's chance for ischemic stroke, independent of all other risk factors.

Blood cholesterol levels High cholesterol levels can contribute to the risk of stroke. Too much cholesterol in the blood is associated with plaque developing in the walls of arteries (atherosclerosis), leading to stenosis of blood vessels. By lowering cholesterol through diet and exercise, a person can lower the risk for atherosclerosis and stroke. Doctors may prescribe cholesterol-lowering medication for people with high cholesterol levels.

Lifestyle changes Many strokes can be prevented with changes in lifestyle. These changes include:

- Stopping smoking
- Avoiding binge drinking and overconsumption of alcohol
- Avoiding illicit drugs: cocaine and crack cocaine can cause stroke, and marijuana may produce wide fluctuations in blood pressure and heart rate, which could contribute to stroke development

Medical measures To prevent stroke, doctors may prescribe medications to lower blood pressure and cholesterol levels. In some cases, particularly if a person has atrial fibrillation, doctors may prescribe regular doses of aspirin, coumadin, or other medications that prevent blood clotting. If carotid (ka-ROT-id) arteries (arteries supplying the brain) are partially blocked by plaque, surgery can clear them and prevent strokes in many cases.

Strokes can happen to people of either sex no matter what their age or racial background. Transient ischemic attacks (TIAs) multiply a person's risk of having a full stroke and should receive immediate medical attention.

▶ *See also* **Aneurysm** • **Heart Disease** • **Hypertension**

Resources

Books and Articles

Butler, Dori Hillestad. *My Grandpa Had a Stroke.* Washington, DC: Magination Press, 2007.

Hreib, Kinan K. *100 Questions and Answers about Stroke: A Lahey Clinic Guide.* Sudbury, MA: Jones and Bartlett, 2008.

Lindley, Richard I. *Stroke.* Oxford, UK: Oxford University Press, 2008.

Organizations

American Heart Association. 7272 Greenville Avenue, Dallas, TX, 75231-4596. Toll free: 800-AHA-USA1. Web site: http://www.americanheart.org.

Heart and Stroke Foundation of Canada. 222 Queen Street, Suite 1402, Ottawa, ON, K1P, 5V9, Canada. Telephone: 613-569-4361. Web site: http://www.hsf.ca/az/atoz-a.htm.

National Institute of Neurological Disorders and Stroke. P.O. Box 5801, Bethesda, MD, 20824, Web site: http://www.ninds.nih.gov/disorders/stroke/stroke.htm.

National Stroke Association. 96 Inverness Drive East, Suite I, Englewood, CO, 80112-5112. Toll free: 800-787-6537. Web site: http://www.stroke.org.

Stupor and Coma

Stupor and coma describe two different altered states of consciousness. Coma is the deeper of the two.

What Are Stupor and Coma?

Stupor and coma describe two different altered states of consciousness. Stupor is a state of unconsciousness from which an individual can only be roused with a forceful, physical stimulus. Coma is an even deeper level of unconsciousness, during which the individual does not have any voluntary movement or behavior. When in a coma, an individual cannot be aroused with verbal, physical, or even physically painful stimuli, and even basic reflexes may be lost.

* **dehydration** (dee-hi-DRAY-shun) is a condition in which the body is depleted of water, usually caused by excessive and unreplaced loss of body fluids, such as through sweating, vomiting, or diarrhea.

ABOUT CONSCIOUSNESS

Consciousness has two components: awareness and arousal. Awareness is the ability to receive and process all the information communicated by the five senses. People who have intact awareness are able to relate to themselves and to the outside world. Awareness itself is made up of two components: the psychological and the physiological realms. The psychological component involves the individual's mind and mental processes, whereas the physiological component refers to the chemical and physical functioning of the individual's brain and nervous system. The cortical areas of the cerebral hemispheres govern awareness. Awareness, then, suggests a higher level of intellectual functioning.

Arousal, however, is a more basic, physiological level of primitive functioning. Arousal is governed by the functioning of the reticular activating system, which is a network of structures (the brainstem, medulla, the thalamus, and variety of nerve pathways) that function together to produce and maintain arousal. Arousal is exemplified by the involuntary but predictable reflexes that are an individual's automatic response to specific stimuli.

The continuum of consciousness, then, ranges from full intellectual engagement at the highest end of functioning to complete brain death at the lowest end of functioning. States between these two extremes include lethargy, obtundation (reduced level of consciousness), and stupor. When in any of these states, an individual will respond in some capacity to stimuli, even though the stimulus may need to be sufficiently intense to garner even a minimal response (as may occur with stupor). In the case of coma, however, even an intense stimulus will fail to provoke a response.

What Causes Stupor and Coma?

Stupor and coma may stem from the same kinds of disorders. In each case, the disorders affect the functioning of the brain's nerve cells, causing them to respond very slowly or to cease responding. Common causes include liver disease, kidney failure, thyroid disorders, hypothermia (abnormally, dangerously low body temperature), hyperthermia (abnormal, dangerously high body temperature), toxic exposures/poisonings, excess alcohol, drugs such as sedatives or opioids, severe dehydration* and electrolyte imbalances, drug reactions, infection (particularly in the elderly), direct trauma (injury) to the brain, strokes, tumors, aneurysms, seizures, brain abscesses, heart attacks, metabolic problems (high blood glucose, low blood glucose, excess or deficient blood sodium), and oxygen deprivation (asphyxiation).

Who Is Likely to go into a Stupor or Coma?

Given the right circumstances, anybody can suffer from stupor or coma, although the elderly are particularly vulnerable. The same level of illness, trauma, or toxic exposure that a younger person might be able to weather successfully, may well produce stupor or coma in an older individual.

What are the Symptoms of Stupor and Coma?

The most notable symptom of stupor is the individual's inability to respond to normal stimuli. Instead, shouting, shaking, or painful stimuli are necessary to provoke a response. The individual's eyes may be open, but clearly not focusing. In coma, intense stimuli do not provoke a response, and the eyes are closed.

Other features of stupor and coma that may be present include abnormal breathing patterns; unusual contraction or flaccidity of muscles, resulting in odd positioning of limbs and/or head; abnormal dilatation or contraction of the pupils of the eyes; and odd eye movements.

How Are Stupor and Coma Diagnosed?

Impaired consciousness is quite evident upon initial observation, although determining the level and the cause of impairment requires further investigation. Differentiating between stupor and coma requires simple maneuvers to see whether the individual will arouse to intense stimuli (as in stupor) or whether no arousal is possible (as in coma). Physical examination will also be performed to look for other clues that may point to the reason for the impaired consciousness.

If coma is diagnosed, a rating system called the Glasgow Coma Scale (GCS) may be used to assess the depth of the coma, to monitor the individual's progress over time, and to roughly ascertain the individual's overall prognosis. The Glasgow Coma Scale uses a point system to evaluate three categories of functioning: opening of the eyes, using words or voice to respond, and motor response (moving a part of the body to respond). The highest level of functioning is assigned to individuals who spontaneously open their eyes, can give appropriate verbal responses to questions, and can carry out a simple command to move a part of their body. A GCS score of 3-5 may suggest fatal brain damage; a GCS score of eight or more suggests that the chance of recover is good.

Evaluation of the pupils of the eyes and breathing pattern are also important. Blood and urine tests will probably be performed in order to quickly diagnose the presence of toxins (such as high levels of alcohol, drugs, carbon dioxide, or poisons), abnormalities of blood chemistry (such as sodium, potassium, and glucose), liver or kidney failure, low blood oxygen, or infection. CT scans* or MRI* brain scans may be performed to evaluate the possibility of brain injury due to trauma, stroke, aneurysm, or tumor. Quick, thorough evaluation is necessary, so that the cause of the coma is quickly identified and potentially reversible conditions can be treated immediately.

How Are Stupor and Coma Treated?

Impairment of consciousness is considered a medical emergency. Evaluation and treatment of any abnormalities in respiration or circulation should be attended to immediately. Oxygen is often given, and an intravenous (in the vein) line is placed in case fluids or medications need to be given

* **CT scans** or CAT scans are the shortened name for computerized axial tomography (to-MOG-ra-fee), which uses computers to view structures inside the body.

* **MRI** which is short for magnetic resonance imaging, produces computerized images of internal body tissues based on the magnetic properties of atoms within the body.

* **diuretics** (dye-yoor-EH-tiks) are medications that increase the body's output of urine.

* **obesity** (o-BEE-si-tee)is an excess of body fat. People are considered obese if they weigh more than 30 percent above what is healthy for their height.

quickly. The ultimate treatment will depend on the underlying cause of the coma, although basic measure may include elevation of the head of the bed, use of diuretics* or steroid drugs to decrease swelling in the brain, and/or administration of sedative drugs to decrease muscle contractions. Infections may require antimicrobial drugs; chemical abnormalities may respond to the administration of sodium or glucose; dehydration may improve with fluids; narcotic overdose may be treated with Narcan; and antiepileptics may stop seizures. In severe situations, surgery may be necessary to relieve excess pressure on the brain or to remove or repair abnormalities (such as a tumor or bleeding aneurysm).

If the coma persists, it may become necessary to place a tube for feeding, either through the nose or through an incision in the abdomen into the stomach. Physical therapy may be employed to move the individual through passive range of motion exercises in order to keep joints and muscles as healthy as possible.

What Is the Prognosis of Stupor and Coma?

Prognosis (the prediction of future healing) depends on the underlying condition responsible for the impaired level of consciousness, the patient's original medical condition, the duration of the stupor or coma, how quickly the individual begins to make a recovery, and the degree of structural damage that the brain has suffered. When the impairment is due to sedative overdose, complete recovery is likely, unless oxygen deprivation has caused brain damage. Prognosis for recovery after impairment due to low blood sugar is very good, if the low blood sugar has been corrected in less than an hour. Head injury may have a good prognosis, although coma lasting more than three months reverses this prognosis. A stroke that prompts a coma lasting less than six hours may have a reasonably good prognosis, although coma lasting more than six hours has a poor prognosis. Heart attack or oxygen deprivation share a poor prognosis.

With treatment, stupor or coma due to toxic exposures (such as drug overdoses) has a higher rate of complete recovery than many other causes of impairment. Only about 15 percent of adults who suffer stupor or coma due to other causes and who remain in a coma for more than just a few hours, return to their previous level of functioning. Children and younger adults may return to their expected level of functioning after as long as two months of impairment of consciousness.

Can Stupor and Coma be Prevented?

Although there is no way to prevent stupor and coma, certain basic measures can decrease the risk, including wearing seatbelts and using appropriate protective head gear (helmets while bike riding); avoiding illicit drugs and excess alcohol; using prescription medications exactly as prescribed; and following standard recommendations for avoiding or treating high blood pressure, diabetes, obesity*, high cholesterol, and other medical conditions.

Resources

Books and Articles

Marx, John A., et al. *Rosen's Emergency Medicine,* 6th ed. St. Louis, MO: Mosby, 2006.

Senelick, Richard C., and Karla Dougherty. *Living with Stroke: A Guide for Families,* 3rd ed. Clifton Park, NY: Delmar Cengage Learning, 2001.

Organizations

Brain Injury Association. 1608 Spring Hill Road, Suite 110, Vienna, VA, 20036. Toll free: 800-444-6443. Web sites: http://www.biausa.org; http://www.biausa.org/Pages/coma.html.

National Institute of Neurological Disorders and Stroke. P.O. Box 5801, Bethesda, MD, 20824, Web site: http://www.ninds.nih.gov/disorders/coma/coma.htm.

Stuttering

Stuttering is a speech disorder in which the normal flow of words is broken by sounds that are repeated or held longer than normal, or by problems with starting a word.

What Does Stuttering Sound Like?

People who stutter may repeat a speech sound over and over (st-st-stuttering), or they may hold a sound longer than normal (sssssstuttering). In some cases, they may have trouble starting a word, leading to abnormal stops in their speech (no sound). Yet many people who stutter learn to control the problem. The list of famous people in history who overcame stuttering includes scientists Isaac Newton and Charles Darwin; Clara Barton; George VI of England, Winston Churchill, and Joe Biden; and actors Marilyn Monroe, Bruce Willis, and James Earl Jones.

What Is Stuttering?

Stuttering is a speech disorder in which the normal flow of speech is broken. Along with the effort to speak, some people who stutter also make unusual face or body movements, such as rapid eye blinking or trembling of the lips. Certain situations, such as speaking on the phone, tend to make stuttering worse. By contrast, people usually do not stutter when they sing, whisper, or speak as part of a group, or when they do not hear their own voices. No one is sure why this is so.

Being a Good Listener

People who talk to others who stutter should do the following:

- Be patient. Do not finish sentences or fill in words for the person.

- Make normal eye contact. Try not to look embarrassed or concerned.

- Be understanding. Do not make remarks such as "slow down" or "relax."

- Set a relaxed pace. Try to keep their own speech at a medium speed.

- Be sensible. If they do not understand what the other person says, they should politely ask the person to repeat it.

* **sex-linked** genetic traits involve the chromosomes that determine whether a person is male or female. They usually affect boys, who have only one X chromosome.

* **anxiety** (ang-ZY-e-tee) can be experienced as a troubled feeling, a sense of dread, fear of the future, or distress over a possible threat to a person's physical or mental well-being.

Most children go through a stage of choppy speech when they are first learning to talk. In addition, teenagers and adults often add extra sounds (for example, "uh" and "um") to their speech, and they occasionally repeat sounds. These speech interruptions are perfectly normal. Such problems are considered a disorder only when they last past the age when most children outgrow them and get in the way of communicating clearly. Treating stuttering even in young children may help prevent a lifelong problem. Treatment may be considered for children who stutter longer than six months or for those who seem to struggle when they speak. Sometimes, however, no treatment is the best treatment, especially in the case of children whose stuttering worsens when attention is focused on the problem.

What Causes Stuttering?

Stuttering usually begins between two and six years of age. About 1 percent of children stutter, and boys are three times more likely to do so than girls. The most common form of stuttering is thought to arise when children's developing speech and language abilities are not yet able to keep up with their needs. Stuttering occurs when they search for the right word. This kind of stuttering usually is outgrown.

Another form of stuttering is caused by signal problems between the brain and the nerves or muscles involved in speech. The brain is unable to control all the different parts of the speech system. This kind of stuttering sometimes is seen in people who have had a stroke or brain injury. Yet another, less common form of the disorder is caused by severe stress or some types of mental illness. Some kinds of stuttering seem to run in families, and it is likely that stuttering is sex-linked* (je-NE-tik) in some cases, although no gene for stuttering had been found as of 2009.

How Is Stuttering Linked to Fear?

Contrary to popular belief, there is no evidence that stuttering is caused by anxiety* (ang-ZY-e-tee); an intense, long-lasting feeling of fear; worry; or nervousness. Yet people who stutter may become fearful of meeting new people, speaking in public, or talking on the phone. In such cases, it is the stuttering that causes the fear, not the activity.

How Is Stuttering Diagnosed?

Stuttering usually is diagnosed by a speech-language pathologist (pa-THAH-lo-jist), a professional who is trained to test and treat people with speech, language, and voice disorders. The speech pathologist will ask questions about the problem, such as when it first started and when it is most and least noticeable. The speech pathologist will also test speech and language abilities. In addition, some people may be sent to other professionals for hearing tests and medical tests of the nervous system.

How Is Stuttering Treated?

There are several treatments that may improve stuttering, although none is an instant cure. With young children, the focus often is on teaching parents how to help the child at home. Parents typically are told to have a relaxed attitude and give their children plenty of chances to speak. They may be warned not to criticize their children's speech. They may be urged not to pay attention to the children. Instead, they can be good role models, speaking in a slow, relaxed manner themselves and listening patiently when their children talk.

Speech therapy can help older children, teenagers, and adults relearn how to speak or unlearn faulty ways of speaking. Some people who stutter have fears related to the disorder, such as a fear of speaking in public. Such problems caused by the stuttering can be helped with psychotherapy (sy-ko-THER-a-pea), in which people talk about their feelings, beliefs, and experiences with a mental health professional who can help them work out issues that play a part in their speech problems.

▶ *See also* **Anxiety and Anxiety Disorders • Social Phobia (Social Anxiety Disorder) • Speech Disorders**

Resources

Books and Articles

De Geus, Eelco. *Sometimes I Just Stutter.* Memphis, TN: Stuttering Foundation of America, 1999.

Stuttering and Your Child: Questions and Answers, 3rd ed. Memphis, TN: Stuttering Foundation of America, 2007.

Williams, Dale F. *Stuttering Recovery: Personal and Empirical Perspectives.* Mahwah, NJ: Erlbaum, 2006.

Organizations

American Speech-Language-Hearing Association. 2200 Research Boulevard, Rockville, MD, 20850-3289. Toll free: 800-638-8255. Web site: http://www.asha.org/public/speech/disorders/stuttering.htm.

National Institute on Deafness and Other Communication Disorders, National Institutes of Health. 31 Center Drive, MSC 2320, Bethesda, MD, 20892-2320. Toll free: 800-241-1044. Web site: http://www.nidcd.nih.gov/health/voice/stutter.htm.

National Stuttering Association. 119 W. Fortieth Street, 14th Floor, New York, NY, 10018. Toll free: 800-937-8888. Web site: http://www.nsastutter.org.

Stuttering Foundation of America. P.O. Box 11749, 3100 Walnut Grove Road, Suite 603, Memphis, TN, 38111-0749. Toll free: 800-992-9392. Web site: http://www.stutteringhelp.org.

Substance Abuse

Substance abuse is the unhealthy, even dangerous pattern of over consuming alcohol, tobacco, illegal drugs, prescription drugs, and other substances (such as paint thinners or aerosol gasses) that change how the mind and body work. It is possible to abuse some substances without becoming physically, emotionally, or psychologically dependent on them, but continued abuse tends to make people dependent. Dependency on some substances happens very quickly and is difficult to reverse.

What Is Substance Abuse?

Substance abuse is the unhealthy, even dangerous over consumption of various substances such as alcohol and other drugs that usually leads to frequent, serious problems at home, school, or work. People who abuse substances can get sick, ruin their relationships with other people, destroy their lives and the lives of family members, and even die, and while under the influence, they can injure or kill others. In 2007, 19.9 million Americans age 12 and over said they were current users of illegal drugs. In that same year, more than 17 million Americans age 12 or older reported that they drank alcohol heavily. Heavy drinking means that these people binge drank or they drank five or more drinks on five or more days during the previous month. Substance abuse is a serious problem in the United States.

Substance abuse is not the same as occasional alcohol or other drug use. When people are addicted to a substance, they develop a strong physical or psychological need for that drug. One hallmark of addiction is tolerance (TOL-er-uns), which means that over time, people need more and more of the substance to feel a high. Another symptom is withdrawal,

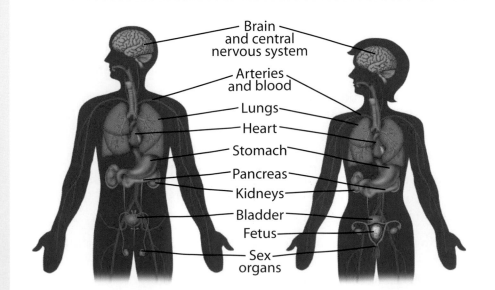

Substance abuse and addiction affect many different parts of the body. *Illustration by Frank Forney. Reproduced by permission of Gale, a part of Cengage Learning.*

which means that people who are addicted have physical symptoms and feel sick if they stop using the substance.

Alcohol and other drugs cause "intoxication" (in-TOK-sih-KAY-shun), the medical term for a temporary feeling of being high or drunk that occurs just after using a drug. Intoxication leads to changes in the way people think and act. For example, people may become angry, moody, confused, or uncoordinated. These changes increase the risk that people will make poor choices, have accidents that hurt themselves or others, or behave in a way that they will later regret.

Different substances have different effects on the body. Substances that are commonly abused in the United States include the following:

- Alcohol
- Amphetamines
- Anabolic steroids
- Cocaine
- Depressants
- Hallucinogens
- Inhalants
- Marijuana
- Narcotics
- Prescription medications
- Nonprescription (over-the-counter) medications
- Tobacco

What Causes Substance Abuse?

People give many reasons for starting to drink alcohol or use other drugs. Some people are looking for an easy way to escape problems at home, school, or work. Others hope that alcohol or other drugs will help them fit in or make them appear to be something better than what they are. Some may use substances to "treat" or "self-medicate" depression or boredom. Still others are initially just curious. Whatever the original reason, no one can say for sure which people will go on to have a serious substance abuse problem. However, certain factors raise the risk that abuse will develop. Risk factors for substance abuse problems include the following:

- Family history of substance abuse
- Using alcohol or tobacco at a young age
- Depression
- Low self-esteem*
- Feeling like an outsider
- Poverty
- Child abuse or neglect
- Family problems

* **self-esteem** is the value that people put on the mental image that they have of themselves.

Cocaine is a mood-altering drug that interferes with normal transport of the neurotransmitter dopamine, which carries messages from neuron to neuron. When cocaine molecules block dopamine receptors, too much dopamine remains active in the synaptic gaps between neurons, creating feelings of excitement and euphoria. *Illustration by Frank Forney. Reproduced by permission of Gale, a part of Cengage Learning.*

Cocaine

Dopamine

Vesicles containing dopamine

Transmitting neuron

Dopamine reuptake transporter functioning normally

Dopamine transporter blocked by cocaine

Synapse

Dopamine receptors

Receiving neuron

The United States and the World

The World Health Organization (WHO) and the U.S. Centers for Disease Control and Prevention (CDC) accumulate statistics about health problems resulting from substance abuse. Notable facts include the following:

In 2004, 19,838 people died as a result of accidental drug overdoses. That number increased from 11,155 in 1999. The abuse of legal drugs among people ages 15 to 24 is likely responsible for the dramatic increase.

In 2007, twice as many males (12.5%) as females (5.7%) were categorized as substance abusers; however, abuse rates among males and females ages 12 to 17 was equal.

In 2007, 12.5 percent of people over the age of 12 reported that they had driven a vehicle while under the influence of alcohol or other drugs.

Some of these factors can be changed or controlled by the people themselves, but others cannot. However, that does not mean that those who come from troubled families or low income neighborhoods are destined to be substance abusers. Certain other factors raise the odds that young people will be able to cope with problems without turning to alcohol or other drugs. These factors include the following:

- Learning to do something well
- Being active at school or in the community
- Having a caring adult or friend to talk to

Addiction is a special type of dependence in which people have a compulsive need to use the substance no matter what the consequences are. People who are psychologically addicted need to keep using the substance to feel satisfied. People who are physically addicted feel sick and have physical withdrawal symptoms if they stop using the substance. The risk and type of dependence varies by substance. Substance abuse occurs among people of all ages, cultures, sexes, and races.

What Are Some Commonly Abused Substances?

People abuse a wide variety of drugs, both legal and illegal. Legally available substances include alcohol, tobacco, chemicals in certain household products, over-the-counter drugs, and medicines prescribed by a doctor. Illegally sold substances include numerous street drugs.

Alcohol Although moderate drinking (two to four drinks a day for men and one to two drinks a day for women and older people) is not normally considered harmful, millions of people in the United States abuse alcohol or are alcoholics (people who are physically dependent on alcohol). A 2007 national survey found that 17 million Americans are heavy drinkers and that 57.8 million people engage in binge drinking (more than five drinks on one occasion).

Alcohol affects virtually every organ in the body, and long-term use can lead to a number of medical problems. The immediate effects of drinking too much include slurred speech, poor coordination, unsteady walking, memory problems, poor judgment, and the inability to concentrate. Drinking too much alcohol at one time can cause alcohol poisoning and sudden death. The recklessness that comes from drinking too much is a leading cause of traffic accidents and other injuries. In addition, alcohol drinking by pregnant women is the cause of the most common preventable birth defect fetal alcohol syndrome*. Long-term risks of heavy drinking include liver damage, heart disease*, neurological effects, reduced cognitive functioning, sexual problems for men, and trouble getting pregnant for women.

Tobacco Tobacco contains nicotine (NIK-o-teen), a highly addictive chemical. Nicotine is readily absorbed from tobacco smoke in the lungs, whether the smoke comes from cigarettes, cigars, or pipes. Smoking is the number one cause of preventable death in the United States. The long-term health risks include cancer, lung disease, heart disease, and stroke*. Smoking by pregnant women has been linked to miscarriage*, stillbirth*, premature birth*, low birth weight*, and infant death. Nicotine is readily absorbed from smokeless tobacco as well. Like smoking, dipping or chewing tobacco can have serious long-term effects, including cancer of the mouth, gum problems, loss of teeth, and heart disease.

Marijuana Marijuana (mar-ih-HWAH-nuh; nicknames: pot, herb, weed, blunts, Mary Jane) is the most widely used illegal drug. It is typically the first illegal drug tried by teenagers. It is a mixture of dried, shredded flowers and leaves from the cannabis plant. Marijuana usually is smoked in a cigarette, pipe, or water pipe, but some users also mix it with foods or use it to brew tea. Short-term effects of marijuana use include euphoria*, sleepiness, increased hunger, trouble keeping track of time, memory problems, inability to concentrate, poor coordination, increased heart rate, paranoia*, and anxiety. Long-term risks include lung disease, changes in hormone levels, lower sperm counts in men, and infertility.

Hallucinogens Hallucinogens (huh-LOO-sih-no-jenz) are drugs that distort a person's view of reality. They include LSD (lysergic acid diethylamide; nickname: acid), PCP (phencyclidine; nicknames: angel dust, loveboat), psilocybin (SY-lo-SY-bin; nickname: magic mushrooms), mescaline (MES-kuh-len), and peyote (pay-YO-tee or pay-YO-tay). People who use

Medicinal Marijuana

Marijuana is an illegal drug. In some states, however, it can legally be prescribed for certain medical purposes. Research indicates that marijuana may help in the treatment of glaucoma*, and it may relieve the nausea and wasting away that people with AIDS and cancer sometimes experience as a side effect of medical treatments. But research also shows that marijuana smoke contains more tar than cigarette smoke and may contain high levels of other cancer-causing agents. As of 2009, further research was needed and public policies regarding marijuana remained controversial.

* **glaucoma** is a group of disorders that cause pressure to build in the eye, which may result in vision loss.

* **fetal alcohol syndrome** which occurs if the fetus is exposed to alcohol, is a condition that can be associated with mental, physical, and behavioral differences. Oppositional behavioral problems, learning difficulties, mental retardation, and retarded growth can occur in the children of women who drink alcohol while they are pregnant.

* **heart disease** is a broad term that covers many conditions that prevent the heart from working properly to pump blood throughout the body.

* **stroke** is a brain-damaging event usually caused by interference with blood flow to the brain. A stroke may occur when a blood vessel supplying the brain becomes clogged or bursts, depriving brain tissue of oxygen. As a result, nerve cells in the affected area of the brain, and the specific body parts they control, do not properly function.

* **miscarriage** (MIS-kare-ij) is the end of a pregnancy through the death of the embryo or fetus before birth.

* **stillbirth** is the birth of a dead fetus.

* **premature birth** (pre-ma-CHUR) means born too early. In humans, it means being born after a pregnancy term lasting less than 37 weeks.

* **low birth weight** means born weighing less than normal. In humans, it refers to a full-term (pregnancy lasting 37 weeks or longer) baby weighing less than 5 pounds.

* **euphoria** (yoo-FOR-ee-uh) is an abnormally high mood with the tendency to be overactive and overly talkative, and to have racing thoughts and overinflated self-confidence.

* **paranoia** (pair-a-NOY-a) refers to either an unreasonable fear of harm by others (delusions of persecution) or an unrealistic sense of self-importance (delusions of grandeur).

these drugs may lose all sense of time, distance, and direction. They may behave strangely or violently, which can lead to serious injuries or death. Users react differently to hallucinogens, and some individuals have bad experiences with them.

LSD is one of the most potent of all mind-altering drugs. It may be taken in the form of paper that has been dipped in the drug, powder, liquid, gelatin, or pills. LSD can last for as long as 12 hours in the body. The physical effects of LSD use include dilated (widened) pupils, increased heart rate, higher blood pressure, sweating, loss of appetite, trouble sleeping, dry mouth, and shaking. The psychological effects are much more dramatic, however. Users may feel several different emotions at once, or they may swing from one emotion to another, from euphoria to paranoia. They may have bizarre or terrifying thoughts, or they may see things that are not really there, like walls melting. Some users later have flashbacks, in which they relive part of what they experienced while taking the drug, even though the drug is no longer active in their bodies. Hallucinogens are not physically addictive, but people using them are at risk for accidents,

SAME PROBLEM, DIFFERENT SOLUTION

In the United States, using and selling drugs such as marijuana and heroin is illegal, and people who break drug laws go to jail. In the Netherlands, the government is trying a different approach that stresses treatment rather than punishment.

In the mid-1970s, the Netherlands was hit by a sharp upswing in heroin use. In response, the government launched a policy called harm reduction, which aims to lower the harmful effects of drug use for both users and other members of society. The policy is based on the belief that so-called soft drugs, such as marijuana and the related drug hashish (hah-SHESH), are less dangerous than so-called hard drugs, such as heroin, cocaine, amphetamines, and methamphetamine. To encourage people not to try hard drugs, the government tolerates the sale of small amounts of marijuana and hashish in adults-only coffee shops, much the way alcohol is sold in bars. Marijuana is still considered a controlled substance, but the government generally does not enforce the law regarding it.

Much debate in the early 2000s surrounded this policy and how well it was perceived to work. However, the number of drug addicts in the Netherlands was lower than in many countries. In addition, the average age of addicts was rising, which suggested that fewer young people were getting hooked. But the rate of marijuana and hashish use increased in the late 1990s and early 2000s, although it remained lower than in the United States. Furthermore, the policy failed to address the impact on international laws. Substances were brought into the Netherlands from and through countries where the sale and use of marijuana was strictly prohibited.

violence, panic attacks*, and other consequences of impaired judgment. All of these substances are illegal to use, make, or sell.

PCP can be snorted, smoked, or eaten. It can cause bizarre and sometimes violent behavior. Other possible effects of PCP use include increased or shallow breathing rate, higher blood pressure, flushing, sweating, numbness, poor coordination, and confused or irrational thinking. High doses can lead to seeing or hearing things that are not really there, paranoia, seizures*, coma*, injuries, and suicidal behavior.

Stimulants Stimulants (STIM-yoo-lunts) are drugs that produce a temporary feeling of euphoria, alertness, power, and energy. As the high wears off, however, depression and edginess set in. Stimulants include cocaine (ko-KANE; nicknames: coke, snow, blow, nose candy), crack cocaine, amphetamine (am-FET-uh-mean), methamphetamine (METH-am-FET-uh-mean; nicknames: speed, meth, crank), and crystallized methamphetamine (nicknames: ice, crystal, glass).

Cocaine is a white powder that is either snorted into the nose or injected into a vein. Crack is a form of cocaine that has been chemically changed so that it can be smoked. Both forms are very addictive. Possible physical effects of cocaine and crack use include increased heart rate, higher blood pressure, increased breathing rate, heart attack, stroke, trouble breathing, seizures, and a reduced ability to fight infection. Possible psychological effects include violent or strange behavior, paranoia, seeing or hearing things that are not really there, feeling as if bugs are crawling over the skin, anxiety, and depression. Eventually, cocaine addicts often wind up losing interest in food, sex, friends, family, everything except getting high.

Amphetamines are human-made stimulants that speed up the central nervous system*, creating a sense of euphoria and increased energy. Amphetamines can be taken orally, injected, smoked, or sniffed. They may be legally prescribed to treat attention deficit hyperactivity disorder (ADHD), to suppress appetite, and to combat fatigue or narcolepsy (a disorder that causes uncontrolled falling asleep). Amphetamines include benzedrine, dexedrine, and methedrine. Street names for amphetamines include black beauties, crystal, hearts, bennies, crank, ice, speed, and meth.

People who abuse amphetamines need more and more of the drug to achieve the same effect or high. When they become dependent, amphetamine users may be jittery, lose weight, feel depressed, anxious, restless, hostile, and lack energy. An overdose may cause tachycardia (very fast heartbeat), high blood pressure, seizures, fever, delirium, paranoia, psychosis*, coma, and cardiovascular collapse.

Narcotics Narcotics (nahr-KOT-iks) are addictive painkillers that produce a relaxed feeling and an immediate high, followed by restlessness and an upset stomach. They can also be deadly. Drugs in this class include heroin (HAIR-oh-in; nicknames: smack, H, skag, junk), morphine (MOR-feen), opium (OH-pee-um), and codeine (KO-deen).

* **panic attacks** are periods of intense fear or discomfort with a feeling of doom and a desire to escape. During a panic attack, a person may shake, sweat, be short of breath, and experience chest pain.

* **seizures** (SEE-zhurs) are sudden bursts of disorganized electrical activity that interrupt the normal functioning of the brain, often leading to uncontrolled movements in the body and sometimes a temporary change in consciousness.

* **coma** (KO-ma) is an unconscious state, like a very deep sleep. A person in a coma cannot be awakened, and cannot move, see, speak, or hear.

* **central nervous system** (SEN-trul NER-vus SIS-tem) is the part of the nervous system that includes the brain and spinal cord.

* **psychosis** (sy-KO-sis) refers to mental disorders in which the sense of reality is so impaired that a patient cannot function normally. People with psychotic disorders may experience delusions (exaggerated beliefs that are contrary to fact), hallucinations (something that a person perceives as real but that is not actually caused by an outside event), incoherent speech, and agitated behavior, but they usually are not aware of their altered mental state.

The Opium Trade

Ancient Chinese medical texts indicated that opium, imported to the West from China by Arab traders in the 8th century, was used originally for medicinal purposes. When tobacco was introduced to China from the Philippines, the mixing of tobacco with opium became popular. British colonial traders recognized the strong demand for opium. Despite an 18th-century edict by the Chinese government banning the sale of opium and the operation of opium houses, the British continued its sale on the black market. During the late 18th century, opium was at times the largest single commodity in trade.

* **HIV** or human immunodeficiency virus (HYOO-mun ih-myoo-no-dih-FIH-shen-see), is the virus that causes AIDS (acquired immunodeficiency syndrome).

* **bone marrow** is the soft tissue inside bones where blood cells are made.

Heroin is made from morphine, a natural substance that comes from the poppy plant. It is a powder that is injected, snorted, or smoked, and it is highly addictive. Immediate effects of heroin use include a heavy feeling in the arms and legs, warm flushing of the skin, dry mouth, clouded thinking, and going back and forth between being wide awake and feeling drowsy. In addition, street heroin varies in strength, and users never know if they are getting a particularly strong dose. If they do, they can overdose (OD) easily, resulting in coma and death. Long-term effects include collapsed veins, infection of the heart lining and valves, liver disease, and HIV*/AIDS from sharing needles.

Sedatives (SED-uh-tivz), sometimes called tranquilizers (TRANK-will-LY-zerz) or sleeping pills, include barbiturates (downers). These drugs produce a calming effect and sleepiness. Physicians prescribe them to relieve anxiety, promote sleep, and treat seizures. When they are abused or taken at high doses, however, many of these drugs can lead to loss of consciousness and death. Combining sedatives with alcohol is particularly dangerous. Possible effects of sedative abuse include poor judgment, slurred speech, staggering, poor coordination, and slow reflexes.

Inhalants

Inhalants are chemical vapors that can be inhaled to produce mind-altering effects. The vapors then enter the lungs. There are three types of inhalants: solvents (such as paint thinners, gasoline, glues, felt-tip marker fluid), gases (such as butane lighters, whipping cream aerosols, spray paints, deodorant sprays, and nitrous oxide or "laughing gas"), and nitrites.

The physical effects of inhalants depend on the chemical being inhaled. Many cause serious, often irreversible health problems, and sometimes cause death. Users can lose consciousness. Other serious, but potentially reversible, effects include liver damage, kidney damage, and depletion of blood oxygen. Irreversible effects of inhalants include hearing loss, loss of muscle control and limb spasms, damage to the central nervous system and brain, damage to the bone marrow*, lung damage, and heart failure.

Club drugs

Club drugs are drugs that are mainly used by young people at parties, clubs, and bars. Although users may think these are harmless, research has shown that they can cause serious health problems and sometimes even death. When combined with alcohol, they can be particularly dangerous. Drugs in this category include MDMA (nicknames: XTC, ecstasy, Adam) GHB (nicknames: liquid ecstasy, Georgia home boy), Rohypnol (nicknames: roofies, roach), and ketamine (nickname: special K).

MDMA combines some of the properties of hallucinogens and stimulants. Possible effects include euphoria, confusion, paranoia, increased heart rate, higher blood pressure, blurred vision, faintness, chills, and sweating. Because this drug is increasingly abused at dances, young people may forget to drink, become dehydrated, and need to be rushed to the emergency room for immediate treatment. Possible psychological effects include confusion, depression, sleep problems, anxiety, and paranoia. Research has linked MDMA to long-term damage in parts of the brain that are critical for thought, memory, and pleasure.

GHB, Rohypnol, and ketamine are often colorless, tasteless, and odorless, which makes it easy for someone to slip one of these drugs into another person's drink. As a result, these substances are sometimes called "date rape" drugs, because they have been used against women who were drugged unknowingly and then raped. To make matters worse, people may be unable to remember what happened to them while they were under the influence of one of these drugs.

Prescription and Over-the-Counter Drugs

People can abuse legal medicines by taking more than prescribed, using them for nonmedical reasons, or using them to treat unrelated illnesses. The most commonly abused prescription and over-the-counter medicines are stimulants, pain relievers, depressants (such as sleeping pills), cough and cold medicines, and laxatives.

Abusing these substances can cause physical and psychological dependence. Some prescription medications contain alcohol and narcotics—such as codeine—that are physically addicting. Combining alcohol with prescription and over-the-counter drugs, or mixing drugs, can change the effectiveness of the drugs and cause harmful side effects.

Anabolic steroids

Anabolic steroids (AN-uh-BOL-ik STER-oidz) are drugs that are related to testosterone (tes-TOS-tuh-rone), the major male sex hormone. Although these drugs have medical uses, many athletes and bodybuilders abuse them because they can increase muscle build-up with weight lifting or strength training. Although steroids may seem like a shortcut to improved sports performance and a more muscular body, they carry serious health risks. In boys and men, steroids can reduce sperm production, shrink the testicles, enlarge the breasts, and cause problems with sexual performance. In girls and women, they can lead to unwanted body hair, a deep voice, and irregular periods. Steroids can damage the heart, liver, and kidneys. In teenagers, they can stunt bone growth, making users reach a shorter final height than they would have otherwise. High doses of testosterone can also cause outbursts of aggressive or violent behavior (steroid rage).

What Are Some Other Risks of Substance Abuse?

Abusing drugs leads to unclear thinking and unpredictable behavior. Many drugs also cause poor coordination and slow reflexes. It is little wonder, then, that substance abuse is closely tied to accidents and injuries. In 2006, 25 percent of drivers ages 15 to 20 who were killed in automobile accidents were under the influence of alcohol at the time their deaths.

In the United States, substance abuse is a major factor in the spread of infection with HIV (human immunodeficiency virus), the virus that

* **outpatient** a medical procedure that is conducted in a doctor's office or hospital for treatment but does not require an overnight stay in a hospital bed.

* **psychotherapy** (sy-ko-THER-a-pea) is the treatment of mental and behavioral disorders by support and insight to encourage healthy behavior patterns and personality growth.

causes AIDS. It is a direct cause, because many drugs are injected into a vein, and people can spread HIV by using or sharing unclean needles. It is also an indirect cause, because people whose thinking is clouded by alcohol or other drugs are more likely to have unsafe sex, which increases their risk of catching HIV from an infected partner.

How Is Substance Abuse Diagnosed and Treated?

Diagnosis Substance abuse often is difficult to diagnose and treat. Doctors can screen for substance abuse through a medical history, a physical exam, and sometimes blood or urine testing, but doctors and family members often have a hard time convincing substance abusers that they need help. In many cases, substance abusers are more afraid of losing the drug and of withdrawal symptoms than of the health and safety consequences of continued use.

Treatment Treatment for substance abuse consists of helping people stop using the substance, treating withdrawal symptoms, and preventing people from returning to substance abuse afterwards. Outpatient* psychotherapy* and self-help groups can be effective. People with severe problems may require residential treatment programs. Treatment often is provided by doctors and organizations that specialize in substance abuse programs. Steps for helping substance abusers are as follows:

- Evaluate people for psychiatric or medical disorders
- Teach them about the effects of the drug and their addiction
- Offer mutual support and self-help groups
- Provide individual and group psychotherapy
- Offer a replacement for the substance being given up
- Emphasize behavior changes that promote not using the substance
- Offer rehabilitation and life skills training

Even people who are successfully treated must guard against starting to use the abused substance again. People with serious medical or psychiatric symptoms, people who overdose on drugs, and people who have toxic reactions to drugs require immediate medical treatment.

▶ *See also* **Alcoholism • Eating Disorders: Overview • Pregnancy • Prematurity • Tobacco-Related Diseases**

Resources

Books and Articles

Freimuth, Marilyn. *Addicted? Recognizing Destructive Behavior before It's Too Late.* Lanham, MD: Rowman and Littlefield, 2008.

Klosterman, Lorrie. *The Facts about Drugs and the Body.* New York: Marshall Cavendish Benchmark, 2008.

Rebman, Renee C. *Addictions and Risky Behaviors: Cutting, Bingeing, Snorting, and Other Dangers.* Berkeley Heights, NJ: Enslow, 2006.

Schwartzenberger, Tina, ed. *Substance Use and Abuse.* New York: Weigl, 2007.

Organizations

Alcoholics Anonymous. Grand Central Station, P.O. Box 459, New York, NY, 10163. Telephone: 212-870-3400. Web site: http://www.aa.org.

National Institute on Alcohol Abuse and Alcoholism. 5635 Fishers Lane, MSC 9304, Bethesda, MD, 20892-9304. Telephone: 301-443-3860. Web site: http://www.niaaa.nih.gov.

National Institute on Drug Abuse–National Institutes of Health. 6001 Executive Boulevard, Room 5213, Bethesda, MD, 20892-9561, Web site: http://www.nida.nih.gov.

Substance Abuse and Mental Health Services Administration. 1 Choke Cherry Road, Rockville, MD, 20857. Toll free: 877-SAMH-SA-7. Web site: http://ncadi.samhsa.gov.

Sudden Infant Death Syndrome

Sudden infant death syndrome (also known as SIDS) refers to the sudden death of an apparently healthy infant under one year of age whose death cannot be explained even after a complete investigation.

Taking Care

Mrs. Wyatt is following all the instructions her doctor gave for the care of her new baby. She puts him to sleep both at night and for daytime naps on his back instead of on his stomach. She makes sure the crib has a mattress that is firm and that no blankets, pillows, or toys are around the baby. She refrains from bundling her baby in thick clothing before putting the baby to bed.

The doctor recommended these precautions because they reduce the risk of sudden infant death syndrome (SIDS), a mysterious disorder that is a leading cause of death for children between the ages of one month and one year.

Since mothers like Mrs. Wyatt started to put their babies to sleep on their backs and began to adopt other preventive strategies, the number of SIDS deaths has dropped substantially. However, SIDS still accounts for about 3,000 deaths per year in the United States, usually while the babies

* **vaccination** (vak-sih-NAY-shun), also called immunization, is giving, usually by an injection, a preparation of killed or weakened germs, or a part of a germ or product it produces, to prevent or lessen the severity of the disease caused by that germ.

are asleep in their cribs. No one knows for sure why these babies die. Most appear to be healthy until their deaths.

Parents often feel guilt mixed with their grief over the death of their baby. They think perhaps they could have done something more for the baby, but SIDS is no one's fault.

What Is Sudden Infant Death Syndrome?

It is easier to say what SIDS is not than what it is. SIDS does not result from suffocation, choking, vomiting, or a fatal reaction to a vaccination*. A baby does not catch it like a cold.

THE BACK TO SLEEP CAMPAIGN

For decades, parents thought it was best to put babies to sleep on their stomachs. They assumed that if babies were on their backs, they might choke on their vomit if they threw up.

Doctors later explained that there was no reason to fear this potential for choking. In 1992 the American Academy of Pediatrics recommended that babies sleep on their backs, and in 1994 the National Institute of Child Health and Human Development and other organizations reiterated that call by launching a national Back to Sleep Campaign to reduce the risk of SIDS. Between 1992 and 1997, the number of children sleeping on their stomachs decreased dramatically, and the death rate from SIDS dropped by 50 percent.

The National Institute of Child Health and Human Development offers a number of ways to lower the risk of SIDS. These include:

- Providing the baby with a firm mattress or other surface for sleeping
- Having the mother avoid smoking during pregnancy
- Having family members avoid smoking around the baby
- Having the baby sleep near, but not with, a parent, sibling, or other person
- Keeping pillows, loose blankets, and soft toys out of the crib
- Dressing a baby in light clothes while the child is sleeping or napping.

Not all babies should sleep on their backs. A few have problems with their airways or with keeping food down. In these rare cases, parents should consult a doctor, who may recommend that the babies be placed on their stomachs on a firm mattress without soft pillows, blankets, or plush toys.

Some parents have misunderstood the intent of the Back to Sleep Campaign. They never put their children on their stomachs, even when they are awake. Doctors say it is important for children's physical and mental development to spend some time on their stomachs while they are awake, so long as an adult is watching.

Doctors assign a baby's death to SIDS when no other cause of death is found after conducting an autopsy*, an investigation of the place where the baby died, and a review of the baby's medical history.

Researchers explored the possible causes of SIDS for years, and many came to believe that it results from a problem in an area of the brain that controls two important functions while infants are asleep: breathing and waking up. In 2006, a research team conducted autopsies* on 31 infants who had died of SIDS, and they found that about three-fourths of the infants had abnormalities in a certain brain chemical called serotonin. The researchers believed the abnormality prevented the infants from responding normally when they were not getting enough oxygen. These responses include turning the head or taking deeper breaths. It was hoped that this finding would lead to tests that could help determine if an infant actually died of SIDS and possibly to medications that might someday identify and prevent the problem.

Several factors can cause a baby to get insufficient oxygen. For example, babies might not get enough oxygen when they breathe air that is trapped in soft beds or in folds of blankets near their mouths. In such circumstances, they are breathing in their own exhaled carbon dioxide, rather than the oxygen available in the air. A normal baby's brain gets the warning about the insufficient oxygen, but a baby with the serotonin abnormality does not.

A baby can also experience breathing difficulties from respiratory infections such as a cold or other ailment. This fact might explain why SIDS is more likely to occur in the winter, when the risk of infection is higher and, at the same time, babies are more likely to be sleeping with extra bedclothes or blankets.

Researchers have investigated other possible physical problems that could contribute to the risk of SIDS. One possible factor is an immune system* disorder that creates too many white blood cells and proteins, which disrupt the brain's control over breathing and heart rate.

SIDS might be caused by a combination of factors, including some that have yet to be identified.

Who Is at Risk for Sudden Infant Death Syndrome?

SIDS can happen any time within the first year, but it occurs most often between the second and fourth month after birth. It seldom occurs the first two weeks following birth or after six months. The vast majority of babies do not experience SIDS even if they sleep on their stomachs, have infections, or sleep with blankets in their cribs. Others who sleep on their backs in ideal conditions still die of SIDS. No warning signs of SIDS are evident before a baby dies. Doctors only diagnose it after ruling out other possible causes of death.

Although research is beginning to suggest causes for SIDS, no test is yet available to predict who will die of the disorder.

* **autopsy** (AW-top-see) is an examination of a body after death to look for the cause of death or the effects of a disease.

* **autopsies** (AW-top-seez) are examinations of bodies after death to look for causes of death or the effects of diseases.

* **immune system** (im-YOON SIS-tem) is the system of the body composed of specialized cells and the substances they produce that helps protect the body against disease-causing germs.

What Are the Risk Factors for Sudden Infant Death Syndrome?

A baby is more likely to die of SIDS if the baby has:

- A mother who smoked during pregnancy
- A mother younger than 20 years of age
- A mother who did not receive proper medical care before her baby was born
- A birth before the full nine months of a normal pregnancy
- A lower than normal birth weight
- Family members who smoked around the baby

In addition, babies who are strictly bottle-fed have a higher risk of SIDS. One possible reason is that breast-feeding helps reduce the risk of the types of infections that may contribute to breathing problems.

▶ *See also* **Prematurity • Tobacco-Related Diseases**

Resources

Books and Articles

Horchler, Joani. *SIDS and Infant Death Survival Guide: Information and Comfort for Grieving Family and Friends and Professionals Who Seek to Help Them,* 3rd ed. Hyattsville, MD: SIDS Educational Services, 2003.

Parks, Peggy J. *SIDS.* Detroit, MI: Lucent Books, 2009.

Organizations

Eunice Kennedy Shriver National Institute of Child Health and Human Development. 31 Center Drive, Building 31, Room 2A32, MSC 2425, Bethesda, MD, 20892-2425. Toll free: 800-370-2943. Web site: http://www.nichd.nih.gov/sids/sids.cfm.

First Candle. 1314 Bedford Avenue, Suite 210, Baltimore, MD, 21208. Toll free: 800-221-7437. Web site: http://www.sidsalliance.org.

National Sudden Infant Death Resource Center. 2115 Wisconsin Ave., NW, Washington, DC, 20007. Toll free: 866-866-7437. Web site: http://www.sidscenter.org.

Sudden Infant Death Syndrome Network, Inc.. PO Box 520, Ledyard, CT, 06339. Web site: http://sids-network.org.

Suicide

Suicide is the intentional taking of a person's own life.

Shocking Statistics

There are more suicides than murders and more than twice as many suicides as deaths from acquired immunodeficiency syndrome (AIDS*) in the United States every year, yet suicide gets far less press attention than murder or AIDS. Talking about suicide makes people uncomfortable, perhaps because there are religious prohibitions against suicide, because suicide is thought of as a shameful act, or because many people simply cannot imagine why someone would intentionally take his or her own life.

Who Commits Suicide?

Suicide results from many factors, some of which are complicated and not well understood. It is not clear or predictable why the setbacks, losses, or difficulties that would lead one person to feel unhappy may push another person to consider suicide.

It is estimated that more than 30,000 Americans die as the result of suicide each year, whereas about 20,000 people are murdered. Some experts, however, believe that the number of suicides is even higher. Many so-called accidents, such as self-inflicted gunshot wounds or single-car crashes, actually may be unrecognized or unreported suicides. Although no official record is kept of suicide attempts, it is estimated that there are 25 attempts for each completed suicide. Overall, suicide is ranked eleventh as a cause of death in the United States, but among the young, suicide ranks third.

Although more women than men attempt suicide, about four times more men die, because they use more deadly means. Men of European ancestry committed 69 percent of all suicides in 2005, whereas women of European ancestry accounted for about 18 percent of these deaths. The rate of suicide among people of Native American ancestry is particularly high (about 12 per 100,000). The suicide rate among men of African ancestry fell steadily between 1996 and the early 2000s. Age is another factor in suicide. Among people 65 years of age and older, the rate of suicide among men of European heritage increases steadily with age. Elderly men (older than 85) of European heritage have a suicide rate that is 2.5 times the national male average. Various factors explain why the rate of suicide is among people of different ethnic backgrounds, gender, and ages. Factors include increased rates of alcoholism, poverty, loneliness, and violence for particular groups at particular stages of life.

Young people have a higher than average rate of suicide. Suicide is the third leading cause of death among people 15 to 24 years old. The 2003 Youth Risk Behavior Surveillance Survey found that 16.9 percent of high school students reported seriously considering suicide. Meanwhile, the number of children ages 10 to 14 committing suicide increased sharply between 1981 and the early 2000s. The most common methods of committing suicide are by intentionally taking a drug overdose (prescription or over-the-counter medicines), inhaling carbon monoxide from car exhausts, or using guns.

* **AIDS** or acquired immunodeficiency (ih-myoo-no-dih-FIH-shen-see) syndrome, is an infection that severely weakens the immune system; it is caused by the human immunodeficiency virus (HIV).

What Factors Make People More Likely to Commit Suicide?

About 90 percent of people who commit suicide have a diagnosed psychiatric disorder. Depression and substance abuse (either alone or in combination) are the two most common factors that play a part in suicide. This does not mean that everyone who has depression or an alcohol or drug problem will consider committing suicide. The majority of people with these problems are not suicidal.

People who are more likely to kill themselves may also have the following:

- Have previously attempted suicide
- Live alone and have no social support network
- Have chronic (long-lasting or recurring) physical pain or a terminal (life-ending) illness
- Have a family history of suicide
- Be unemployed
- Be impulsive
- Keep a gun in the home
- Have spent time in jail
- Have experienced family violence, child abuse, or sexual abuse

What Are the Signs that a Person Is Thinking of Committing Suicide?

People who talk about killing themselves are at risk for committing suicide. Most people who attempt suicide have given clues about their intentions before they acted on them. It is important to take seriously any talk about suicide or any indication that suicide is a possibility.

Common warning signs that a person is thinking about suicide include the following:

- Talking about death or making suicide threats
- Making such statements as "You would be better off without me" or "I'm no good to anybody" (even if these are said jokingly)
- Having any of the symptoms or signs of depression
- Exhibiting major personality changes or unexplainable odd behavior
- Making a will or giving away cherished possessions
- Seeking isolation and becoming uncommunicative
- Being fascinated with death
- Taking a sudden interest in religion if previously not religious or rejecting religion if previously devout

Why Do People Commit Suicide?

No one can explain why some people commit suicide and others do not. One theory is that suicide is an act of rage, an expression of intense anger at oneself and/or others. Another theory is that people may commit suicide because they feel they have no other choice. Hopelessness and distorted thinking may prevent a person from seeing solutions to their problems.

For a mentally healthy person, the idea that a person would have no choice except to commit suicide is absurd. But depression, substance abuse, and other mental illnesses, such as schizophrenia*, alter the healthy mind and cloud people's thinking. People with these problems may feel that they are in a deep, dark hole from which there is no escape and that life is so painful that there are no alternatives except death.

There may be inherited tendencies for depression, schizophrenia, alcoholism, substance abuse, and certain personality disorders*. All of these problems can increase a person's vulnerability to suicidal thoughts when things go wrong. Some studies suggest that the brain chemistry of people who commit suicide is abnormal. Some research has sought to examine the effects of certain medications that alter brain chemistry in a way that could decrease suicidal behavior.

What Should Others Do If Someone Is Suicidal?

People who are thinking about committing suicide need professional help. They have usually sunk so deeply into their mental and emotional black holes that they may be unable to recognize that they are in trouble or to seek help on their own. It is important to pay attention when people talk about wanting to die and to take their words seriously. Having another person approach the subject directly is often a relief to them. It is sometimes thought that speaking to people about their possible wish to commit suicide will "put thoughts in their heads." But people who talk about suicide often are already thinking about suicide.

Professional help is available through suicide prevention and crisis intervention centers, mental health clinics, hospitals and emergency rooms, family doctors, health maintenance organizations, mental health practitioners, and members of the clergy. When a person is possibly suicidal, it is a good idea to talk to another mature, responsible person and ask that person to join in helping to deal with the crisis. Many telephone books have community service sections that list suicide and mental health crisis hotlines. Immediate help can be obtained by calling emergency services (911 in most communities).

Other ways of possibly minimizing the risk of suicide include the following:

- Removing guns and ammunition from the house
- Locking up medications and alcohol
- Staying with the person, because suicide is an act most often performed alone
- Talking calmly, without lecturing, being judgmental, or pointing out all the reasons a person has to continue living

Suicide places an intense emotional burden on the survivors. People who have been close to someone who has attempted or completed suicide

* **schizophrenia** (skit-so-FREE-nee-ah) is a serious mental disorder that causes people to experience hallucinations, delusions, and other confusing thoughts and behaviors, which distort their view of reality.

* **personality disorders** are a group of mental disorders characterized by long-term patterns of behavior that differ from those expected by society. People with personality disorders have patterns of emotional response, impulse control, and perception that differ from those of most people.

might consider mental health counseling to help them to deal with their own emotions.

▶ *See also* **Bipolar Disorder** • **Brain Chemistry (Neurochemistry)** • **Death and Dying** • **Depressive Disorders** • **Substance Abuse**

Resources

Books and Articles

Esherick, Joan. *The Silent Cry: A Teen's Guide to Escaping Self-Injury and Suicide.* Philadelphia, PA: Mason Crest, 2005.

Giddens, Sandra. *Frequently Asked Questions about Suicide.* New York: Rosen, 2009.

Marcovitz, Hal. *Teens and Suicide.* Philadelphia, PA: Mason Crest, 2004.

Powell, Jillian. *Self-Harm and Suicide.* Pleasantville, NY: Gareth Stevens, 2009.

Shannon, Joyce Brennfleck, ed. *Suicide Information for Teens: Health Tips About Suicide Causes and Prevention: Including Facts about Depression, Risk Factors, Getting Help, Survivor Support, and More.* Detroit, MI: Omnigraphics, 2005.

Organizations

American Psychiatric Association. 1000 Wilson Boulevard, Suite 1825, Arlington, VA, 22209. Toll free: 888-35-PSYCH. Web site: http://www.psyh.org.

National Center for Injury Prevention and Control. 4770 Buford Highway NE, Mailstop K65, Atlanta, GA, 30341-3724. Telephone: 770-488-1506. Web site: http://www.cdc.gov/ncipc/dvp/Suicide/default.htm.

National Institute of Mental Health. 6001 Executive Boulevard, Room 8148, MSC 9663, Bethesda, MD, 20892-9663. Telephone: 301-443-4513. Web site: http://www.nimh.nih.gov.

Supraglottitis *See Epiglottitis.*

Swimmer's Ear *See Otitis (Ear Infections).*

Syncope *See Fainting (Syncope).*

Syphilis

Syphilis (SIH-fih-lis) is a sexually transmitted disease that, if untreated, can lead to serious lifelong physical problems, including blindness and paralysis*.

What Is Syphilis?

Syphilis is a disease that is caused by the bacterium *Treponema pallidum* (treh-puh-NEE-muh PAL-ih-dum). The disease develops in three distinct phases. The first, or primary, stage is marked by a chancre*. In the secondary stage, a rash develops. There can be an interval of months to years for late syphilis to develop, if early stages are not detected and treated. By the third stage, also known as the tertiary stage, the disease can cause widespread damage to the body, affecting the brain, nerves, bones, joints, eyes, heart, and other organs. Syphilis does not advance to this point in all infected people, and it does so only if it has not been treated adequately during either of the two earlier stages.

Without treatment, syphilis can be fatal. It can also have serious consequences for the fetus* of an infected woman. If a pregnant woman has syphilis, she can pass it to her unborn offspring, a condition known as congenital* syphilis. Because the immune system* of a baby is not developed fully until the infant is well into the first year of life, infection with syphilis bacteria can lead to severe complications. Among pregnant women who are infected but are not treated, up to 80 percent of their fetuses may become infected, and up to 40 percent may die before or shortly after birth.

How Common Is Syphilis?

Syphilis was rampant in the United States until the antibiotic penicillin was introduced in the 1940s. After that, the number of syphilis cases dropped. The reduction in the rate of primary and secondary syphilis in the United States was particularly noticeable between 1990 and 2000, when it fell nearly 90 percent. By 2000 the rate was at its lowest level since reporting began in 1941, according to the Centers for Disease Control and Prevention (CDC). After that, syphilis cases rose. Between 2001 and 2006, the CDC reported a particular increase among men, going from a rate of 3.0 cases per 100,000 to 5.7 cases per 100,000 population. The CDC reported that more than 60 percent of new infections occurred in men who have sex with men. Among women, the rate also rose, although much more slowly. The rate was 0.8 cases per 100,000 in 2004, 0.9 cases per 100,000 in 2005, and 1.0 case per 100,000 in 2006.

The CDC launched a "National Plan to Eliminate Syphilis," which worked on many fronts to reduce the numbers. Some of these included enhancing public health services and assisting in syphilis-prevention efforts directed at targeted cultural groups.

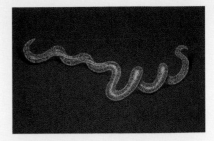

The corkscrew-shaped bacterium *Spirochete Treponema pallidum* causes syphilis. *Chris Bjornberg/Photo Researchers, Inc.*

A Pox of Many Names

Over the centuries, the disease syphilis has been called by many names. The term "great pox" was used to differentiate syphilis from smallpox. The name "syphilis" seems to have originated in a 1530 poem about a shepherd named "Syphilis," which was written by the Italian physician Girolamo Fracastoro (Fracastorius) (1478–1553). The poem was titled "Syphilis, sive morbus Gallicus" (meaning "Syphilis, the French disease").

In his play *Timon of Athens*, William Shakespeare (1564–1616) refers to syphilis as the "infinite malady."

Cultural embarrassment caused many nations to refer to syphilis as the disease of another national group. The English and Germans called it the "French pox." The Russians suffered from the "Polish sickness." The Poles identified syphilis as the "German sickness." The French named it the "Neapolitan sickness" (meaning Italian or from the area around Naples, Italy). The Flemish, Dutch, Portuguese, and North Africans caught the "Spanish" or "Castilian sickness." Meanwhile, the Japanese referred to syphilis as the "Canton rash" or the "Chinese ulcer."

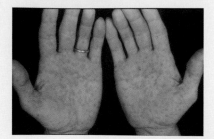

Secondary syphilis. If syphilis is not treated in its first phase, it can progress to its second stage a month or two later in which a rash may appear on the palms of the hands and the soles of the feet. *Custom Medical Stock Photo, Inc. Reproduced by permission.*

Is Syphilis Contagious?

Syphilis is a sexually transmitted disease (STD) that spreads from person to person through vaginal*, oral*, or anal* sexual intercourse. A pregnant female can also pass the disease to her fetus. Syphilis is contagious during its first and second stages, and sometimes in the early latent period, which is described below. People are most contagious, however, during the second stage of the infection.

What Are the Signs and Symptoms of Syphilis Infection?

Syphilis has been called "the great imitator," because its symptoms can resemble those of many other diseases. Not all people have obvious symptoms, but in those who do, signs of disease appear 10 to 90 days after being infected. The first symptom is a small, usually painless sore known as a chancre that appears where the syphilis bacterium entered the body, such as on the penis or the lips of the vagina*. Without treatment, chancres heal on their own within six weeks. A person who is infected may never even notice a chancre, especially if it is inside the vagina or the rectum*.

HOW SYPHILIS CHANGED THE FACE OF MEDICAL RESEARCH

During the middle decades of the 20th century syphilis was the subject of what became known as the most infamous public health study ever carried out in the United States. From 1932 to 1972, the U.S. Public Health Service conducted a study in Macon County, Alabama, to learn more about the long-term consequences of the disease. Six hundred poor African American men, 399 of them infected with syphilis, participated in the study in exchange for free medical exams, free meals, and burial insurance.

The Tuskegee Syphilis Study became notorious because local doctors who participated in the study were instructed not to treat the men's infections, even after an easy cure with penicillin became widely available in 1947. Although the men had agreed to be part of the project, they were never told they would not be treated fully for their condition. They were simply told that they were part of a study of "bad blood," a local term used for several illnesses.

Public outrage erupted in 1972 when it became known that men with syphilis in the study had been allowed to remain untreated so that doctors could investigate the progression of the disease, and the project was stopped. That came too late for the men, however, and many had already been disabled permanently or had died. In the wake of the study, the government moved quickly to adopt policies that protect people who take part in research programs. In 1974, a new law created a national commission to set basic ethical standards for research. New rules also required that participants in government-funded studies must be made fully aware of how a study will proceed and must voluntarily agree to take part in it. In addition a review process ensures that any study involving humans meets ethical standards before it begins.

Of course, these changes could not reverse the physical and emotional harm done to the men in the Tuskegee Syphilis Study and to their families. In recognition of that harm, President Bill Clinton in 1997 offered an apology to the survivors, families, and descendants of those men on behalf of the U.S. government.

One to two months after the chancre fades, the disease moves to its second stage. In this phase, a rash of rough, reddish or brownish spots appears on the body, including the soles of the feet and the palms of the hands. The rash may be so faint that it is barely noticeable. Second-stage symptoms of syphilis may also include fever, headache, extreme tiredness, sore throat, muscle aches, swollen lymph nodes*, weight loss, hair loss, and ulcers* on mucous membranes* in the mouth and on the genitals*. Wart-like lesions* may appear on the vagina or anus. These symptoms also disappear on their own, fooling many people into thinking that they have had a common viral illness.

After the second-stage symptoms clear up, the disease enters a latent, or hidden, period in which the patient shows no signs of illness. The latent period can last for many years, and in some infected people the bacteria do no further damage. In about one-third of people who reach the latent period, the disease progresses to its final stage. This phase has no symptoms at first, but as the bacteria invade and damage nerves, bones, and the heart and other organs, the patient may experience dizziness, headaches, seizures*, dementia*, loss of coordination, numbness, increasing blindness, and paralysis. The disease also can eat away at tissue in the mouth and nose, disfiguring the face. This last stage of the disease can begin two to 40 years after a person is first infected.

Babies who are born with syphilis may have symptoms right away or may show signs of the disease within a few weeks or months. These symptoms include so-called failure to thrive*, or a failure to gain weight and grow at the expected rate; irritability; fever; rash; a nose without a bridge (known as saddle nose); bloody fluid from the nose; and a rash on the palms, soles, or face. As these children grow older, they may become blind and deaf, and may have notched teeth (called Hutchinson teeth). Bone lesions may arise, and lesions and scarring may appear around the mouth, genitals, and anus.

How Do Doctors Diagnose Syphilis?

If a patient has a chancre or other lesion, the doctor collects a sample of fluid from the sore to examine under a special microscope. Syphilis bacteria in the fluid are visible under magnification. The doctor also may take a blood sample to look for antibodies* to the bacterium. If neurosyphilis (nur-o-SIH-fih-lis), which is syphilis that has progressed to the point that it affects the brain, spinal cord, and nerves, is suspected, the doctor may also order tests of the spinal fluid to look for antibodies. Routine prenatal care for pregnant women includes a screening for syphilis.

How Is Syphilis Treated?

Even though visible signs of the infection clear up on their own, doctors provide treatment for syphilis. Doing so prevents the disease from progressing to the late, potentially much more harmful stage, and in pregnant women, prevents infants from suffering damage caused by the infection.

* **paralysis** (pah-RAH-luh-sis) is the loss or impairment of the ability to move some part of the body.

* **chancre** (SHANG-ker) is a usually painless sore or ulcer that forms where a disease-causing germ enters the body, such as with syphilis.

* **fetus** (FEE-tus) is the term for an unborn human after it is an embryo, from 9 weeks after fertilization until childbirth.

* **congenital** (kon-JEH-nih-tul) means present at birth.

* **immune system** (im-YOON SIS-tem) is the system of the body composed of specialized cells and the substances they produce that helps protect the body against disease-causing germs.

* **vaginal** (VAH-jih-nul) refers to the canal in a woman that leads from the uterus to the outside of the body.

* **oral** means by mouth or referring to the mouth.

* **anal** refers to the anus, the opening at the end of the digestive system through which waste leaves the body.

* **vagina** (vah-JY-nah) is the canal, or passageway, in a woman that leads from the uterus to the outside of the body.

* **rectum** is the final portion of the large intestine, connecting the colon to the outside opening of the anus.

* **lymph nodes** (LIMF) are small, bean-shaped masses of tissue containing immune system cells that fight harmful microorganisms. Lymph nodes may swell during infections.

* **ulcers** are open sores on the skin or the lining of a hollow body organ, such as the stomach or intestine. They may or may not be painful.

* **mucous membranes** are the thin layers of tissue found inside the nose, ears, cervix (SER-viks) and uterus, stomach, colon and rectum, on the vocal cords, and in other parts of the body.

* **genitals** (JEH-nih-tuls) are the external sexual organs.

* **lesions** (LEE-zhuns) is a general term referring to a sore or a damaged or irregular area of tissue.

* **seizures** (SEE-zhurs) are sudden bursts of disorganized electrical activity that interrupt the normal functioning of the brain, often leading to uncontrolled movements in the body and sometimes a temporary change in consciousness.

* **dementia** (dih-MEN-sha) is a loss of mental abilities, including memory, understanding, and judgment.

* **failure to thrive** is a condition in which an infant fails to gain weight and grow at the expected rate.

* **antibodies** (AN-tih-bah-deez) are protein molecules produced by the body's immune system to help fight specific infections caused by microorganisms, such as bacteria and viruses.

Doctors can easily treat early-stage syphilis with antibiotics. They advise people who are infected with syphilis to notify all their recent sexual partners so that these people can be tested for the disease. Patients with advanced cases of the disease often need hospitalization. They also receive antibiotics, although medications cannot reverse damage already done to the body.

How Long Does Infection Last?

A single dose of antibiotics can clear up syphilis infections that are less than a year old. Longer-term cases require longer courses of treatment. Congenital syphilis also needs a longer course of treatment. Without treatment, the disease can last for years or even decades.

Does the Disease Have Complications?

Untreated cases of syphilis can lead to destructive tissue lesions known as gummas (GOOM-ahz) on the skin, bones, and organs; seizures; damage to the spine that can result in paralysis; heart problems; damage to blood vessels that can lead to stroke*; and death. According to the CDC, a person with syphilis has a two- to five-fold greater risk of acquiring human immunodeficiency (ih-myoo-no-dih-FIH-shen-see) virus (HIV), the virus that causes acquired immunodeficiency syndrome (AIDS), an infection that weakens the immune system. The reason for this increased risk is that open sores make an easy entry for HIV during sexual contact. Also, people infected with HIV are more likely to experience neurological* complications of syphilis. In infants, syphilis can lead to hearing loss, blindness, neurological problems, and death.

Can Syphilis Be Prevented?

Using latex condoms or not having sex, especially with someone who is known to be infected, can prevent the spread of syphilis and other STDs. To be effective, the condom has to cover all syphilis sores. Contact with sores in the mouth or on other uncovered areas, such as the rectum, can spread the disease. Doctors advise pregnant women to be tested and, if needed, treated for syphilis to minimize the risk of passing the disease to the developing fetus.

▶ *See also* **Gonorrhea • Sexually Transmitted Diseases (STDs)**

Resources

Books and Articles

Hayden, Deborah. *Pox: Genius, Madness, and the Mysteries of Syphilis.* New York: Basic Books, 2003.

Parascandola, John. *Sex, Sin, and Science: A History of Syphilis in America.* Westport, CT: Praeger, 2008.

Winters, Adam. *Syphilis.* New York: Rosen, 2007.

Organizations

American Social Health Association. P.O. Box 13827, Research Triangle Park, NC, 27709. Telephone: 919-361-8400. Web site: http://www.ashastd.org/learn/learn_syphilis_facts.cfm.

Centers for Disease Control and Prevention. 1600 Clifton Road, Atlanta, GA, 30333. Toll free: 800-232-4636. Web site: http://www.cdc.gov/std/syphilis/STDFact-Syphilis.htm.

National Women's Health Information Center. 8270 Willow Oaks Corporate Drive, Fairfax, VA, 22031. Toll free: 800-994-9662. Web site: http://womenshealth.gov/faq/syphilis.cfm.

Systemic Lupus Erythematosus *See Lupus.*

---

* **stroke** is a brain-damaging event usually caused by interference with blood flow to the brain. A stroke may occur when a blood vessel supplying the brain becomes clogged or bursts, depriving brain tissue of oxygen. As a result, nerve cells in the affected area of the brain, and the specific body parts they control, do not properly function.

* **neurological** (nur-a-LAH-je-kal) refers to the nervous system, which includes the brain, spinal cord, and the nerves that control the senses, movement, and organ functions throughout the body.

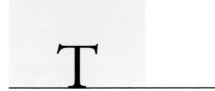

Tapeworm

A tapeworm is a long, flat, intestinal worm found in humans and many other animals.

What Are Tapeworms?

Tapeworms are long, flat, intestinal worms called cestodes, found in humans and many other animals. Tapeworms do not have an intestinal tract, they absorb nutrients through their body surface. Human tapeworm infestations may be caused by eating meat or fish contaminated with tapeworm larvae* but also by ingesting soil or water contaminated with human fecal matter containing the eggs. Meat contaminated with tapeworm larvae has larvae enclosed in cyst* form within the meat. The larvae are worms at an intermediate stage of the life cycle between eggs and adulthood. They burrow into the animal tissue and form fluid-filled cysts, which are protective capsules. Like other intestinal parasites*, these worms frequently cause infestations in areas with poor sanitation, where livestock animals are exposed to contaminated soil or fish to contaminated water, and have the parasites within their body tissues. Humans are either infested through ingestion of eggs or larvae. The tapeworms mature within the intestinal tract of the human and lay new eggs, which are released into the fecal matter and passed out of the body to begin the cycle again. Tapeworm infection may be prevented by thoroughly cooking meat until juices run clear and the centers are no longer pink or raw. Doing so ensures that any tapeworm cysts in the meat are destroyed.

What Are the Types of Tapeworm?

There are three common species of tapeworms: *Taenia saginata* (beef tapeworm), *Taenia solium* (pork tapeworm), and *Diphyllobothrium latum* (freshwater fish tapeworm). After ingesting contaminated tapeworm encysted meat or fish, the larvae travel to the intestines*, where they latch onto the lining of the intestines and gradually grow into adults. Symptoms of a tapeworm infestation are often mild or nonexistent but

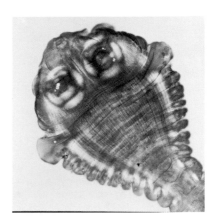

▲

The head of the beef tapeworm *Taenia saginata*, which is where the worm attaches to the intestine. *Alfred Pasieka/ Photo Researchers, Inc.*

* **larvae** (LAR-vee) are the immature forms of an insect or worm that hatches from an egg.

* **cysts** (SISTS) are shell-like enclosures that contain small organisms in a resting stage.

* **parasites** (PAIR-uh-sites) organisms such as a protozoan (one-celled animals), worm, or insect that must live on or inside a human or other organism to survive. An animal or plant harboring a parasite is called its host. A parasite lives at the expense of the host and may cause illness.

* **intestines** are the muscular tubes that food passes through during digestion after it exits the stomach.

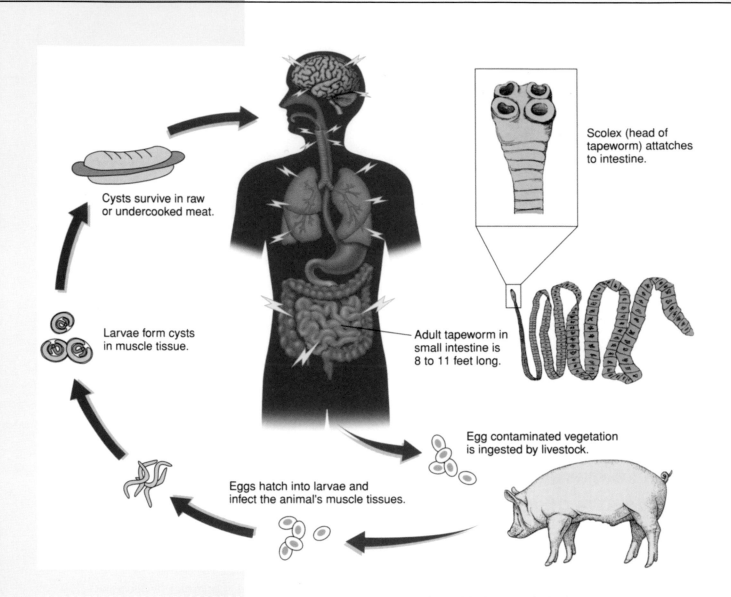

Cysts survive in raw or undercooked meat.

Larvae form cysts in muscle tissue.

Eggs hatch into larvae and infect the animal's muscle tissues.

Egg contaminated vegetation is ingested by livestock.

Adult tapeworm in small intestine is 8 to 11 feet long.

Scolex (head of tapeworm) attaches to intestine.

▲

Life cycle of the pork tapeworm.
Illustration by Frank Forney. Reproduced by permission of Gale, a part of Cengage Learning.

* **central nervous system** (SEN-trul NER-vus SIS-tem) is the part of the nervous system that includes the brain and spinal cord.

* **seizures** (SEE-zhurs) are sudden bursts of disorganized electrical activity that interrupt the normal functioning of the brain, often leading to uncontrolled movements in the body and sometimes a temporary change in consciousness.

can include abdominal pain, loss of appetite, diarrhea, tiredness, weight loss, and malnutrition. In individuals without symptoms tapeworm infestation is often not noted until pieces of worm are found in the stool or undergarments.

Beef, fish, and pork tapeworms Beef and fish tapeworms generally remain limited to the human gastrointestinal tract and usually only migrate to further tissues in animals. The pork tapeworm is unique because it is known for leaving the human gastrointestinal tract in larval form and migrating to other parts of the human body to create cysts of worm larvae in human body tissues. Whereas cysts may form in any body tissue, the most commonly affected part of the body is the central nervous system*, including the brain. The condition of having a tapeworm cyst in body tissues is called cysticercosis. Having one in the brain is known as neuro-cysticercosis and may cause seizures*, blindness, or other nervous system abnormalities. Cysts may also form in the heart, eye, or other locations. If the encysted larvae die, the body may calcify (deposit calcium salts in) the region as part of the healing process. Calcified cysts may also cause health problems.

The fish tapeworm is often noted for causing vitamin B12 deficiencies. In the human body, vitamin B12 is absorbed in the end portion of the small intestines known as the ileum. The closer the fish tapeworm physically is to the ileum, the more severe the vitamin B12 deficiency in the person serving as its host. This vitamin is necessary for red blood cells to function. Vitamin B12 deficiency causes a type of anemia, or red blood cell deficiency, known as pernicious anemia. Because the body tissues are not getting enough oxygen, the individual with pernicious anemia feels tired and weak and may even have nerve damage if the anemia is bad enough. Pernicious anemia responds well to vitamin therapy.

The largest tapeworms can reach an amazing size, measuring more than 45 feet long in some cases. The adult beef tapeworm is usually 15 to 30 feet long (4.5 to 9 meters). An infected person usually has only one or two worms. The tapeworms use their head, called the scolex, to attach themselves to the intestinal wall. They have 1,000 to 2,000 body segments, called proglottids, each containing 80,000 to 100,000 eggs. The eggs can survive for months or years in the environment outside the human body. If humans eat raw or undercooked beef containing cysts, the cysts develop over a two-month period into adult tapeworms. Adult beef tapeworms can live for more than 30 years.

The adult pork tapeworm is about half as long as the beef tapeworm, usually eight to 11 feet (2.5 to 3.5 meters) long. It also has a scolex for attaching to the intestinal wall and a body of about 1,000 proglottids. Each proglottid contains about 50,000 eggs. Adult pork tapeworms can live up to 25 years.

The adult fish tapeworm is from 3 to 49 feet long (one to 15 meters) and is the longest human tapeworm. They have 3,000 to 4,000 proglottids that are wider than they are long, giving this tapeworm the name broad tapeworm. The fish tapeworm affects freshwater fish as well as some saltwater fish that have a freshwater component to their lifecycle (such as salmon). Fish tapeworm infestations are most common in societies that consume large amounts of raw or pickled fish.

How Is Tapeworm Infestation Diagnosed and Treated?

Eggs and proglottids can be seen in stool samples by microscopic examination. In order to differentiate between a beef, pork, or fish tapeworm, a scolex has to be removed and examined. This is seldom done, as doctors usually can prescribe the same medication for all types of tapeworm infestation. Stool is checked at three and six months after treatment to ensure that the parasite is gone.

Cysticercosis is diagnosed by examining the muscles or brain with a CT scan*, which uses x-rays and computers to view structures inside the body that contain cysts. Blood tests for antibodies, which are specific

* **CT scans** or CAT scans are the shortened name for computerized axial tomography (to-MOG-ra-fee), which uses computers to view structures inside the body.

proteins the body makes to fight the tapeworm infestation, can confirm the diagnosis. Tapeworm infestations are treated with one of various types of anti-worm drug called anthelmintics (ant-HEL-min-tics). Some anthelmintics work only in the gastrointestinal tract while others affect body tissues. Cysticercosis can be treated with some types of anthelmintics, but in rare instances cysts may be removed surgically.

▶ *See also* **Parasitic Diseases: Overview • Worms: Overview**

Resources

Books and Articles

Allman, Toney. *Parasites! Tapeworms.* San Diego, CA: KidHaven Press, 2003.

Organizations

Centers for Disease Control and Prevention. 1600 Clifton Road,Atlanta, GA, 30333. Toll free: 800-311-3435. Web site: http://www.cdc.gov.

National Library of Medicine. 8600 Rockville Pike,Bethesda, MD, 20894. Toll free: 888-346-3656. Web site: http://www.nlm.nih.gov/ medlineplus/ency/article/001391.htm; http://www.nlm.nih.gov/ medlineplus/ency/article/001378.htm.

Tay-Sachs Disease

Tay-Sachs disease is a rare inherited disorder that results in slow destruction of the central nervous system (brain and spinal cord).

People inherit Tay-Sachs disease when they inherit a defective gene from both parents, resulting in two defective genes that make the body unable to produce Hex-A correctly. People who have only one defective gene are called carriers. Carriers do not have the disease, because they have inherited one healthy gene to code for Hex-A, but they may pass the defective gene on to their children. If both parents are carriers, each child born to them has a 1 in 4 likelihood of having the disease. *Illustration by Frank Forney. Reproduced by permission of Gale, a part of Cengage Learning.*

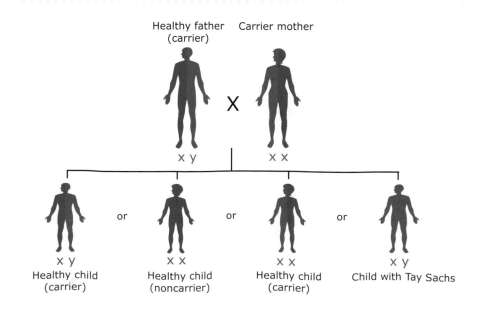

What Is Tay-Sachs Disease?

Tay-Sachs disease is a rare metabolic* disorder with severe neurologic (nervous system) symptoms. The term "metabolic" refers to the body's chemical processes that produce protein and other substances and break down nutrients to release energy. Tay-Sachs disease is a metabolic disorder because it is caused by the absence of the enzyme* (a type of protein) hexosaminidase A (Hex-A). Hex-A is necessary for breaking down fatty substances called lipids. Without Hex-A, these lipids build up in, and eventually destroy, the nerve cells in the brain. Ultimately, the nervous system stops functioning properly.

How Does Tay-Sachs Disease Affect the Body?

Classical Tay-Sachs   The most common form of Tay-Sachs disease (classical Tay-Sachs) affects children and usually is fatal. It is caused by a complete lack of Hex-A. Destruction of nerve cells begins before birth, but affected babies do not begin to lose nerve function until they are about six months old. By age two, the child may have seizures* and begins to lose skills such as crawling, sitting, turning over, and reaching for objects. Eventually, the child will be blind, paralyzed, and mentally retarded. Children with this form of Tay-Sachs disease do not live past five years of age.

A variation of this scenario occurs when children develop symptoms between the ages of two and five years of age rather than as an infant. The same symptoms emerge, but the disease progresses more slowly. Children with this form usually die by age 15.

Late onset Tay-Sachs (LOTS)   Late onset Tay-Sachs disease (LOTS) is less common than the infantile form. It affects teenagers and adults in their twenties and thirties by causing a gradual loss of nerve function. People with LOTS have low levels of Hex-A rather than a complete lack of it. As LOTS develops, people affected by it may grow clumsy, uncoordinated, and moody. They may experience muscle weakness, twitching, slurred speech, and intellectual impairment. The symptoms vary in type and severity from person to person. Because this form develops so gradually, life expectancy of affected people seems to be similar to that of unaffected people.

How Do People Get Tay-Sachs Disease?

Tay-Sachs disease is caused by a mutation (abnormal change) in the gene that codes for Hex-A. It is a recessive trait, which means that people will have the disease if they have two copies of the defective gene, but they will not have the disease if they have at least one unaffected copy. People with one normal copy and one defective copy are called carriers, because they can pass the disease on to their children.

Just about anyone can be a carrier of the gene for Tay-Sachs disease. In the general population, about 1 in 250 people carries the gene. However, some populations of people include more carriers than others. For

* **metabolic** (meh-tuh-BALL-ik) pertains to the process in the body (metabolism) that converts food into energy and waste products.

* **enzyme** (EN-zime) is a protein that helps speed up a chemical reaction in cells or organisms.

* **seizures** (SEE-zhurs) are sudden bursts of disorganized electrical activity that interrupt the normal functioning of the brain, often leading to uncontrolled movements in the body and sometimes a temporary change in consciousness.

WHAT'S IN A NAME?

Tay-Sachs disease was named for two scientists working on opposite sides of the Atlantic Ocean.

Warren Tay (1843–1927) was a British eye doctor. In 1881 he described a patient with a cherry red spot on the retina (the structure inside the eye that receives light) of the eye. This spot is characteristic of the classical form of the disease.

The American neurologist (nerve and brain specialist) Bernard Sachs (1858–1944) described the changes in cells caused by the disease. He also recognized that it was an inherited condition that ran in families and that most babies with the disease were of eastern European Jewish descent.

example, 1 in 27 people of eastern European Jewish (Ashkenazi) descent in the United States is a carrier. People of French-Canadian ancestry from one part of Quebec and the Cajun population in Louisiana also have a higher than usual risk of carrying the Tay-Sachs gene.

Is There a Cure for Tay-Sachs Disease?

Although researchers look for a way to prevent or treat Tay-Sachs disease, as of 2009 no treatment or cure was known. However, tests have been developed that allow people to find out if they carry the defective gene. Blood tests can determine the level of Hex-A in people's blood (carriers have about half as much as noncarriers), and DNA tests may find evidence of mutations in the Hex-A gene. Testing is particularly useful for people who have had relatives with Tay-Sachs disease and for people in high-risk populations. Finding out about risk before having a baby can prevent an afflicted child from suffering and prevent the parental anguish of watching a child develop and then die from Tay-Sachs disease.

Prenatal tests also exist for women who already are pregnant. The amniotic fluid (the fluid in which the fetus develops) or the chorionic villus (structures inside the mother's uterus) both contain fluid from the developing baby that can be sampled and tested for the presence of Hex-A. If Hex-A is present, that means that the fetus does not have Tay-Sachs disease.

▶ *See also* **Genetic Diseases • Metabolic Disease**

Resources

Books and Articles

Walker, Julie. *Tay-Sachs Disease.* New York: Rosen, 2007.

Organizations

March of Dimes. 1275 Mamaroneck Avenue, White Plains, NY, 10605. Telephone: 914-997-4488. Web site: http://www.marchofdimes. com/pnhec/4439_1227.asp.

National Tay-Sachs and Allied Diseases Association. 2001 Beacon Street, Suite 204, Brookline, MA, 02146. Toll free: 800-906-8723. Web site: http://www.ntsad.org.

National Institute of Neurological Disorders and Stroke. P.O. Box 5801, Bethesda, MD, 20824. Toll free: 800-352-9424. Web site: http://www.ninds.nih.gov/disorders/taysachs/taysachs.htm.

National Library of Medicine. 8600 Rockville Pike, Bethesda, MD, 20894. Toll free: 888-346-3656. Web site: http://ghr.nlm.nih.gov/condition=taysachsdisease.

TB *See Tuberculosis.*

Teeth, Impacted *See Impacted Teeth.*

Temperature *See Fever.*

Temporomandibular Joint (TMJ) Syndrome

Temporomandibular (tem-po-ro-man-DIB-yoo-lar) joint syndrome refers to symptoms caused by problems with the joint that joins the jawbone to the skull.

What Is Temporomandibular Joint Syndrome?

The temporomandibular joint (TMJ) is the name for the jaw joint, one of which is located on each side of the head. These joints connect the lower jaw, or mandible (MAN-di-bul), to the temporal (TEM-po-ral) bone, which is one of a pair of bones that form the lower part of the skull. The temporomandibular joint acts as both a hinge and a gliding joint; together the pair of joints allow the jaw to open and close and to slide from side to side.

Side view of a temporomandibular joint. *Illustration by Frank Forney. Reproduced by permission of Gale, a part of Cengage Learning.*

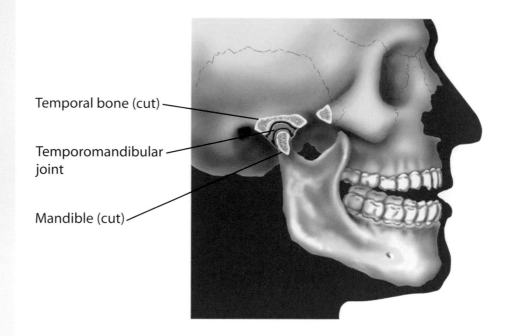

Temporal bone (cut)

Temporomandibular joint

Mandible (cut)

* **whiplash injuries** describe general injuries to the spine and spinal cord at the junction of the fourth and fifth vertebrae (VER-te-bray) in the neck occurring as a result of rapid acceleration or deceleration of the body.

* **arthritis** (ar-THRY-tis) refers to any of several disorders characterized by inflammation of the joints.

Temporomandibular joint syndrome refers to cases in which the joints do not function properly. This syndrome may cause pain, difficulty opening and closing the mouth, or problems with chewing and swallowing, as well as other symptoms.

What Are the Causes of Temporomandibular Joint Syndrome?

TMJ syndrome can be caused by dislocated temporomandibular joints or by inherited problems with the joints. In the condition called bruxism (BRUK-siz-um), some people grind their teeth during sleep or times of stress, which can lead to TMJ syndrome. Malocclusion (mal-o-KLOO-zhun), when teeth do not fit together properly; whiplash injuries* from car accidents; being hit on the head or jaw; and arthritis* are other causes of TMJ syndrome.

What Are the Symptoms of Temporomandibular Joint Syndrome?

Because the TMJ is located near many important nerves going between the brain and many parts of the body, the symptoms can be felt in parts of the body that do not seem related to the TMJ. Millions of Americans report some of the following symptoms:

- Frequent headaches
- Pain in the face, sinuses, ears, eyes, teeth, neck, and back
- Clicking sounds in the jaw
- Difficulty in opening or closing the mouth
- Trouble chewing or swallowing

How Is Temporomandibular Joint Syndrome Diagnosed and Treated?

Doctors or dentists ask the patient to describe the symptoms and then they examine the patient. Sometimes, x-rays and MRIs* are used to examine the joints to diagnose TMJ syndrome.

Hot compresses and over-the-counter pain medications may help relieve TMJ syndrome. Stress management and mouth guards worn at night can help eliminate teeth grinding and its effects.

▶ See also **Arthritis** • **Headache**

Resources

Organizations

National Institute of Dental and Craniofacial Research. 45 Center Drive, MSC 6400, Bethesda, MD, 20892. Telephone: 301-496-4261. Web site: http://www.nidcr.nih.gov/OralHealth/Topics/TMJ.

TMJ Association. P.O. Box 26770, Milwaukee, WI, 53226-0770. Telephone: 262-432-0350. Web site: http://www.tmj.org.

Tendinitis *See Repetitive Stress Syndrome.*

Tennis Elbow *See Repetitive Stress Syndrome.*

Testicular Cancer

Testicular (tes-TIK-yoo-lar) cancer occurs when cells in the testicle (TES-ti-kul), one of the two male sex glands located in the scrotum* below the penis, divide without control or order, forming a tumor*. Over time, these cancer cells can spread to other parts of the body.

Lance Armstrong's Story

In 1996, champion bicyclist Lance Armstrong (b. 1971) noticed that one of his testicles was enlarged. When he began coughing up blood, he went to his doctor. After discovering that he had cancer* in his testicle, he underwent an operation to remove the testicle. During the operation, doctors performed a CT scans*, which showed that the cancer had metastasized

* **MRI** which is short for magnetic resonance imaging, produces computerized images of internal body tissues based on the magnetic properties of atoms within the body.

* **scrotum** (SKRO-tum) is the pouch on a male body that contains the testicles.

* **tumor** (TOO-mor) is an abnormal growth of body tissue that has no known cause or physiologic purpose. A tumor may or may not be cancerous.

* **cancer** is a condition characterized by abnormal overgrowth of certain cells, which may be fatal.

* **CT scans** or CAT scans are the shortened name for computerized axial tomography (to-MOG-ra-fee), which uses computers to view structures inside the body.

Anatomy of the human male reproductive system showing the position of the testis. *Illustration by Frank Forney. Reproduced by permission of Gale, a part of Cengage Learning.*

▶

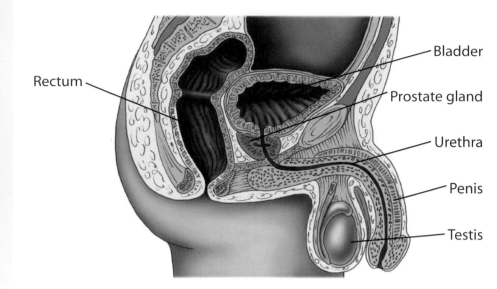

Rectum

Bladder

Prostate gland

Urethra

Penis

Testis

* **chemotherapy** (KEE-mo-THER-a-pee) is the treatment of cancer with powerful drugs that kill cancer cells.

* **hormones** are chemical substances that are produced by various glands and sent into the bloodstream carrying messages that have certain effects on other parts of the body.

(spread) to his abdomen, lungs, and brain. Lance immediately began an alternative chemotherapy* regimen to destroy the cancerous cells. He was given a 50 percent chance of survival.

For the next several months, Armstrong underwent chemotherapy in the hope that it would destroy the cancer. Fortunately, Armstrong was declared cancer free in 1997. Over the next year, Armstrong trained hard to get back into shape for cycling, and in 1998, he made his comeback by finishing fourth in the Vuelta a Espana, a three-week race in Europe. A year later, Armstrong won the Tour de France, which he went on to win every year following until 2005, shattering records.

In 1997, before he even knew if he would survive cancer, Armstrong established the Lance Armstrong Foundation, a nonprofit intended to inspire and empower all people who are affected by cancer. As of 2009, it had raised more than $250 million for cancer awareness, research, prevention, screening, and treatment.

"Livestrong," the motto of the Lance Armstrong Foundation, became a symbol of hope and perseverance worldwide. The simple yellow logo printed on wristbands, clothing, and even laptop computers.

What Is Testicular Cancer?

The testicles, also called the testes or male gonads, are the male sex glands located below the penis in a pouch of skin called the scrotum. The testicles are the body's main source of male hormones*, which control the development of the reproductive organs and male sex characteristics such as body and facial hair, low voice, and muscular arms. They also produce and store sperm (the tiny, tadpole-like cells that fertilize the female egg).

Testicular cancer usually begins when cells begin to divide without control or order, forming a tumor. Cells can break away from the tumor and enter the blood or the lymph, an almost colorless fluid produced by tissues all over the body. The fluid passes through lymph node*, the bean-shaped organs that filter the lymph, fight infection, and produce certain kinds of blood cells. When testicular cancer spreads, cancer cells usually are found in the nearby lymph nodes, the liver*, or the lungs.

What Makes Early Detection Important?

Like most types of cancer, testicular cancer can be treated most easily when it is found early. That is why doctors encourage all teenage boys and men to perform monthly testicular self-examination (TSE), which involves rolling each testicle between the fingers and thumb. The testicles are smooth, oval-shaped, and rather firm, and men who examine themselves regularly become familiar with the way their testicles feel. If any change occurs, it should be reported to a doctor. For many men, it takes time to get comfortable with doing TSE, but it is the best way to find a lump early. This usually is the first sign of testicular cancer.

Other possible symptoms of testicular cancer include the following:

- Any enlargement of a testicle
- A feeling of heaviness in the scrotum
- A dull persistent ache in the lower abdomen or the groin
- A sudden collection of fluid in the scrotum
- Pain or discomfort in a testicle or in the scrotum

It is important for all men to be aware of these symptoms, because doctors cannot predict who will get testicular cancer and who will not. As of 2009, the cause of testicular cancer was not known. Boys who are born with undescended testicles (located in the lower abdomen, rather than in the scrotum) have a higher risk of developing testicular cancer later in life. However, it usually develops for no apparent reason.

How Is Testicular Cancer Diagnosed?

Doctors begin by examining the scrotum and testes carefully and ordering urine and blood tests. These tests can help determine whether an infection or some other disorder might be causing the symptoms. Also, if a tumor is present, certain substances in the blood may be found at elevated levels. These substances are called tumor markers, because they often are found in abnormal amounts in patients with some types of cancer. The doctor may also order tests that create images of the inside of the body, such as a CT scan or an ultrasound*.

After all of these tests, the doctor can be reasonably certain about the diagnosis. However, the only sure way to determine whether cancer is present is to examine a sample of tissue under a microscope. In an operation, surgeons remove the affected testicle.

Once cancer is diagnosed, doctors need to figure out whether it has spread to other parts of the body and formed metastases*. They may perform other tests to look for cancer elsewhere. Because the cancer frequently

lymph node (LIMF) a small, bean-shaped mass of tissue containing immune system cells that fight harmful microorganisms. The lymph node may swell during infections.

liver is a large organ located beneath the ribs on the right side of the body. The liver performs numerous digestive and chemical functions essential for health.

ultrasound also called a sonogram, is a diagnostic test in which sound waves passing through the body create images on a computer screen.

metastases (me-TAS-ta-seez) are new tumors formed when cancer cells from a tumor spread to other parts of the body.

* **prosthesis** (pros-THEE-sis) is an artificial substitute for a missing body part. It can be used for appearance only or to replace the function of the missing part (as with a prosthetic leg).

spreads through the lymph nodes in the abdomen, these may be removed and then checked for cancer cells.

How Is Testicular Cancer Treated?

The removal of the testicle, which is necessary to diagnose the cancer, is also the first step in treating it. In addition, tumors that have spread to other parts of the body may be removed partly or entirely by surgery. In most cases, surgery will be followed by radiation therapy, which focuses high-energy rays on the remaining tumor to kill cancer cells and stop their growth.

In some cases, chemotherapy may be used either before or after surgery. During chemotherapy, anticancer drugs are given by mouth or by injection into a muscle or vein.

Life after Testicular Cancer

Fortunately, this disease responds well to treatment, even when it has spread from the testicle to other parts of the body. Men who have had testicular cancer need to see their doctors for regular follow-up appointments to make sure that the cancer has not returned.

A man with one healthy testicle can still have sex and father children. Radiation therapy and chemotherapy may cause a temporary drop in sperm production, but it usually returns to normal within a few months. Patients who are concerned about how they look can also have an artificial testicle, called a testicular prosthesis*, placed in the scrotum. It looks and feels just like a normal testicle.

▶ *See also* **Cancer: Overview • Prostate Problems**

Resources

Books and Articles

Armstrong, Lance, and Sally Jenkins. *It's Not about the Bike: My Journey Back to Life.* New York: Penguin, 2001.

Johanson, Paula. *Frequently Asked Questions about Testicular Cancer.* New York: Rosen, 2008.

Verville, Kathleen. *Testicular Cancer.* New York: Chelsea House, 2009.

Organizations

Lance Armstrong Foundation. P.O. Box 161150, Austin, TX, 78716. Telephone: 512-236-8820. Web site: www.livestrong.org.

National Cancer Institute. Public Inquiries Office, 6116 Executive Boulevard, Room 306A, Bethesda, MD, 20892. Toll free: 800-4-CANCER. Web site: http://www.cancer.gov/cancertopics/types/testicular.

Testing and Evaluation

Evaluation (ee-val-yoo-AY-shun) is the process of examining a problem or condition so that it can be understood and diagnosed. Testing is one of the ways to evaluate possible behavioral and mental health problems. Tests also can be used to measure normal abilities, such as intelligence, personality, certain brain functions, learning capabilities, and school progress.

Neal's Story

Neil was glad that he had remembered to bring an extra pencil with him to school today. He tapped it nervously on the desk while the teacher passed out booklets for the standardized test his class was about to take. Even though he knew this test did not count for his report card, he wanted to do well. As soon as the teacher finished giving the instructions, Neil opened the test booklet and began to read the first question.

What Are Standardized Tests?

A standardized test is a test that is given under the same conditions to everyone who takes it. The questions on the test, the instructions, the time allowed for taking the test, and the rules for scoring it are the same every time the test is given and for every person who takes it. For example, students in classrooms across the country may take the same standardized test to measure school progress. At each school the same test booklets, answer sheets, and instructions are used.

Standardized tests make it possible to compare the scores of a large group of people. For example, the math scores of all sixth grade students in the United States can be compared using a standardized test. It would not be possible to make such comparisons with the tests teachers make separately for their own classes, because those tests most likely would differ in ease or difficulty or might include different material. Using such tests, it would not be possible to make fair comparisons among students in different classes.

What Does a Score on a Standardized Test Mean?

The results of a standardized academic (schoolwork) test can show how well a student scored in certain subjects, such as reading comprehension (com-pree-HEN-shun) or math problem solving, compared with other students in the same grade throughout the country. Scores usually are given as percentiles in this type of test. For example, a student may score in the 86th percentile in reading comprehension, which means that the student can read and understand the readings as well as, or better than, 86 percent of all the students in the same grade who were tested.

What Do Standardized Tests Measure?

There are many types of standardized tests. Different tests measure different factors. There are standardized tests that can measure students regarding their academic progress, intelligence, memory, and behavior capabilities. Some standardized tests are given to a whole group of people at once, whereas others are given individually. Group tests generally are given in a classroom, such as tests that measure school progress. Scores show how well a student is doing in academic subjects compared with all other students in the same grade. A typical standardized test to measure academic progress consists of a test booklet with multiple-choice questions and a separate answer sheet on which the student fills in a circle to mark the correct answer.

Group standardized tests can measure academic progress at every level. Colleges and universities often use these tests to help decide whether to accept an individual as a student. For example, colleges and universities often require applicants to take the standardized test called the Scholastic Aptitude Test (SAT), graduate schools may require the standardized test called the Graduate Record Exam (GRE), and medical schools usually require the standardized test called the Medical College Admission Test (MCAT). Scores from these tests help a college or university compare the abilities of students who are applying and decide which students to accept. These tests measure how much a student has learned in school and how well a student can solve problems, as well as other learned skills or natural aptitudes that may predict that a given applicant will be a good student. Tests are just one measure of someone's capabilities, and they are generally just one of several factors used in evaluating an applicant for a college or university.

What Are Psychological Tests?

Some tests are given only by psychologists (sy-KAH-lo-jists), and they are called psychological (sy-ko-LAH-ji-kal) tests. Among the most common psychological tests are those that measure intelligence. Intelligence tests are examples of standardized psychological tests. Some other psychological tests are not standardized, but they can still provide important information about a person's personality, feelings, ideas, and concerns and can help evaluate and diagnose problems they may have. Most psychological tests are given individually and involve a face-to-face meeting with the psychologist during testing.

One commonly used psychological test to measure intelligence (IQ) in childhood is the Wechsler Intelligence Scale for Children (ages 6–16). There is also the Wechsler Adult Intelligence Scale, which can be given to anyone over 16 years of age. Intelligence tests also can help evaluate a person for possible learning disabilities, attention problems, and mental retardation. These tests can accurately measure a person's intelligence under most circumstances, but some factors may prevent individuals from scoring their best, such as not feeling well or being extremely nervous about taking the test. The psychologist takes these possibilities into account and decides whether the test on that day should be considered an accurate reading of the person's true capabilities.

Placing Students in the Right Classroom

Paula was not sure what to expect when it came time for her to meet with Dr. James, the school psychologist. She knew there would be tests, but she did not know what type. As she walked from her classroom to Dr. James's office, she felt just a little nervous. But as Dr. James showed her what to do, Paula felt more at ease. Paula found that taking the tests was interesting. Some parts were easy, and others were more difficult. There were vocabulary words, number problems, puzzle pieces to put together, and pictures to arrange in order. There were about a dozen tests in all. Dr. James asked Paula to work quickly but carefully, and she used a stopwatch to time how long it took Paula to do certain parts of the test, such as arranging blocks to match a design. Paula was excited when, a few weeks later, she found out that she had done well enough on the tests to be placed next year in a class for gifted students. The test Paula had taken was the Wechsler Intelligence Scale for Children.

Paula's best friend, Kim, took the same tests, as well as some others, with Dr. James, but for a different reason. Kim had been having trouble with her schoolwork and was finding it hard to remember what she read. In Kim's case, the tests helped Dr. James diagnose a learning disability. The tests showed that although Kim was quite intelligent, her learning disability was preventing her from doing her best work. Kim started to go to a learning support class and knew it was helping when she got a B+ on her reading test.

What Are Personality Tests?

Certain psychological tests assess personality. Some personality tests are standardized, whereas others are not. An example of a standardized personality test is the Myers-Briggs Type Indicator (MBTI), which can measure a person's usual personality style. Although this test is designed for adults, it can be used for teens, and there are variations designed for younger children. Another standardized personality test for older teens and adults is the Minnesota Multiphasic Personality Inventory—Adolescent (MMPI-A), which helps identify problems with personality.

Projective tests also give information about someone's personality. Projective tests are not standardized, but psychologists follow certain guidelines for scoring and interpreting them. Projective tests usually include pictures that could have many possible meanings. People are asked to say what they see in the picture or to tell a story about it. Examples are the Thematic Apperception Test (TAT) for older teens and adults and the Children's Apperception Test (CAT) for younger children. The Rorschach Test is a projective test in which individuals are shown a series of inkblot designs on cards and asked what they see in the inkblot. These tests

* **reaction speed** is the time it takes to respond to a stimulus.

* **dementia** (dih-MEN-sha) is a loss of mental abilities, including memory, understanding, and judgment.

* **battery** in this case refers to a group of related tests that are given together.

* **vocational** (vo-KAY-shun-al) means relating to training in a particular job skill.

* **attention deficit hyperactivity disorder**, or ADHD, is a condition that makes it hard for a person to pay attention, sit still, or think before acting.

are called projective tests because people project their own imagination, ideas, and personality onto the inkblots or pictures.

What Are Neuropsychological Tests?

A specialized group of psychological tests measure brain capacities that can affect a person's behavior. These tests can help evaluate brain damage. These neuropsychological (nur-o-sy-ko-LAW-ji-kal) tests can measure such brain functions as memory, attention, eye-hand coordination, mental processing, and reaction speed*. Neuropsychological tests may be used to evaluate the effects of a brain injury, brain infection, or stroke or to assess individuals who have problems with memory, balance or learning or people who might have dementia*. Examples of neuropsychological test batteries include the Halstead-Reitan and the Luria-Nebraska tests. Each battery* includes a number of tests that are analyzed to find a pattern of functions. For example, some tests might examine language functions (left brain activities), some might compare motor coordination with each hand (comparing how each side of the brain works), and some might evaluate rapid decision making and problem solving (examining frontal brain regions).

Other Tests

Adaptive behavior tests can measure people's capabilities to care for themselves and carry out other types of behavior important for daily living, such as counting money, shopping, and taking public transportation. They also can assess various job skills. Adaptive behavior tests often are used to evaluate the strengths, capabilities, and needs of individuals who have a developmental disability.

Vocational* tests can assess people's interests, skills, and aptitudes for particular jobs. There are also many kinds of tests that allow people to choose words or phrases that best describe themselves. Such "self-report" tests include checklists about behavior, feelings, or problems. These checklists can help identify important issues and start a discussion with a mental health professional who may be evaluating individuals' needs and how best to help them. For example, a self-report measure to examine possible attention deficit hyperactivity disorder* might include symptoms of hyperactivity, impulsivity, and poor concentration. Scores are rated against how others self-report to give an indication of how significant the symptom pattern might be within a person's age group.

Evaluation Interviews

Tests are not the only means of finding out about a person. In fact, the most commonly used method of evaluation by psychologists and other mental health professionals is the interview. Interviewing, which consists of questions and answers and in-depth discussion, is an important and effective way to evaluate a person's emotional and behavioral condition. Mental health professionals are trained to use interviews to understand the many aspects of someone's situation and to begin to diagnose possible problems.

How Can Evaluation and Testing Help?

Evaluation, which sometimes includes testing, is the first step toward diagnosing a person's mental health condition and possible behavioral, emotional, or learning problems. Evaluation and testing lead to a greater understanding of a problem or condition and pave the way for effective treatment. Evaluation and testing also can provide greater understanding of a person's intelligence, vocational interests, aptitudes, and learning needs, so that an educational plan can be put in place that is best suited to that person's strengths and needs.

What Are the Limitations of Evaluation and Testing?

The limitations of evaluation and testing begin with the expressed purpose through which each method has been designed. A method that may be quite effective for one analysis may be highly inaccurate for a related concern. For example, the Stanford-Binet Intelligence Test is accurate for identifying how one's intellectual ability relates to the average. However, the Stanford-Binet could not identify the presence of a learning disability if someone was scoring below average. The validity of the test is compromised if the test is used in a way that is not intended for its use. Most tests are not designed to be administered too often in a short period of time. If a child were sick on the day of the first administration, a second administration can be scheduled shortly after the first. However, if someone were taking the test over and over trying to improve his/her score, the results would not be accepted as valid. The results could be skewed in a higher direction because the student became more familiar with the content. By contrast, the results could be skewed in a lower direction if the student became bored with the constant administrations.

The results of the evaluation and testing could be limited by unfounded assumptions regarding the constructs being tested. For example, the traditional view of intelligence has been that it is a fixed capability. If someone were to use the results of the intelligence test to promote this misconception, it would greatly limit the use of the test results. The practical application of the construct is, of course, a better measure of the construct than any test. The best validation of any intelligence test is its correlation with a student's adaptation to school. Adaptation to school has many influences. Changing any of these influences can help the student better adapt to school. Therefore, the practical application of intelligence would be improved.

How Well Do These Techniques Perform in Terms of Outcomes?

Evaluation and testing instruments are constantly updated and revised as their common use and expectations change. If some instrument was not producing the expected outcomes, it would surely be rejected as the problems become identified. Many research projects rely on the effectiveness of these instruments and techniques and are constantly reporting how they can be modified or under what conditions they should be used. In spite of this constant research and evaluation of the effectiveness of tests and techniques, there are still some general concerns.

Tests that rely on a high predictive value include the SAT, the GRE, and the MCAT. These tests have the goal of predicting how well a student will do in college as part of the college's evaluation of the student for admission. The evidence for the test's sole effectiveness is inconclusive. However, using the scores from these tests in coordination with other predictive measures such as the student's current Grade Point Average appears to be an effective means of predicting the student's first semester as a freshman for the SAT or the first semester in graduate school for the GRE or MCAT. Most colleges and university do not use the scores from these tests alone for determining admissions but find that they do contribute to the effectiveness of the overall decision-making process.

In the early 2000s the Myers-Briggs remained a popular personality test, even though it was designed originally in 1962. The purpose of the Myers-Briggs is different from many other tests as the results are meant to be used by the person taking the test. The result of the Myers-Briggs is one of 16 personality types, each with a description of preferences. Recognizing one's preferences can help in developing relationships with others and in exploring possible careers. The debatable value of the Myers-Briggs is that its concept of personality is different from the traditional view of personality. The Myers-Briggs test produces mutually exclusive types whereas the traditional personality types are based on a continuum of various traits. The Myers-Briggs approach sees personalities as qualitatively different whereas the traditional approach sees personalities as quantitatively different.

In general, projective techniques are accepted as being just as accurate for what they are meant to produce as standardized tests are. However, there are conflicting reports of the validity of projective techniques. One perceived threat in using the projective techniques with children is that children may fake their responses, thus hiding their true self. Also, the situation and the examiner's manner may influence the child's responses. Moreover, the lack of norms for these types of tests leads clinicians to rely on an individualized interpretation.

In spite of these weaknesses, the projective techniques remained popular with clinicians in the early 2000s. One reason is that the techniques work well as an "ice breaker" to therapy. Using these techniques helps to build rapport between the clinician and the children being evaluated. Another reason is that many clinicians use these techniques as part of a structured interview. The clinicians who use these techniques are looking for broad information while recognizing the low precision of the measures. The results then are treated like clues that can be further pursued later in therapy. No serious decision or immediate action would be based solely on the results of any one of these tests.

How Are These Evaluations Evaluated?

These evaluations need to be evaluated through constant monitoring and observation. Every testing instrument is evaluated through research efforts such as replicating the original research that developed the instrument. However, the reliability and validity established relate only to the instrument and not to its use or result in any given situation. No matter how well the evaluation of the test or technique might be in general, the test cannot guarantee an accurate evaluation for any individual. Each diagnosis has to be accepted as a hypothesis that is tested through constant updates of the student's situation or condition.

What Kind of Biases Have Been Found in These Methods?

Standardized tests are developed through constant updating of statistics for a specified population through a process called "norming." These tests are expected to be free from bias for the population for which it has been normed. However, the degree to which the normed population is described varies among the many tests available. For instance, if the population is given as American students in specified grade or range of grades, there should be some recognition for the diversity of ethnic groups among modern American students. Because there was no serious recognition of gender differences before the 1980s, if the test has not been normed since the early 1980s, there may be some gender bias.

There are other chances of bias in standardized tests, even the ones that have been normed properly. Most tests rely on questions that present an example or small story, often with a character's gender or ethnicity identified in some way. If these examples or stories promote gender or ethnic stereotypes, certain test takers may feel that the test was not meant for someone like them. Such stereotypes could be promoted if all the female characters are depicted as involved in traditional feminine roles or if every minority character is depicted as in trouble.

Another source of bias is called item bias in which the wording of the test question leads students of the same minority backgrounds to choose the same specific wrong answer over the right answer that they would have chosen had the wording been different. An example of item bias would be if a question on a standardized test required the test-taker to quickly recognize if the wife of a duke is a "duchess" or a "dutchess". Otherwise knowledgeable students from Dutchess County, New York, may not recognize the misspelling in the time allowed. They would have to ignore the spelling that is common to them in a way that students in other parts of the country would not. Therefore, the question would be testing something different for the Dutchess County students than for the other students taking the same standardized test. Similarly, the test question could use a term that may have a different meaning for members of a minority group. Usually the test publisher will catch these incidents of item bias for each administration of the test. There are some basic analytical methods to determine if all (or most) of the high test takers of a specific minority are choosing the same wrong answer on a particular question.

The use of standardized tests also may introduce a bias in comparing people with different test-taking skills. Students with limited English proficiency may not do as well on the test as an English-speaking student with similar characteristics (e.g. intelligence or achievement). The limited-English students will need more time to demonstrate their capability. Similarly, using a standardized test to compare students who are currently in school with adults who have been out of school for years may not be appropriate. The adults would not be as practiced in answering test questions as the students would be. This can be seen in the results of cross-sectional studies of age-related differences in intelligence. Young people were compared with middle-age and elderly people. The results demonstrated that the older the participant was, the more likely the intelligence score would be low. This reduction in intelligence has not been seen in other studies of age-related differences. Therefore, the difference must be a function of the testing situation or the test used to measure intelligence.

Projective tests are not free from cultural or gender bias; however, they have a new set of biases not seen in the standardized tests. Because the interpretation of the test rests on the judgment of the test administrator, there are openings for various subjective biases. The first bias is researcher bias, which occurs when test interpreters believe that they know what the outcome will be. Test interpreters may make small recording errors that lead the results to support the pre-established judgment. Additionally, test interpreters may pay more attention to those results that coincide with the pre-established judgment and ignore those results that go against it. If test interpreters are the same individuals as the test administrators, they may ask leading questions or give subtle hints to what the "correct" response is.

Another source of bias in the administration of projective tests is the social desirability on the part of individuals being tested. Social desirability occurs when individuals who are being tested respond with what they think are the socially acceptable response and not what they truly feel or think. Individuals may also think that the testing is leading to a predetermined end and may respond in a way that they believe will bring about that end. If individuals being tested perceive that the test administrator or interpreter has already decided what the results are, they may infer cues from the administrator and respond accordingly.

Resources

Books and Articles

Braaten, Ellen, and Gretchen Felopulos. *Straight Talk about Psychological Testing for Kids.* New York: Guilford, 2004.

Gregory, Robert J. *Psychological Testing: History, Principles, and Applications,* 5th ed. Boston: Pearson/Allyn and Bacon, 2007.

Organizations

American Psychological Association. 750 First Street NE,
Washington, DC, 20002-4242. Toll free: 800-374-2721.
Web site: http://www.apa.org/topics/topictest.html.

Association for Psychological Science. 1133 Fifteenth Street NW,
Suite 1000, Washington, DC, 20005. Telephone: 202-293-9300.
Web site: http://www.psychologicalscience.org.

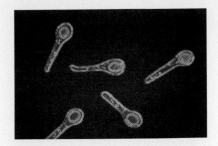

▲

Clostridium tetani spores magnified
2,000 times. *Peter Arnold, Inc./Alamy.*

Tetanus (Lockjaw)

Tetanus (TET-nus) is a serious bacterial infection that affects the body's central nervous system*. Tetanus, also known as lockjaw, can lead to muscle rigidity, convulsions*, and death.

What Is Tetanus?

Tetanus is a disease caused by infection with *Clostridium tetani* (klos-TRIH-dee-um teh-TAH-nye) bacteria, which are found all over the world in soil, dust, and some animal feces (FEE-seez, or bowel movements) and even on human skin. The bacteria can enter the body through any type of wound, such as a scratch or deep cut. Infection begins after bacterial spores* have moved deep within the body and become active. *Clostridium tetani* bacteria are anaerobic (ah-nuh-RO-bik), meaning that they grow best in places with very little oxygen—so the deeper they travel into the body, the better their chances of survival.

Once tetanus spores become active, the bacteria begin producing a toxin (a poisonous substance) called tetanospasmin (teh-tuh-no-SPAZ-min), which attaches to the nerves around the area of the wound. The tetanus toxin also can spread to the spine and attach to the ends of nerves of the spinal cord and at neuromuscular junctions (where nerves meet muscles). The toxin blocks the release of a neurotransmitter (nur-o-trans-MIH-ter), a chemical that carries a signal from nerves to other nerves or muscles. This block affects the messages that the muscles receive, resulting in severe muscle spasms* that can be powerful enough to tear muscles apart.

There are three types of tetanus infection. Local tetanus is limited to the area of the wound; cephalic (seh-FAH-lik) tetanus is an uncommon form that affects the nerves of the face after a head injury or, rarely, a long-lasting ear infection; and generalized tetanus affects much of the body and accounts for the majority of tetanus cases. Neonatal* tetanus is a generalized form of the infection that occurs in newborns. It is caused by bacteria contaminating the stump of the umbilical cord*,

* **central nervous system** (SEN-trul NER-vus SIS-tem) is the part of the nervous system that includes the brain and spinal cord.

* **convulsions** (kon-VUL-shuns), also called seizures, are involuntary muscle contractions caused by electrical discharges within the brain and are usually accompanied by changes in consciousness.

* **spores** are a temporarily inactive form of a germ enclosed in a protective shell.

* **spasms** (SPAH-zumz) are involuntary muscular tightening or contractions.

* **neonatal** (ne-o-NAY-tal) means pertaining to the first 4 weeks after birth.

* **umbilical cord** (um-BIH-lih-kul) is the flexible cord that connects a baby to the placenta, the organ that unites the unborn child to the mother's uterus, the organ in which the baby develops.

* **sterilize** (STAIR-uh-lyze) is to eliminate all live bacteria or microorgranisms from something, usually through the use of heat, pressure, chemicals, or other antimicrobial agents.

* **vaccination** (vak-sih-NAY-shun), also called immunization, is giving, usually by an injection, a preparation of killed or weakened germs, or a part of a germ or product it produces, to prevent or lessen the severity of the disease caused by that germ.

* **intravenous** (in-tra-VEE-nus) or IV, means within or through a vein. For example, medications, fluid, or other substances can be given through a needle or soft tube inserted through the skin's surface directly into a vein.

* **abdominal** (ab-DAH-mih-nul) refers to the area of the body below the ribs and above the hips that contains the stomach, intestines, and other organs.

* **culture** (KUL-chur) is a test in which a sample of fluid or tissue from the body is placed in a dish containing material that supports the growth of certain organisms. Typically, within days the organisms will grow and can be identified.

* **immune globulin** (ih-MYOON GLAH-byoo-lin), also called gamma globulin, is the protein material that contains antibodies.

* **respiratory system** or respiratory tract, includes the nose, mouth, throat, and lungs. It is the pathway through which air and gases are transported down into the lungs and back out of the body.

* **respirator** is a machine that helps people breathe when they are unable to breathe adequately on their own.

particularly if the cord has been cut with an instrument that has not been sterilized*.

How Common Is It?

Tetanus occurs around the world but is found frequently in densely populated areas that have hot, damp climates. The disease is rare in the United States primarily because of vaccination*. Nearly all reported cases of tetanus occur in people who have never been vaccinated or who have not had a booster shot in the previous 10 years. Neonatal tetanus infection is rare in developed countries because of improved surgical techniques, but there are hundreds of thousands of deaths from tetanus annually worldwide, mostly in developing countries. Intravenous* drug abusers, such as people who inject heroin, are at a higher risk of contracting the disease.

Is Tetanus Contagious?

Tetanus is not spread from person to person. Bacterial spores must enter a wound for the infection to spread.

What Are the Signs and Symptoms of Infection?

Symptoms of tetanus appear from 3 to 21 days or longer after infection, but usually they develop within seven days. In about 50 percent of generalized cases of tetanus, the first sign is trismus, or stiffness in the jaw muscles (also known as lockjaw), followed by a stiff neck, shoulder, or back; trouble swallowing; and fever. Spasms can soon spread to the abdominal* muscles, upper arms, and thighs. Other symptoms include sweating, high blood pressure, and periods of rapid heartbeat. The closer the infection is to the central nervous system, the sooner the symptoms appear. The earlier the symptoms begin to appear, the greater the risk of death.

How Do Doctors Make the Diagnosis?

The diagnosis is made based on the presence of symptoms and the patient's history (for example, getting a wound by stepping on a soil-contaminated nail). Laboratory tests are not useful in determining whether a patient has tetanus. A culture* of the wound can be done, but these cultures generally do not show the bacteria.

What Is the Treatment for Tetanus?

Typically, tetanus infection is treated in a hospital. Treatment begins with giving the patient tetanus immune globulin* to control or reverse the effects of toxin that has not yet attached itself to nerve endings. Penicillin or other antibiotics also may be given to kill the bacteria. Cleaning the wound and removing dead tissue, in some cases by surgery, is important in ridding the body of invading bacteria. Muscle spasms can be treated with muscle relaxants. Respiratory system* support, provided by a respirator* may be necessary to help maintain breathing if the respiratory muscles have been affected.

How Long Does Tetanus Last?

Symptoms may last three to four weeks, although complete recovery can take several months. Tetanus can be mild, but in most cases the illness is severe and death may occur even after treatment has begun. Tetanus usually requires a long stay in the intensive care unit of the hospital.

What Are the Complications?

Complications of the illness include spasms of the vocal cords and the muscles that control breathing, which can lead to difficulty breathing; fractures in the long bones or the spine from severe muscle spasms and convulsions; high blood pressure; abnormal heart rhythm; secondary infections, such as sepsis* and pneumonia (inflammation of the lung); a blood clot* in the lungs; and death. In the United States, 10 to 20 percent of reported tetanus cases are fatal. Unvaccinated children and the elderly are at greater risk of dying if they become infected with tetanus bacteria.

Can Tetanus Be Prevented?

Immunization is the best means of preventing tetanus. The vaccination usually is given in combination with other vaccines: the DTaP (diphtheria*/tetanus/acellular/pertussis*) form for children and the Td (tetanus/diphtheria) form for adults. A series of shots is required to develop immunity to tetanus toxin, followed by booster shots every 10 years. In some cases of unclean wounds, a booster is given after the injury to help prevent tetanus.

▶ See also **Skin and Soft Tissue Infections**

Resources

Books and Articles

Guilfoile, Patrick. *Tetanus.* New York: Chelsea House, 2008.

Organization

Centers for Disease Control and Prevention. 1600 Clifton Road, Atlanta, GA, 30333. Toll free: 800-311-3435. Web site: http://www.cdc.gov/vaccines/vpd-vac/tetanus/default.htm.

* **sepsis** is a potentially serious spreading of infection, usually bacterial, through the bloodstream and body.

* **blood clot** is a thickening of the blood into a jelly-like substance that helps stop bleeding. Clotting of the blood within a blood vessel can lead to blockage of blood flow.

* **diphtheria** (dif-THEER-e-uh) is an infection of the lining of the upper respiratory tract (the nose and throat). It is a serious disease that can cause breathing difficulty and other complications, including death.

* **pertussis** (per-TUH-sis) is a bacterial infection of the respiratory tract that causes severe coughing.

Thalassemia

Thalassemia is a genetic blood disorder. People with thalassemia have too few red blood cells and lower-than-normal hemoglobin.

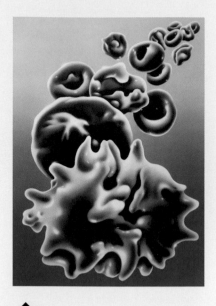

▲

Distorted red blood cells in the inherited blood disorder thalassemia. Affected red blood cells are variously shaped and fragile; they rapidly break up as they move through the body. *John Bavosi/ Photo Researchers, Inc.*

* **hemoglobin** (HE-muh-glo-bin) is the oxygen-carrying pigment of the red blood cells.

* **immune system** (im-YOON SIS-tem) is the system of the body composed of specialized cells and the substances they produce that helps protect the body against disease-causing germs.

* **platelets** (PLATE-lets) are tiny disk-shaped particles within the blood that play an important role in clotting.

* **anemia** (uh-NEE-me-uh) is a blood condition in which there is a decreased hemoglobin in the blood and, usually, fewer than normal numbers of red blood cells.

* **genes** (JEENS) are chemical structures composed of deoxyribonucleic acid (DNA) that help determine a person's body structure and physical characteristics. Inherited from a person's parents, genes are contained in the chromosomes found in the body's cells.

What Is Thalassemia?

Thalassemia is a blood disorder that runs in families. People who have thalassemia have too few red blood cells and lower hemoglobin* than normal.

What Causes Thalassemia?

The type of thalassemia that individuals develop depends on which chain of the hemoglobin is affected. If the alpha chain is defective, alpha-thalassemia results; if the beta chain is defective, beta-thalassemia results. The severity and specifics of the disease also depend on how many defective genes individuals have.

In the case of alpha-thalassemia, one defective gene does not cause individuals to develop any of the symptoms of thalassemia, although they can go on to pass that same defective gene on to offspring. Inheriting two defective genes results in a condition called alpha-thalassemia minor, with only very mild symptoms. Three defective genes results in a condition called hemoglobin H disease, which causes moderately severe symptoms. Four defective genes is termed alpha-thalassemia major or hydrops fetalis, which is fatal to offspring in utero or within a short time after birth.

In the case of beta-thalassemia, one defective gene results in beta-thalassemia minor, which causes mild symptoms; two defective genes results in beta-thalassemia major (also known as Cooley's anemia), which causes moderately severe symptoms. Babies with this condition are usually

ABOUT THE BLOOD AND HEMOGLOBIN

Blood is made up of a watery substance called plasma, in which circulate the various types of blood cells: red blood cells (mainly responsible for delivering oxygen to the tissues), white blood cells (involved in immune system* response), and platelets*.

Red blood cells contain hemoglobin, a complex, iron-rich protein that is responsible for picking up oxygen molecules from the lungs, delivering oxygen to all of the tissues throughout the body, picking up carbon dioxide (a waste product) from all of the tissues, and taking the carbon dioxide back to the lungs where it can be dissipated during exhalation. Too little hemoglobin in the bloodstream is called anemia*.

Hemoglobin is made up of two types of protein chains, called alpha and beta chains. Defects in alpha chains result in alpha-thalassemia; defects in beta chains result in beta-thalassemia. The production of alpha chains requires four different genes* (two from each parent), whereas production of beta chains requires only two different genes (one from each parent).

asymptomatic at birth but develop symptoms of the disease during their first year.

Who Gets Thalassemia?

Thalassemia is one of the most common genetic* conditions. It occurs worldwide, but most commonly affects people of Greek, Italian, Middle Eastern, Asian, and African descent. Alpha-thalassemia is particularly common among descendents of people who come from Southeast Asia, China, and the Philippines. People who already know that family members have the disease are obviously at very high risk of having the condition themselves or of passing it on to their offspring.

Some experts believe that the genetic defects of thalassemia have persisted because the abnormal red blood cell configurations actually provide some protection against malaria*, because the shape of the thalassemic red blood cells inhibits the entry of the malarial parasite into the cells. Malaria is a serious problem in all the geographic areas where thalassemia has the highest frequency.

What Are the Symptoms of Thalassemia?

Symptoms of thalassemia are those of anemia, including pallor, weakness, severe fatigue, shortness of breath, dizziness, fast heart rate, decreased appetite, unintentional weight loss, failure to thrive* in babies or poor growth and development in children. Other symptoms may include jaundice*, dark urine, bloated abdomen, fevers, diarrhea, smooth swollen tongue, and abnormalities of the facial bones.

How Is Thalassemia Diagnosed?

Thalassemia may be suspected based on the presence of characteristic symptoms, as well as due to knowledge of individuals' family history. A physical examination will reveal some of the characteristic signs of thalassemia. Blood tests can be done to demonstrate red blood cell abnormalities (in shape, size, and quantity), decreased levels of hemoglobin and iron, which is a major component of hemoglobin. Genetic testing may be performed to reveal the abnormal genes that are responsible for thalassemia.

How Is Thalassemia Treated?

Minor forms of thalassemia may have such mild symptoms that no treatment is required. In some cases, illness, stress, surgery, childbirth, or severe infections may prompt the need for a blood transfusion*.

Major forms of thalassemia may require regular blood transfusions. Unfortunately this treatment puts recipients at high risk of accumulating too much iron in the blood, which can be damaging to multiple organs, including the heart and liver. Drugs may be required to decrease the amount of iron in the blood (called iron chelators or chelating agents). Very severe complications from thalassemia may require a bone marrow* transplant or stem cell transplant.

* **genetic** (juh-NEH-tik) refers to heredity and the ways in which genes control the development and maintenance of organisms.

* **malaria** (mah-LAIR-e-uh) is a disease spread to humans by the bite of an infected mosquito.

* **failure to thrive** is a condition in which an infant fails to gain weight and grow at the expected rate.

* **jaundice** (JON-dis) is a yellowing of the skin, and sometimes the whites of the eyes, caused by a buildup in the body of bilirubin, a chemical produced in and released by the liver. An increase in bilirubin may indicate disease of the liver or certain blood disorders.

* **blood transfusion** is the process of giving blood (or certain cells or chemicals found in the blood) to a person who needs it due to illness or blood loss.

* **bone marrow** is the soft tissue inside bones where blood cells are made.

* **chorionic villus sampling** (KOR-ee-on-ik VIL-lus sampling) is a test in which a small tube is inserted through the cervix and a small piece of the placenta supporting the fetus is removed for genetic testing.

* **amniocentesis** (am-nee-o-sen-TEE-sis) is a test in which a long, thin needle is inserted in the mother's uterus to obtain a sample of the amniotic fluid from the sac that surrounds the fetus. The fetal cells in the fluid are then examined for genetic defects.

* **in vitro** in the laboratory or other artificial environment rather than in the living body.

* **oral** means by mouth or referring to the mouth.

* **yeast** (YEEST) is a general term describing single-celled fungi that reproduce by budding.

Can Thalassemia Be Prevented?

People who know that thalassemia runs in their families can undergo genetic counseling to ascertain their own risk of passing the condition on to their offspring. Once a baby has been conceived, prenatal tests can determine whether the fetus has the disease. Tests include chorionic villus sampling* or amniocentesis*

Assisted reproductive technology can also be used to try to avoid conceiving babies who have the genes for thalassemia. This technology requires in vitro* fertilization. Blastoplasts (cell masses that can develop into embryos) are tested for the presence of the thalassemia-causing genes, and only those without these genes (usually two) are then implanted into the woman's uterus.

▶ See also **Anemia, Bleeding, and Clotting**

Resources

Organizations

Cooley's Anemia Foundation. 330 Seventh Avenue, No. 900, New York, NY, 10001. Toll free: 800-522-7222. Web site: http://www.thalassemia.org.

March of Dimes. 1275 Mamaroneck Avenue, White Plains, NY, 10605. Toll free: 914-997-4488. Web site: http://search.marchofdimes.com.

Thrombosis *See Phlebitis and Venous Thrombosis.*

Thrush

Thrush is a fungal infection of the oral* cavity. It usually manifests as raised white patches in the mouth and throat that may have the appearance of cottage cheese. The infection is usually caused by a Candida fungus (a fungus of the genus Candida), of which Candida albicans is the most common. Candida is also the type of fungus that causes most diaper rash and vaginal yeast* infections. Thrush may also be caused by a fungus of the genus Monila.

What Is Thrush?

Thrush is an oral fungal infection. The most common causative agent, Candida albicans, is a single-celled fungus (single-celled fungi, or yeasts, reproduce by budding) that is a natural inhabitant of the mouth. Usually, the body maintains a natural balance of microbes* in the mouth. If that natural balance has been disturbed, however, *Candida* and other fungi may begin to grow in the warm moist environment of the mouth and throat. Other names for thrush are oral candidiasis (kan-di-DY-a-sis) and oral moniliasis (mon-i-LY-a-sis).

Thrush and the immune system   Thrush is common in newborns. In older children, and adults, it may be a sign of an immune system* disorder. People whose immune systems have been damaged by HIV*, human immunodeficiency virus, the virus that causes AIDS*, for example, may develop thrush, as a properly functioning immune system is needed to maintain the natural balance of microbes in the mouth. Others at risk for thrush include individuals who are treated with antibiotics* for bacterial infections and people who use steroid inhalers for asthma*.

Neonatal thrush   Infants may become infected during the birth process if their mothers have vaginal yeast infections, or they may get thrush from bottles or rubber nipples that have not been handled carefully, or from a family member or caregiver whose hands have been poorly washed. Thrush usually appears as whitish, smooth (even velvety) patches on the tongue, palate (roof of the mouth), inner cheeks, or throat. The whitish patches should not be scraped, as this will hurt the infant and leave behind an inflamed and possibly bleeding area, and infants may refuse to suck because of pain in the mouth. Candida also causes diaper rash, but the rash is reddish rather than white.

How Is Thrush Diagnosed and Treated?

A doctor can almost always diagnose thrush just by looking at the mouth and tongue. If uncertain, however, the doctor may perform a culture of one of the lesions. Thrush may be a sign of an immune system deficiency, and people with thrush or with suspected thrush should visit a doctor or dentist, who will be able to identify the yeast under a microscope if necessary, check for possible causes, and suggest ways to prevent its recurrence. For thrush in neonates and infants, treatment is often unnecessary. Doctors usually treat thrush with antifungal drugs* that is either taken orally or applied directly to the affected areas. They will also recommend careful hygiene, which includes frequent hand washing, frequent diaper changes, and the use of certain mouth washes.

In some people, thrush may progress to a full systemic disease, which is generally severe. This includes persons with HIV/AIDS, persons receiving chemotherapy* or immunosuppressant drugs, or persons with some other immune system disorder. The treatment for this type of often-severe

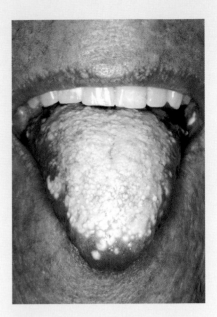

▲

Candida albicans coats the tongue of a person with thrush. ©*Medical-on-Line/Alamy.*

* **microbes** (MY-krobes) are microscopic living organisms, such as bacteria, viruses and fungi.

* **immune system** (im-YOON SIS-tem) is the system of the body composed of specialized cells and the substances they produce that helps protect the body against disease-causing germs.

* **HIV** or human immunodeficiency virus (HYOO-mun ih-myoo-no-dih-FIH-shen-see), it the virus that causes AIDS (acquired immunodeficiency syndrome).

* **AIDS** or acquired immunodeficiency (ih-myoo-no-dih-FIH-shen-see) syndrome, is an infection that severely weakens the immune system; it is caused by the human immunodeficiency virus (HIV).

* **antibiotics** (an-tie-by-AH-tiks) are drugs that kill or slow the growth of bacteria.

* **asthma** (AZ-mah) is a condition in which the airways of the lungs repeatedly become narrowed and inflamed, causing breathing difficulty.

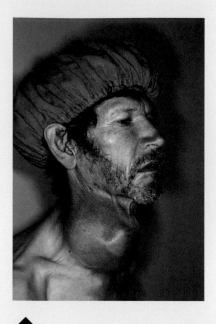

Bolivian man suffering from thyroid cancer. ©PHOTOTAKE Inc./Alamy.

* **antifungal drugs** (an-ty-FUNG-al drugs) are medications that kill fungi.

* **chemotherapy** (KEE-mo-THER-a-pee) is the treatment of cancer with powerful drugs that kill cancer cells.

* **intravenous** (in-tra-VEE-nus) or IV, means within or through a vein. For example, medications, fluid, or other substances can be given through a needle or soft tube inserted through the skin's surface directly into a vein.

* **endocrine** (EN-do-krin) refers to a group of glands, such as the thyroid, adrenal, and pituitary glands, and the hormones they produce. The endocrine glands secrete their hormones into the bloodstream, and the hormones travel to the cells that have receptors for them. Certain hormones have effects on mood and sometimes cause emotional swings.

candidiasis is intravenous* antifungal medication, which is administered in a hospital setting.

▶ See also **Oral Infections**

Resources

Organizations

Centers for Disease Control and Prevention. 1600 Clifton Road, Atlanta, GA, 30333. Toll free: 800-232-4636. Web site: http://www.cdc.gov/nczved/dfbmd/disease_listing/candidiasis_gi.html.

University of Michigan Health System. 1500 E. Medical Center Drive, Ann Arbor, MI, 48109. Telephone: 734-936-4000. Web site: http://www.med.umich.edu/1libr/pa/pa_thrush_hhg.htm.

Thyroid Cancer

Thyroid cancer is a cancer that begins in the thyroid gland, one of the largest endocrine glands in the human body.

What is the Thyroid Gland?

The thyroid gland is a large, butterfly shaped gland that regulates the endocrine* (Ehn-doh-crin) system. It is located in the front of the throat, just below the Adam's apple. Normally, the thyroid cannot be seen or felt under the skin.

The thyroid gland has two kinds of cells: follicular cells and parafollicular cells, also called C cells. The follicular cells make thyroid hormones (T3 and T4), and the C cells make another hormone called calcitonin, which is involved with the regulation of calcium in the blood. The pituitary* gland, which is located in the brain, releases TSH, or thyroid stimulating hormone*. This hormone stimulates the follicular and C cells in the thyroid to create important hormones for the rest of the body. These hormones control factors that are regulated by metabolism, such as heart rate, blood pressure, body temperature, and energy consumption.

What Is Thyroid Cancer?

To understand thyroid cancer*, it is important to understand what cancer is. Cancer occurs when the cells in a certain part of the body undergo abnormal changes and start dividing without control or order, forming tumors*. A tumor found on the thyroid is called a nodule. Nodules are usually felt under the skin by the patient or by a doctor during a routine exam. Sometimes, nodules can cause neck pain or a change in voice.

There are about 37,000 new cases of thyroid cancer every year in the United States. It is much more common in women than men. Up to 95 percent of thyroid nodules are noncancerous, or benign*, but a small percentage are cancerous, or malignant*. If detected early, thyroid cancer treatment is usually very successful. Thyroid cancer is one of the least deadly cancers.

What Are The Three Types of Thyroid Cancer?

There are three types of thyroid cancer:

- Papillary and follicular (fole-ik-U-lar) thyroid cancers make up the vast majority of thyroid cancer (80–90%). These types of cancers both begin in the follicular cells of the thyroid. These cancers tend to grow slowly and are therefore very treatable.

- Medullary thyroid cancers make up about 5 to 10 percent of all thyroid cancers. This type of cancer begins in C cells. If medullary thyroid cancer is found early, it is usually very treatable.

- Anaplastic thyroid cancer is the rarest form of the disease, and it makes up only about 1 to 2 percent of all cases. This cancer tends to metastasize (meh-tas-tah-size), or spread to other parts of the body, very quickly, making it much more difficult to treat.

What Are the Symptoms of Thyroid Cancer?

Sometimes, people who have thyroid cancer may not even know that there is anything wrong. Over time nodules may grow bigger. The vast majority of cases are detected when a patient feels a nodule in the neck. Most of these nodules (95 percent) are benign. Once thyroid cancer progresses, it may cause a variety of symptoms. These may include a change in voice, a lump on the thyroid that can be felt in the neck, enlarged lymph nodes*, pain or discomfort in the neck or ears, frequent coughing, or difficulty eating, swallowing, or breathing.

What Causes Thyroid Cancer?

As of 2009, scientists had not pinpointed what exactly causes thyroid cancer. There are, however, several known risk factors. These include the following:

- Gender. Thyroid cancer is about three times more likely to occur in women than in men.

- Age. Most cases of thyroid cancer are found in people between the ages of 20 and 60.

- Race. White people are more likely to be diagnosed with thyroid cancer than African Americans.

Did You Know?

Over 95 percent of all thyroid nodules are benign. Most people who are diagnosed with thyroid cancer have an excellent prognosis. The 5-year survival rate for thyroid cancer is about 97 percent.

* **pituitary** (pih-TOO-ih-tare-e) is a small oval-shaped gland at the base of the skull that produces several hormones—substances that affect various body functions, including growth.

* **hormone** is a chemical substance that is produced by a gland and sent into the bloodstream carrying messages that have certain effects on other parts of the body.

* **cancer** is a condition characterized by abnormal overgrowth of certain cells, which may be fatal.

* **tumors** (TOO-morz) are abnormal growths of body tissue that have no known cause or physiologic purpose. Tumors may or may not be cancerous.

* **benign** (be-NINE) refers to a condition that is not cancerous or serious and will probably improve, go away, or not get worse.

* **malignant** (ma-LIG-nant) refers to a condition that is severe and progressively worsening.

* **lymph nodes** (LIMF) are small, bean-shaped masses of tissue containing immune system cells that fight harmful microorganisms. Lymph nodes may swell during infections.

* **genes** (JEENS) are chemical structures composed of deoxyribonucleic acid (DNA) that help determine a person's body structure and physical characteristics. Inherited from a person's parents, genes are contained in the chromosomes found in the body's cells.

* **endocrinologist** (en-do-krin-OL-o-jist) is a doctor who specializes in treating patients with hormone-related disorders.

* **ultrasound** also called a sonogram, is a diagnostic test in which sound waves passing through the body create images on a computer screen.

* **biopsy** (BI-op-see) is a test in which a small sample of skin or other body tissue is removed and examined for signs of disease.

* **aspiration** (as-puh-RAY-shun) is the sucking of fluid or other material out of the body, such as the removal of a sample of joint fluid through a needle inserted into the joint.

■ Diet. Thyroid cancer is most common in areas where people tend to eat foods that are very low in iodine, which is often not a problem in people who follow standard American diets.

■ Heredity. Some people may be predisposed to thyroid cancer by inheriting a gene*called RET. But not all people who have the RET gene develop thyroid cancer.

■ Radiation. People who are exposed to high doses of radiation may be at a higher risk of developing thyroid cancer.

How Is Thyroid Cancer Diagnosed?

Most thyroid cancers are detected when a patient or doctor feels nodules on the front of the neck. The doctor may request further testing to determine exactly what the nodule is. After nodules are found, patients are usually referred to a specialist called an endocrinologist*, who will do the following:

■ Order tests such as x-rays, ultrasound*, and other imaging tests, which produce images of the thyroid gland and are used to determine the size and amount of nodules present on the thyroid.

■ Order lab tests that can determine the amount of thyroid stimulating hormone (TSH), calcitonin, and calcium that is present in the blood.

■ Perform a biopsy* to determine if the thyroid nodules are benign or malignant. A biopsy usually entails taking sample tissue and cells from the nodules with a needle, a process called needle aspiration*. Another doctor, called a pathologist, then looks at the tissue and cells under a microscope to determine whether they are cancerous.

What Are The Stages of Thyroid Cancer?

Using some of the same tests that are used during diagnosis, doctors are able to assign a stage to thyroid cancer. Staging is used to give patients a treatment plan and prognosis. There is a standard staging system that is used for all types of cancer called TNM. *T* refers to the size of the tumor and whether it has spread to nearby areas. *N* describes how much the tumor has spread to areas such as the lymph nodes. *M* indicates whether the cancer has spread to other major body organs, such as the lungs or brain.

The American Cancer Society uses the following chart on its web site to explain the complex staging system for thyroid cancer.

T categories for thyroid cancer:

■ TX: Primary tumor cannot be assessed.

■ T0: No evidence of primary tumor.

■ T1: The tumor is 2cm (slightly less than an inch) across or smaller.

■ T2: Tumor is between 2cm and 4cm (slightly less than 2 inches) across.

- T3: Tumor is larger than 4cm or has begun to grow into nearby tissues outside the thyroid.
- T4a: Tumor of any size and has grown extensively beyond the thyroid gland into nearby tissues of the neck.
- T4b: Tumor has grown either back toward the spine or into nearby large blood vessels.

For anaplastic thyroid cancers:

- T4a: Tumor is still within the thyroid and may be resectable (removable by surgery).
- T4b: Tumor has grown outside the thyroid and is not respectable.

N categories for thyroid cancer:

- NX: Regional (nearby) lymph nodes cannot be assessed.
- N0: No spread to nearby lymph nodes is noted.
- N1: Spread to nearby lymph nodes is noted.
- N1a: Spread to lymph nodes around the thyroid in the neck (cervical) is noted.
- N1b: Spread to lymph nodes in the sides of the neck (lateral cervical) or the upper chest (upper mediastinal) is noted.

M categories for thyroid cancer:

- MX: Presence of distant metastasis (spread) cannot be assessed.
- M0: No distant metastasis is noted.
- M1: Distant metastasis is present, involving distant lymph nodes, internal organs, bones.

By considering several specific aspects of TNM, a patient's age, and the type of thyroid cancer the individual has, doctors can assign a stage from I (1) through IV (4). As with most types of cancer, those that are detected in early stages before they have spread have a better prognosis.

How Is Thyroid Cancer Treated?

Once a diagnosis of thyroid cancer has been made, patients undergo a series of procedures. In order to get rid of the cancer, doctors must get rid of all of the cells that have been affected by the cancer. Doing so almost always includes the removal of the thyroid gland, which is called a thyroidectomy. Sometimes, doctors also remove nearby lymph nodes.

A few weeks after the thyroid has been removed surgically, patients may also be given treatment with radioactive iodine to destroy any remaining tissue of the thyroid that may have cancerous cells.

If thyroid cancer is diagnosed as advanced, patients may need to undergo chemotherapy* or radiation therapy.

Because the thyroid produces important hormones that the body needs to function properly, patients who undergo a thyroidectomy are placed on hormone replacement therapy for the rest of their lives.

* **chemotherapy** (KEE-mo-THER-a-pee) is the treatment of cancer with powerful drugs that kill cancer cells.

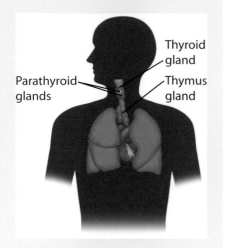

Anatomy of the thyroid glands, parathyroids, and thymus. *Illustration by Frank Forney. Reproduced by permission of Gale, a part of Cengage Learning.*

* **hormone** is a chemical substance that is produced by a gland and sent into the bloodstream carrying messages that have certain effects on other parts of the body.

What Is the Prognosis for Thyroid Cancer?

Patients who are diagnosed with thyroid cancer are usually given an excellent prognosis. If treated quickly and appropriately, most cases of thyroid cancer have more than a 97-percent treatment success rate.

▶ *See also* **Cancer: Overview**

Resources

Books and Articles

Quickfacts Thyroid Cancer: What You Need to Know Now. Atlanta, GA: American Cancer Society, 2009.

Rosenthal, M. Sara. *The Thyroid Cancer Book* 2nd ed. Canada: Your Health Press, 2006.

Van Nostrand, Douglas, Gary Bloom, and Leonard Wartofsky, eds. *Thyroid Cancer: A Guide for Patients.* Pasadena, MD: Keystone Press, 2004.

Organizations

American Thyroid Association. 6066 Leesburg Pike, Suite 550, Falls Church, VA, 22041. Telephone: 703-998-8890. Web site: www.thyroid.org.

ThyCa: Thyroid Cancer Survivors' Association. P.O. Box 1545, New York, NY, 10159. Toll free: 877-588-7904. Web site: www.thyca.org.

Thyroid Disease

Thyroid disease is an impairment in the normal functioning of the thyroid, an important gland located below the chin at the base of the neck. A major function of the thyroid is to regulate metabolism, the biochemical processes in the body. Thyroid disease may speed up or slow down metabolism, producing a wide range of physical and mental symptoms.

What Is the Thyroid?

The thyroid is an H-shaped gland that has two main parts, or lobes, that lie on either side of the trachea (TRAY-key-a), or windpipe. The lobes are connected by a narrow segment called the isthmus. The principal hormone* produced by the thyroid is thyroxine. Production of this hormone is in turn controlled by another hormone, called thyroid-stimulating hormone (TSH), secreted by the pituitary gland located at the base of the brain. Thyroxine is released into the bloodstream and controls the rate of metabolism*. In children, thyroid hormones are essential for normal growth and development.

What Is Thyroid Disease?

Disorders of the thyroid can cause overproduction of thyroid hormones (hyperthyroidism) or underproduction of thyroid hormones (hypothyroidism). Sometimes the thyroid becomes enlarged, a condition known as goiter.

Hyperthyroidism: a revving engine   The most common type of hyperthyroidism, or thyrotoxicosis (thy-ro-tox-i-KO-sis), is Graves' disease, an autoimmune disease*, a disturbance of the immune system*. Antibodies* stimulate the thyroid to produce excessive quantities of hormone, thereby raising the rate of metabolism. Graves' disease can occur in people of any age, but the highest incidence is in women between 20 and 40 years of age.

Symptoms of Graves' disease include an increased heart rate, nervousness and irritability, tremor, loss of weight, enlarged thyroid gland (goiter), abnormalities of the menstrual periods, sweating and heat intolerance, restless overactivity, and sleeplessness. Sometimes there is also exophthalmos (eks-off-THAL-mus), a condition in which the eyeballs protrude (bulge outward).

Less commonly, hyperthyroidism results from a form of thyroiditis (thy-roid-EYE-tus), an inflammation of the thyroid caused by a viral infection or by thyroid nodules (lumps or growths) that may produce excess hormones.

Hypothyroidism: a slowing down   Whereas hyperthyroidism abnormally raises the metabolic rate, hypothyroidism slows it down too much. Many of the symptoms of hypothyroidism are thus the reverse of those seen in hyperthyroidism. The most common cause of hypothyroidism is Hashimoto's thyroiditis, which occurs most often in young and middle-aged women.

Hashimoto's thyroiditis, like Graves' disease, is an autoimmune disease. The immune system damages the thyroid rather than stimulating it, resulting in an underproduction of hormone. Symptoms of Hashimoto's thyroiditis include a slow heart rate, tiredness, muscular weakness, weight gain, abnormal menstrual periods, intolerance of cold, dry skin, hair loss, hoarseness, enlarged thyroid (goiter), and mental dullness. In more severe cases, there may be myxedema (mik-se-DEE-ma), a thickening and puffiness of the skin most noticeable in the face.

Less often, hypothyroidism is caused by surgical removal of part or all of the thyroid gland to treat other thyroid conditions, or by insufficient iodine in the diet, which is rare in developed countries.

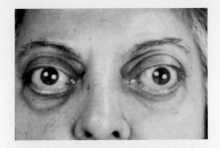

▲

Graves' disease causes exophthalmos or bulging of the eyes. *Chet Childs/ Custom Medical Stock Photo, Inc. Reproduced by permission.*

* **metabolism** (meh-TAB-o-liz-um) is the process in the body that converts foods into the energy necessary for body functions.

* **autoimmune disease** (aw-toh-ih-MYOON) is a disease in which the body's immune system attacks some of the body's own normal tissues and cells.

* **immune system** (im-YOON SIS-tem) is the system of the body composed of specialized cells and the substances they produce that helps protect the body against disease-causing germs.

* **antibodies** (AN-tih-bah-deez) are protein molecules produced by the body's immune system to help fight specific infections caused by microorganisms, such as bacteria and viruses.

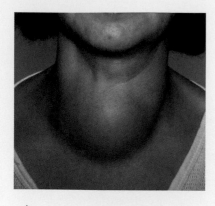

Goiter of the neck. *Custom Medical Stock Photo, Inc. Reproduced by permission.*

* **inflammation** (in-fla-MAY-shun) is the body's reaction to irritation, infection, or injury that often involves swelling, pain, redness, and warmth.

* **benign** (be-NINE) refers to a condition that is not cancerous or serious and will probably improve, go away, or not get worse.

* **puberty** (PU-ber-tee) is the period during which sexual maturity is attained.

IODIZED SALT

Goiter and other thyroid disorders sometimes result from too little iodine in the diet. In ancient Greece, iodine-rich seaweed was eaten to treat enlarged thyroid glands. In 1811, the French chemist Courtois identified iodine, which began being used internally in the treatment of thyroid disorders in 1821.

In 1922, the Swiss Goiter Commission introduced the first program of adding iodine to salt as a preventive measure against goiter in Switzerland. Also in 1922, Michigan physician David Murray Cowie (1872–1940) expressed interest in eliminating goiter by means of iodized salt. Cowie worked with the Michigan State Medical Society to have iodized salt placed on Michigan grocery shelves and, eventually, in stores across the United States. In areas with such programs, iodine deficiency is rarely seen.

When hypothyroidism occurs in infancy and is not treated, cretinism (KREET-in-izm) results. A child with cretinism has stunted growth and mental deficiency. Older children who have hypothyroidism show slowing of growth and delayed sexual maturation.

Goiter Goiter is not itself a disease. The term simply refers to enlargement of the thyroid, sometimes visible as a swelling in the front of the neck. Enlargement of the thyroid can be a sign of hyperthyroidism or hypothyroidism. It even can occur when thyroid function is normal.

A goiter can be seen in hyperthyroidism of Graves' disease, in which the thyroid enlarges due to stimulation of the gland by the malfunctioning immune system. In hypothyroidism, it enlarges as part of the body's attempt to produce enough hormone to compensate for damage done to it by the disease, or because of inflammation* caused by the disease, or both.

Goiter can also occur in parts of the world where there is inadequate iodine in the diet. Found in seafood and most table salt preparations, iodine is an element essential for the formation of thyroid hormones in the body.

Nodules Distinct swellings or lumps within the thyroid are called nodules. They are most common in women and their incidence increases with age. The large majority of thyroid nodules are benign*, but some may be cancerous. Thus they require prompt medical evaluation.

Sometimes the thyroid temporarily enlarges slightly during puberty* or pregnancy, without impairing its function or causing any other symptoms.

How Are Thyroid Diseases Diagnosed and Treated?

Diagnosis To diagnose a suspected thyroid disorder, the doctor takes a medical history and performs a physical examination. Blood samples usually are taken to measure the levels of thyroid hormones and TSH, the pituitary hormone that stimulates the thyroid. The thyroid also may be checked using various scanning techniques. If a thyroid tumor is suspected, a sample of thyroid tissue may be removed for examination.

Treatment Most thyroid diseases are highly treatable. Hyperthyroidism may be treated with a single dose of radioactive iodine, which destroys overactive thyroid cells. Alternatively, antithyroid medications may be prescribed to suppress formation of thyroid hormones. Surgical removal of most of the thyroid is another treatment. Hypothyroidism is treated with hormone replacement medication, which typically is continued for life.

A goiter of uncertain cause may disappear on its own, or it may be small and not need treatment. Goiters caused by thyroid disease usually shrink with treatment. Occasionally, surgery is needed for removing a very large goiter. Thyroid disease is not contagious. It often runs in families, and there is no way a person can prevent it. People who live in parts of the world where seafood is scarce and table salt is not iodized, however, need to make sure they take in sufficient amounts of iodine to avoid hypothyroidism and goiter.

▶ *See also* **Dietary Deficiencies • Growth and Growth Disorders • Metabolic Disease**

Resources

Books and Articles

Burch, Warner M. *100 Q&A about Thyroid Disorders.* Sudbury, MA: Jones and Bartlett, 2008.

Vanderpump, Mark P. J, and W. Michael G. Tunbridge. *Thyroid Disease: The Facts,* 4th ed. New York: Oxford University Press, 2008.

Wood, Lawrence C., David S. Cooper, and E. Chester Ridgway. *Your Thyroid: A Home Reference,* 4th ed. New York: Ballantine Books, 2006.

Organizations

American Thyroid Association. 6066 Leesburg Pike, Suite 550, Falls Church, VA, 22041. Telephone: 703-998-8890. Web site: http://www.thyroid.org.

National Graves' Disease Foundation. P.O. Box 1969, Brevard, NC, 28712. Telephone: 828-877-5251. Web site: http://www.ngdf.org.

New York Thyroid Center, Herbert Irving Pavilion. 161 Fort Washington Avenue, 8th Floor, New York, NY, 10032. Telephone: 212-305-0442. Web site: http://cpmcnet.columbia.edu/dept/thyroid/index.html.

George and Barbara Bush

When George H. W. Bush was president of the United States (1989–1993), he and his wife, Barbara, both were diagnosed with Graves' disease, a type of hyperthyroidism (overactive thyroid).

Because only one or two of every 100 women, and even fewer men, get Graves' disease, the likelihood of a husband and wife having the disorder at the same time is extremely rare. Because one person cannot catch Graves' disease from another, this was an amazing medical coincidence.

* **neurological** (nur-a-LAH-je-kal) refers to the nervous system, which includes the brain, spinal cord, and the nerves that control the senses, movement, and organ functions throughout the body.

* **motor** relates to body movement.

TIA (Transient Ischemic Attack) *See Stroke.*

Tic Disorders

Tic disorders are neurological* conditions characterized by sudden, rapid movements (for example, neck jerking) or sounds (words or other types of sounds, such as grunting or sniffing) that are repeated in a consistent way many times per day.

What Are Tics?

Tics have been described as brain-activated "involuntary" movements or sounds, meaning that the person does not produce them intentionally. People with tics often can suppress them, sometimes for up to hours at a time, just as one might suppress a cough or a sneeze for a period of time. A parallel can be drawn between suppressing a tic and trying to suppress a cough in the middle of a concert. To avoid interrupting the musicians, people might try very hard not to cough until the intermission. When they finally cough, however, they might cough several times instead of just once or twice. The experience of trying to suppress a tic is similar. After a tic is suppressed, it may erupt with even greater force or frequency.

Tics tend to get worse when people feel anxious or tired and get better when they are calm and focused on an activity. One interesting aspect of the condition is that tics usually lessen around strangers and are expressed more freely among family members and other trusted people. This does not mean that a person is producing the tics purposely around family members. It probably reflects the fact that individuals work harder to suppress them in less comfortable situations, whereas they are naturally relax their suppression when they are in more familiar surroundings. It is not uncommon for a child to be taken to a doctor to diagnose the problem, only to have the child be unable to produce tics "on command." Just as tics are experienced as uncontrollable, they cannot be voluntarily brought on. While tics may appear in individuals as early as two years of age, the average age at onset is about seven.

What Are the Symptoms of Tics?

Simple tics   Simple tics involve a single movement, such as eye blinking or repeatedly sticking out the tongue. Tics also may be vocal, made up of a single sound, such as throat clearing or snorting, stuttering, or sniffing. The most common type of tics, and often the first to appear, are simple facial tics. Over time, more complex motor* tics may appear.

Complex tics   Complex motor tics involve several coordinated muscle movements, such as touching or smelling an object, jumping or twirling, or making deep knee bends while walking. These tics may include neck stretching, foot stamping, body twisting and bending, or mimicking the gestures of other people. Complex vocal tics can range from combining "simple" throat clearing or grunting with other vocal behaviors, to repeating a long but meaningless string of words at regular intervals.

With complex tics, the repeated phrase or gesture at first may seem meaningful, even when it is not. For example, the person with a complex motor tic may feel a need to do and then redo or undo the same action several times (for example, stretching out one arm ten times before writing or retracing the same letter or repeating the same word) before proceeding to another activity. Such forms of behavior can interfere with a person's ability to accomplish school- or work-related tasks.

Researchers have identified more than 80 tics, which are a mix of simple and complex motor and vocal tics. Recognizable tic patterns include:

- Echopraxia (EK-o-PRAX-ee-a): imitating other people's movements or gestures
- Copropraxia (KO-pro-PRAX-ee-a): making obscene, rude, or socially unacceptable gestures
- Palilalia (PA-li-LAY-lee-a): repeating a person's own words
- Echolalia (EK-o-LAY-lee-a): repeating someone else's words
- Coprolalia (KO-pro-LAY-lee-a): shouting obscenities or impolite and offensive language
- Repetition: repeating words or phrases out of context (for example, "Look before you leap").

What Are Tic Disorders?

Doctors usually classify tic disorders into four categories: Tourette's syndrome, chronic motor or vocal tic disorder, transient (TRAN-shent) tic disorder, and tic disorder (not otherwise specified).

Tourette's syndrome   Tourette's syndrome is the best known of the tic disorders, and it is characterized by a frequent and long-lasting pattern of both vocal and motor tics.

Chronic motor or vocal tic disorder   In contrast to Tourette's syndrome, chronic* motor or vocal tic disorder involves only one of these two basic types of tics (either motor or vocal). In other respects, chronic tic disorder has many of the same symptoms as Tourette's syndrome:

- The tics occur many times per day, nearly every day, and the condition lasts for more than a year.
- The tics may disappear for a time, but that period never exceeds more than three months in a row.
- The tics first appear in individuals before the age of 18.

* **chronic** (KRAH-nik) lasting a long time or recurring frequently.

* **genetically** (je-NE-ti-klee) means stemming from genes, the material in the body that helps determine a person's characteristics, such as hair or eye color.

- The tics are not the result of a medication or another medical condition.
- The tics cause significant impairment at school or work.

Transient tic disorder   In contrast to chronic motor or vocal tic disorder, transient tic disorder refers to a briefer problem with tics. Transient tics may be motor or vocal or both. For a condition to be considered transient tic disorder, the tics must begin before a person reaches the age of 18; occur several times per day; occur nearly every day for at least four weeks; but for no longer than 12 months in a row. As with the other tic disorders, transient tics are not the result of another medical condition or a medication.

Tic disorder (not otherwise specified)   This category for tic disorders is used when the disorders do not fit into any of the other three groups, usually because the tics last less than four weeks or because they begin when a person is older than 18.

How Are Tic Disorders Diagnosed?

While there are clear differences between tic disorders, a doctor may find it difficult to make a diagnosis because tics often change in type or frequency over time. Transient tics, for example, are short-lived tics that last for less than a year. But a child may experience a series of transient tics over several years. Neck jerking may last for several months and then be replaced by finger snapping or stamping in place. Chronic tics, by contrast, last longer than a year and tend to remain stable and constant over time.

Transient tics that change over time are believed to affect as many as one-fourth of all school-aged children. While they last, these tics may be quite odd. They might range from sticking out the tongue again and again to repeating a word or phrase a set number of times to poking or pinching various parts of the body. These strange kinds of behavior are more common than was once believed, but often they disappear as a child matures.

Distinguishing transient tics from chronic tics often requires careful evaluation by a physician over a period of years. In addition, it is important for a doctor to gather information about other members of the family (including parents, grandparents, and siblings) who also may have tics or related conditions. It is now known that the tendency for tics to develop is passed on genetically* (inherited) from generation to generation. Because a person may inherit the genetic tendency to tics without ever experiencing tics, it is possible for the disorder to skip several generations in one family. Researchers have attempted to identify the specific gene (or genes) for tic disorders and to understand other factors that may influence whether a person at risk actually will experience tics.

Related Conditions

For most people who have tics, the real threat may not be the tics themselves but the sense of shame and social isolation that can result from this odd behavior. A child may have great difficulty dealing with these embarrassing, unwanted behaviors. It also may be hard for teachers, fellow students, and family members to understand that a person with tic disorder is not making these strange gestures and sounds intentionally, to gain attention or to avoid working. Other people can easily get that impression if the pattern of tics changes from day to day, as it often does. It can make matters even more difficult when tic disorders in children are associated with attention disorders, hyperactivity, impulsive behavior, obsessive-compulsive disorder*, irritability, or aggressiveness.

It is estimated that as many as half of the children with Tourette's syndrome also have the attention and impulse-control problems that are seen in attention deficit hyperactivity disorder. Children with Tourette's syndrome also have higher than average rates of learning disabilities that cause reading or language problems.

How Are Tics Treated?

There are several therapies to help children with tics cope with the frightening feelings of being out of control and with the specific types of behavior related to their condition. These include relaxation and stress-reduction techniques and biofeedback. Often medication is an important part of the treatment plan. Because of associated stress, anxiety, and self-esteem and relationship issues, working with a mental health professional when concerns begin to interfere with the quality of life is particularly important. A combination of treatment approaches is often required when tics and associated mental health problems are serious.

▶ See also **Attention Deficit Hyperactivity Disorder (ADHD) • Learning Disabilities • Obsessive-Compulsive Disorder • Tourette Syndrome**

Resources

Books and Articles

Chowdhury, Uttom. *Tics and Tourette Syndrome: A Handbook for Parents and Professionals.* New York: Jessica Kingsley, 2004.

Moe, Barbara. *Coping with Tourette Syndrome and Tic Disorders,* rev. ed. New York: Rosen, 2004.

Organizations

American Academy of Child and Adolescent Psychiatry. 3615 Wisconsin Avenue, NW, Washington, DC, 20016-3007. Telephone: 202-966-7300. Web site: http://www.aacap.org/cs/root/facts_for_families/tic_disorders.

American Academy of Pediatrics. 141 Northwest Point Boulevard, Elk Grove Village, IL, 60007-1098. Telephone: 847-434-4000. Web site: http://www.aap.org/publiced/BK5_Tics.htm.

* **obsessive-compulsive disorder** is a condition that causes people to become trapped in a pattern of repeated, unwanted thoughts, called obsessions (ob-SESH-unz), and a pattern of repetitive behaviors, called compulsions (kom-PUL-shunz).

How to Remove a Tick

Using thin-tipped tweezers, grasp the tick as close to the person's skin as possible.

Pull straight upward firmly and steadily until the tick lets go (do not squeeze or twist the tick body).

Clean the skin with soap and warm water, alcohol, or other antiseptic.

Save the tick for identification.

Petroleum jelly, lit matches, nail polish or other products do not help in tick removal and should not be used.

* **host** is an organism that provides another organism (such as a parasite or virus) with a place to live and grow.

Tick-borne Illnesses

A tick-borne illness is an infection that is transmitted through the bite of a tick.

What Are Tick-borne Infections?

Ticks can spread bacteria or parasites through their bites. A tick becomes infected when it bites an infected animal, and then the tick can pass the infection to humans when it bites them. Tick-borne infections cannot pass from human to human; they need time in the host* animal to develop.

Ticks can spread a number of different diseases, including Rocky Mountain spotted fever, ehrlichiosis (air-lik-e-O-sis), Lyme (LIME) disease, and babesiosis (bah-bih-sye-OH-sis).

Rocky Mountain spotted fever Despite its name, most cases of Rocky Mountain spotted fever (RMSF) are not found in the Rocky Mountains but in the southeastern states. Cases also appear throughout the continental United States and in Canada, Mexico, and Central and South America. RMSF is one of the most dangerous tick-borne infections because it can be difficult to diagnose and has severe complications. Caused by the *Rickettsia rickettsii* (rih-KET-see-uh rih-KET-see-eye) bacterium, the disease spreads to humans through bites from the wood tick, dog tick, and Lone Star tick.

Symptoms of RMSF include high fever, headache, aching in the muscles, nausea (NAW-zee-uh), vomiting, and diarrhea (dye-uh-REE-uh). A rash may appear first at the wrists, ankles, palms, and soles and then on the forearms, neck, face, and trunk. RMSF is fatal in about 5 percent of cases, probably because of delays in diagnosing and treating the disease.

Ehrlichiosis Several types of bacteria in the genus *Ehrlichia* (air-LIH-kee-uh) cause ehrlichiosis. In the United States, the Lone Star tick, the blacklegged tick, and the western blacklegged tick spread the illness. People have long known that ehrlichiosis causes disease in animals, but the first case in humans in the United States was not identified until the 1980s. Ehrlichiosis is found in most parts of the country.

Symptoms of ehrlichiosis resemble those of the flu: fever, chills, extreme tiredness, headache, muscle and joint pain, nausea, and vomiting. There is usually no rash in adults, but many children develop a rash. Some people have no symptoms or only mild symptoms. Complications, although rare, can occur in the elderly and people with weakened immune systems.

Lyme disease Lyme disease gets its name from the town in Connecticut where doctors discovered the disease in 1975. It is the most common tick-borne illness in the United States. The majority of cases appear in the northeastern, north central, and northwestern states.

The life cycle of a tick takes 2 years to complete. In the spring, eggs hatch into larvae, which feed on mice, birds, and small mammals until the fall, when they become dormant. The following spring they molt into nymphs, which feed through the summer and then become adults in the fall. At any of these stages of growth, ticks may become infected with Lyme disease bacteria by feeding on infected animals; as adults they may feed on humans and transmit the bacteria that cause the disease. *Illustration by Molly A. Moore Blessington. Reproduced by permission of Gale, a part of Cengage Learning.*

* **disseminated** describes a disease that has spread widely in the body.

* **meningitis** (meh-nin-JY-tis) is an inflammation of the meninges, the membranes that surround the brain and the spinal cord. Meningitis is most often caused by infection with a virus or a bacterium.

* **radiculitis** (ruh-dih-kyoo-LYE-tis) is numbness, tingling, or burning sensation along the course of a nerve due to irritation or inflammation of the nerve.

* **Bell's palsy** (PAWL-zee) is a condition in which there is weakness or loss of function of muscles on one side of the face.

* **malaria** (mah-LAIR-e-uh) is a disease spread to humans by the bite of an infected mosquito.

* **anemia** (uh-NEE-me-uh) is a blood condition in which there is a decreased hemoglobin in the blood and, usually, fewer than normal numbers of red blood cells.

The bacterium *Borrelia burgdorferi* (buh-REEL-e-uh burg-DOR-fe-ree), transmitted through deer ticks, causes Lyme disease. In most cases, the first sign of infection is the erythema migrans (air-uh-THEE-muh MY-granz) rash. It usually appears at the site of the tick bite, although it can develop anywhere on the body. The rash can be round, oval, or shaped like a bull's-eye with a red center surrounded by a clear area and then by a ring of red. Other early signs of the disease, such as extreme tiredness, headache, muscle aches, and fever, are similar to those of many infections, making diagnosis difficult. Not everyone who has Lyme disease develops the rash, and some people never show any symptoms.

The early disseminated* stage of the disease typically comes weeks to months later in people who have not received treatment. Symptoms at this stage include multiple rashes, meningitis*, radiculitis*, Bell's palsy*, and in some cases abnormalities of the heart rhythm. Lyme disease is not usually fatal, but if the illness remains untreated it can cause symptoms even years later. They can include arthritis, confusion, lack of coordination, difficulty in sleeping, and mood changes.

Babesiosis Babesiosis is a rare disease that appears mainly in the northeastern United States. It spreads through the bite of a deer tick that has been infected with a *Babesia* (buh-BE-she-uh) parasite, which attacks red blood cells. Because the deer tick also can spread Lyme disease, some people become infected with both diseases at the same time.

In healthy people, babesiosis infection may cause no symptoms. In others, early symptoms are extreme tiredness, lack of appetite, and a general feeling of being sick. Later symptoms include high fever, sweating, muscle aches, headache, and dark urine. The symptoms of babesiosis are similar to those of malaria*. Infected people also may have anemia* because of the parasite's attack on their red blood cells. The disease is not often fatal, but it can cause complications in the elderly, pregnant women, people with weakened immune systems, and people who have had their spleen removed.

How Common Are Tick-borne Infections?

Close to 20,000 cases of Lyme disease occur in the United States each year. RMSF is the second most common type of tick-borne illness, with the Centers for Disease Control and Prevention receiving as many as 1,200 reports of RMSF cases each year.

In contrast to these diseases, both ehrlichiosis and babesiosis are rare, with about 1,200 reports of ehrlichiosis over an 11-year period and several hundred cases of babesiosis since it was first reported in 1966.

How Are Tick-borne Infections Diagnosed and Treated?

Diagnosing a tick-borne illness can be difficult because the symptoms of many of the illnesses resemble those of the flu or other infections. One of the best clues is a recent tick bite, but many people do not remember being bitten.

Doctors often diagnose these diseases based on the patient's history of symptoms and activities, where the patient lives or became sick, and a physical examination that includes looking for rashes. A doctor may order a blood test to check for antibodies* to the organism causing the infection, but these tests usually are not helpful in the early stages of the illness. Skin biopsy* from a rash area may confirm a diagnosis.

Antibiotics are effective against the bacterial infections. Anti-parasitic medicines work well for babesiosis. In most cases, patients recover at home. Sometimes, however, especially in cases of RMSF, patients may need hospitalization for more intensive antibiotic therapy and supportive care.

What Should People Expect if They Have a Tick-borne Infection?

In almost all cases of tick-borne illnesses, quick treatment brings a complete cure, although it may take several months before all symptoms disappear. Untreated cases of Lyme disease can cause problems years after the tick bite.

Complications, while rare, can occur. Examples of complications are as follows:

- RMSF can cause paralysis*, hearing loss, and nerve damage.
- Ehrlichiosis can cause kidney* failure, respiratory problems, seizures*, and coma*.
- Long-term complications from Lyme disease include chronic* arthritis and nervous system problems.
- Babesiosis can cause respiratory problems, seizures, kidney failure, and other organ failure.

Can People Prevent Tick-borne Infections?

Avoiding areas where ticks are found is the best way to prevent the diseases they carry. If people venture into areas where ticks are likely to live, experts suggest that they wear long pants and long-sleeved shirts in light colors (to make it easier to find ticks) when going outside and that they tuck their pant legs into their socks. Applying insect repellents containing DEET* can also be helpful. Checking for ticks after being outside is wise. Studies show that ticks may not infect people until they have been attached for two days, so quickly removing ticks can help prevent illness. When ticks are found, they should be removed with tweezers and the area of the bite should be washed carefully with soap and water and alcohol, and people should watch for signs of infection, such as rash or fever.

▶ *See also* **Babesiosis • Ehrlichiosis • Lyme Disease • Rickettsial Infections • Rocky Mountain Spotted Fever**

* **antibodies** (AN-tih-bah-deez) are protein molecules produced by the body's immune system to help fight specific infections caused by microorganisms, such as bacteria and viruses.

* **biopsy** (BI-op-see) is a test in which a small sample of skin or other body tissue is removed and examined for signs of disease.

* **paralysis** (pah-RAH-luh-sis) is the loss or impairment of the ability to move some part of the body.

* **kidney** is one of the pair of organs that filter blood and remove waste products and excess water from the body in the form of urine.

* **seizures** (SEE-zhurs) are sudden bursts of disorganized electrical activity that interrupt the normal functioning of the brain, often leading to uncontrolled movements in the body and sometimes a temporary change in consciousness.

* **coma** (KO-ma) is an unconscious state, like a very deep sleep. A person in a coma cannot be awakened, and cannot move, see, speak, or hear.

* **chronic** (KRAH-nik) lasting a long time or recurring frequently.

* **DEET** (abbreviation for N,N-Diethyl-meta-toluamide) is the active ingredient in many insect repellants.

Resources

Books and Articles

Colligan, L. H. *Tick-Borne Illnesses.* New York: Marshall Cavendish Benchmark, 2009.

Vanderhoof-Forschner, Karen. *Everything You Need to Know about Lyme Disease and Other Tick-Borne Disorders,* 2nd ed. Hoboken, NJ: Wiley, 2003.

Organizations

American Lyme Disease Foundation. P.O. Box 466, Lyme, CT, 06371, Web site: http://www.aldf.com/majorTick.shtml.

Centers for Disease Control and Prevention. 1600 Clifton Road, Atlanta, GA, 30333. Toll free: 800-311-3435. Web site: http://www.cdc.gov/niosh/topics/tick-borne.

Lyme Disease Foundation. P.O. Box 332, Tolland, CT, 06084-0332. Telephone: 860-870-0070. Web site: http://www.lyme.org.

National Institute of Allergy and Infectious Diseases. Office of Communications and Public Liaison, 6610 Rockledge Drive, MSC 6612, Bethesda, MD, 20892-66123. Toll free: 866-284-4107. Web site: http://www3.niaid.nih.gov/topics/tickborne.

Tics *See Tic Disorders; Tourette Syndrome.*

Tinnitus

Tinnitus (ti-NY-tus) is the sense of ringing, whistling, or similar noise in the ear when no external sound is present.

What Is Tinnitus?

Tinnitus is a mysterious disorder that affects as many as 50 million Americans. People with tinnitus often describe the sound they hear as a ringing, but they sometimes say it resembles whistles, sizzles, clicks, roars, or other sounds too complex to explain easily. Some people experience the noise only at certain times or notice it only when it is quiet, such as at bedtime. Others, however, live with a constant unpleasant sound.

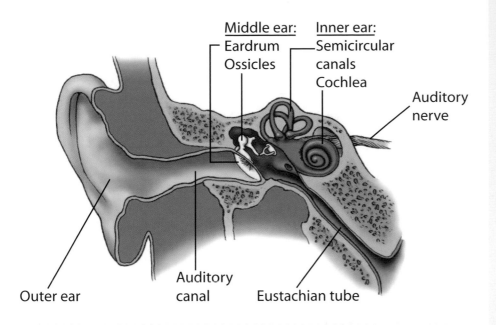

Middle ear:
Eardrum
Ossicles

Inner ear:
Semicircular
canals
Cochlea

Auditory
nerve

Outer ear

Auditory
canal

Eustachian tube

Anatomy of the ear. *Illustration by Frank Forney. Reproduced by permission of Gale, a part of Cengage Learning.*

The noise can be high-pitched like a baby's whine or low like a rumbling train. It might sound like a continuous tone or cycle in a rhythm, often in time with the heartbeat.

What Causes Tinnitus?

Tinnitus is sometimes a symptom of other problems, such as too much earwax* or an ear or nasal infection. Other causes include cardiovascular disease, tumors, jaw misalignment, anemia, and neck and head injuries. Certain medicines, such as aspirin and some antibiotics, as well as carbon monoxide and alcohol, can also cause tinnitus. Long-term exposure to loud sounds such as a jet plane or loud music can also lead to tinnitus.

In some cases, a person may have problems with a part of the hearing pathway, such as the cochlea, which is a bony, coil-shaped part of the inner ear. Some evidence suggests another portion of the hearing pathway may be involved in many cases of tinnitus, the dorsal cochlear nucleus, which is basically a relay point between the nerves in the ear and the brain. Researchers have studied the dorsal cochlear nucleus in the hopes of one day developing a treatment for tinnitus.

What Can a Doctor Do?

First, a doctor looks for the cause. If a doctor can find the cause and determine that it can be corrected through a straightforward measure, such as removing earwax or treating an infection, the tinnitus usually goes away.

Sometimes a doctor cannot easily correct tinnitus, and people must find ways to live with it. Hearing aids are a common way to help, if the cause is related to hearing loss. Sometimes the person uses a device such as a hearing aid that covers the tinnitus with another sound that is less noticeable or less disturbing.

* **ear wax** also known as cerumen (se-ROO-men), is the wax-like substance in the ear that traps dust and other particles to prevent them from damaging the inner ear.

* **stroke** is a brain-damaging event usually caused by interference with blood flow to the brain. A stroke may occur when a blood vessel supplying the brain becomes clogged or bursts, depriving brain tissue of oxygen. As a result, nerve cells in the affected area of the brain, and the specific body parts they control, do not properly function.

* **cancer** is a condition characterized by abnormal overgrowth of certain cells, which may be fatal.

▶ *See also* **Deafness and Hearing Loss • Otitis (Ear Infections) • Vertigo**

Resources

Books and Articles

Bauman, Neil G. *When Your Ears Ring! Cope with Your Tinnitus—Here's How,* 4th ed. Stewartstown, PA: GuidePost, 2005.

Tyler, Richard S., ed. *The Consumer Handbook on Tinnitus.* Sedona, AZ: Auricle Ink, 2008.

Organization

American Tinnitus Association. P.O. Box 5, Portland, OR, 97207-0005. Toll free: 800-634-8978. Web site: http://www.ata.org.

TJM *See Temporomandibular Joint (TMJ) Syndrome.*

Tobacco-Related Diseases

Tobacco-related diseases, including lung disease, heart disease, stroke*, and cancer*, are illnesses caused by tobacco use, the leading preventable cause of death in the United States.

▶

Parts of the body affected by tobacco in men and women. *Illustration by Frank Forney. Reproduced by permission of Gale, a part of Cengage Learning.*

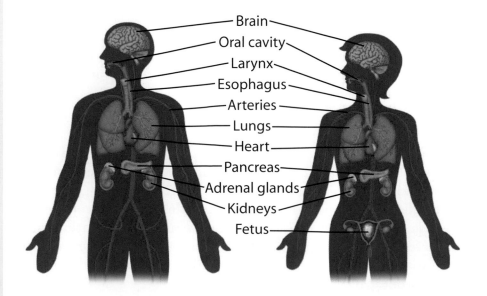

Brain
Oral cavity
Larynx
Esophagus
Arteries
Lungs
Heart
Pancreas
Adrenal glands
Kidneys
Fetus

What Are Tobacco-Related Diseases?

Where there is smoke, there is disease. Hundreds of studies have found that cigarette smoking can cause lung disease, heart disease, stroke, cancer and many other diseases. Smoking as few as one to four cigarettes per day is enough to cause serious health problems. About 6 percent of all the money spent on health care each year in the United States is spent to treat tobacco-related diseases and health problems.

Tobacco use eventually leads to death or disability for half of all regular users. In fact, it is the leading cause of preventable death in the United States. Tobacco use is responsible for more than 430,000 deaths each year, or one in every five deaths. It kills more people than AIDS* (acquired immune deficiency syndrome), alcohol, drug abuse, car crashes, murders, suicides, and fires combined. The following are some of the disease and health conditions that are linked to tobacco use.

Chronic bronchitis   Bronchitis (brong-KY-tis) refers to inflammation* of the bronchial (BRONG-kee-al) tubes, the airways that connect the windpipe to the lungs. This condition leads to a cough that brings up lots of thick, sticky mucus*. About 9 million Americans have chronic* bronchitis, and smoking is by far the most common cause.

Emphysema   Emphysema (em-fe-ZEE-ma) is a chronic lung disease in which the air sacs of the lungs are overly large. This condition makes the lungs work less efficiently and leads to shortness of breath. About 3.6 million Americans have emphysema, and most of these cases are caused by smoking.

Heart disease   A heart attack occurs when the blood supply to part of the heart muscle is decreased or stopped. This situation happens when one of the large blood vessels that bring blood to the heart is blocked, usually by a buildup of fatty deposits inside the vessel. More than 325,000 Americans die each year from a heart attack. Smokers are twice as likely as nonsmokers to have a heart attack, and two to four times as likely to die suddenly of heart problems.

Stroke   A stroke occurs when a blood vessel to the brain is blocked or bursts, which can damage the brain. Strokes are the leading cause of serious, long-term disability in the United States. Strokes also kill more than 150,000 people per year. Smoking raises the risk of having a stroke.

Lung cancer   Lung cancer kills more people than any other kind of cancer. Each year, more than 174,000 people are diagnosed with lung cancer in the United States, and about 162,000 people die from it. Smoking is the direct cause of almost 90 percent of all lung cancers.

Other cancers   Cigarette smoke contains more than 4,000 different chemicals, and more than 60 of these have been shown to cause cancer in humans and animals. Smokers are more likely to get several kinds of cancer, including that of the mouth, larynx*, esophagus*, bladder*, cervix*, pancreas*, and kidney*.

* **AIDS** or acquired immunodeficiency (ih-myoo-no-dih-FIH-shen-see) syndrome, is an infection that severely weakens the immune system; it is caused by the human immunodeficiency virus (HIV).

* **inflammation** (in-fla-MAY-shun) is the body's reaction to irritation, infection, or injury that often involves swelling, pain, redness, and warmth.

* **mucus** (MYOO-kus) is a thick, slippery substance that lines the insides of many body parts.

* **chronic** (KRAH-nik) lasting a long time or recurring frequently.

* **larynx** (LAIR-inks) is the voice box (which contains the vocal cords) and is located between the base of the tongue and the top of the windpipe.

* **esophagus** (eh-SAH-fuh-gus) is the soft tube that, with swallowing, carries food from the throat to the stomach.

* **bladder** (BLAD-er) is the sac that stores urine produced by the kidneys prior to discharge from the body.

* **cervix** (SIR-viks) is the lower, narrow end of the uterus that opens into the vagina.

* **pancreas** (PAN-kree-us) is a large gland located behind the stomach that secretes various hormones and enzymes necessary for digestion and metabolism (me-TAB-o-liz-um), notably insulin.

* **kidney** is one of the pair of organs that filter blood and remove waste products and excess water from the body in the form of urine.

Healthy lung of a nonsmoker (left);
damaged lung of a smoker (right).
*St. Bartholomew's Hospital/Photo
Researchers, Inc.*

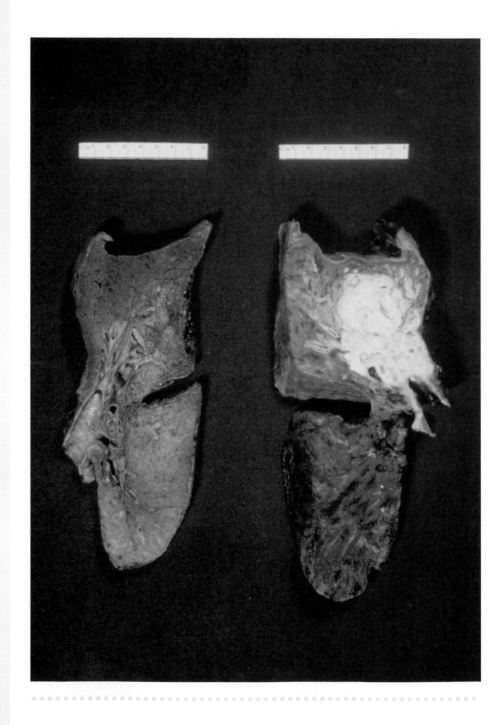

* **miscarriage** (MIS-kare-ij) is the
end of a pregnancy through
the death of the embryo or fetus
before birth.

* **stillbirth** is the birth of a dead
fetus.

* **premature birth** (pre-ma-CHUR)
means born too early. In humans,
it means being born after a
pregnancy term lasting less than
37 weeks.

Pregnancy problems Smoking by pregnant women is linked to
miscarriage*, stillbirth*, premature birth*, low birth weight*, and infant
death. Women who smoke are also more likely to have trouble getting
pregnant.

Dental problems Use of smokeless tobacco can lead to gum problems and tooth loss.

Smoking has also been linked to a variety of other health problems,
including asthma*, high blood pressure, gum disease*, cataracts*, bone

thinning, pneumonia*, peripheral artery disease (disease of the blood vessels outside the heart, such as those of the legs, hips and kidneys), and peptic ulcers*.

What Are Other Risks of Tobacco Use?

Smoking causes shortness of breath and reduces the amount of oxygen that is available for the muscles and other body tissues to use. These changes can limit people's ability to engage in various activities. In young people, sports performance can suffer as a result. For example, many smokers cannot run as far or as fast as nonsmokers. Tobacco use also makes people less attractive. It stains teeth and causes bad breath, yellowed fingers, and smelly clothes. Research has found that two-thirds of teenagers say that seeing someone smoke turns them off, and more than four-fifths say they would rather date nonsmokers. Over the years, smoking causes skin to wrinkle more than normal aging does among nonsmokers.

Are All Forms of Tobacco Harmful?

No form of tobacco use is safe. In addition to smoking cigarettes, using smokeless tobacco (also called oral, spitting, or chewing tobacco, and snuff), can have deadly results. It can cause bleeding gums, tooth loss, and sores of the mouth that never heal. Eventually, smokeless tobacco can cause cancer of the mouth, larynx, and esophagus. Young people who use smokeless tobacco are also more likely to start using cigarettes.

Pipe and cigar smokers, like cigarette smokers, have higher death rates from heart disease than nonsmokers. They are more likely to get cancer of the mouth, larynx, and esophagus, too. The use of any tobacco product, even ones that are labeled "low tar," "naturally grown," or "additive free,", as well as hand-rolled cigarettes and smoking using a hookah (water pipe), can cause addiction and health problems.

What about Secondhand Smoke?

In addition to harming the health of the smoker, smoking harms non-smokers. Each year in the United States, about 3,400 nonsmokers die from lung cancer and more than 22,000 nonsmokers die from heart disease caused by exposure to secondhand smoke*. Secondhand smoke also causes infections of the lower airways and lungs in up to 300,000 children and makes asthma worse in as many as 1 million children with asthma each year.

Why Does Tobacco Harm the Body?

Cigarette smoke is a mixture of several thousand chemicals; some are present naturally in the tobacco, and some are added by cigarette manufacturers to enhance the flavor and make smoking more pleasant. Tar, ammonia, carbon monoxide, and nicotine (NIK-o-teen) are some of these chemical compounds. The carbon monoxide in smoke attaches to

* **low birth weight** means born weighing less than normal. In humans, it refers to a full-term (pregnancy lasting 37 weeks or longer) baby weighing less than 5.

* **asthma** (AZ-mah) is a condition in which the airways of the lungs repeatedly become narrowed and inflamed, causing breathing difficulty.

* **gum disease** is an infection caused by bacteria that affect the tissues surrounding and supporting the teeth.

* **cataracts** (KAH-tuh-rakts) are areas of cloudiness of the lens of the eye that can interfere with vision.

* **pneumonia** (nu-MO-nyah) is inflammation of the lungs.

* **ulcer** is an open sore on the skin or the lining of a hollow body organ, such as the stomach or intestine. It may or may not be painful.

* **secondhand smoke**, also called environmental tobacco smoke or passive smoke, is smoke that is inhaled passively or involuntarily by someone who is not smoking. It is a mixture of gases and particles from a burning cigarette, cigar, or pipe and the smoke exhaled by smokers.

Butting Out

The following tips can help smokers to quit the habit:

- Pick a quit date. Write it down. Make a commitment to yourself and stick to your quit date.

- Tell your friends and family members that you plan to quit. Ask them not to smoke around you or leave cigarettes around.

- Stop smoking completely on the quit date. Do not just cut back on smoking. People who try to smoke fewer cigarettes usually wind up smoking the same amount again soon.

- Think about past attempts to quit. Try to figure out what worked and what did not.

- Do something other than smoking to reduce stress. Exercise, take a hot bath, or listen to soothing music.

- Try to distract yourself from the urge to smoke. Call a friend, go for a walk, or take up a new hobby.

- Be ready for short-term symptoms. Quitting smoking can lead to a dry mouth, cough, scratchy throat, and feelings of edginess.

- Get professional help, if needed. A doctor, dentist, therapist, or school nurse may be a good source of advice and support.

---

* **immune system** (im-YOON SIS-tem) is the system of the body composed of specialized cells and the substances they produce that helps protect the body against disease-causing germs.

* **addiction** (a-DIK-shun) is a strong physical or psychological dependence on a physical substance.

compounds in the blood that normally carry oxygen. As a result, less oxygen is able to reach body tissues. Smoke contains at least 60 chemicals that harm the genetic material inside cells, triggering changes that lead to cancer. Other chemicals in smoke cause inflammation in body tissues, damage the lining of the airways, or harm the body's immune system*. Nicotine damages blood vessels, causing changes that can eventually lead to heart disease and stroke. Cigarettes and tobacco products contain compounds that damage the body in many other ways.

How Do Tobacco Users Become Addicted?

The nicotine in tobacco is the chemical that causes people who smoke to become addicted (hooked). Nicotine is absorbed easily from tobacco smoke in the lungs. Within seconds, nicotine travels through the bloodstream to the brain. There, it signals the brain to release chemicals that make people want to smoke more. The effect is very powerful. Smokers can become addicted to nicotine, which means they can become dependent on it physically and suffer unpleasant symptoms when it is taken away. The ability of nicotine to cause addiction* is as strong as that of heroin or cocaine. Users of smokeless tobacco can also become addicted because nicotine is absorbed through the inner lining of the mouth.

One hallmark of any addiction is tolerance (TAH-le-rans), which means that over time people start to need more and more of a substance to feel its effects. When people first start smoking, one cigarette may make them queasy and dizzy; some first-time smokers even vomit with their first inhalation. Soon these individuals can smoke several cigarettes without any symptoms, however, and most smokers are up to a pack or more each day by age 25.

Another sign of addiction is withdrawal symptoms, which means that people have physical symptoms and feel sick if they stop using the substance to which they are addicted. When people are forced to stop smoking even for a short time, they may have unpleasant symptoms. Many rush to light up as soon as they leave a place where smoking is not allowed.

Who Uses Tobacco?

About 45 million adults in the United States smoke cigarettes, including people of all ethnic groups. Among adults in 2005, the highest rates of smoking were among Native American and Native Alaskans (32%), non-Hispanic whites (22%), and African Americans (22%). Hispanics and Asian Americans are less likely to smoke. Although fewer women than men smoke, the gap has been steadily decreasing; in the early 2000s, nearly as many women as men smoke.

Tobacco use during the teenage years is of special concern because nicotine is highly addictive at this age. Four out of five adults who smoke began smoking by age 18. Young people who stay smoke-free through high school have a good chance of never lighting up. The 2004

National Youth Tobacco Survey reported that about 8 percent of middle school students and 22 percent of high school students smoked cigarettes. About 3 percent of middle school students and 6 percent of high school students used smokeless tobacco. Sizeable numbers of students also smoked cigars, kreteks (clove cigarettes), or bidis (small, flavored cigarettes from India). Although the rate of smoking among African-American students nearly doubled in the 1990s, it decreased in the early 2000s, and as of 2008 they were far less likely to smoke than white or Hispanic students.

Young people who start smoking are more likely to get low grades in school than nonsmokers. These students often have low self-esteem, and they may turn to smoking because they think it will make them more attractive or popular. Because such teenagers lack self-confidence, they may have trouble saying no to tobacco.

How Can Tobacco-Related Problems Be Prevented?

The best way to prevent tobacco-related diseases is never to start smoking. For people who already are smokers, there is good news, though. Those who quit, no matter how old they are, live longer than those who keep smoking. Quitting is hard. It usually takes people two or more tries to succeed. However, studies have shown that each time a person tries to quit, he or she learns more about what works and what does not. Eventually, all people can succeed if they really want to stop smoking. Half of all people who have ever smoked have quit.

Quitting the Habit   Most smokers say they do not plan to be smoking in five years. But in fact, more than 70 percent of smokers continue to smoke. The main reason it is so tough for them to quit is the discomfort of withdrawal. When smokers suddenly stop or sharply cut back on their tobacco use, a host of distressing symptoms quickly set in. People are tempted to start smoking again to relieve the distress. Common symptoms of tobacco withdrawal include the following:

- Bad mood
- Depression
- Trouble sleeping
- Irritability
- Anger
- Anxiety
- Short attention span
- Increased appetite
- Weight gain

Three strategies have been shown to best help people quit smoking: using medications, getting support and encouragement, and learning to handle the urge to smoke.

Teen Smoking

- Each day, more than 4,000 teenagers try their first cigarette and 2,000 start smoking regularly.

- However, most young people, 88 percent to be exact, do not use tobacco.

- More than four in five teenagers say that they would rather date a nonsmoker.

- About two-thirds of teenagers say that seeing someone smoke turns them off.

- Some problems, such as coughing, shortness of breath, nausea, and dizziness, begin with a person's first cigarette.

- Problems such as coughing and wheezing have been found in young people who smoke as little as one cigarette a week.

- About two in five young people who smoke say they have tried to quit but failed.

* antidepressant medications are used for the treatment and prevention of depression.

Using medications   Research shows that almost all smokers can benefit from temporarily wearing a small nicotine patch or chewing gum that contains nicotine. The nicotine passes through the skin and reduces the craving for this substance. Nicotine patches, gum, and lozenges are available without a prescription, but people should talk to their doctor before using them. A prescription nicotine inhaler and nasal spray are also approved for use in the United States. Bupropion and verenicline are other prescription drugs approved for use in smoking cessation. Antidepressant medications*, such as nortriptyline, have also been shown to help smokers quit. Using any of these products doubles a person's chances of success.

Getting support and encouragement   Personal counseling or a quit-smoking program can help someone learn how to live life as a nonsmoker. Studies have shown that the more counseling people have, the greater their chances of success. A quit-smoking program that offers at least four to seven sessions over a period of at least two weeks and devotes a satisfactory amount of time and attention to the problem. Friends and family members can also give support. In addition, self-help books and telephone hotlines may be helpful.

Learning to handle the urge to smoke   People benefit from becoming aware of the situations or problems that make them want to smoke. For example, many people like to smoke when they are around other smokers or are feeling sad or frustrated. It is a good idea to avoid these situations as much as possible when trying to quit. Engaging in physical enjoyable and healthy activities, such as going for a walk or bike ride, can reduce stress. People who want to quit need to keep their minds busy, too, to help control thoughts of smoking.

Avoiding Passive Smoke   Choosing not to smoke goes a long ways toward preventing tobacco-related diseases, but it is not enough. Studies have shown that smoke from the cigarettes of others contains carcinogens (car-SIN-o-jenz), cancer-causing chemicals that can affect people who are around smoke often. The secondhand smoke from cigarettes contains more tars and other chemicals than does the smoke exhaled by the smoker. Most cigarettes are filtered and remove at least some of the harmful chemicals. Protecting oneself and others requires taking the following steps:

- Avoiding places where people are smoking whenever possible

- Encouraging smokers to quit for their health and the health of others

- Preventing children from regularly being exposed to smoke

- Encouraging restaurants, stores, and other social settings to provide no-smoking areas or to change their policy so the building is smoke free.

▶ *See also* **Addiction • Asthma • Bronchiolitis and Infectious Bronchitis • Cancer: Overview • Environmental Diseases • Halitosis • Heart Disease • Hypertension • Kidney Cancer • Lung Cancer • Oral Cancer • Pancreatic Cancer • Pregnancy • Substance Abuse • Sudden Infant Death Syndrome • Uterine Cancer**

Resources

Books and Articles

Cowan, David, and Susanna Palomares. *Don't Get Hooked: Tobacco Awareness and Prevention Activities.* Austin, TX: PRO-ED, 2005.

Organizations

American Academy of Family Physicians. P.O. Box 11210, Shawnee Mission, KS, 66207-1210. Toll free: 800-274-2237. Web site: http://www.aafp.org.

American Cancer Society. 250 Williams Street NW, Atlanta, GA, 30303. Toll free: 800-ACS-2345. Web site: http://www.cancer.org.

American Heart Association. 7272 Greenville Avenue, Dallas, TX, 75231-4596. Toll free: 800-AHA-USA1. Web site: http://www.americanheart.org.

American Lung Association. 1301 Pennsylvania Ave. NW, Suite 800, Washington, DC, 20004. Toll free: 800-LUNG-USA. Web site: http://www.lungusa.org.

Campaign for Tobacco-Free Kids. 1400 Eye Street NW, Suite 1200, Washington, DC, 20005. Telephone: 202-296-5469. Web site: http://www.tobaccofreekids.org.

Centers for Disease Control and Prevention. 1600 Clifton Road, Atlanta, GA, 30333. Toll free: 800-311-3435. Web site: http://www.cdc.gov/tobacco.

Office of the Surgeon General. 5600 Fishers Lane, Room 18-66, Rockville, MD, 20857. Telephone: 301-443-4000. Web site: http://www.surgeongeneral.gov/tobacco.

QuitNet. Web site: http://www.quitnet.org.

Smoke-Free.gov. Web site: http://www.smokefree.gov.

Tonail, Ingrown *See Ingrown Toenail.*

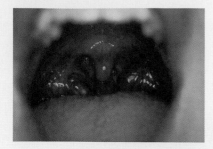

A case of tonsillitis caused by a streptococcal infection. The bacterium is spread by respiratory droplets and the illness primarily affects children between five and fifteen years of age. *Dr. P. Marazzi/Photo Researchers, Inc.*

* **lymphatic tissue** is tissue where white blood cells fight invading germs.

* **pharyngitis** (far-in-JI-tis) is inflammation of the pharynx, part of the throat.

* **respiratory** (RES-pi-ra-tor-ee) refers to the breathing passages and lungs.

Tonsillitis

Tonsillitis is an infection of the tonsils, which are two lumps of tissue located at the back of the mouth on either side of and near the opening of the throat.

Tonsillectomy's Cool Cure

Until the last part of the 20th century, the removal of tonsils (tonsillectomy) was very common in childhood. Many adults in the early 2000s recall the unlimited ice cream they were given as children to soothe throat pain after surgery. In the early 2000s, however, it is uncommon to remove the tonsils unless they become infected repeatedly or are large enough to obstruct breathing.

What Is Tonsillitis?

The tonsils are collections of lymphatic tissue* involved in helping the body to prevent and fight infection. Sometimes, however, the tonsils themselves become infected with viruses or bacteria. The tonsils swell and sometimes become coated with whitish spots or pus. This condition commonly occurs with pharyngitis*, influenza, or other respiratory* infections.

The first symptom of tonsillitis is usually a sore throat. Fever and chills may follow, and the lymph nodes (glands) under the jaw and in the neck may become swollen and sore. Tiredness and loss of appetite are common. Swallowing may become difficult. Sometimes there is also a middle ear infection because the eustachian (yoo-STAY-ke-an) tube, which connects the throat and middle ear, becomes blocked by the swelling of the tonsils.

Who Gets Tonsillitis?

Tonsillitis can happen to anyone, but it is more common in children. A doctor will try to determine whether a virus or a bacterium is causing the tonsillitis. A cotton swab is touched to the tonsillar area and used to test for the presence of streptococci bacteria, which cause strep throat and can be killed with antibiotics. If, however, a virus is causing the tonsillitis, then antibiotics will not work. The body's own defenses must fight the virus.

A non-aspirin pain reliever can lessen soreness in the throat. Soft food, soups, milkshakes, and ice pops also help. Getting adequate rest is important, as is drinking enough liquid. Most people start to feel better within five days after the sore throat starts. It might take longer if the tonsillitis is the result of a viral infection.

Can Tonsillitis Be Prevented?

The best way to avoid a bout of tonsillitis is to avoid close contact with people who have respiratory infections. This is especially important for people who have had tonsillitis before. It is important not to share cups or utensils with people who have sore throats or who are coughing and sneezing. It is always important to wash the hands frequently to help prevent the spread of this and other infections.

* **adenoids** (AH-din-oyds) are the fleshy lumps of tissue behind the nose that contain collections of infection-fighting cells of the immune system.

Will the Doctor Cut Out the Problem?

Recurrent bouts of tonsillitis may cause a doctor to recommend tonsillectomy (ton-si-LEK-to-mee), which means surgery to remove the tonsils. Often, the surgeon removes the adenoids* (also lymphatic tissue near the tonsils) at the same time. Surgery may be considered when a child has had many infections. This surgery was common for many years, although in the early 2000s it is done less frequently. In some cases, the tonsils are removed to help people with sleep apnea, which is a disorder that causes breathing to stop for brief periods during sleep.

▶ See also **Otitis (Ear Infections)** • **Sleep Apnea**

Resources

Books and Articles

Zelinger, Laurie. *The "O, My" in Tonsillectomy & Adenoidectomy: How to Prepare Your Child for Surgery, a Parent's Manual.* Ann Arbor, MI: Loving Healing Press, 2009.

Organization

University of Virginia Health System. P.O. Box 800224, Charlottesville, VA, 22908. Telephone: 434-924-3627. Web site: https://www.med.virginia.edu/uvahealth/adult_ent/tonsillitis.cfm; http://www.healthsystem.virginia.edu/UVAHealth/adult_respire/pharyn.cfm.

Tooth Decay *See Cavities.*

Tourette Syndrome

Gilles de la Tourette (ZHEEL de la too-RETT) syndrome is a neurological disorder that causes a person to make sudden movements or sounds, which are called tics. Many scientists think Tourette syndrome is caused by a chemical imbalance in the brain.

Daniel's Story

When Daniel yelped out loud like a dog, and his classmates erupted with laughter, Ms. Jones sent him to the school office. The teacher knew Daniel was being treated for hyperactivity, but recently he had been blinking his eyes, twitching his nose, and shuffling his feet. Ms. Jones decided she could no longer tolerate his interruptions. She also was concerned about Daniel. Was he just showing off, or could he have a more serious condition? She had read about Tourette syndrome, which causes strange movements and sounds. Was that Daniel's problem?

What Is Tourette Syndrome?

Gilles de la Tourette syndrome is named after the French physician Georges G. A. B. Gilles de la Tourette (1857–1904), who first described the disorder in 1885. It is commonly referred to as Tourette syndrome (TS). The symptoms are tics: abrupt, rapid, and repeated movements or vocal sounds. Researchers have identified more than 80 tics associated with this syndrome, including grunts, barks, babbling, eye movements, head or neck motions, throat clearing, grimaces, shrugging, sniffing, leg and mouth motions, and motions of the torso.

Tics are categorized as either simple or complex. Simple motor tics include twitching of an eye or a jerking movement of the arm. Simple vocal tics include grunts, barks, or other noises. Complex tics involve several coordinated muscle movements, including twirling or doing deep knee bends when walking. Complex vocal tics include stuttering, babbling, uttering profanities, or echoing sounds. The more common tics in Tourette syndrome are:

- Echolalia (eh-koh-LAY-lee-uh): echoing other people's words
- Palilalia (pal-ee-LAY-lee-uh): repeating one's own last words, sounds, or sentences
- Coprolalia (ko-pro-LAY-ee-uh): literally "babbling about feces," but also includes use of explicit and obscene language or sounds
- Echopraxia (eh-koh-PRAK-see-uh): imitating other people's movements
- Copropraxia (ko-pro-PRAK-see-uh): making obscene and socially unacceptable gestures

People with more severe tics may mutilate themselves by biting their lips or banging their heads. Others may exhibit obsessive-compulsive behavior such as excessive hand washing. In addition to tics, a person with Tourette syndrome may show signs of hyperactivity, poor coordination, or attention deficit hyperactivity disorder (ADHD).

People with TS can sometimes control their tics for minutes, but like a suppressed sneeze, the tic returns inevitably. Tics get worse when a person is tired or anxious; they get better when a person is focused and concentrating on something. Severe tics can be more pronounced around family and close friends and less pronounced in the presence of strangers. Tics are less pronounced in the morning, worse at night, and, generally, not evident when a person is sleeping.

The disorder usually begins in childhood. Symptoms appear around age seven, and 90 percent of cases develop before age 10. Boys are four

LITERARY GIANT: SAMUEL JOHNSON

Samuel Johnson (1709–1784) is a towering figure in English literature. He wrote essays, poetry, and in 1755 the monumental *Dictionary of the English Language.* Johnson's friends recognized that he was a brilliant writer. They also thought he was quite eccentric.

Johnson was always in motion, rocking or swerving. He twitched and grunted and blew out his breath like a whale. His friends noticed he had obsessive-compulsive behaviors. For example, when he walked outside, he maneuvered so that he never walked on cracks in the paving stones, and he touched every post he passed. If he missed a post, he would go back to touch it. He also would scrape his fingernails and joints with a knife until they were raw.

When Samuel Johnson died in 1784, a physician examined his brain, looking for evidence of disease. He found none. Based on the observations and letters of his friends, most modern scholars believe Johnson had Tourette syndrome.

times more likely to develop TS than girls. About one person in 2,000 has Tourette syndrome.

At least 25 percent of all children display a simple tic. However, these tics go away within a year and are not a sign of TS. A person with Tourette syndrome may have tics for a lifetime, although the frequency and type of tic may change. About 35 percent of people with TS experience an easing of symptoms in adolescence; most others find that, even if they do not disappear, tics become less frequent and less severe in adulthood. The reverse can also be true: Some people with mild symptoms develop severe tics in their twenties or early thirties.

People with Tourette syndrome may suffer social embarrassment or emotional stress due to their tics. The disorder does not affect their intelligence or ability to lead a full life.

What Causes Tourette Syndrome?

In the Middle Ages, people who displayed movement and vocal tics were thought to be possessed by demons. Gilles de la Tourette, the French physician who studied the disorder in the 1800s, thought TS had a physiological basis, which means that its cause was physical, not mental. Modern scientists think Gilles de la Tourette was right.

Scientists believe TS is caused by an abnormality in the brain's neurotransmitters, which are chemicals that carry signals from one nerve cell to another. The affected neurotransmitter is dopamine, a chemical that controls movement. Research indicates that some forms of TS are inherited, which means they are passed down from parent to child.

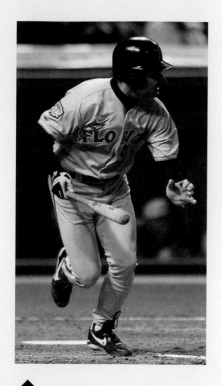

Jim Eisenreich, Major League Baseball player from 1982 to 1984 and 1987 to 1998, has Tourette Syndrome. Eisenreich was the Florida Marlins designated hitter when they won the World Series in 1997. *AP Images.*

HOME RUN HITTER: JIM EISENREICH

Jim Eisenreich (b. 1959) was different from other children. His body was constantly in motion, but not in the same way as other active children. His head twitched from side to side, and his shoulders jerked and shrugged. He often grunted, suddenly, for no apparent reason. His classmates laughed at his odd behavior. Doctors said Eisenreich was hyperactive and nervous and would outgrow the behavior. He did not.

Because he was embarrassed by his behavior, Eisenreich kept to himself and concentrated on baseball. He was a terrific baseball player, and in 1982, he won a spot on the Minnesota Twins.

Baseball in the big leagues was competitive and stressful. Much to his embarrassment, Eisenreich began to experience tics on the field in front of thousands of fans. His neck and shoulders twitched. His face twitched. One day, deeply embarrassed, Eisenreich walked off the field.

Eisenreich retired from baseball for four years. During those years, he sought medical help and discovered the reason for the tics: He had Tourette syndrome. Medication helped ease the tics and counseling helped Eisenreich accept himself.

Eisenreich returned to baseball and became a star hitter and outfielder for the Philadelphia Phillies. In the second game of the 1993 World Series, he smacked a three-run home run that helped Philadelphia beat the Toronto Blue Jays. Eisenreich had returned to baseball with a new outlook on life and on a condition known as TS.

How Do Doctors Treat Tourette Syndrome?

An accurate and prompt diagnosis is important to a person with Tourette syndrome, especially if the symptoms surface during childhood. People with TS often are misunderstood or ridiculed, and children may be punished for behavior that is out of their control.

Most people with Tourette syndrome do not need medication. Medication is reserved for people with severe or disruptive cases of TS. For those with severe tics, medication can reduce the frequency and severity of their symptoms so they can function at school, at work, and in social settings.

▶ *See also* **Tic Disorders**

Resources

Books and Articles

Chowdhury, Uttom. *Tics and Tourette Syndrome: A Handbook for Parents and Professionals.* London: Jessica Kingsley, 2004.

Hollenbeck, Peter. *Treating Tourette Syndrome and Tic Disorders: A Guide for Practitioners.* New York: Guilford Press, 2007.

Marsh, Tracy. *Children with Tourette Syndrome: A Parents' Guide,* 2nd ed. Bethesda, MD: Woodbine House, 2007.

Woods, Douglas. *Managing Tourette Syndrome: A Behavioral Intervention for Children and Adults.* New York: Oxford University Press, 2008.

Organizations

American Academy of Child and Adolescent Psychiatry. 3615 Wisconsin Avenue NW, Washington, DC, 20016-3007. Telephone: 202-966-7300. Web site: http://www.aacap.org/cs/root/resources_for_families/glossary_of_symptoms_and_illnesses/tourettes_syndrome.

American Academy of Family Physicians. P.O. Box 11210, Shawnee Mission, KS, 66207-1210. Toll free: 800-274-2237. Web site: http://www.aafp.org.

American Academy of Neurology. 1080 Montreal Avenue, St. Paul, MN, 55116. Telephone: 651-695-1940. Web site: http://www.aan.org.

Mayo Clinic. 200 First Street SW, Rochester, MN, 55905. Web site: http://www.mayoclinic.com/health/tourette-syndrome/DS00541.

National Institute of Neurological Disorders and Stroke. P.O. Box 5801, Bethesda, MD, 20824. Web site: http://www.ninds.gov/patients/Disorder/tourette/tourette.htm.

National Library of Medicine. 8600 Rockville Pike, Bethesda, MD, 20894. Web site: http://www.nlm.nih.gov/medlineplus/tourettesyndrome.html.

Tourette Syndrome Association. 42-40 Bell Boulevard, Suite 205, Bayside, NY, 11361. Toll free: 800-237-0717. Web site: http://www.tsa-usa.org.

Toxemia of Pregnancy *See Pregnancy.*

Toxic Inhalation Injuries

Toxic inhalation injuries occur when individuals are harmed by breathing toxic materials, which may include gas, dust, mist, fumes, smoke, or aerosols.

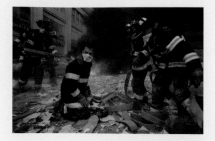

Firefighters and other first responders like these at the site of the collapsed World Trade Center on September 11, 2001, are at risk for toxic inhalation disorders. *AP Images.*

What Are Toxic Inhalation Injuries?

A toxic inhalation injury is damage that results from breathing in toxic materials. Toxic inhalations can be acute. Acute inhalations happen when a person has symptoms soon after breathing in toxic materials, such as gas, dust, mist, fumes, smoke, or aerosols. Chronic inhalations are longer-term exposures to a toxin and may not result in symptoms until many months or even years later. Toxic inhalation injuries may be accidental or intentional. Accidental injuries occur when individuals have inhaled a toxin by mistake or have knowingly inhaled a toxin but did not intend to do any harm to themselves. Individuals who work on cars, for instance, may know that the spray from a certain can of cleaning product is dangerous, but they may ignore warnings on the can that recommend the use of a breathing mask. Intentional injuries occur when individuals inhale a toxin with the intent to harm themselves. For instance, individuals may purposely breathe toxic chemicals in an attempt to commit suicide.

Generally, toxic inhalations cause injury in several different ways:

- Irritant gases may dissolve in water present on the mucous membrane of the trachea (windpipe) or other parts of the respiratory tract and cause inflammation of respiratory tract due to their acidity or alkalinity
- Toxic materials can damage cells of multiple organ systems
- Toxins can cause asphyxiation, which is a dangerous drop in oxygen available to the body

What Are the Symptoms of Toxic Inhalation Injuries?

The symptoms of toxic inhalation injuries vary depending on the inhaled toxin and the duration of exposure. In general, these injuries have the following symptoms: coughing, shortness of breath, wheezing, a burning sensation, and increased phlegm or other respiratory secretions. Some examples of common inhaled toxins include the following:

- Carbon monoxide
- Chlorine gas
- Vinyl chloride
- Asbestos
- Cyanide
- Hydrocarbons

Carbon monoxide One of the most common and dangerous of toxic materials carbon monoxide is a chemical compound made of one carbon atom bonded to one oxygen atom. When individuals breathe in carbon monoxide with regular air, the carbon monoxide removes oxygen from the air so that the body takes in less oxygen with every breath. As a result, even though they continues to breathe in and out, they are becoming asphyxiated because less oxygen is available.

Carbon monoxide poisoning can be acute or chronic. Symptoms of acute carbon monoxide poisoning include: flu-like symptoms, such as headache, dizziness, nausea, and/or vomiting; shortness of breath during activity; problems walking; memory loss, which may be mild or severe; confusion and sometimes hallucinations; chest pain; anxiety; depression; abdominal pain; fainting; a fast heartbeat; an increase in blood pressure; seizure; and unconsciousness. Occasionally, a patient may have noticeable reddening of the cheeks, but this so-called cherry-red appearance often does not occur. A particular danger with carbon monoxide poisoning is that people may at first have only the flu-like symptoms and, therefore, mistake their symptoms for the flu. Because carbon monoxide gas is colorless, odorless, and tasteless, they may be unaware they are breathing it in. If they then go to sleep in the place where the gas is located, their symptoms may get worse while they are asleep, and they may die. Occasionally, entire families die overnight because of exposure in their home to carbon monoxide poisoning. Such poisoning in homes is often the result of faulty appliances, such as furnaces, or the improper use of appliances, such as operating a space heater without proper ventilation. Fortunately, inexpensive home detectors are available to alert family members to the presence of carbon monoxide before it becomes a problem.

Carbon monoxide poisoning is quite common. The Centers for Disease Control and Prevention reports that more than 20,000 people visit the emergency room each year due to carbon monoxide poisoning. Of those 20,000, more than 4,000 are hospitalized and more than 400 Americans die from accidental CO poisoning. The CDC also notes that fetuses, infants, and people 65 years old and older, as well as people with chronic heart disease, anemia, or respiratory problems, are especially susceptible to the effects of carbon monoxide poisoning.

Individuals who may experience chronic carbon monoxide poisoning include firefighters, because carbon monoxide is present in smoke; certain automotive workers because carbon monoxide is present in car exhaust; warehouse or factory employees who work in buildings where propane-powered fork lifts or other equipment is used; and welders, who are exposed to shielding gas, which breaks down into carbon monoxide. Symptoms of chronic carbon monoxide poisoning include repeated and lasting headaches; lightheadedness; nausea and sometimes vomiting; depression; and confusion.

In addition, carbon monoxide is one of the compounds found in cigarette smoke. Both habitual cigarette smokers and those exposed to second-hand smoke can be affected by chronic carbon monoxide poisoning.

Chlorine Gas When a person mixes the commonly used cleaning products ammonia and chlorine bleach (or bleach-containing products), dangerous chlorine gas can result. Inhalation of this gas can cause choking and severe breathing problems. It can also be fatal.

* **convulsions** (kon-VUL-shuns), also called seizures, are involuntary muscle contractions caused by electrical discharges within the brain and are usually accompanied by changes in consciousness.

Vinyl Chloride   Vinyl chloride is a colorless, somewhat sweet-smelling gas that is used in building and construction products, such as electrical wiring and polyvinyl chloride (PVC) plastic; for the automotive and other industries; for various industrial and household equipment; and in medical supplies. Vinyl chloride is also known by such names as chlorethene, chlorethylene, and monovinyl chloride (or MVC). The Environmental Protection Agency lists vinyl chloride as a dangerous carcinogen (kar-SIN-o-jen), which means that has been linked to cancer. Symptoms of acute exposure to high levels of vinyl chloride in the air include dizziness, drowsiness, and headaches. Repeated exposure over a long period of time can result in liver damage and also increases the risk of liver angiosarcoma (an-gee-o-sar-CO-muh), which is a type of liver cancer. Regulations are in place in the United States to help protect workers who are employed in at-risk jobs from exposure to vinyl chloride.

Asbestos   Asbestos, which was once used in many building products, is one of several types of minerals that contain microscopic fibers. When asbestos is disturbed, such as during building renovations, these tiny fibers become airborne and are easily inhaled. Once breathed into the lungs, they can become lodged in the respiratory tract and produce health problems many years after the initial exposure. These health problems include lung cancer; mesothelioma (me-zoe-thee-lee-O-muh), which is a type of cancer of the lung and the lining surrounding the lungs; and asbestosis (az-bess-TOE-sis), which is breathing disorder.

Cyanide   Cyanide is present in smoke from the burning of plastics, rubber, and other common household products. It is also present in certain plastic-manufacturing, metal-processing, and other industries. Workers in these industry factories are most at risk for cyanide poisoning. Symptoms from acute exposure include one or more of the following: headache, weakness and/or fatigue, confusion, vertigo (an unsettling dizzy feeling), anxiety, shortness of breath, nausea sometimes with vomiting, bluish skin, convulsions*, unconsciousness, and sometimes death. Symptoms from chronic exposure are similar to those for acute exposure, but also may include thyroid problems and itchy, irritated skin.

Hydrocarbons   Medical professionals have become alarmed by the practice—often among teenagers—of purposely breathing in toxins to become high. This practice is known as huffing, sniffing, or bagging, and involves a variety of dangerous substances, especially those containing hydrocarbons. These substances include petroleum products, numerous cleaning products, and many glues. Typical symptoms of acute poisoning include: drowsiness, lightheadedness, dizziness, hallucinations, and impaired judgment. Chronic hydrocarbon abusers can suffer depression, weight loss, a decrease in motor skills, weakness, and changes in mood, often including irritability. In both acute and chronic poisoning, however, some individuals experience permanent damage to the brain, heart, or other organs, and some of them die. In some cases, teens who inhale hydrocarbons die after trying it only once.

How Are Toxic Inhalation Injuries Treated?

Treatment of acute exposures depends on the specific toxin but always includes removing of the victim from the area of exposure, giving the victim oxygen, and decontaminating the area as needed. Victims often spend time in a hospital or other clinical setting where they are monitored 24 hours to keep watch for the development of a severe lung condition, called acute respiratory distress syndrome (ARDS), that can be fatal without immediate treatment.

Diagnosing chronic exposures to toxins is often much more difficult. In many cases, medical professionals are able to treat the symptoms but cannot determine the exact cause of the patient's health problems.

Major Disasters and Their Prevention

Accidental exposures sometimes happen in industrial settings, and such accidents may be devastating. An example is the release of the deadly gas methyl isocyanate from a chemical plant in Bhopal, India, in 1984. More than 500,000 people were exposed to the gas, and at least 3,000 of them died shortly thereafter.

In the United States, strict rules are in place to protect workers and the general public from exposure to airborne and other toxic chemicals. Two groups that create the rules and monitor workplace safety are the Occupational Safety and Health Administration (OSHA) and the National Institute for Occupational Safety and Health.

Weapons of Mass Destruction

Several toxic gases have been developed as weapons of mass destruction. In World War I, for instance, soldiers on all sides used different toxins, including a yellow substance known as mustard gas. Shortly after exposure to mustard gas, victims experienced intense blistering and itching of the skin, and those who inhaled a substantial amount of the gas had severe breathing problems. In addition, exposed individuals who survived exposure faced an increased the risk of cancer later in life.

Whereas most developed nations have signed the Geneva Protocol that bans the use of chemical weapons, many countries have developed and stockpiled chemical weapons and chemical responses to the possible use of those weapons.

▶ *See also* **Carbon Monoxide Poisoning • Liver and Biliary Tract Cancers • Lung Cancer • Mesothelioma**

Resources

Organizations

Agency for Toxic Substances and Disease Registry. 1600 Clifton Road, Atlanta, GA, 30333. Toll free: 800-232-4636. Web site: http://www.atsdr.cdc.gov.

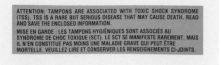

ATTENTION: TAMPONS ARE ASSOCIATED WITH TOXIC SHOCK SYNDROME (TSS). TSS IS A RARE BUT SERIOUS DISEASE THAT MAY CAUSE DEATH. READ AND SAVE THE ENCLOSED INFORMATION.
MISE EN GARDE : LES TAMPONS HYGIÉNIQUES SONT ASSOCIÉS AU SYNDROME DE CHOC TOXIQUE (SCT). LE SCT SE MANIFESTE RAREMENT, MAIS IL N'EN CONSTITUE PAS MOINS UNE MALADIE GRAVE QUI PEUT ÊTRE MORTELLE. VEUILLEZ LIRE ET CONSERVER LES RENSEIGNEMENTS CI-JOINTS.

▲

The outer packaging of a tampon box shows a warning about Toxic Shock Syndrome. *Leonard Lessin/Peter Arnold, Inc.*

* **tampon** is a plug of cotton or other material placed in the vagina during menstruation to absorb menstrual blood and other fluids.

* **vagina** (vah-JY-nah) is the canal, or passageway, in a woman that leads from the uterus to the outside of the body.

American Cancer Society. 1599 Clifton Road NE, Atlanta, GA, 30329-4251. Toll free: 800-227-2345. Web site: http://www.cancer.org.

Centers for Disease Control and Prevention. 1600 Clifton Road, Atlanta, GA 30333. Toll free: 800-232-4636. Web site: http://www.cdc.gov.

National Institute for Occupational Safety and Health. 1600 Clifton Road, Atlanta, GA, 30333. Toll free: 800-232-4636. Web site: http://www.cdc.gov/NIOSH.

Occupational Safety and Health Administration. 200 Constitution Avenue NW, Washington, DC, 20210. Web site: http://www.osha.gov.

Toxic Shock Syndrome (TSS)

Toxic shock syndrome (TSS) is a sometimes life-threatening form of bacterial poisoning usually associated with Staphylococcus *or* Streptococcus *bacteria. Very few people get TSS. On average, it affects approximately three of every 100,000 men, women, and children in the United States, and most of them recover without any lingering problems.*

What Is Going On?

Between October 1979 and May 1980, doctors all over the United States began reporting a new illness to the Centers for Disease Control and Prevention (CDC) in Atlanta, Georgia. Fifty-five women between the ages of 13 and 52 had shown up in doctors' offices and in hospitals with symptoms of serious infections. The cooperation of doctors, health officials, epidemiologists, and laboratory scientists in the months that followed revealed a surprising coincidence: All the women were menstruating and used tampons*. This discovery led to recommendations that reduced the risk for the illness.

What Is Toxic Shock?

Bacteria are microscopic, one-celled organisms found all over the Earth. Many bacteria play a beneficial role in producing antibiotics and nutrients such as vitamins for use by humans, plants, and animals. Bacteria are also essential ingredients in foods such as yogurt and sauerkraut. In addition, however, bacteria can cause disease. *Staphylococcus aureus* (staf-i-lo-KOK-us AW-ree-us) is a bacterium that normally lives harmlessly on the skin and in the nose, armpit, groin, or vagina*, but can cause disease under certain circumstances.

For reasons scientists continued to try to understand, certain forms of bacteria sometimes produce, or secrete, poisonous substances called toxins. People whose bodies are not equipped to fight these toxins may develop a severe reaction to them called toxic shock syndrome. In humans, the toxin does not poison the cells directly. Instead, it stimulates the immune cells (the body's defenders against disease) to secrete huge amounts of cytokines (SI-to-kines), which are proteins that act on other cells. The action of these cytokines produces the symptoms of TSS.

In 1987 experts recognized a second kind of TSS, which is caused by *Streptococcus* (strep-to-KOK-us) bacteria and called STSS. This illness behaves similarly to TSS, but it is much rarer and is related to injured skin and wounds. It is not associated with tampon use.

How Does a Person Get Toxic Shock?

Anyone can get TSS. TSS is not contagious like the cold or flu, but a person who has the bacteria on his or her hands can infect areas of broken skin or wounds anywhere on the body. Half of TSS cases occur in women who use tampons during menstruation* or who have had injuries to the vagina from other causes, and half are related to infections arising from burns, insect bites, chickenpox blisters, or wounds resulting from surgery.

Signs and Symptoms

Symptoms for TSS are vomiting, a high fever, diarrhea, and muscle aches. A sunburn-like rash develops over the body during the first two days of illness. Curiously, the place on the body where the bacteria are multiplying and producing toxin may appear perfectly normal. The early signs and symptoms of TSS go away within a few days. As the rash heals, the skin on the torso, face, hands, and feet begins to peel. Later symptoms may include low blood pressure and heart and kidney failure.

Most people with TSS recover in 7 to 10 days, but 3 percent of people who get TSS die from it, mainly because they do not get treatment for it. People are more likely to die from TSS that is unrelated to menstruation.

Diagnosis

The early symptoms of TSS may resemble those of severe allergic drug reactions or other illnesses. Lacking any other explanation, a doctor will suspect TSS in certain patients, such as women who use vaginal methods of birth control (for example, a diaphragm) or anyone who has recently had an operation. A blood test can confirm the diagnosis.

How Is TSS Treated?

Hospitalization is usually recommended for TSS. Doctors treat TSS with antibiotics and anti-inflammatory drugs, and they disinfect the place on the body where the toxin is being produced. During the worst part of the illness, treatment typically includes fluids to maintain normal blood

Introducing
Staphylococcus aureus

The staphylococci were among the first human disease-causing organisms to be discovered. They grow in various shapes, including irregular bulky clusters from which they get their name (the Greek word *staphulé* means "grapelike"). Staphylococci are the most common causes of the infections that people get in hospitals. In fact, they are at the root of about 2 million hospital infections each year. Various kinds of staphylococci exist. Some are particularly dangerous to people whose systems are already weak from other diseases.

Staphylococcus aureus, a bacterium that causes toxic shock syndrome, is a major public health worry because it is very destructive, and the infections it causes can be hard to treat.

---

* **menstruation** (men-stroo-AY-shun) is the discharge of the blood-enriched lining of the uterus. Menstruation normally occurs in females who are physically mature enough to bear children. Most girls have their first period between the age of 9 and 16. Menstruation ceases during pregnancy and with the onset of menopause. Because it usually occurs at about four-week intervals, it is often called the monthly period.

Naming Bacteria

Bacteria, like all other organisms, have a two-word scientific name. The scientific name is a pair of Latin words that identify the species in the same way that a person's name identifies the person. The first word is the genus name and the second word is the species name. One genus can have many species in it. For example, some members of the genus *Staphylococcus* are named *Staphylococcus aureus, Staphylococcus epidermidis,* and *Staphylococcus saprophyticus* to distinguish them from one another. Like members of a family, they are all related, but each acts in a different way.

* **dialysis** (dye-AL-uh-sis) is a process that removes waste, toxins (poisons), and extra fluid from the blood. Usually dialysis is done when a person's kidneys are unable to perform these functions normally.

* **cutaneous** (kyoo-TAY-nee-us) related to or affecting the skin.

pressure. A patient may also need a breathing machine (ventilator), and if the kidneys fail, may require dialysis* to remove waste products from the blood.

Can Toxic Shock Syndrome Be Prevented?

On average, toxic shock syndrome affects approximately three of every 100,000 men, women, and children in the United States. No sure way exists to prevent TSS, but women can take precautions against it. Menstruating women should avoid using superabsorbant tampons; they should change tampons frequently and never leave a tampon inserted overnight. They also should wash their hands before and after inserting tampons. Girls and women who have had TSS should check with their doctor before using tampons again.

▶ *See also* **Bacterial Infections** • **Shock**

Resources

Books and Articles

Sheen, Barbara. *Toxic Shock Syndrome.* San Diego, CA: Lucent Books, 2006.

Sommers, Michael. *Yeast Infections, Trichomoniasis, and Toxic Shock Syndrome.* New York: Rosen Central, 2008.

Organizations

Centers for Disease Control and Prevention. 1600 Clifton Road, Atlanta, GA, 30333. Toll free: 800-311-3435. Web site: http://www.cdc.gov/ncidod/dbmd/diseaseinfo/toxicshock_t.htm.

TSS Information Service. P.O. Box 450, Godalming, Surrey, GU7 1GR, UK, Web site: http://www.toxicshock.com.

Toxocariasis

Toxocariasis (TOK-so-ka-RY-a-sis) is an infection that occurs in people, and most commonly affects young children who come in contact with contaminated dirt. It is caused by parasitic roundworms found in the intestines of cats and dogs.

What Is Toxocariasis?

Toxocariasis comes in two forms: visceral larva migrans (VIS-er-ul LAR-vuh MY-granz) and cutaneous* larva migrans. Visceral larva migrans is a syndrome that usually results from infection with certain worms. Many cats and dogs, especially kittens and puppies, have intestinal worms called *Toxocara canis* (in dogs) or *Toxocara cati* (in cats). The culprit in visceral larva migrans is usually *Toxocara canis* and sometimes *Toxocara cati*. In rare instances, a pig roundworm called *Ascaris suum* or a raccoon roundworm called *Baylisascaris procyonis* may cause visceral larva migrans. This syndrome occurs when eggs from one of these worms pass with the stools from infected cats and dogs and then contaminate the soil. When children play in these contaminated areas, the eggs can stick to their hands or toys, and the children may then put their hands or the toys in their mouths and swallow the eggs. Those children who eat dirt are especially at risk. Adults may become infected, too, especially if they eat unwashed, contaminated vegetables.

When the eggs enter the digestive system, they hatch. The larvae* burrow through the intestinal wall and move to the liver, lung, and sometimes to other sites, including the central nervous system*, heart, kidney, and eye. (When it affects the eye, the syndrome is sometimes called ocular [OK-yoo-lur] larva migrans.) The larvae may stay alive for many months and cause damage to tissues or organs. Because the larvae are cat or dog parasites, they do not complete their life cycle in humans, so the larvae do not grow into egg-producing adults in humans.

Cutaneous larva migrans, which sometimes goes by the name of ground itch or creeping eruption, results from infection with various roundworm species, especially *Ancylostoma braziliense*, which occurs in dogs and cats in North America (usually from the central United States and South) and South America; *Ancylostoma caninum*, which affects dogs in Australia; and *Uncinaria stenocephala*, which affects dogs in Europe. In addition, people occasionally, although rarely, get cutaneous larva migrans from roundworms that occur in other animals, such as cows, horses, sheep, and goats. People can become infected when the larvae of these worms burrow into the skin. For instance, the larvae may infect the buttocks of a child who is sitting in contaminated dirt, or they may infect the bare feet of a beachgoer who is walking upon contaminated sand. A few days to a few months after they have burrowed into the skin, the larvae start to move beneath the skin, traveling an inch or more per day. Their movements are evident in red lines that appear on the skin. The larvae eventually reach and enter the bloodstream. From there, they typically travel to the lungs.

What Are the Symptoms of Toxocariasis?

Most people with visceral larva migrans have no symptoms. Those that do have symptoms may experience one or more of the following: fever, cough or wheezing, abdominal pain, enlarged liver or spleen, loss of appetite and weight loss, rash, and enlarged lymph nodes*. Some patients may experience seizures* or behavioral disorders, and in rare instances, an individual may die from heart, lung, or nerve problems associated with the syndrome. When an infection affects the eye, it can cause decreased vision, swelling around the eyes, and a cross-eyed appearance.

* **larvae** (LAR-vee) are the immature forms of an insect or worm that hatches from an egg.

* **central nervous system** (SEN-trul NER-vus SIS-tem) is the part of the nervous system that includes the brain and spinal cord.

* **lymph nodes** (LIMF) are small, bean-shaped masses of tissue containing immune system cells that fight harmful microorganisms. Lymph nodes may swell during infections.

* **seizures** (SEE-zhurs) are sudden bursts of disorganized electrical activity that interrupt the normal functioning of the brain, often leading to uncontrolled movements in the body and sometimes a temporary change in consciousness.

* **pneumonia** (nu-MO-nyah) is inflammation of the lungs.

* **anemia** (uh-NEE-me-uh) is a blood condition in which there is a decreased hemoglobin in the blood and, usually, fewer than normal numbers of red blood cells.

* **hormones** are chemical substances that are produced by various glands and sent into the bloodstream carrying messages that have certain effects on other parts of the body.

* **inflammation** (in-fla-MAY-shun) is the body's reaction to irritation, infection, or injury that often involves swelling, pain, redness, and warmth.

Some patients with cutaneous larva migrans have no symptoms. Others, however, will notice a puffy, red area at the site where the larvae have burrowed into the skin. This symptom appears within hours of the penetration. When the larvae start to move beneath the skin, red lines appear. The lines become extremely itchy, and sometimes blisters appear. After the larvae have entered the bloodstream and reached the lungs, they can cause additional symptoms, including pneumonia*, coughing, and anemia*.

How Is Toxocariasis Diagnosed and Treated?

To diagnose visceral larva migrans, a doctor will typically order a blood test to determine whether the patient has a higher than normal number of certain white blood cells, called eosinophils (e-o-SIN-o-filz), which is a sign of this syndrome. In some cases, the doctor may also request that the blood be examined with a test called ELISA, which stands for enzyme-linked immunosorbent assay. ELISA is a very sensitive technique that can scan for signs of the body's own, very specific immune response (its defense system) to the larvae. In addition, the doctor will look for or ask the patient about other symptoms, including lung or eye problems. Visceral larva migrans often goes away on its own. When doctors feel treatment is necessary, they frequently prescribe the drug albendazole, which kills the larvae. If a patient is having severe, infection-related heart, nervous-system, or lung problems, the doctor may prescribe hormones* known as glucocorticoids that reduce inflammation* in these organs.

To diagnose cutaneous larva migrans, a doctor will look for the characteristic red lines, which the patient will typically report as extremely itchy. Doctors can also take a very close look at the red lines with a microscope using a technique called epiluminescence (eh-pih-loom-in-ES-sens) to verify that the lines were made by the larvae. Cutaneous larva migrans usually goes away on its own without treatment. Sometimes, however, doctors will prescribe albendazole or ivermectin to help eliminate the larvae.

How Can Toxocariasis Be Prevented?

As with other infections, good hygiene and frequent hand-washing are essential. Important safety measures include the following:

■ Keeping children from playing in areas that may be contaminated by cat or dog feces, such as the damp area under a porch

■ Teaching children not to put their hands and toys in their mouths after playing with cats and dogs

■ Keeping pets away from sandboxes, which should be covered when not in use

■ Prohibiting pets from public areas, such as beaches and parks, where people are likely to come into contact with sand or dirt

■ Having a veterinarian periodically check pets for parasites, and if parasites are present, treat the pets

- Keeping an especially close watch on children who are known to eat dirt
- Teaching children to wash their hands thoroughly after playing outside, after playing with pets, and before eating
- Washing raw vegetables before eating them

▶ *See also* **Parasitic Diseases: Overview • Worms: Overview • Zoonoses**

Resources

Organizations

Centers for Disease Control and Prevention. 1600 Clifton Road, Atlanta, GA, 30333. Toll free: 800-311-3435. Web site: http://www.cdc.gov/ncidod/dpd/parasites/toxocara/default.htm.

National Library of Medicine. 8600 Rockville Pike, Bethesda, MD, 20894. Web site: http://www.nlm.nih.gov/medlineplus/ency/article/000633.htm.

Toxoplasmosis

Toxoplasmosis (tok-so-plaz-MO-sis), often called toxo, is an infection caused by the Toxoplasma gondii *parasite that animals can transmit to people. It usually causes no symptoms in healthy people, but it can be serious in people with weak immune systems and in unborn babies.*

What Is Toxoplasmosis?

Toxoplasmosis is a disease caused by the microscopic parasite* *Toxoplasma gondii.* This parasite lives in the soil and can infect humans and many species of animals. It is particularly common in cats, and the parasite's eggs pass from their bodies in their feces (FEE-seez, or bowel movements). Touching dirty litter from a cat's litter box is one common way that people contract the parasite. The eggs can stick to a person's hands and may eventually end up in the mouth, where the person can inadvertently swallow them. People also become infected by accidentally eating contaminated soil or by eating raw or undercooked meat, especially pork, lamb, and venison, containing the parasite's cysts*. Thorough cooking kills the parasite.

In addition, pregnant women can pass the disease to their unborn babies, leading to congenital* toxoplasmosis, a condition that can range from mild to severe, and may involve developmental problems and mental retardation, seizures*, and vision problems.

In rare cases, blood transfusions*, organ transplants, and laboratory accidents also can cause toxoplasmosis.

* **parasite** (PAIR-uh-site) is an organism such as a protozoan (one-celled animals), worm, or insect that must live on or inside a human or other organism to survive. An animal or plant harboring a parasite is called its host. A parasite lives at the expense of the host and may cause illness.

* **cysts** (SISTS) are shell-like enclosures that contain small organisms in a resting stage.

* **congenital** (kon-JEH-nih-tul) means present at birth.

* **seizures** (SEE-zhurs) are sudden bursts of disorganized electrical activity that interrupt the normal functioning of the brain, often leading to uncontrolled movements in the body and sometimes a temporary change in consciousness.

* **blood transfusions** (trans-FYOO-zhunz) are procedures in which blood or certain parts of blood (such as specific cells) are given to a person who needs them due to illness or blood loss.

* **immune system** (im-YOON SIS-tem) is the system of the body composed of specialized cells and the substances they produce that helps protect the body against disease-causing germs.

* **miscarriage** (MIS-kare-ij) is the end of a pregnancy through the death of the embryo or fetus before birth.

* **stillbirth** is the birth of a dead fetus.

* **AIDS** or acquired immunodeficiency (ih-myoo-no-dih-FIH-shen-see) syndrome, is an infection that severely weakens the immune system; it is caused by the human immunodeficiency virus (HIV).

* **lymph nodes** (LIMF) are small, bean-shaped masses of tissue containing immune system cells that fight harmful microorganisms. Lymph nodes may swell during infections.

Toxoplasmosis is a life-long infection, although usually it is latent (inactive). Most people with toxoplasmosis have no symptoms or symptoms that are very mild. The disease can be life-threatening, however, for people with weakened immune systems* and for babies born with the disease. Toxoplasmosis also may cause miscarriage* or stillbirth*.

How Common Is Toxoplasmosis?

The Centers for Disease Control estimates that *T. gondii* infects more than 60 million Americans, but cases of actual disease are much less common. Most people who carry the parasite have no symptoms of illness.

What Are the Symptoms of Toxoplasmosis?

Most people with toxoplasmosis, including pregnant women, have no symptoms. When symptoms do appear, they usually appear within 10 days of exposure, and they vary with the person's age and the response of his or her immune system. Children with toxoplasmosis fall into three groups:

- Babies born with toxoplasmosis: Congenital infection occurs when babies get toxoplasmosis before birth from their mothers. Most of these babies (85 percent) appear normal at birth but later have learning disabilities, movement disorders, mental retardation, and loss of vision.

- Healthy children who become infected: These children may have no symptoms, or they may have swollen glands, fever, general tiredness, and weakness.

- Children with immune disorders such as AIDS* or cancer: These children may have severe infections, which attack the central nervous system, brain, lungs, and heart. Symptoms may include fever, seizures, headache, psychosis (severe mental disturbance), and problems in vision, speech, movement, or thinking.

For most people who get toxoplasmosis after birth, symptoms may include:

- fever
- night sweats
- weight loss
- general tiredness
- sore throat
- muscle pain
- swollen lymph nodes*
- calcium deposits in the brain

For people with weakened immune systems (especially those with AIDS), toxoplasmosis can cause major infections of the brain or, less commonly, the lungs or heart. Severe disease can be fatal.

How Is Toxoplasmosis Diagnosed?

If toxoplasmosis is suspected, the doctor draws a blood sample and tests it for evidence of the parasite. For people who have weakened immune systems and are therefore more likely to develop a severe infection, a doctor may order a magnetic resonance imaging* (MRI), a computerized tomography* (CT) scan of the head, or rarely, a brain biopsy (removing a small sample of brain tissue to examine) to look for signs of damage caused by the parasite.

The doctor may also suggest a visit to an ophthalmologist for an eye exam, which may include the use of a special lamp called a slit lamp to check for signs of the disease in the eyes. These signs may include reduced, hazy, or blurred vision; pain when looking into bright light; eye redness; tearing; inflammation in the back of the eye; swelling in part of the retina*; and lesions (injuries) in the retina and/or an adjacent membrane called the chorioid. Ophthalmologists sometimes prescribe medicine to treat an active disease. Occasionally, an eye doctor may find signs of a prior infection with the *Toxoplasma gondii* parasite during a routine eye exam, even though the patient never experienced or noticed any symptoms. This is not a cause for alarm, but pregnant women and those with weakened immune systems should discuss the findings with their regular doctor to determine whether they should take any additional precautions to prevent repeat infection.

What is the Treatment for Toxoplasmosis?

People who have symptoms from toxoplasmosis but are otherwise healthy do not need any treatment, and their symptoms will likely only last a few days. Doctors treat with medication pregnant women, newborns with the congenital infection, and people with weak immune systems. Patients with AIDS often continue taking the medicine even after the infection clears up to keep it from returning. In newborns and patients with unhealthy immune systems, the illness can last for weeks or months, and it can cause permanent disability.

How Is Toxoplasmosis Prevented?

Toxoplasmosis can be prevented by careful attention to hygiene and sanitation. Preventive steps include:

- Thoroughly cooking meat, which means heating it to an internal temperature of 160 degrees Fahrenheit, and until it is no longer pink in the center or until the juices run clear.
- Washing hands, utensils, and food preparation surfaces after handling meats.
- Washing fruits and vegetables before eating them
- Keeping flies and cockroaches away from food
- Washing hands after petting cats and changing litter boxes
- Wearing gloves when working in the garden or cleaning sandboxes.
- Keeping outdoor sandboxes covered when not in use so that they will not be used as litter boxes by cats who roam outdoors

* **magnetic resonance imaging** or MRI, uses magnetic waves, instead of X-rays, to scan the body and produce detailed pictures of the body's structures.

* **computerized tomography** (kom-PYOO-ter-ized toe-MAH-gruh-fee) or CT, also called computerized axial tomography (CAT), is a technique in which a machine takes many X rays of the body to create a three-dimensional picture.

* **retina** (RET-i-na) is the tissue that forms the inner surface of the back of the eyeballs; it receives the light that enters the eye and transmits it through the optic nerves to the brain to produce visual images.

In addition, pregnant women and people whose immune systems are weak can take additional precautionary measures, including being tested for the parasite. This allows the doctor to discover the infection and begin treatment even if the individual does not have any symptoms. Even if people in these groups do not have an infection, they should be especially careful to avoid contact with soil, uncooked meat, and strange or stray cats. In addition, they should keep their own cats indoors and on a diet of canned or dried cat food because cats can pick up the parasite from eating raw meat.

▶ *See also* **AIDS and HIV Infection • Cancer: Overview • Parasitic Diseases: Overview • Pregnancy • Zoonoses**

Resources

Books and Articles

Subauste, Carlos S. *Toxoplasmosis and HIV.* HIV InSite Knowledge Base Chapter available at http://hivinsite.ucsf.edu/InSite?page=kb-05-04-03.

Organizations

American Academy of Family Physicians. P.O. Box 11210, Shawnee Mission, KS, 66207-1210. Toll free: 800-274-2237. Web site: http://familydoctor.org/online/famdocen/home/women/pregnancy/illness/180.html.

Centers for Disease Control and Prevention. 1600 Clifton Road, Atlanta, GA, 30333. Toll free: 800-311-3435. Web site: http://www.cdc.gov/toxoplasmosis.

Medical College of Wisconsin. 8701 Watertown Plank Road, Milwaukee, WI, 53226, Web site: http://healthlink.mcw.edu/article/955156433.html.

Trachoma *See Chlamydial Infections.*

Transgender Health *See Gay, Lesbian, Bisexual, and Transgender Health.*

Transient Ischemic Attack (TIA) *See Stroke.*

Trauma

Trauma occurs when a person experiences a sudden or violent injury. Safety should be foremost in people's minds because preventing a trauma is easier than treating it.

Seat Belts Saved Marcus

Marcus was 16 years old and in a car with four other teenagers. The driver was going too fast, missed a curve, and smashed into a tree. The compact car flipped over, tossing out the teens who were not wearing seat belts. Marcus was not one of them. Paramedics found him conscious and still belted in the back seat with only a broken arm and leg. The four other passengers died. "Without them," Marcus said of seat belts, "I'd be dead."

What Is Trauma?

Physical trauma is an injury or wound caused by external force or violence: motor vehicle accidents, falls, burns, drowning, electric shock, stabbings, gunshots, and other physical assaults. Physical trauma may cause permanent disability. It is the leading cause of death for people below age 45 in the United States and is responsible for 73 percent of deaths in those persons aged between 15 and 24 years of age. In all, more than 100,000 Americans die every year as a result of trauma.

The majority of deaths occur in the first several hours after trauma. Trauma also may cause psychological shock that produces confusion, disoriented feelings and behaviors, and long-term aftereffects.

Trauma Emergencies

Traumatic injuries may include broken bones, severe sprains, head injuries, burns, and internal or external bleeding. They may occur at any time, and they are medical emergencies, meaning they require immediate treatment.

Doctors often try to evaluate the severity of a patient's injuries using numerical scales. These scales help the patient and/or the patient's family understand just how damaging the injuries are and assist in making difficult decisions about options for a patient who will likely not survive regardless of treatment. In addition, medical professionals use these scales to help them quickly evaluate the injuries of multiple patients during a disaster, such as a bus accident or factory explosion, so they can do the most good in a hectic situation. Some of the commonly used scales include the Abbreviated Injury Scale (AIS), the Injury Severity Score (ISS), the Acute Physiology and Chronic Health Evaluation (APACHE), and the Simplified Acute Physiology Score (SAPS).

Burns   A burn is tissue damage that results from scalds, fires, flammable liquids, gases, chemicals, heat, electricity, sunlight, or radiation. In the

* **dehydration** (dee-hi-DRAY-shun) is a condition in which the body is depleted of water, usually caused by excessive and unreplaced loss of body fluids, such as through sweating, vomiting, or diarrhea.

* **epilepsy** (EP-i-lep-see) is a condition of the nervous system characterized by recurrent seizures that temporarily affect a person's awareness, movements, or sensations. Seizures occur when powerful, rapid bursts of electrical energy interrupt the normal electrical patterns of the brain.

* **coma** (KO-ma) is an unconscious state, like a very deep sleep. A person in a coma cannot be awakened, and cannot move, see, speak, or hear.

United States each year, more than 1 million people receive burns severe enough that they need medical attention, and 45,000 of them require hospitalization. In addition to the 4,500 Americans who die each year from the burns themselves, as many as 10,000 more die from burn-related infections, particularly pneumonia.

The symptoms of burns vary. Burns may cause one or more of the following: swelling, blistering, dehydration*, infection, and destruction of skin and other body organs. Depending on the severity of the burn, its treatment may require antibiotics, transfusions, and/or surgery.

Traumatic brain injury   Traumatic brain injury is the form of trauma most likely to result in permanent disability or death. According to the National Center for Injury Prevention and Control, about 1.4 million Americans sustain traumatic brain injuries (TBIs), and most of the injuries result from falls (28%) and motor-vehicle accidents (20%). For active duty military personnel in war zones, blasts are a leading cause of TBI. Adolescents and young adults between the ages of age 15 and 24 have the highest incidence of these injuries out of any age group, and males incur nearly twice as many TBIs as females do. About 50,000 Americans die from these injuries each year, and according to the Centers for Disease Control and Prevention, another 5 million Americans have long-term consequences, including a need for assistance in performing normal daily activities.

Traumatic brain injuries affect many different parts of the body, and they may impair vision, memory, mood, concentration, strength, coordination, and balance. These injuries sometimes cause epilepsy* and coma*, and they may increase the risk for other diseases, such as Parkinson's or Alzheimer's.

Shock   In some cases, a trauma patient may go into shock, a condition in which the body's circulatory system shuts down. Shock may result from internal or external bleeding, dehydration, vomiting, other loss of body fluids, burns, drug overdoses, severe allergic reactions, bacteria in the bloodstream (septic shock), and severe emotional upset. The symptoms of shock include cold and sweaty skin, weak and rapid pulse, dilated pupils, and irregular breathing.

Doctors who treat trauma patients often take action to avert shock even before they treat the injury itself. One way they do so is by ordering a transfusion of salt solution to maintain fluid levels and blood pressure.

Preventing Trauma

Trauma is one of the most preventable causes of death. Reducing traumatic injury requires individual, group, and government attention to public health and safety. Some important preventive measures for individuals are as follows:

■ Using vehicle seatbelts, restraints, and airbags
■ Installing child-safety seats in cars and using them correctly

- Wearing bicycle helmets
- Installing home smoke detectors and keeping them stocked with fresh batteries

The Trauma May Last

Survivors of traumatic events are at risk for psychological problems. These include post-traumatic stress disorder, which can interfere with activities of daily living long after physical wounds have healed. Emotional support and counseling can provide assistance. Signs and symptoms of ongoing psychological trauma include the following:

- Dreams, flashbacks, or intrusive thoughts during which people re-experience the traumatic event
- The avoidance of places and people the victim associates with the trauma
- Insomnia* or difficulty concentrating
- Anxiety or depression
- Physical problems that did not exist before the trauma

▶ *See also* **Broken Bones (Fractures) • Burns • Concussion • Post-Traumatic Stress Disorder • Seizures • Shock • Strains and Sprains**

Resources

Organizations

American Trauma Society. 7611 South Osborne Road, Suite 202, Upper Marlboro, MD, 20772. Toll free: 800-556-7890. Web site: http://www.amtrauma.org.

Centers for Disease Control and Prevention. 1600 Clifton Road, Atlanta, GA, 30333. Toll free: 800-311-3435. Web site: http://www.cdc.gov.

National Institute of General Medical Sciences. 45 Center Drive, MSC 6200, Bethesda, MD, 20892-6200. Telephone: 301-496-7301. Web site: http://www.nigms.nih.gov/Publications/trauma_burn_facts.htm.

Travel-related Infections

When people travel to other countries, they are at increased risk for travel-related infections.

* **insomnia** abnormal inability to get adequate sleep.

* **parasite** (PAIR-uh-sites) is an organism such as a protozoan (one-celled animals), worm, or insect that must live on or inside a human or other organism to survive. An animal or plant harboring a parasite is called its host. A parasite lives at the expense of the host and may cause illness.

* **anemia** (uh-NEE-me-uh) is a blood condition in which there is a decreased hemoglobin in the blood and, usually, fewer than normal numbers of red blood cells.

* **seizures** (SEE-zhurs) are sudden bursts of disorganized electrical activity that interrupt the normal functioning of the brain, often leading to uncontrolled movements in the body and sometimes a temporary change in consciousness.

* **kidney** is one of the pair of organs that filter blood and remove waste products and excess water from the body in the form of urine.

* **endemic** (en-DEH-mik) describes a disease or condition that is present in a population or geographic area at all times.

What Are Travel-related Infections?

When Americans travel to other countries, they may be exposed to many bacterial, viral, parasitic, and fungal infections that they would not come into contact with in the United States. With different climates, sanitation, and hygiene practices (such as bathing and defecating in the same water source), some diseases that are rarely or never seen in the United States are common in other parts of the world. The risk of infectious disease is greatest in tropical and subtropical countries because warm, moist climates offer an ideal environment for the survival and growth of certain organisms. Visiting developing regions of the world, particularly Africa (especially sub-Saharan Africa), Southeast Asia, and Central and South America, also puts people from northern developed countries such as those in Europe and North America at higher risk for travel-related infections. One of the most common ailments is "traveler's diarrhea" (dye-uh-REE-uh), which can be caused by a variety of bacterial, parasitic, and viral infections. According to the Centers for Disease Control and Prevention (CDC), between 20 and 50 percent of these travelers experience diarrhea.

How Are Travel-related Infections Spread?

Some travel-related infections are spread through the bites of insects, such as mosquitoes, which carry malaria and yellow fever, or flies, for example, the tsetse (SET-see) fly, which can carry trypanosomiasis (trih-pan-o-so-MY-uh-sis). Other diseases, including schistosomiasis (shis-tuh-so-MY-uh-sis), can be contracted from swimming, wading, or bathing in contaminated water. Eating or drinking contaminated food or water is another common way of contracting disease, especially traveler's diarrhea.

What Are Some Common Travel-related Infections?

Malaria   Malaria is a disease that is transmitted through a mosquito bite. It is a public health problem throughout many countries and affects 300 to 500 million people each year, according to the World Health Organization (WHO). When an infected mosquito bites a human, the *Plasmodium* (plaz-MO-dee-um) parasite* causes fever and symptoms similar to those of the flu, such as extreme tiredness, muscle aches, nausea (NAW-zee-uh), and chills. The *Plasmodium* parasite typically invades red blood cells. Many symptoms of the disease are related to the destruction of infected red blood cells and resulting anemia*. If left untreated, malaria can cause seizures*, kidney* failure, and death. Medications can treat malaria and prevent this disease in travelers. Malarial prophylaxis (medicine that prevents malaria) is strongly recommended for individuals traveling to endemic* areas. The specific medications to be used vary regionally, depending on resistance patterns of the parasite. For those residing in malaria hot spots, extensive trials of a potentially effective anti-malarial vaccine was initiated in 2008.

Cholera Cholera (KAH-luh-ruh) is a gastrointestinal* disease that causes watery diarrhea, vomiting, and other symptoms. Without treatment, it can lead to dehydration* and even death. People develop cholera by eating food or drinking water that has been contaminated with the cholera bacterium, *Vibrio cholerae* (VIH-bree-o KAH-luh-ray). Eating contaminated shellfish or coming into contact with the feces* of an infected person also can infect someone. A person with cholera is treated to replace fluids lost through vomiting or diarrhea; some antibiotics may reduce the severity and length of the illness.

Dengue fever Dengue (DENG-gay) fever is caused by a virus from the *Flavivirus* (FLAY-vih-vy-rus) group transmitted to humans via the bite of an infected mosquito. According to the CDC, up to 100 million people worldwide develop symptoms of dengue fever each year, such as fever, severe headaches, joint pain, and rashes. Dengue hemorrhagic (heh-muh-RAH-jik) fever is a severe form of dengue that is associated with bruising easily, bleeding from the nose or gums, and bleeding internally, in addition to the other symptoms of dengue fever. No medication can treat either form of the illness. Doctors recommend that people who have dengue fever drink plenty of fluids to avoid dehydration and take acetaminophen* for pain relief.

Filariasis A bite from an infected mosquito can transmit filariasis (fih-luh-RYE-uh-sis), a parasitic disease that affects the lymphatic system*. When the infected mosquito feeds, tiny worms pass from it to the person, where they travel to and grow in the lymph vessels. Someone with this disease may not have noticeable symptoms, but filariasis can lead to permanent damage to the kidneys and lymphatic system. It can also progress to a condition called elephantiasis (eh-luh-fan-TIE-uh-sis), in which fluid builds up in parts of the body and causes swelling and disfigurement. The condition can be treated with medication.

Viral hepatitis Viral hepatitis (heh-puh-TIE-tis) is a viral infection of the liver* that leads to inflammation of the organ. Infections caused by the hepatitis B and C viruses are contracted sexually or through contact with contaminated blood or other body fluids, but hepatitis A virus is more contagious and is the hepatitis virus that more commonly infects travelers. It can spread through person-to-person contact or through contaminated water and food, especially shellfish and raw vegetables and fruits. A person with hepatitis may have symptoms similar to those of the flu, such as fever, chills, and weakness. People with hepatitis A may need extra fluids and rest, but most recover without medication.

Leishmaniasis Travelers who are bitten by an infected sand fly can develop leishmaniasis (leesh-muh-NYE-uh-sis), a disease caused by *Leishmania* (leesh-MAH-nee-uh) parasites that can affect the skin or the internal organs. People with the skin disease often have skin sores that may spread to cause facial disfigurement. Those with the internal form of

* **gastrointestinal** (gas-tro-in-TES-tih-nuhl) means having to do with the organs of the digestive system, the system that processes food. It includes the mouth, esophagus, stomach, intestines, colon, and rectum and other organs involved in digestion, including the liver and pancreas.

* **dehydration** (dee-hi-DRAY-shun) is a condition in which the body is depleted of water, usually caused by excessive and unreplaced loss of body fluids, such as through sweating, vomiting, or diarrhea.

* **feces** (FEE-seez) is the excreted waste from the gastrointestinal tract.

* **acetaminophen** (uh-see-teh-MIH-noh-fen) is a medication commonly used to reduce fever and relieve pain.

* **lymphatic system** (lim-FAH-tik) is a system that contains lymph nodes and a network of channels that carry fluid and cells of the immune system through the body.

* **liver** is a large organ located beneath the ribs on the right side of the body. The liver performs numerous digestive and chemical functions essential for health.

* **spleen** is an organ in the upper left part of the abdomen that stores and filters blood. As part of the immune system, the spleen also plays a role in fighting infection.

* **lymph nodes** (LIMF) are small, bean-shaped masses of tissue containing immune system cells that fight harmful microorganisms. Lymph nodes may swell during infections.

* **shock** is a serious condition in which blood pressure is very low and not enough blood flows to the body's organs and tissues. Untreated, shock may result in death.

* **paralysis** (pah-RAH-luh-sis) is the loss or impairment of the ability to move some part of the body.

* **coma** (KO-ma) is an unconscious state, like a very deep sleep. A person in a coma cannot be awakened, and cannot move, see, speak, or hear.

* **urinary tract** (YOOR-ih-nair-e TRAKT) is the system of organs and channels that makes urine and removes it from the body. It consists of the urethra, bladder, ureters, and kidneys.

* **systemic** (sis-TEM-ik) a problem affecting the whole system or whole body, as opposed to a localized problem that affects only one place on the body.

the disease experience fever and an enlarged spleen* or liver and may need to be hospitalized.

Plague   Fleas that bite rodents infected with the bacterium *Yersinia pestis* (yer-SIN-e-uh PES-tis) can transmit plague (PLAYG) to humans. Two to six days after becoming infected with plague, a person may have swollen and tender lymph nodes*, fever, cough, chills, and belly pain. The plague can lead to severe respiratory illness, shock*, and death if a person is not treated with antibiotics.

Rabies   Although rabies (RAY-beez) in humans is rare in the United States, people who travel to certain other countries may be at higher risk for infection. The virus that causes rabies, from the Rhabdoviridae (rab-doh-VEER-ih-day) family, is transmitted to humans through a bite from an infected animal, and without treatment rabies can cause paralysis*, seizures, coma*, and death. A person who has been bitten by an animal suspected of having rabies has to receive injections of the rabies vaccine to prevent the infection from developing.

Schistosomiasis   Schistosomiasis is a disease caused by parasitic *Schistosoma* (shis-tuh-SO-mah) worms that infect humans when they come into contact with contaminated water. The worms must spend part of their life cycle growing in freshwater snails before they enter and infest humans. Common symptoms include rash, fever, muscle aches, and chills. Years later, if left untreated, schistosomiasis can lead to permanent liver damage or damage to the urinary tract*. In certain areas of the world, the free swimming larvae of Schistosoma that primarily infect aquatic birds may penetrate the skin of humans and lead to an itchy rash, called swimmer's itch. This symptom resolves over a short period of time and does not lead to systemic* infection.

Typhoid fever   According to the CDC, typhoid (TIE-foyd) fever affects up to 16 million people worldwide each year, although only about 400 cases occur in the United States (and the majority of those are among individuals who contracted it while traveling abroad). A person who has contact with water or food contaminated with *Salmonella typhi* (sal-muh-NEH-luh TIE-fee) bacteria may develop symptoms such as fever, weakness, rash, stomach pain, or headache. Typhoid fever is treatable with antibiotics.

Typhus   Typhus (TY-fis) is transmitted by the bites of fleas or lice infected with Rickettsiae (rih-KET-see-eye) bacteria. Symptoms of typhus include an extremely high fever, rash, nausea, joint pain, and headache. Patients often become very sick, and without treatment the disease can be life threatening. However, it is treatable with antibiotics.

Viral hemorrhagic fevers   Viral hemorrhagic (heh-muh-RAH-jik) fevers (VHF) are a group of rare but potentially life-threatening viral illnesses that cause symptoms ranging from fever, extreme tiredness, and dizziness to bleeding from the eyes and ears, kidney failure, and seizures. Humans contract VHF after exposure to people or animals that have been infected with one of a variety of viruses. Examples of VHF include Ebola virus infection and Lassa fever.

Yellow fever   The yellow fever virus (from the flavivirus group) is transmitted to humans by a mosquito bite. Within a week of being infected, a person may experience fever, muscle aches, nausea, or vomiting. Most people recover within three to four days, but according to WHO about 15 percent of people with yellow fever develop a more serious form of the disease that can cause bleeding, kidney failure, and death. An effective vaccine is available for yellow fever and is often recommended for travelers who will be visiting areas where the disease is found.

Trypanosomiasis   African trypanosomiasis is a parasitic illness commonly known as sleeping sickness. The *Trypanosoma* (trih-pan-o-SO-mah) parasite is transmitted to humans through a bite from the tsetse fly, after which a person may develop a skin sore, high fever, extreme tiredness, swollen lymph nodes, and swelling around the eyes. The disease is called sleeping sickness because people who have an advanced form of it can have an uncontrollable urge to sleep. If untreated, trypanosomiasis can cause the brain and membranes around the brain to swell and become inflamed. The disease can be treated with hospitalization and medication.

American trypanosomiasis is found in the western hemisphere. It is also known as Chagas' disease. It is transmitted to humans by the bite of the Reduviid (kissing bug) The disease is caused by the protozoan parasite, *Trypanosoma cruzi*. WHO estimates that 16 to 18 million persons are infected with *Trypanosoma cruzi* every year. Acute infections are usually mild but repeated infections can lead to damage to the digestive tract or heart.

Tuberculosis   Tuberculosis (TB) reemerged as a major public health problem in the early 2000s. Experts estimate that up to one-third of the world population has been infected by a TB bacterium at some point. The reemergence of this disease is becoming even more troubling because multiple-drug resistant strains of TB were also emerging. Therefore, travelers who develop any symptoms suspicious of TB (low-grade fevers, weakness, night sweats, cough, and weight loss) should see a doctor as soon as the symptoms are observed.

Avian influenza   Avian influenza is largely confined to birds such as chickens, ducks and geese. However, people experiencing prolonged close contact with infected birds have developed the disease. As of early 2009, sustained human-to-human transmission had not occurred.

Although primarily affecting birds, a relatively small number of human cases have been reported. The mortality (death) rate among humans as of

* **pandemic** (pan-DEH-mik) is a worldwide outbreak of disease, especially infectious disease, in which the number of cases suddenly becomes far greater than usual.

* **prophylaxis** (pro-fih-LAK-sis) means taking specific measures, such as using medication or a device (such as a condom), to help prevent infection, illness, or pregnancy.

* **vaccinations** (vak-sih-NAY-shunz), also called immunizations, are the giving of doses of vaccines, which are preparations of killed or weakened germs, or a part of a germ or product it produces, to prevent or lessen the severity of the disease that can result if a person is exposed to the germ itself.

late 2008 was approximately 60 percent. Many experts predicted that avian influenza would mimic the influenza pandemic* of 1918 and 1919. Global travel is seen as a major potential factor in the possible spread of this virus, especially with marked increase in travel to the Far East, Indonesia, and the Indian subcontinent.

How Can Travelers Protect Themselves from Illness?

Travelers can take precautions to reduce their risk of contracting a disease while abroad. Experts offer the following tips for staying healthy:

- Do not swim, wade, or bathe in freshwater sources, the ocean near beaches that are contaminated with human feces, or pools that are not chlorinated.

- Use only bottled water or water that has been boiled for drinking and brushing teeth.

- Avoid drinks containing ice, as the ice may be from unsafe water. Canned or bottled beverages are the safest drinks. Carefully wiping the top of the can or bottle before drinking from it may help remove disease-causing agents.

- Do not eat raw foods, particularly meat and salad. Avoid raw fruits and vegetables unless you peel them yourself.

- Avoid shellfish and other fish, which can be toxic at certain times of the year even if they have been cooked.

- Do not eat foods that are bought from street vendors.

- Avoid unpasteurized milk (milk that has not been processed with heat to kill parasites and bacteria) and dairy products.

- Prevent insect bites by wearing long sleeves and long pants in light colors so the insects can be seen easily.

- Use repellent and sleep under mosquito netting.

- Stay inside at times when biting insects are most active, mostly dawn and dusk.

Vaccination   Prophylaxis* is especially important for preventing certain illness, such as malaria. Individuals traveling to areas of the world that are considered to be high-risk for contracting malaria, typically take prophylactic medication to prevent malaria. Special travel medicine clinics provide advice on specific disease patterns depending on the destination and offer appropriate vaccinations* and prophylaxis.

Depending on the destination and the length of the planned trip, travelers may receive immunizations for hepatitis, meningococcal infection, typhoid fever, or yellow fever, as well as any vaccinations in the regular immunization schedule that the person may have missed or may need to renew, such as those for diphtheria and tetanus. If someone plans to travel abroad, it is important to discuss travel plans with a doctor so that any necessary vaccinations can be given.

See also **Cholera • Dengue Fever • Ebola Hemorrhagic Fever • Filariasis • Hepatitis • Lassa Fever • Leishmaniasis • Malaria • Plague • Rabies • Schistosomiasis • Severe Acute Respiratory Syndrome (SARS) • Trypanosomiasis • Typhoid Fever • Typhus • Vaccination • Yellow Fever**

Resources

Books and Articles

Jong, Elaine. *The Travel and Tropical Medicine Manual,* 4th ed. Philadelphia, PA: Saunders, 2008.

Keystone, Jay. *Travel Medicine: Expert Consult,* 2nd ed. St. Louis: Mosby, 2008.

Steffen, Robert. *Manual of Travel Health and Medicine,* 3rd ed. Hamilton, Ontario: BC Deckcr, 2007.

Organizations

American Academy of Family Physicians. P.O. Box 11210, Shawnee Mission, KS, 66207-1210. Toll free: 800-274-2237. Web site: http://www.aafp.org/afp/980800ap/dick.html.

American College of Occupational and Environmental Medicine. 55 West Seegers Road, Arlington Heights, IL, 60005. Telephone: 708-228-6850. Web site: http://www.acoem.org.

Centers for Disease Control and Prevention. 1600 Clifton Road, Atlanta, GA, 30333. Toll free: 800-311-3435. Web site: http://www.cdc.gov/travel.

International Society of Travel Medicine. 2386 Clower Street, Suite A-102, Snellville, GA, 30078. Telephone: 770-736-7060. Web site: http://www.istm.org.

Pan American Health Organization. 525 Twenty-third Street NW, Washington, DC, 20037. Telephone: 202-974-3000. Web site: http://www.paho.org.

Trichinosis

Trichinosis (trih-kih-NO-sis) is a parasitic infection that comes from eating raw or undercooked meat. It is caused by species of the roundworm Trichinella (trih-kih-NEH-luh).

What Is Trichinosis?

Also called trichinellosis (trih-kih-neh-LO-sis), trichinosis can occur when people eat meat that is infected with the larvae* of *Trichinella* roundworms (also called nematodes, NEE-muh-todes); *Trichinella spiralis* (spy-RAL-is)

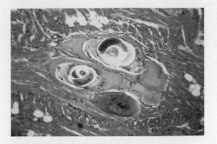

The larvae of the *Trichinella* worm after they have become embedded in muscle causing trichinosis as seen under the microscope. *Custom Stock Medical Photos, Inc. Reproduced by permission.*

* **larvae** (LAR-vee) are the immature forms of an insect or worm that hatches from an egg.

* **cysts** (SISTS) are shell-like enclosures that contain small organisms in a resting stage.

* **small intestine** is the part of the intestines—the system of muscular tubes that food passes through during digestion—that directly receives the food when it passes through the stomach.

* **biopsy** (BI-op-see) is a test in which a small sample of skin or other body tissue is removed and examined for signs of disease.

* **antibodies** (AN-tih-bah-deez) are protein molecules produced by the body's immune system to help fight specific infections caused by microorganisms, such as bacteria and viruses.

is the most common species that causes trichinosis. People can become infected only by eating infected meat; the disease is not spread through human contact. The parasite also can spread when animals eat the infected flesh of other animals. Most often, meat infected with the parasite comes from pigs or wild game, such as bear, horse, wolf, and fox.

Trichinella larvae form cysts* in meat. When an animal eats this meat, the animal's stomach acid dissolves the cysts, and the worms are released into the body. They travel to the small intestine*, where they grow into adult worms and mate. After about a week, the mature female worm releases larvae, which travel through the bloodstream to the muscles. There they form the hard cysts that began the cycle. The cysts remain in the muscles, and people become infected when they eat these cysts in animal meat.

How Common Is Trichinosis?

According to the Centers for Disease Control and Prevention, approximately 12 cases of trichinosis per year have been reported to them since the late 1990s. The cases of so few because people became more aware of the dangers of eating raw or undercooked meat; better storage and freezing methods of meat were being used; and laws prohibiting the feeding of raw meat to pigs were passed. Most trichinosis cases in the early 2000s were associated with eating wild game.

How Do People Know They Have Trichinosis?

The length of the period between eating the infected meat and the first symptoms of illness depends on the number of parasites in the meat and how much a person ate. The time before symptoms occur can range from 1 to 45 days, but symptoms often surface in 10 to 14 days. Symptoms can be mild and even go unnoticed, but they usually start with fever, diarrhea (dye-uh-REE-uh), stomach pain, nausea (NAW-zee-uh), vomiting, and extreme tiredness. Other symptoms may follow, such as headache, cough, chills, muscle and joint pain, eye swelling, and constipation. If the infection is severe, a person may have trouble with coordination as well as heart and breathing problems.

How Do Doctors Diagnose and Treat Trichinosis?

A blood test or muscle biopsy* can be done to determine whether a person has trichinosis. The blood test can detect antibodies* working to destroy the parasite, and the biopsy shows the presence of cysts in the muscles. Asking if a person has recently eaten game or traveled outside the United States may provide information useful in making the diagnosis.

The infection can be treated with various medications to kill the worms in the intestine, but the medication does not get rid of the larvae that have produced cysts in the muscles. These larvae remain in a dormant (inactive) state in the muscle tissue. If the infection is mild, symptoms usually go away after a few months. Muscle aches and weakness may last longer. Some people require only bed rest; others need to be hospitalized and receive oxygen and intravenous (in-tra-VEE-nus) fluids (fluids injected directly into a vein). Severe complications of trichinosis include inflammation of the heart muscle, heart failure, lung problems, delirium*, and coma*. The disease can be fatal if it is not treated.

How Can Trichinosis Be Prevented?

The best way to prevent infection is to eat only thoroughly cooked meat. Curing, drying, salting, and microwaving meat may not kill *Trichinella* larvae. Meat is thoroughly cooked when the juices are clear (not bloody), and the meat has reached an internal temperature of 170 degrees Fahrenheit. Freezing meat at subzero temperatures for several weeks also should kill any larvae in cysts. Raw meat can contaminate work surfaces, so it must not touch surfaces used to prepare food, and grinders and other utensils used with raw meat must be cleaned thoroughly and not used to prepare cooked meat.

▶ *See also* **Intestinal Parasites • Zoonoses**

Resources

Books and Articles

Gittleman, Ann Louise. *Guess What Came to Dinner? Parasites and Your Health,* 2nd ed. New York: Avery, 2001.

Organizations

Centers for Disease Control and Prevention. 1600 Clifton Road, Atlanta, GA, 30333. Toll free: 800-311-3435. Web site: http://www. cdc.gov/ncidod/dpd/parasites/trichinosis/factsht_trichinosis.htm.

National Institute of Allergy and Infectious Diseases. Office of Communications and Public Liaison, 6610 Rockledge Drive, MSC, 6612, Bethesda, MD, 20892-66123. Toll free: 866-284-4107. Web site: http://www3.niaid.nih.gov/topics/trichinosis/default.htm.

Trichomoniasis

Trichomoniasis (trih-ko-mo-NYE-uh-sis) is a common sexually transmitted disease (STD) that occurs in women and men.

What Is Trichomoniasis?

Trichomoniasis (also known as "trich") is an infection caused by the parasite* *Trichomonas vaginalis* (trih-koh-MO-nas vah-jih-NAL-is). It usually affects the urethra* in men and the vagina* or urethra in women.

* **delirium** (dih-LEER-e-um) is a condition in which a person is confused, is unable to think clearly, and has a reduced level of consciousness.

* **coma** (KO-ma) is an unconscious state, like a very deep sleep. A person in a coma cannot be awakened, and cannot move, see, speak, or hear.

* **parasite** (PAIR-uh-sites) is an organism such as a protozoan (one-celled animals), worm, or insect that must live on or inside a human or other organism to survive. An animal or plant harboring a parasite is called its host. A parasite lives at the expense of the host and may cause illness.

* **urethra** (yoo-REE-thra) is the tube through which urine passes from the bladder to the outside of the body.

* **vagina** (vah-JY-nah) is the canal, or passageway, in a woman that leads from the uterus to the outside of the body.

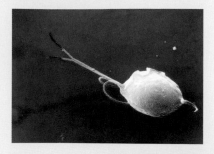

Scanning electron micrograph of *trichomonas vaginalis*, the parasite that causes the sexually transmitted disease trichomoniasis. *BSIP/Photo Researchers, Inc.*

* **abdominal** (ab-DAH-mih-nul) refers to the area of the body below the ribs and above the hips that contains the stomach, intestines, and other organs.

* **ejaculation** (e-jah-kyoo-LAY-shun) is the discharge of semen, a whitish fluid containing sperm, from the penis.

* **pelvic exam** is an internal examination of a woman's reproductive organs.

* **cervix** (SIR-viks) is the lower, narrow end of the uterus that opens into the vagina.

* **Pap smear** is a common diagnostic test used to look for cancerous cells in the tissue of the cervix.

* **cultured** (KUL-churd) means subjected to a test in which a sample of fluid or tissue from the body is placed in a dish containing material that supports the growth of certain organisms. Typically, within days the organisms will grow and can be identified.

* **antibiotics** (an-tie-by-AH-tiks) are drugs that kill or slow the growth of bacteria.

The disease spreads from person to person through sexual contact and infects primarily women between the ages of 16 and 35. It is one of the most common STDs in young sexually active women, and the Centers for Disease Control and Prevention estimates that 7.4 million new cases occur each year among women and men in the United States. As with all STDs, people who have had many sexual partners are more likely to contract trichomoniasis.

What Are the Signs and Symptoms of Trichomoniasis?

Women who contract trichomoniasis are more likely to have symptoms than men who become infected, although many people who have trichomoniasis experience no symptoms at all. If a person has symptoms, they usually appear within six months of becoming infected. Women often have a strong-smelling yellow-green or gray foamy vaginal discharge and itching in or around the vagina. They may feel pain or burning during sex or urination and, rarely, lower abdominal* pain. Men typically have no symptoms. When they do, they may feel irritation inside the penis and burning after urination or ejaculation*. They may have a discharge from the penis as well.

How Do Doctors Diagnose Trichomoniasis?

If a woman has symptoms of the disease, the doctor will perform a pelvic exam* to look for the telltale signs of inflammation on the cervix* and inner walls of the vagina. The doctor will take a sample of fluid from the vagina to look at under the microscope for evidence of the parasite. In some instances, *Trichomonas* infection may be found during a routine Pap smear* or when vaginal fluid is cultured* to diagnose infection caused by other organisms. Most cases of trichomoniasis that cause symptoms can be diagnosed in the doctor's office by examining the vaginal fluid under a microscope.

When trichomoniasis is suspected in a man, the doctor may take a sample of fluid from the man's urethra to confirm the diagnosis. If the doctor diagnoses trichomoniasis in any patient, tests for other STDs will likely be done as well, because it is common for a person to have more than one STD at the same time.

What Is the Treatment for Trichomoniasis?

Most cases of trichomoniasis are treated with a single-dose of the oral antibiotic* metronidazole. Doctors recommend that people who are infected not have sex until they have completed treatment, to limit the risk of spreading the infection. Treating all sexual partners of someone who has trichomoniasis, even if they have no symptoms, also is suggested as a way to prevent a new round of infection or the spread of the disease.

Does the Disease Have Complications?

In a pregnant woman, the infection can bring about early rupture of the amniotic sac* and premature delivery*. Trichomoniasis may also increase the risk of becoming infected with human immunodeficiency (ih-myoo-no-dih-FIH-shen-see) virus (HIV), the virus that causes acquired immunodeficiency syndrome (AIDS), which severely weakens the immune system.

Can Trichomoniasis Be Prevented?

The risk of trichomoniasis can be lowered or prevented by taking the following precautions:

- Practicing abstinence (not having sex)
- Practicing safe sex by using a male latex condom
- Reducing the number of sexual partners

▶ See also **AIDS and HIV Infection • Chlamydial Infections • Gonorrhea • Sexually Transmitted Diseases (STDs)**

Resources

Books and Articles

Holmes, King. *Sexually Transmitted Diseases,* 4th ed. New York: McGraw Hill, 2007.

Marr, Lisa. *Sexually Transmitted Diseases: A Physician Tells You What You Need to Know,* 2nd ed. Baltimore, MD: Johns Hopkins University Press, 2007.

Sommers, Michael. *Yeast Infections, Trichomoniasis, and Toxic Shock Syndrome.* New York: Rosen Central, 2008.

Organizations

American Academy of Family Physicians. P.O. Box 11210, Shawnee Mission, KS, 66207-1210. Toll free: 800-274-2237. Web site: http://www.aafp.org.

American College of Obstetricians and Gynecologists. 409 12th Street SW, P.O. Box 96920, Washington, DC, 20090-6920. Telephone: 202-638-5577. Web site: http://www.acog.org.

American College of Physicians. 190 N. Independence Mall West, Philadelphia, PA, 19106. Toll free: 800-523-1546. Web site: http://www.acponline.org.

American Social Health Association. P.O. Box 13827, Research Triangle Park, NC, 27709. Telephone: 919-361-8400. Web site: http://www.ashastd.org/learn/learn_vag_trich_tri.cfm.

Centers for Disease Control and Prevention. 1600 Clifton Road, Atlanta, GA, 30333. Toll free: 800-311-3435. Telephone: Hotline 800-227-8922. Web site: http://www.cdc.gov/std/Trichomonas/STDFact-Trichomoniasis.htm.

* **amniotic sac** (am-nee-AH-tik SAK) is the sac formed by the amnion, the thin but tough membrane that lines the outside of the embryo in the uterus and is filled with fluid to cushion and protect the embryo as it grows.

* **premature delivery** is when a baby is born before it has reached full term.

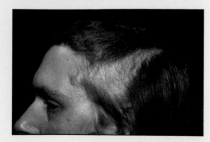

▲

About 75 percent of people with trichotillomania pull hair from the scalp. In some cases trichotillomania is a response to stress at home or school, while in others it results from a hair-pulling habit developed during childhood. *Custom Medical Stock Photos, Inc. Reproduced by permission.*

Trichotillomania

Trichotillomania (trik-o-til-o-MAY-nee-a) is a condition that involves compulsive (kom-PUL-siv) hair pulling, usually the hair on the scalp or the eyebrows or eyelashes.

Penny's Story

Penny put on her favorite baseball cap and headed out the door for school. The cap hid the bald spot on the side of her head pretty well. She envied the girls who could wear barrettes and ponytails to school, and she remembered the days when she had worn them, too. Over the previous two years, Penny had started to pull out her hair and her eyebrows. It began gradually at first, but pretty soon her eyebrows were gone, and she had bald patches on her head. She did not want to pull the hair, but she felt a powerful urge to do it. She just could not stop. No one understood why she was doing it, not even Penny. The boys in her class teased her. She pretended not to listen to them, but their unkind comments made her cry when she was alone. Even the nice kids asked her why she did not have any eyebrows. Until recently, Penny did not really know what to say. Then Penny began to see a therapist, who helped her understand that she had trichotillomania.

What Is Trichotillomania?

Trichotillomania is a condition that involves strong urges to pull hair. People with this condition pluck or pull the hair on their heads, their eyelashes, their eyebrows, or hair on other body parts. For people with trichotillomania, the hair pulling is more than a habit. It is a compulsive behavior, which means the behavior is irrational and very hard to stop. A person with trichotillomania feels a strong urge to pull hair, an impulse that is so powerful that it seems impossible to resist.

Pulling the hair often provides a brief feeling of relief, like the feeling of finally scratching an itch but much more intense. But after the feeling of relief, which lasts only a moment, the person usually feels distressed and unhappy about having pulled the hair. Soon the urge to pull hair returns. People with trichotillomania wish they could stop, and they may feel ashamed or embarrassed. Many people who have this condition try to keep it secret.

What Causes Trichotillomania?

The condition trichotillomania was first described in 1889 by the French physician François Hallopeau (1842–1919). The term "trichotillomania" comes from the Greek words "thrix," meaning "hair," and "tillein," meaning "to pull." "Mania," the Greek word for "madness" or "frenzy," was used in the 19th century for any condition that affected human behavior. Hallopeau wrote that his patients with hair-pulling compulsions were, in fact, quite emotionally healthy.

Although the exact cause of trichotillomania is unknown, in the early 2000s there was growing evidence that suggested it is a biological disorder of neurotransmitter* function in the brain. Trichotillomania has some similarities to obsessive-compulsive disorder* (OCD), but in trichotillomania there are no obsessions*, and hair pulling is the only compulsion. Both trichotillomania and OCD fall into the larger category of anxiety disorders*. Some people with trichotillomania have other forms of anxiety as well. Trichotillomania can affect children, adolescents, and adults. Both males and females can have trichotillomania, but it seems to be more common among females.

How Is Trichotillomania Diagnosed?

When individuals lose their hair or eyebrows, doctors may first check for other conditions that might cause a person's hair to fall out, such as ringworm*, alopecia areata*, or other skin diseases. But if the person tells the doctor about the hair pulling, it is probably trichotillomania. Penny's doctor sent her to see a therapist, a mental health specialist who listens to people talk about their experiences and feelings and who can help people work out ways to deal with behavior problems. The therapist explained Penny's condition to her and told her about the urges, habits, and anxiety that are part of the problem. She helped Penny understand that the hair pulling was not her fault. Penny felt relieved to know that she was not the only person with this problem and that she could do something about it.

How Is Trichotillomania Treated?

One common treatment for trichotillomania is a behavior therapy* technique called habit reversal. In habit reversal, the person first learns to notice the urge before the compulsion to pull hair becomes too strong to resist. Then the person learns to do something else instead of hair pulling until the urge grows weaker and passes. This shift in behavior can be more difficult than it sounds, because the person may feel increasing, uncomfortable tension and anxiety while trying to resist the urge to pull hair. With time and practice, the brain can begin to react differently to the urges, and the person can start to control the compulsive behavior. Some people may also take medication that helps with the compulsions and decreases the strength of the urges, making them easier to resist. After a few weeks of practice, coaching from her therapist, and support from her parents, Penny began to get better at resisting the urges she felt. Penny started to see results; her hair began to grow back in.

What Is It Like to Live with Trichotillomania?

Now that Penny's hair and eyelashes are growing in, she feels better about herself and more hopeful about coping with trichotillomania. Now and then, Penny may continue to feel urges to pull her hair and eyebrows, but she knows what to do to resist them. She knows that these impulses can be stronger in times of stress, but they can also arise on their own during

* **neurotransmitter** (NUR-o-tranz-mit-er) is a brain chemical that lets brain cells communicate with each other and therefore allows the brain to function properly. In other words, a neurotransmitter transmits (carries) a chemical message from neuron to neuron.

* **obsessive-compulsive disorder** is a condition that causes people to become trapped in a pattern of repeated, unwanted thoughts, called obsessions (ob-SESH-unz), and a pattern of repetitive behaviors, called compulsions (kom-PUL-shunz).

* **obsessions** (ob-SESH-unz) are repeated disturbing thoughts or urges that a person cannot ignore and that will not go away.

* **anxiety disorders** (ang-ZY-e-tee dis-OR-derz) are a group of conditions that cause people to feel extreme fear or worry that sometimes is accompanied by symptoms such as dizziness, chest pain, or difficulty sleeping or concentrating.

* **ringworm** is a fungal infection of the skin or scalp that appears as a round, red rash.

* **alopecia areata** (al-o-PEA-shah a-ree-AH-ta) is a condition that leads to sudden hair loss, often in small, round patches on the scalp. The cause is not known.

* **behavior therapy** is a type of counseling that works to help people change their actions.

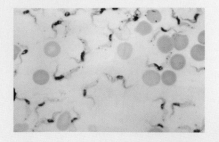

Blood infected with the protozoa that cause trypanosomiasis seen under a microscope. The disease is known as sleeping sickness in Africa and Chagas' disease in Latin America. *Custom Stock Medical Photos, Inc. Reproduced by permission.*

* **parasite** (PAIR-uh-sites) is an organism such as a protozoan (one-celled animals), worm, or insect that must live on or inside a human or other organism to survive. An animal or plant harboring a parasite is called its host. A parasite lives at the expense of the host and may cause illness.

* **protozoa** (pro-tuh-ZOH-uh) are single-celled microorganisms (tiny organisms), some of which are capable of causing disease in humans.

times when Penny is bored or just relaxed. Her therapist helped Penny learn and practice ways to cope with normal stresses, to stop the urges before they get too strong, and to control her compulsive pulling.

▶ *See also* **Anxiety and Anxiety Disorders • Obsessive-Compulsive Disorder**

Resources

Books and Articles

Golomb, Ruth Goldfinger, and Sherrie Mansfield Vavrichek. *The Hair Pulling "Habit" and You: How to Solve the Trichotillomania Puzzle.* Silver Spring, MD: Writers' Cooperative of Greater Washington, 2000.

Penzel, Fred. *The Hair-Pulling Problem: A Complete Guide to Trichotillomania.* New York: Oxford University Press, 2003.

Organizations

Mental Health America. 2000 N. Beauregard Street, 6th Floor, Alexandria, VA, 22311. Toll free: 800-969-6642. Web site: http://www.mentalhealthamerica.net.

Trichotillomania Learning Center. 207 McPherson Street, Suite H, Santa Cruz, CA, 95060-5863. Telephone: 831-457-1004. Web site: http://www.trich.org.

Truancy *See School Avoidance.*

Trypanosomiasis

Trypanosomiasis (trih-pan-o-so-MY-uh-sis) is a disease found in Africa and the American continents that is caused by infection with a parasite*. Forms of the disease may persist for many years and have several phases, with symptoms that can vary from one stage to the next.

What Is Trypanosomiasis?

Trypanosomiasis is the name for three types of infections caused by protozoa* and spread to humans through insect bites. There are two kinds of African trypanosomiasis, East African and West African. Both of these varieties also are known as sleeping sickness. The disease can affect people living on the African continent south of the Sahara Desert. American trypanosomiasis is also called Chagas' (SHAH-gus) disease. It occurs only on the American continents, from Mexico to Argentina.

What Causes Trypanosomiasis?

The bite of an infected tsetse (SET-see) fly usually transmits the organisms that cause the African forms of trypanosomiasis. These flies live in the countryside in Africa, especially in bushes and thick vegetation near rivers and lakes. Tsetse flies infected with the protozoan *Trypanosoma brucei rhodesiense* (trih-pan-o-SO-mah BRU-see-eye ro-dee-see-EN-see) spread East African trypanosomiasis, the most severe form of the disease, to humans. The West African variety comes from a fly infected with *Trypanosoma brucei gambiense* (trih-pan-o-SO-mah BRU-see-eye gam-be-EN-see).

Reduviid (rih-DO-vee-id) bugs (also called assassin, cone-nose, or kissing bugs) carry the *Trypanosoma cruzi* (trih-pan-o-SO-mah KROO-zee) protozoa that cause the American variety of trypanosomiasis, or Chagas' disease, named for the Brazilian physician Carlos Chagas (1879–1934) who discovered it in 1909. These bugs hide during the day in the cracks in mud and adobe homes. At night they crawl across sleeping people and bite them, usually on the face but sometimes on the arms, legs, or trunk. They also leave behind their feces*, which contain the protozoa. Without knowing it, people can rub the infected feces into the bite, a cut, or open sore, or even into their noses, mouths, or eyes.

How Common Is Trypanosomiasis?

Trypanosomiasis can infect people of every age and race, although it is uncommon in the United States. Since the late 1960s, fewer than 30 cases have been reported among U.S. citizens traveling to areas where the infection is found. In other parts of the world, however, the disease affects thousands of people. The World Health Organization estimates that as many as 500,000 people could have African trypanosomiasis, but because of poor monitoring most of these cases are not reported. Between 16 million and 18 million people in the Americas in the early 2000s had Chagas' disease. Approximately 50,000 may die from the disease each year.

Is Trypanosomiasis Contagious?

People cannot catch any form of trypanosomiasis in the same way that they catch a cold or the flu from other people. Only the tsetse fly spreads the African varieties, and the reduviid bug spreads Chagas' disease. Rarely, a mother infected with the West African variety of trypanosomiasis or with Chagas' disease can pass the illness to her unborn child. People who receive a transfusion* of blood or an organ transplant from an infected person also may contract the disease; this form of transmission tends to happen more often with Chagas' disease than with the African types.

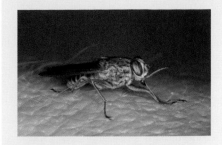

▲

The tsetse fly is responsible for transmitting trypanosomiasis in Africa. *©Ray Wilson/Alamy.*

* **feces** (FEE-seez) is the excreted waste from the gastrointestinal tract.

* **transfusion** (trans-FYOO-zhun) is a procedure in which blood or certain parts of blood, such as specific cells, is given to a person who needs it due to illness or blood loss.

Global Warming

The bite of an insect can transmit bacteria, protozoa, or even worms into a person's bloodstream, leading to a variety of illnesses. Trypanosomiasis is just one example of a tropical insect-borne disease. A few others, along with the insects that spread them, are:

- Malaria (mah-LAIR-e-uh) mosquitoes

- Yellow fever mosquitoes

- Elephantiasis (eh-luh-fan-TIE-uh-sis) mosquitoes

- Leishmaniasis (leesh-muh-NYE-uh-sis) sandflies

- Onchocerciasis, (on-koh-sir-KYE-us-sis) or river blindness black flies

These diseases are common to the tropics because the hot and often rainy climate makes the tropics an ideal breeding ground for insects. Greenpeace, among other organizations dedicated to protecting the environment, has warned that global warming could create new breeding grounds for insects throughout the world. At the same time, rising temperatures could raise insect reproductive rates, increasing their numbers. As the climate in the United States and Europe becomes more "tropical," diseases such as yellow fever and malaria may become more common, bringing the tropics into the backyards of people living in northern areas.

* **lymph nodes** (LIMF) are small, bean-shaped masses of tissue containing immune system cells that fight harmful microorganisms. Lymph nodes may swell during infections.

What Are the Symptoms of the Disease?

African trypanosomiasis People who contract the African varieties of trypanosomiasis may start sleeping more, although this usually does not happen until the later stages of the disease. Sleeping sickness may start with the appearance of a sore called a chancre (SHANG-ker) at the spot where the person received the tsetse fly bite. Later symptoms include fever, extreme tiredness, severe headaches, rashes, itching, joint pain, and swelling of the hands and feet. The lymph nodes* on the back of the neck may become swollen as well. These signs typically appear two to four weeks after infection with East African trypanosomiasis.

Other symptoms can follow quickly, as the protozoa cross the blood-brain barrier* and start affecting a patient's mental functions. The later stages of sleeping sickness may bring mental confusion, changes in personality, problems with walking and talking, weight loss, and seizures*. The spleen and liver may become enlarged. Sleeping sickness gets its name from the later part of the disease, when the sick person has night-time insomnia* but sleeps for long periods during the day. If the person does not receive treatment, the heart muscles may become inflamed or weakened, causing death from heart failure.

The early symptoms in West African trypanosomiasis are similar but may take longer to appear. Months or years may pass before an infected person becomes sick, and the disease develops more slowly, although it can still cause death if it is left untreated. The gap between infection and the start of symptoms can make this form of sleeping sickness difficult to diagnose.

Chagas' disease The first sign of Chagas' disease may show up a few hours after infection, when a raised red spot called a chagoma (chuh-GO-mah) appears at the site of the insect bite. Most people have no other symptoms during the early, or acute, phase of the disease, which begins a few weeks later. People who experience symptoms may have fevers, rashes, extreme tiredness, vomiting, loss of appetite, or swollen lymph nodes. The side of the face where the infected feces were rubbed into an eye or a bug bite may swell. In most people these symptoms usually disappear within four to eight weeks without causing problems, but infants can die in this early stage from brain swelling. About 10 to 20 years after this first phase, approximately one-third of infected people can show symptoms of the chronic* phase of Chagas' disease. They may become constipated and experience trouble swallowing. The heart may become enlarged, and patients may have altered heart rhythms or heart failure leading to death.

How Do Doctors Diagnose Trypanosomiasis?

Because all types of trypanosomiasis are rare in the United States, it is important for people who have any symptoms of the disease to let their doctor know right away if they have been traveling in areas where the disease is common. To diagnose sleeping sickness or Chagas' disease, a doctor orders blood tests to look for protozoa or antibodies* to the organism. In cases in which the doctor suspects sleeping sickness, a sample drawn from fluid surrounding the brain and spinal cord or tissue from swollen lymph nodes may be examined for evidence of the disease. If a patient has a suspicious-looking skin lesion*, a biopsy* is performed to test for *Trypanosoma cruzi* protozoa.

Can Trypanosomiasis Be Treated Successfully?

There are medications available to treat all types of the disease. Doctors recommend that people with trypanosomiasis receive treatment as soon as possible. Treatment is given in a hospital. After leaving the hospital, patients typically are watched closely by a doctor for at least two years to see whether they show any signs that they still have the infection.

What Happens to People with Trypanosomiasis?

East African sleeping sickness can move through the body quickly, progressing in just weeks or months to the most serious phase of illness. West African sleeping sickness takes longer to develop. People may not reach the critical phase for months or even years. People who do not receive treatment for African trypanosomiasis can die from heart failure, and those who wait to start treatment may have permanent brain damage. Long-term complications of Chagas' disease, which may not appear for 20 or more years after infection, include damage to the digestive and nervous systems, heart problems, and sudden death.

Can Trypanosomiasis Be Prevented?

There is no vaccine or medication that can prevent any form of the disease, so it is wise for people who travel in areas where the disease is common to take precautions. In Africa precautions include wearing clothes of thick material, with long sleeves and long pants. Neutral colors, such as tan, are best because tsetse flies are attracted to dark and bright colors. Doctors recommend that travelers to Africa sleep under netting and avoid riding in the backs of open trucks because dust from moving vehicles attracts the flies. It is also advisable not to walk through brush. In areas where Chagas' disease is found, it is a good idea for people to avoid sleeping in mud, adobe, or thatch houses; to sleep under netting; and to use insect repellent.

▶ *See also* **Chagas' Disease • Leishmaniasis • Travel-related Infections**

Resources

Books and Articles

Kruel, Donald. *Trypanosomiasis.* New York: Chelsea House, 2007.

* **blood-brain barrier** is a biological shield in the body that helps prevent germs or other potentially harmful materials in the blood from entering the brain and spinal cord.

* **seizures** (SEE-zhurs) are sudden bursts of disorganized electrical activity that interrupt the normal functioning of the brain, often leading to uncontrolled movements in the body and sometimes a temporary change in consciousness.

* **insomnia** abnormal inability to get adequate sleep.

* **chronic** (KRAH-nik) lasting a long time or recurring frequently.

* **antibodies** (AN-tih-bah-deez) are protein molecules produced by the body's immune system to help fight specific infections caused by microorganisms, such as bacteria and viruses.

* **lesion** (LEE-zhun) is a general term referring to a sore or a damaged or irregular area of tissue.

* **biopsy** (BI-op-see) is a test in which a small sample of skin or other body tissue is removed and examined for signs of disease.

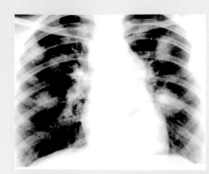

X-ray of lungs infected with *Mycobacterium tuberculosis,* the bacterium that causes tuberculosis. This disease has infected humans for thousands of years. *Custom Medical Stock Photo, Inc. Reproduced by permission.*

* **immune system** (im-YOON SIS-tem) is the system of the body composed of specialized cells and the substances they produce that helps protect the body against disease-causing germs.

Organizations

Centers for Disease Control and Prevention. 1600 Clifton Road, Atlanta, GA, 30333. Toll free: 800-311-3435. Web site: http://www.cdc.gov/ncidod/dpd/parasites/trypanosomiasis/default.htm; http://www.cdc.gov/chagas.

World Health Organization. Avenue Appia 20, CH - 1211 Geneva 27, Switzerland. Telephone: +41 22 791 2111. Web site: http://www.who.int/topics/trypanosomiasis_african/en; http://www.who.int/tdr/diseases/chagas/default.htm.

Tuberculosis

Tuberculosis (too-ber-ku-LO-sis) is a bacterial infection that spreads through the air and usually affects the lungs. Worldwide, it kills more people than any other infectious disease.

An Ancient Disease

Hippocrates (*c.*460–*c.*377 B.C.E.), a Greek physician who in modern times is called "the father of medicine," accurately described tuberculosis (TB) about 2,400 years ago when he coined the term "phthisis," which means to melt and to waste away. In later years, tuberculosis was called consumption because people with TB tended to waste away as if they were being slowly consumed.

What Is Tuberculosis?

Tuberculosis is a potentially serious infection caused by *Mycobacterium tuberculosis* bacteria. The bacteria are spread mainly through the air from an infected person to others nearby. TB usually infects the lungs, but it can also cause symptoms that affect the whole body.

Not everyone who is infected with tuberculosis bacteria (called primary infection) gets sick or infects other people. About 10 million people in the United States are infected with tuberculosis, but only 1 out of every 10 of these people develops active TB (called secondary infection). Of the 10 percent of infected people who ultimately develop active disease, about one-third to one-half manifest illness in the first two months to two years after they are initially infected; the remainder develop active TB later in life.

People with primary TB infection are protected from developing active TB by their body's immune system*, but they still carry the bacteria in their bodies. As long as the infection is inactive, they cannot spread TB. They can, however, develop active (secondary) TB years later if their immune systems are weakened by other diseases such as HIV/AIDS or diabetes, or by alcohol or drug abuse. Most people with active TB who are treated can be cured. If left untreated, however, TB is fatal 40 to 60 percent of the time. Importantly, individuals discovered to have TB infection can be given preventive therapy, which can reduce the lifetime risk of developing active disease by at least 70 percent.

How Is Tuberculosis Spread?

When people with active tuberculosis of the lungs or throat cough or sneeze, they spread bacteria through the air. Other people who breathe

---

THE UNITED STATES AND THE WORLD

- In the United States, tuberculosis is a serious disease, but it is not a leading cause of death or illness. In 2004, for instance, there were about 14,500 new cases of TB and about 662 deaths. It is estimated that 10 million people in the United States have primary (in other words, nonactive) TB infection. Of these about 1 in 10 eventually become ill with the disease.

- In the United States, TB is most common among people with HIV, people in homeless shelters and prisons, other poor people who live in big cities, and elderly people. Rates are higher for men than for women and far higher for people of African ancestry than for people of European ancestry, which may be because a higher proportion of African Americans are poor. Another factor may be that, over the centuries, TB was largely a European disease and Europeans who survived it may have developed resistance to it.

- In the United States, tuberculosis was on the decline until the mid-1980s, when it began to make a comeback. A main reason was the rise of HIV, the AIDS virus, which weakens the immune system. HIV-infected people are more likely to get new TB infections and to have old, inactive infections become active and cause illness. Health officials responded to the upsurge with better TB control programs, and rates of TB went down again. By the late 1990s, the number of new U.S. illnesses was the lowest ever and was dropping each year.

- Worldwide, TB causes more deaths than any other infectious disease. In 2004, it was estimated to cause about 9 million new cases of illness and 1.7 million deaths, on top of nearly 15 million existing cases of illness.

- It is estimated that one-third of the world's people have primary (inactive) TB infection. That means more than 2 billion people are infected.

- Worldwide, most tuberculosis cases occur in Asia. About 4.5 million of the 9 million new cases each year occur in India, China, Bangladesh, Pakistan, Indonesia, and the Philippines. But the rates—the number of cases that occur for each 100,000 people—tend to be highest in some African countries. That is because HIV is particularly common there and HIV-infected people are more likely to get sick with TB. Many cases of tuberculosis also occur in the Middle East and South America. In the developing world, TB is most common among young men and women of reproductive age.

- Worldwide as well, the spread of TB has been fueled by the rise of HIV, and it has not been brought under control. The World Health Organization has been trying to get countries to use the kind of TB control measures that worked in the United States in the 1990s. But the control measures are expensive and difficult to do on the large scale that is needed, and the countries that need them most are not as wealthy as the United States.

- The measures advocated by the World Health Organization are called DOTS, for "directly observed treatment—short course." Under this system, health workers watch patients take their medicines each day for six months to a year, either at a clinic or on visits to the patient's home. This ensures that the patients complete their treatment, rather than stopping whenever they feel better. That cuts down on the spread of the illness and on the emergence of drug-resistant strains.

HIV and TB: A Lethal Combination

Because HIV/AIDS weakens the immune system, patients who have HIV/AIDS are at high risk for contracting TB. Approximately 13 million people around the globe are infected with both HIV and TB. TB is more likely to spread to other areas of the body in people with HIV, and multidrug-resistant (MDR) TB is much more dangerous in these patients. TB infection in patients who have HIV/AIDS can be cured if found and treated early.

* **lymph nodes** (LIMF) are small, bean-shaped masses of tissue containing immune system cells that fight harmful microorganisms. Lymph nodes may swell during infections.

* **peritoneum** is the membrane that lines the abdominal cavity.

* **sputum** (SPYOO-tum) is a substance that contains mucus and other matter coughed out from the lungs, bronchi, and trachea.

the same air may become infected with the bacteria, which can lodge in the lungs and begin to grow. From there, the bacteria can move through the blood and settle in almost any other part of the body, including the urinary tract, brain, kidneys, lymph nodes*, bones, joints, peritoneum*, and heart.

Spending lots of time in close quarters with a person who has untreated active TB is the most common way to becoming infected. Even with close contact, however, only one-third of people who are exposed to TB infection become infected. Within a few weeks of the start of effective treatment, patients are no longer contagious. TB in parts of the body other than the lungs and throat usually is not contagious. People who have primary tuberculosis cannot spread it to others.

Who Gets Tuberculosis?

Tuberculosis can strike anyone, but some people are more likely to get it than others:

- Babies and young children who have weak immune systems
- People with medical problems, such as HIV (the virus that causes AIDS) infection, alcohol or drug abuse, poor nutrition, diabetes, certain types of cancer, or severe kidney diseases that weaken their immune systems
- People who take certain medications, such as corticosteroid drugs that weaken their immune systems
- People who have had organ transplants and take drugs to suppress their immune systems
- People who do not get good medical care due to poverty or homelessness.

What Are the Symptoms of Tuberculosis?

Primary tuberculosis does not cause any symptoms. The symptoms of secondary (active) tuberculosis depend on where in the body the tuberculosis bacteria are growing.

Tuberculosis of the lungs may cause a cough that does not go away, pain in the chest, and coughing up blood or sputum*. Other common symptoms include feeling tired all the time, weight loss, lack of appetite, fever, chills, and sweating at night. People with secondary TB may feel sick quickly or develop symptoms gradually over weeks or months, and they may be highly contagious until treated. However, some people with active TB feel well and only cough occasionally.

Tuberculosis bacteria typically infect the lungs, but they can infect almost any part of the body:

- Urinary tract. Symptoms may include repeated urinary tract infections, repeated fevers, or pus or blood in the urine for which there is no other explanation.

TUBERCULOSIS TIMELINE

Archeologists have found evidence of tuberculosis in skeletons from Peru that are 1,300 years old and in Egyptian skeletons dating back 3,400 years. But TB apparently did not emerge as a major killer until the 1600s in Europe.

By the 1800s the Industrial Revolution had created ideal conditions for TB to spread—overworked, underfed people crowded together in tenements and factories with poor ventilation. TB became the leading killer in many European and U.S. cities. It even took on an aura of romance, as it sapped the life from many literary figures, both real (British poet John Keats, 1795–1821) and fictional (Mimi, the heroine of the opera *La Boheme*).

It was unclear whether TB was inherited or infectious until the 1880s, when the German physician Robert Koch (1843–1910) identified the TB bacterium. Treatment consisted of rest, rich food, and fresh air, often provided in special TB hospitals called sanatoriums that were built in mountain areas.

Streptomycin, an antibiotic that kills TB bacteria, was introduced in the 1940s. Isoniazid, another effective antibiotic, came into use in the 1950s. These drugs dramatically lowered the number of TB cases over the next few decades. Both remained in use in the early 2000s, along with other drugs. As drug-resistant strains of TB continued to emerge, research toward better treatment continued.

- Brain. Tuberculosis bacteria can infect the membranes surrounding the brain and spinal cord (the meninges), especially in babies and young children. Symptoms of tuberculosis meningitis may include headaches, seizures, or abnormal behavior.

- Lymph nodes. Tuberculosis bacteria can infect the small organs commonly known as lymph nodes. Symptoms may include inflammation and swelling of the nodes anywhere in the body, including in the neck.

- Bones and joints. Tuberculosis bacteria can infect the skeleton, especially in the elderly. Symptoms may include fever; pain; and stiff, swollen joints. The lower spine and weight-bearing joints are most often affected.

- Peritoneum. Tuberculosis bacteria can infect the inner lining of the abdomen. Symptoms may include a fever and buildup of fluid inside the abdomen, which often goes along with a buildup of fluid around the lungs.

- Heart. Tuberculosis bacteria can infect the sac enclosing the heart. Although this is extremely rare, the death rate is high when it does occur. Symptoms may include shortness of breath, chest pain, and fever.

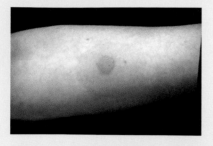

▲

The red spot on the arm indicates a positive skin test for TB.
©PHOTOTAKE Inc./Alamy.

Germs that Resist Arrest

Multi-drug resistant (MDR) tuberculosis, caused by bacteria that cannot be killed by regular tuberculosis drugs, is very dangerous. Even with treatment, 40 to 60 percent of people with MDR tuberculosis die. People with MDR tuberculosis must take special medications that do not work as well as the usual tuberculosis drugs and that have more side effects.

MDR tuberculosis occurs when TB patients stop taking their prescribed medications or do not take them as directed. Patients often stop taking the drugs when they begin to feel better. However, TB bacteria can survive inside the body for several months during treatment and are ready to spring back into activity when the medication disappears.

One way to fight this problem is through directly observed therapy (DOT). In DOT, patients must take their medications regularly in the presence of a health professional. Home visits by health professionals to supervise the taking of medications or free transportation and meals often are provided to encourage patients to take part in this type of program.

MDR tuberculosis is common in some parts of the world, including Southeast Asia, Latin America, Haiti, and the Philippines.

How Is Tuberculosis Diagnosed?

A skin test known as the Mantoux or PPD (purified protein derivative) test is used to diagnose primary tuberculosis. For this test, a small amount of testing fluid is injected with a fine needle just beneath the skin on the lower part of the arm. Two to three days later, a healthcare professional checks the arm to see if a bump has formed at the site of the injection. If a bump wider than a certain size is present (for most people, 10 to 15 millimeters of a half inch), the patient most likely has been infected by TB bacteria; this is known as a positive test. Doctors may order more tests, such as a chest x-ray and a test of sputum that is coughed up, to see if secondary (active) tuberculosis is present.

How Is Tuberculosis Treated?

Primary tuberculosis People with primary tuberculosis who are in high-risk groups for developing active TB may be given medication to help ward off the illness. This treatment is called preventive therapy. People under age 35 with primary tuberculosis who are not in high-risk groups also may benefit from preventive therapy. The goal is to kill the bacteria that are not doing any harm now but that could cause active TB in the future. The medication usually given for this purpose is called isoniazid (INH). To kill these bacteria, however, INH must be taken every day for 6 to 12 months.

Secondary (active) tuberculosis Secondary (active) tuberculosis can often be cured with medication. People with secondary TB usually take several different drugs because doing so is more effective at killing all the bacteria and preventing the formation of resistant bacteria that cannot be killed by drugs.

Although they usually feel better after a few weeks of treatment, people with active TB must continue to take their medication correctly for the full length of the treatment or they can become sick again. Because people with tuberculosis of the lungs or throat can spread the infection to others, they need to stay home from school or work until they are no longer infectious to others, which usually takes several weeks.

People with tuberculosis who are sick enough to go to the hospital may be put in a special room with an air vent system that keeps the bacteria from spreading. Doctors, nurses, and others who work in such rooms must wear special facemasks to protect themselves from breathing the bacteria.

How Can the Spread of Infection Be Stopped?

The Centers for Disease Control and Prevention recommends that certain people at risk for getting tuberculosis get the skin test yearly so that treatment can begin immediately if they are found to have TB. These include:

- People who have spent a lot of time with other people who are infected with TB
- People who think they may have caught the disease for other reasons

- People who have HIV infection or other medical problems that put them at high risk for getting tuberculosis
- People who inject street drugs
- People who come to the United States from countries where tuberculosis is more common (most countries in Latin America and the Caribbean, Africa, and all of Asia except for Japan)
- People who live in the United States in environments in which tuberculosis is common (homeless shelters, migrant farm camps, prisons, and some nursing homes)

People who have tuberculosis can keep from spreading the infection by taking all their medication exactly as prescribed; visiting their doctors regularly; staying away from people until they are no longer infectious to others; covering their mouths with a tissue when they cough, sneeze, or laugh; and airing out the room often.

Tuberculosis bacteria can only be spread through the air. Other people cannot be infected by shaking hands, sitting on toilet seats, or sharing dishes or personal items with people who have tuberculosis. If close contact with someone who has TB is necessary, a special type of facemask (called a respirator) should be worn.

Bacillus Calmette-Guerin (BCG) is a vaccine* that can help protect people against tuberculosis infection. It does not always work and may cause a positive reaction to the tuberculosis skin test, making it harder to tell if people become infected despite the vaccine. BCG is not widely used in the United States, but it often is given to babies and young children in countries where tuberculosis is common.

▶ *See also* **AIDS and HIV Infection • Bacterial Infections • Pneumonia**

Resources

Books and Articles

Yancey, Diane. *Tuberculosis.* Minneapolis: Twenty-First Century Books, 2008.

OrganizationsS

American Lung Association. 1301 Pennsylvania Ave. NW, Suite 800, Washington, DC, 20004. Toll free: 800-LUNG-USA. Web site: http://www.lungusa.org.

Centers for Disease Control and Prevention, National Center for HIV/AIDS, Viral Hepatitis, STD, and TB Prevention. 1600 Clifton Road, Atlanta, GA, 30333. Toll free: 800-311-3435. Web site: http://www.cdc.gov/tb/default.htm.

National Institute of Allergy and Infectious Diseases. Office of Communications and Public Liaison, 6610 Rockledge Drive, MSC

* **vaccine** (vak-SEEN) is a preparation of killed or weakened germs, or a part of a germ or product it produces, given to prevent or lessen the severity of the disease that can result if a person is exposed to the germ itself. Use of vaccines for this purpose is called immunization.

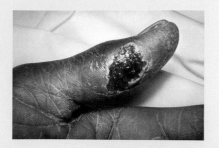

Hand with tularemia ulcer. *Photo Researchers, Inc.*

* **mucous membranes** are the thin layers of tissue found inside the nose, ears, cervix (SER-viks) and uterus, stomach, colon and rectum, on the vocal cords, and in other parts of the body.

6612, Bethesda, MD, 20892-66123. Toll free: 866-284-4107. Web site: http://www3.niaid.nih.gov.

World Health Organization. Avenue Appia 20, CH - 1211 Geneva 27, Switzerland. Telephone: +41 22 791 2111. Web site: http://www. who.int/en.

Tularemia

Tularemia (too-lah-REE-me-uh), sometimes called rabbit fever, is an infection caused by bacteria that can spread from wild animals to humans.

Do Rabbits Cause Rabbit Fever?

The bacterium *Francisella tularensis* (fran-sih-SEL-uh too-lah-REN-sis) causes tularemia. Most cases of tularemia in people in the United States result from contact with infected rabbits and deer, although the bacterium can also live in other small mammals and birds and in the soil.

Tularemia bacteria enter the body through the mucous membranes*, the skin, the lungs, or the digestive system. Seven different forms of the disease exist:

- **Ulceroglandular tularemia** comes from handling an infected animal or from the bite of an infected tick, fly, or mosquito. An ulcer (an open sore) forms on the skin. Some symptoms include headache, fever, chills, and lack of energy.

- **Glandular tularemia** causes symptoms similar to those of the ulceroglandular form but an ulcer does not form. The bacteria may enter the body through small cuts in the skin. Most cases of rabbit fever in the United States are glandular or ulceroglandular tularemia.

- **Oculoglandular tularemia** comes from touching the eye with infected fingers. The eye becomes red and painful and has a discharge.

- **Oropharyngeal tularemia** arises from eating the undercooked meat of an infected animal or from drinking water contaminated by the bacterium. It causes digestive system symptoms, such as vomiting or diarrhea.

- **Pneumonic tularemia** results from inhaling spores (an inactive form of the germ enclosed in a protective shell) in dust from a contaminated area into the lungs. Other types of tularemia may also spread to the lungs.

- **Typhoidal tularemia** affects many organs of the body. This rare form of the disease occurs without any previous signs of infection in any specific part of the body.

- **Septic tularemia** is a severe form of the disease that affects the whole body. Someone with this form may go into shock* and experience serious complications.

How Do People Contract Rabbit Fever?

People cannot catch tularemia from one another. Most cases in the United States occur when someone gets a bite from a tick, fly, or mosquito that has previously bitten an infected rabbit or deer. If a person is in contact with infected animals, the bacterium may be able to enter that person's body through small cuts on the skin. Hunters contract tularemia from handling carcasses or from eating undercooked, contaminated meat. In rare cases, people may breathe in bacterial spores that have been released into the air from the soil where the bacteria live. Drinking contaminated water is another rare but possible way to contract the disease.

Is Tularemia Common?

Tularemia occurs in the United States, Europe, and Asia, mainly in rural areas. Tularemia is highly infectious, but fewer than 200 cases in the United States are reported each year (mostly from Missouri, Arkansas, and Oklahoma). Some additional cases may occur but remain unrecognized or unreported.

Tularemia affects people of every age, sex, and race. In spring and summer months, it occurs most often in children who become infected when playing outside. In fall and winter, hunters are more likely to contract the infection.

What Are the Symptoms of Tularemia?

Symptoms of tularemia depend on the form of the disease. Most infected people have a red spot at the site of the insect bite or the cut where the bacterium entered the body. This spot may become an ulcer.

Other signs and symptoms appear within one to 14 days (most frequently in two to five days) and may come on suddenly. They can include extreme tiredness, muscle aches, fever, headache, sweating, chills, and weight loss. Lymph nodes* in the groin and armpits may become swollen.

People who contract tularemia from inhaled bacteria usually have pneumonia*-like symptoms, such as a dry cough, shortness of breath, or discomfort in the chest area. This form can progress to shock and respiratory failure*.

People who drink contaminated water or eat contaminated meat may experience nausea (NAW-zee-uh), vomiting, pain in the abdomen, diarrhea, sore throat, and sometimes gastrointestinal* bleeding.

Tularemia—the Next Anthrax?

As few as 10 spores of the *Francisella tularensis* bacterium are enough to infect someone and cause tularemia. The bacterium is hard to destroy and the spores are easily released into the air, which also makes it a potent weapon. The United States stockpiled the bacteria as a biological weapon during the 1960s but destroyed its stores in the 1970s at the order of the president. Russia, too, stockpiled and produced the bacteria through the mid-1990s. Experts on biological weapons have warned that other groups could possibly use the bacteria as a weapon, noting that an aerosol release of the bacteria in a city of five million would result in severe symptoms to 250,000 people.

No tularemia vaccine was available in the United States as of 2009, but other countermeasures were. In 2001 a group of 25 health experts, government agency representatives, and others issued a report with recommendations about how to react to an intentional release of the bacteria. If the release was discovered before people began to fall ill, the recommendations called for the swift and widespread use of the antibiotics doxycycline or ciprofloxacin to dampen the effects of the bacteria. If people were already developing symptoms, the recommendations emphasized the use of the antibiotics streptomycin and gentamicin.

* **shock** is a serious condition in which blood pressure is very low and not enough blood flows to the body's organs and tissues. Untreated, shock may result in death.

Tularemia

* **lymph nodes** (LIMF) are small, bean-shaped masses of tissue containing immune system cells that fight harmful microorganisms. Lymph nodes may swell during infections.

* **pneumonia** (nu-MO-nyah) is inflammation of the lungs.

* **respiratory failure** is a condition in which breathing and oxygen delivery to the body are dangerously altered. This may result from infection, nerve or muscle damage, poisoning, or other causes.

* **gastrointestinal** (gas-tro-in-TES-tih-nuhl) means having to do with the organs of the digestive system, the system that processes food. It includes the mouth, esophagus, stomach, intestines, colon, and rectum and other organs involved in digestion, including the liver and pancreas.

* **antibodies** (AN-tih-bah-deez) are protein molecules produced by the body's immune system to help fight specific infections caused by microorganisms, such as bacteria and viruses.

* **immunity** (ih-MYOON-uh-tee) is the condition of being protected against an infectious disease. Immunity often develops after a germ has entered the body. One type of immunity occurs when the body makes special protein molecules called antibodies to fight the disease-causing germ. The next time that germ enters the body, the antibodies quickly attack it, usually preventing the germ from causing disease.

* **meningitis** (meh-nin-JY-tis) is an inflammation of the meninges, the membranes that surround the brain and the spinal cord. Meningitis is most often caused by infection with a virus or a bacterium.

How Is Tularemia Diagnosed?

Doctors use blood tests to check for tularemia. Some tests look for antibodies* to the *Francisella tularensis* bacterium. Doctors also may look for evidence of the bacterium in the blood, fluid from the nose and mouth, and lymph nodes. If the person has symptoms of pneumonia, the doctor will also order a chest x-ray.

How Is Tularemia Treated?

Tularemia responds well to antibiotics, and most people can receive treatment at home. Because tularemia is not contagious, people who have it do not have to be isolated.

In more severe cases, when the disease attacks the lungs or other organs, people may require hospitalization and closer monitoring.

Most people who receive treatment recover from tularemia, but the septic and pneumonic forms of the disease can be life-threatening. Symptoms of tularemia can last for several weeks. Most people do not experience any lasting damage from the disease and may develop some degree of immunity* to it.

Complications of tularemia can include pneumonia, meningitis*, osteomyelitis*, kidney problems, lung abscesses*, pericarditis (inflammation of the sac surrounding the heart), shock, and, rarely, death. Approximately 1.4 percent of all cases in the United States are fatal.

Can Tularemia Be Prevented?

In the past, laboratory workers at risk for contracting tularemia due to frequent contact with laboratory animals received vaccinations against the disease. That vaccine was unavailable for public use in the United States as of 2009. The Food and Drug Administration was, however, continuing its review of a potential vaccine for use by the general public.

The best way to avoid contracting tularemia is to prevent tick and insect bites by using repellent and by wearing light-colored clothing that covers the arms and legs. Another prevention measure is to avoid contact with certain wild animals, such as rabbits. Experts recommend that hunters wear rubber gloves when handling animals and that they cook all meat thoroughly. In addition, people should avoid swimming in or drinking water that might be contaminated.

▶ *See also* **Bioterrorism • Meningitis • Osteomyelitis • Pneumonia • Tick-borne Illnesses • Zoonoses**

Resources

Books and Articles

Friend, Milton. *Tularemia.* Reston, VA: Department of the Interior, Geological Survey, 2006.

Siderovski, Susan Hutton. *Tularemia.* Philadelphia, PA: Chelsea House, 2006.

Organizations

Centers for Disease Control and Prevention. 1600 Clifton Road, Atlanta, GA, 30333. Toll free: 800-311-3435. Web site: http://www.bt.cdc.gov/agent/tularemia.

National Institute of Allergy and Infectious Diseases. Office of Communications and Public Liaison, 6610 Rockledge Drive, MSC 6612, Bethesda, MD, 20892-6612. Toll free: 866-284-4107. Web site: http://www.niaid.nih.gov/factsheets/tularemia.htm.

Tumor

A tumor (TOO-mor) is an abnormal growth of new tissue that can occur in any of the body's organs. Many people automatically associate tumors with the disease called cancer*, but cancer is not always present when someone has a tumor.

What Is a Tumor?

The human body is made up of many types of cells that are constantly dividing to produce new, younger cells that can "take over" for aging or damaged cells. Through this process, the body heals its injuries and keeps tissues healthy. Sometimes, this process gets out of control, and new cells continue to be produced even when they are not needed, forming a clump of extra tissue, a tumor.

There are two types of tumors:

- malignant (ma-LIG-nant), or cancerous, tumors are made up of abnormally shaped cells that grow quickly, invade nearby healthy tissues, and often make their way into the bloodstream. When these cells travel to other parts of the body, they form additional tumors in other locations.
- Benign (be-NINE) tumors are not cancerous. They grow slowly and are self-contained; that is, they do not invade and destroy the tissue around them, nor do they spread to other parts of the body. Their cells are usually normally shaped.

Who Gets Tumors?

People of all ages can develop tumors, but generally they are more common as people grow older. Researchers believe that malignant tumors result from a combination of causes, the most important being genetic

* **osteomyelitis** (ah-stee-o-my-uh-LYE-tis) is a bone infection that is usually caused by bacteria. It can involve any bone in the body, but it most commonly affects the long bones in the arms and legs.

* **abscesses** (AB-seh-sez) are localized or walled off accumulations of pus caused by infection that can occur anywhere within the body.

* **cancer** is a condition characterized by abnormal overgrowth of certain cells, which may be fatal.

* **colon** (KO-lin), also called the large intestine, is a muscular tube through which food passes as it is digested, just before it moves into the rectum and out of the body through the anus.

* **ultrasound** also called a sonogram, is a diagnostic test in which sound waves passing through the body create images on a computer screen.

* **CT scans** or CAT scans are the shortened name for computerized axial tomography (to-MOG-ra-fee), which uses computers to view structures inside the body.

* **MRI** which is short for magnetic resonance imaging, produces computerized images of internal body tissues based on the magnetic properties of atoms within the body.

and environmental. People may inherit a tendency to develop certain kinds of tumors from their parents. Also, repeated exposure to harmful substances such as cigarette smoke, pollutants, and too much sunlight can damage cells and trigger the process of tumor formation.

When a tumor first starts to develop, it is so small that it does not cause symptoms. As it grows, it usually causes symptoms that vary according to its location. For instance, a tumor in the lung may cause a feeling of irritation or a nagging cough. People with brain tumors may experience headaches, dizziness, blurry vision, or loss of coordination. A person with a tumor in the colon* may notice that going to the bathroom is painful or produces blood.

How Are Tumors Diagnosed and Treated?

A doctor can usually diagnose a tumor with one of many tests that create images of the inside of the body, such as x-rays, ultrasound*, CT scans*, or MRIs*. The next step is to figure out whether the tumor is benign or malignant through a process called biopsy (BY-op-see). Surgeons remove part or all of the tumor and examine a sample under the microscope. The appearance of the cells indicates whether a tumor is cancerous.

Even though a benign tumor is not harmful, it may have to be removed if it causes pain, pressure, or other symptoms. In many cases of a malignancy, the tumor and any affected surrounding tissue will be removed. Sometimes, radiation therapy (directed high-energy x-rays) or chemotherapy (cancer-fighting drugs) may be used to shrink the tumor.

▶ *See also* **Cancer: Overview • Tobacco-Related Diseases**

Resources

Books and Articles

Dempsey, Sharon. *My Brain Tumour Adventures: The Story of a Little Boy Coping with a Brain Tumour.* London: Jessica Kingsley, 2003.

Organizations

National Cancer Institute Public Inquires Office. Public Inquiries Office, 6116 Executive Boulevard, Room 3036A, Bethesda, MD, 20892-8322. Toll free: 800-4-CANCER. Web site: http://www.cancer.gov.

National Library of Medicine. 8600 Rockville Pike, Bethesda, MD, 20894, Web site: http://www.nlm.nih.gov/medlineplus/benigntumors.html; http://www.nlm.nih.gov/medlineplus/cancer.html.

Turner's Syndrome

Turner's syndrome (also called Turner syndrome) is a genetic disorder caused by a missing or partially missing X chromosome. It affects only females and typically causes a variety of physical abnormalities. Girls and women with Turner's syndrome usually are short, their ovaries and breasts fail to develop normally, and they are almost always infertile.

What Is Turner's Syndrome?

Turner's syndrome is a genetic disorder that occurs when one of a girl's X chromosomes is partially or completely missing. Almost every cell in a person's body (except for eggs and sperm cells) has 23 pairs of chromosomes. One pair, the sex chromosomes, makes a person male or female: Boys have an X and a Y chromosome (XY), whereas girls have two X chromosomes (XX). The chromosomes contain all of the information the body needs to function and to develop properly. If part of a chromosome is missing, as in Turner's syndrome, the important information on that chromosome is also missing.

How a girl's body is affected physically by Turner's syndrome depends on how much of the chromosome is missing. Some girls have a mild form of the syndrome that is not detected until they are teenagers or adults. If untreated, nearly all girls with Turner's syndrome grow slowly and reach a short adult height, and their breasts do not enlarge, and they do not have menstrual periods as is normal for adolescent girls. Some may have additional problems, including the following:

- abnormalities in appearance
- hearing loss
- obesity
- heart disorders
- kidney disorders
- thyroid disorders

Most of the physical conditions are treatable, and with good consistent medical care, a person with Turner's syndrome can have a fully productive life and normal life span. Most people with Turner's syndrome have normal intelligence, but some may have specific learning problems, especially with math.

It is believed that approximately 98 percent of pregnancies in which the mother is carrying a fetus with the genetic defect that would become Turner's syndrome will spontaneously end in miscarriage*.

What Causes Turner's Syndrome?

About 1 in 2,500 female babies is born with Turner's syndrome, and doctors do not know why. Researchers have tried to find a link between Turner's syndrome and environment, race, geography, and socioeconomic status, but as of 2009 these factors had not been proven to play a role.

* **miscarriage** (MIS-kare-ij) is the end of a pregnancy through the death of the embryo or fetus before birth.

Living with Turner's Syndrome: Carol's Life

Because of physical abnormalities and feeling "different," life might not be easy for a girl with Turner's syndrome. Carol was born with swollen hands and feet, extra skin at the back of her neck (a webbed neck), oddly shaped ears, and arms that tilted outward from the elbows. Based on her appearance, her doctor suspected that she had Turner's syndrome. A test in which Carol's chromosomes were studied confirmed that she was missing one of her X chromosomes.

Carol was teased about her appearance in elementary school, but she was most miserable during her teenage years. She was the shortest person in her class. When other girls started developing breasts and getting their period, Carol still looked and felt like a little girl. After Carol's doctor prescribed the hormone estrogen to promote sexual development, she finally got her period.

How Do Doctors Treat Turner's Syndrome?

Many of the problems associated with Turner's syndrome, such as the failure of the ovaries to develop normally, cannot be prevented, but there are a number of medical treatments that can be performed to improve an affected person's quality of life:

- Plastic surgery for the neck, face, or ears can improve appearance and self-esteem, if necessary.
- Growth rate and adult height may be increased by treatment with injections of growth hormone.
- Taking the female hormone estrogen promotes sexual development in girls with Turner's syndrome.
- Support groups can help girls with Turner's syndrome develop into confident, successful, and productive adults.
- In some cases, women with Turner's syndrome may be able to become pregnant if a fertilized donor egg is inserted into their uterus.

▶ *See also* **Genetic Diseases • Growth and Growth Disorders • Menstruation and Menstrual Disorders**

Resources

Books and Articles

Gizel, Kayli. *All about Me: Growing Up with Turner Syndrome and Nonverbal Learning Disabilities.* Wallingford, VT: Maple Leaf Center, 2004.

Organizations

Eunice Kennedy Shriver National Institute of Child Health and Human Development. Turner Unit, 10 Center Drive, CRC 1-3330, Bethesda, MD, 20892-1103. Toll free: 800-370-2943. Web site: http://turners.nichd.nih.gov/clinical.html#Anchor.

Turner Syndrome Society of the United States. 10960 Millridge North Drive, No. 214A, Houston, TX 77070. Toll free: 800-365-9944. Web site: http://www.turnersyndrome.org/index.php.

Twins *See Conjoined Twins.*

Typhoid Fever

Typhoid fever is a bacterial infection that is common in many parts of the world. It is spread by contaminated water and food and primarily affects the digestive system.

What Is Typhoid?

In many developing countries, typhoid fever is a major problem. An estimated 16 million are infected and more than 500,000 die each year worldwide. The disease is especially common in parts of Asia, Africa, and South America where pure water is not readily available and sewage treatment is inadequate. In many countries, children are the most likely to get typhoid.

Typhoid used to be a serious problem in the United States as well. Early in the twentieth century, before clean water supplies and sewage systems to dispose of human waste were widely available, about 35,000 people contracted typhoid fever each year. Technological advancements in sewage and water treatment made typhoid fever rare in industrialized countries. Only about 400 cases are reported each year in the United States. In most of these cases, the individuals had acquired the disease while traveling abroad.

What Causes Typhoid Fever?

Typhoid fever is caused by a bacterium called *Salmonella typhi.* It is related to the salmonella bacteria that cause food poisoning, but they are not exactly the same.

Salmonella typhi bacteria are present in the solid wastes (stool) of infected people, including some "healthy carriers" who have no symptoms of illness. The bacteria can spread if human waste gets into water that is used for drinking, irrigating crops, or washing food. Typhoid is also occasionally transmitted through an infected person who is working in food preparation. Once swallowed, the bacteria move from the digestive tract into the bloodstream and then to the liver, spleen, gall bladder, and lymph nodes.

The United States and the World

About 21.5 million cases of typhoid fever occur each year worldwide, and more than 200,000 people die from this disease.

The disease is common in many underdeveloped nations, especially in parts of Asia and in South America, with unsanitary water and food preparation. The situation is made more difficult because the disease shows resistance to some of the traditional antibiotics used to treat those who are infected.

About 400 cases a year are reported in the United States, but about 70 percent of them involve people who have traveled internationally.

In 1998 and 1999, 13 people in Florida contracted typhoid fever when they drank shakes made with a frozen tropical fruit containing *Salmonelli typhi.*

Typhoid fever is suspected in the deaths of such famous people as Alexander the Great, Wilbur Wright of the Wright Brothers, and poet Gerard Manley Hopkins.

* **constipation** is the sluggish movement of the bowels, usually resulting in infrequent, hard stools.

TYPHOID MARY

Some people, called carriers, can be infected with *Salmonella typhi* but not develop typhoid fever. If they prepare food for others, however, they may contaminate the food they handle and pass the bacteria on to other people who eat it and then may get sick.

The most famous typhoid carrier was Mary Mallon (1869–1938), also known as Typhoid Mary, who worked as a cook in homes in New York and New Jersey in the early 1900s. Fifty-one cases of typhoid fever resulting in three deaths were traced to her. Mallon never was sick herself, however, and she never accepted that she had infected anyone else.

Against her will, the authorities confined Mallon to a hospital on North Brother Island in New York's East River. Three years later, in 1910, they released her on condition that she never work as a cook again. But in 1915 typhoid struck a maternity hospital in Manhattan, and it turned out that Mallon had cooked there. She spent the rest of her life, 23 years, as a captive on North Brother Island.

What Happens When People Have Typhoid Fever?

Symptoms The symptoms of typhoid fever come on gradually. At first, people may get a headache, stomachache, and constipation*. The people develop a fever and lose their appetite. In some cases, they may get rose spots, a rash mostly on the chest and abdomen. As symptoms worsen, their fever may rise as high as 103 to 104 degrees Fahrenheit. People often develop bloody diarrhea, become dehydrated (lose fluids faster than they are replaced), and start acting confused or disoriented. In severe cases, people may go into a coma, a state of deep unconsciousness, and die.

Diagnosis and Treatment A blood or urine test usually can detect the presence of the bacterium that causes typhoid fever. Antibiotic drugs that fight the bacterial infection can make the illness shorter and milder and prevent complications. Fluids may be given as well to counter the effects of diarrhea. Severe infections can lead to a perforation (hole) in the intestine that requires surgery to repair.

How Is Typhoid Fever Prevented?

Clean water supplies and effective waste disposal systems are the best ways of preventing typhoid, but these are lacking in many countries. A vaccine is available in the early 2000s that is about 70-percent effective for several years.

Travelers to countries where typhoid fever is common should drink only boiled or bottled water. They should eat only food that has been properly cooked or fruit that they peel themselves and that has not been washed with tap water. The Centers for Disease Control and

Prevention sums up advice for travelers this way: "Boil it, cook it, peel it, or forget it."

▶ *See also* **Bacterial Infections • Fever • Gastroenteritis • Salmonellosis**

Resources

Books and Articles

Emmeluth, Donald. *Typhoid Fever.* Philadelphia, PA: Chelsea House, 2004.

Organizations

Centers for Disease Control and Prevention. 1600 Clifton Road, Atlanta, GA, 30333. Toll free: 800-311-3435. Web site: http://www.cdc.gov/ncidod/dbmd/diseaseinfo/typhoidfever_g.htm.

World Health Organization. Avenue Appia 20, CH - 1211 Geneva 27, Switzerland. Telephone: +41 22 791 2111. Web site: http://www.who.int/en.

Typhus

Typhus (TI-fus) is the name for a group of infections caused by bacteria called rickettsiae that are spread by parasites such as lice that live on people or on other warm-blooded animals such as rats and mice.

War, Famine, and Typhus

Throughout history, war and famine have brought outbreaks of typhus, a group of infections spread by parasites that live on people or animals such as rats and mice. During World War II, typhus spread through Europe, North Africa, and the Pacific Islands, and it killed thousands of prisoners in German concentration camps. Epidemic typhus can still be a serious threat in parts of the world where a breakdown in society or a natural calamity such as an earthquake leads to unhealthy living conditions.

What Is Typhus?

Typhus is a group of infections caused by rickettsiae, a group of unusual bacteria. Rickettsiae are like other bacteria in that they can be killed by antibiotics. They are also like viruses, however, in that they must invade living cells in order to grow. There are three main types of typhus: epidemic, murine, and scrub.

■ Epidemic typhus, caused by *Rickettsia prowazekii,* is a severe form of the disease spread by human body lice. In the United States,

---

TYPHUS EPIDEMICS

It is likely that typhus existed in ancient times, although the first specific historical description of typhus comes from the 11th century, when an outbreak took place in a monastery in Sicily. Typhus reached epidemic proportions in 1489, during a siege in Granada. Typhus then spread throughout Europe.

Typhus also was present in the Americas, although there is some controversy as to whether Spanish explorers brought the disease in the 16th century or whether the disease already was present in Aztec and other pre-Columbian societies.

In the early 19th century, typhus increased dramatically in Europe. In the 20th century, typhus spread through Europe, North Africa, and the Pacific Islands. During World War II, typhus killed thousands of prisoners in German concentration camps.

---

this type of typhus occasionally is also spread by lice and fleas on flying squirrels. Sometimes the symptoms of typhus become active again years after the individual suffered the original attack; this reoccurrence is called Brill's disease. Brill's disease is milder than epidemic typhus.

- Murine typhus, caused by *Rickettsia typhi,* is a milder form of the disease and is spread by fleas on rats, mice, and other rodents.

- Scrub typhus, caused by *Rickettsia tsutsugamushi,* is a form of the disease found in the Asian-Pacific area bounded by Japan, Australia, and the Indian subcontinent. It is spread by mites on rats, field mice, and other rodents.

Who Gets Typhus?

Both epidemic and murine typhus are found around the world. However, epidemic typhus is most common in situations where poor hygiene and crowded living conditions exist. Epidemic typhus is rare in the United States. Murine typhus is most common in rat-infested areas. It is the only type of typhus that occurs regularly in the United States, but fewer than 100 cases a year are reported, mainly in Texas and California.

What Happens When People Have Typhus?

Symptoms   The symptoms of typhus include fever, headache, chills, and general aches that are followed by a rash. The rash spreads to most of the body but usually does not affect the face, palms of the hands, or soles of the feet. In murine typhus, the symptoms are similar but milder. In epidemic and scrub typhus, the fever may rise as high as 104 to 105 degrees Fahrenheit and stay high for about two weeks. The headache is intense.

In severe cases of typhus, blood pressure may drop dangerously. Severe illness also may lead to confusion, seizures, coma*, or even death. The disease's name comes from the Greek word "typhos," meaning smoke, a cloud, or a stupor arising from a fever.

Diagnosis and Treatment   Blood tests are used to show if people are infected with typhus rickettsiae. People with typhus who are treated with antibiotics generally recover. If treatment is begun early, they usually get better quickly. If treatment is delayed, however, the improvement usually is slower, and the fever lasts longer. If left untreated, typhus can damage organs, lead to coma, and even to death.

Prevention   Prevention of typhus is based on avoiding the unsanitary conditions in which it spreads. It is always wise to avoid contact with animals such as rats and mice that may carry disease. Travelers to areas where typhus is common should be especially cautious. To prevent the spread of typhus, body lice must be destroyed by removing them from people with the disease and by boiling or steaming the clothes of infected individuals.

▶ *See also* **Bacterial Infections • Lice • Rickettsial Infections • Rocky Mountain Spotted Fever**

Resources

Books and Articles

Zinsser, Hans. *Rats, Lice and History: A Study in Biography.* New Brunswick, NJ: Aldine Transaction, 2007.

Organizations

Centers for Disease Control and Prevention. 1600 Clifton Road, Atlanta, GA, 30333. Toll free: 800-311-3435. Web site: http://wwwn.cdc.gov/travel/yellowBookCh4-Rickettsial.aspx.

* **coma** (KO-ma) is an unconscious state, like a very deep sleep. A person in a coma cannot be awakened, and cannot move, see, speak, or hear.

U

Ulcer *See Bedsores (Pressure Sores); Canker Sores (Aphthous Ulcers); Helicobactor Pylori Infection.*

Ulcerative Colitis *See Inflammatory Bowel Disease.*

Urethritis, Nonspecific *See Nonspecific Urethritis.*

Urinary Tract Infections

A urinary (YOOR-ih-nair-e) tract infection, or UTI, is an infection that occurs in any part of the urinary tract. The urinary tract is made up of the urethra*, bladder*, ureters*, and kidneys*.

What Are Urinary Tract Infections?

A UTI usually is caused by bacteria that under normal circumstances should never be present in the urine. The bacterium most often responsible for UTIs is *Escherichia coli* (eh-sher-IH-she-ah KOH-lye). Many kinds of *E. coli* bacteria normally are found in human intestines*, but sometimes they are able to make their way into the urethra. When this happens, the bacteria can spread up into other parts of the urinary tract and cause an infection. Other types of bacteria from the intestines and some viruses also can produce infections in the urinary tract. The bacteria *Chlamydia* (kla-MIH-dee-uh) and *Mycoplasma* (my-ko-PLAZ-muh) can cause UTIs as well, but these types of infections usually stay in the urethra or reproductive system.

The type of UTI that a person contracts depends on which part of the urinary system is infected with bacteria. If bacteria grow in the urethra and cause inflammation, the condition is called urethritis (yoo-ree-THRY-tis). If the infection involves the bladder, the condition is called cystitis (sis-TIE-tis). If infection has spread to the kidneys, the condition is called pyelonephritis (py-uh-lo-nih-FRY-tis).

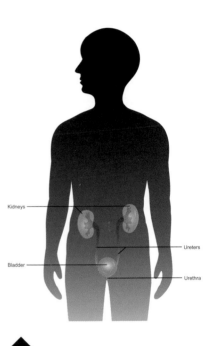

Kidneys

Ureters

Bladder

Urethra

▲

The organs of the urinary tract, any of which may become the site of infection. *Illustration by Frank Forney. Reproduced by permission of Gale, a part of Cengage Learning.*

* **urethra** (yoo-REE-thra) is the tube through which urine passes from the bladder to the outside of the body.

* **bladder** (BLAD-er) is the sac that stores urine produced by the kidneys prior to discharge from the body.

* **ureters** (YOOR-eh-ters) are tube-like structures that carry urine from the kidneys to the bladder.

* **kidneys** are the pair of organs that filter blood and remove waste products and excess water from the body in the form of urine.

* **intestines** are the muscular tubes that food passes through during digestion after it exits the stomach.

1745

* **anus** (A-nus) is the opening at the end of the digestive system, through which waste leaves the body.

* **kidney stone** is a hard structure that forms in the urinary tract. This structure is composed of crystallized chemicals that have separated from the urine. It can obstruct the flow of urine and cause tissue damage and pain as the body attempts to pass the stone through the urinary tract and out of the body.

* **prostate** (PRAH-state) is a male reproductive gland located near where the bladder joins the urethra. The prostate produces the fluid part of semen.

* **urinary catheters** are thin tubes used to drain urine from the body.

* **rectum** is the final portion of the large intestine, connecting the colon to the outside opening of the anus.

* **nitrates** (NYE-trayts) are chemical substances that can be produced by the breakdown of proteins by certain bacteria.

How Common Are Urinary Tract Infections?

Urinary tract infections are very common: Millions of people, especially women, have them every year. It is estimated that one in five women have at least one UTI in her lifetime, and some women have them repeatedly. UTIs are not uncommon in children; by the time children reach their eleventh birthday, 3 in 100 girls and 1 in 100 boys have had a UTI. Women and girls are at a higher risk of UTIs because the female urethra is much shorter than the male urethra. A shorter urethra means a shorter distance for bacteria to travel to enter the urinary tract. Also, because the opening of the urethra is much closer to the anus* in females, if a girl has a bowel movement and any bacteria are left on the skin nearby, it is easy for them to invade the urethra.

Males may have UTIs too, but these infections usually result from something in the urinary tract that blocks the normal flow of urine from the body, such as a kidney stone* or an enlarged prostate* in older men. In fact, anyone who has a problem with the structure of the urinary tract or the way it functions is more likely to have UTIs. Urinary catheters* can cause UTIs in either men or women because bacteria can enter the urinary tract more easily when a catheter is present. For this reason, UTIs can be a serious problem among patients in hospitals, where catheters are used frequently. UTIs are not contagious, which means that a person cannot catch a UTI from someone who has one. *Chlamydia* and *Mycoplasma* bacteria, however, can be transmitted through sexual intercourse.

What Are the Signs and Symptoms of a Urinary Tract Infection?

Some people may not have any symptoms of a UTI, but when the infection occurs, it usually brings with it a burning or stinging feeling during urination. People with UTIs may feel as if they have to urinate more frequently and more urgently than usual, but when a person does urinate, sometimes very little urine comes out. A UTI can make a person feel very tired or feverish; it also can produce a feeling of pressure in the lower belly in women and a sensation of pressure or fullness in the rectum* in men. The urine itself can be cloudy or have a bit of blood in it, and it may smell bad. If the bacteria spread to the kidneys and cause pyelonephritis, the person typically feels very ill, with fever, chills, nausea (NAW-zee-uh), vomiting, and sharp pain in the back or side.

How Do Doctors Diagnose Urinary Tract Infections?

If a doctor suspects that a patient has a UTI, he or she will ask about the person's symptoms to rule out other conditions. For example, an allergic reaction to a soap may cause irritation of the urethra that could lead to stinging when a person urinates, mimicking a UTI. The doctor may take a urine sample and then dip a special strip of paper into it, testing for infection-fighting white blood cells, protein, nitrates*, and blood, which can all be signs that a UTI might be present. The urine sample may be examined under a microscope for bacteria and types of white blood cells that might point to infection. To confirm the presence of a UTI, the urine sample may be cultured*. Any bacteria that grow are tested to see which antibiotics will kill them, which helps the doctor choose a medication for treating the UTI.

If an infant has a UTI or if an adult or child has repeated UTIs, the doctor may want to see if there are any problems in the urinary tract that may be causing or contributing to the infections. The doctor may order tests (such as special x-rays or ultrasound* images of the urinary tract) to take a better look at the shape and function of the kidneys, bladder, and ureters. If there are any problems, the patient may be referred to a urologist, a doctor who specializes in diagnosing and treating problems of the urinary tract. The urologist can examine the urethra and bladder with a cystoscope (SIS-tuh-skope), a special lighted tube with lenses that is inserted into the urethra.

What Is the Treatment for Urinary Tract Infections?

Once a doctor confirms that a bacterial UTI is present, antibiotics are prescribed, which usually clear up the infection. If the UTI involves the kidneys, the condition can be more serious. Patients with a kidney infection usually need to be treated in a hospital. Antibiotics and fluids may be given intravenously* until fever disappears and the patient begins to feel better. Even if they have no symptoms, all men typically are treated if they are found to have a UTI, and so are women who are pregnant and those who have diabetes* or abnormalities of the urinary tract. Treatment is necessary in these cases because there is a higher risk of pyelonephritis. Young women who have bacteria in the urine but who do not have symptoms of a UTI usually do not need treatment.

A person taking antibiotics for urethritis or cystitis usually feels much better soon after starting the medication. During the first few days of treatment, a heating pad can help soothe some of the lower belly pain that may come with UTIs. There are also medicines that ease discomfort during urination. It is important to remember that these medicines do not treat the infection; they treat only the symptoms of stinging and burning. Doctors advise people with UTIs to take all prescribed antibiotics, which usually are given for about a week. Taking all of the prescribed medication is necessary even if a patient begins to feel better right away. Stopping the antibiotics early can mean that the infection will come back, because all the bacteria may not have been killed. A person with pyelonephritis typically can expect a longer recovery time, possibly up to several weeks. It is very important that kidney infections be cured completely because they can lead to serious problems, such as permanent kidney damage, high blood pressure*, and even kidney failure later in life.

Can Urinary Tract Infections Be Prevented?

When it comes to preventing UTIs, practicing good hygiene is a major part of keeping bacteria from entering the urinary tract. It is wise for men and women to keep the genital*, urinary, and anal areas clean. It is recommended that women wipe from front to back, from the urinary tract opening to the anus, after going to the toilet.

* **cultured** (KUL-churd) means subjected to a test in which a sample of fluid or tissue from the body is placed in a dish containing material that supports the growth of certain organisms. Typically, within days the organisms will grow and can be identified.

* **ultrasound** also called a sonogram, is a diagnostic test in which sound waves passing through the body create images on a computer screen.

* **intravenously** (in-tra-VEE-nus-lee) means given or injected directly through a vein.

* **diabetes** (dye-uh-BEE-teez) is a condition in which the body's pancreas does not produce enough insulin or the body cannot use the insulin it makes effectively, resulting in increased levels of sugar in the blood. This can lead to increased urination, dehydration, weight loss, weakness, and a number of other symptoms and complications related to chemical imbalances within the body.

* **high blood pressure** also called hypertension, is a condition in which the pressure of the blood in the arteries is above normal.

* **genital** (JEH-nih-tul) refers to the external sexual organs.

* **malformation** (mal-for-MAY-shun) is an abnormal formation of a body part.

* **uterus** (YOO-teh-rus) is the muscular, pear-shaped internal organ in a woman where a baby develops until birth.

* **fetus** (FEE-tus) is the term for an unborn human after it is an embryo, from 9 weeks after fertilization until childbirth.

Doctors advise that people who want to keep UTIs at bay drink plenty of water, which helps flush out the urinary tract. Going to the bathroom when a person feels the need to go, instead of holding urine in, also can help deter UTIs. Finally, some foods or drinks (such as spicy foods or foods or drinks that contain caffeine) can irritate the bladder; it is a good idea for a person with a UTI to avoid them if they cause irritation. Some research suggests that drinking cranberry juice may have a beneficial effect in preventing UTIs.

Infants, children, and adults who have UTIs as a result of a malformation* or other problems in the urinary tract are at increased risk of contracting UTIs. Their doctors may prescribe small doses of antibiotics to take every day for several months or longer to help prevent infections and possible damage to the kidneys over time.

▶ *See also* **Pinworm Infestation • Schistosomiasis • Sexually Transmitted Diseases (STDs)**

Resources

Books and Articles

Ross, Jonathan H., and Robert Kay. "Pediatric Urinary Tract Infection and Reflux" in *American Family Physician* 59, no. 6 (March 15, 1999): 1472–1488. Also available at http://www.aafp.org/afp/990315ap/1472.html.

West, Krista. *Urinary Tract Infections.* New York: Rosen, 2007.

Organizations

Healthcommunities.com, Inc. 136 West Street, Northampton, MA, 01060. Toll free: 888-950-0808. Web site: http://www.urologychannel.com.

National Kidney and Urologic Diseases Information Clearinghouse. 3 Information Way, Bethesda, MD, 20892-3580. Toll free: 800-891-5390. Web site: http://kidney.niddk.nih.gov/Kudiseases/pubs/utiadult.

National Women's Health Information Center. 8270 Willow Oaks Corporate Drive, Fairfax, VA, 22031. Toll free: 800-994-9662. Web site: http://www.4woman.gov/faq/Easyread/uti-etr.htm.

Uterine Cancer

Uterine (YOO-te-rin) cancer occurs in the tissue of the uterus, part of the reproductive tract of women.

What Is the Uterus?

The uterus* is the hollow, pear-shaped organ in which a fetus* develops when a woman is pregnant.

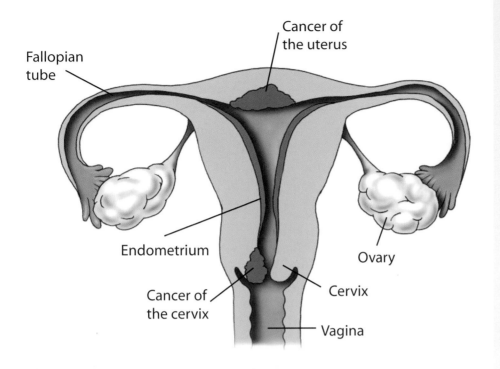

Fallopian tube

Cancer of the uterus

Endometrium

Ovary

Cancer of the cervix

Cervix

Vagina

Anatomy of the female reproductive system showing uterine and cervical cancers. *Illustration by Frank Forney. Reproduced by permission of Gale, a part of Cengage Learning.*

◀

What Is Uterine Cancer?

Uterine cancer is the fourth most common type of cancer among women. It occurs when cells in a woman's uterus undergo abnormal changes and start dividing without control or order, forming tumors*.

Uterine cancer* usually begins in the cells of the endometrium (en-do-MEE-tree-um), the thin layer of tissue that lines the inside of the main part of the uterus. That is why it is sometimes called endometrial (en-do-MEE-tree-al) cancer.

Uterine cancer is more common in women who have gone through menopause* (usually 50 years old or older), but it can occur earlier. It usually develops gradually, with some of the cells first undergoing precancerous changes. These cells are not yet cancerous, but they have undergone some abnormal changes that indicate that they could turn into cancer.

What Causes Uterine Cancer?

Although the cause of uterine cancer is not fully understood, cancer of the uterus occurs more frequently in those women who have an imbalance of reproductive hormones*, particularly estrogen (ES-tro-jen). Researchers as of 2009 were exploring the connection between estrogen and uterine cancer. There are several known risk factors associated with uterine cancer. These include:

- A high fat diet
- Obesity
- Hypertension (elevated blood pressure)
- Diabetes (increased sugar in the blood)

* **tumors** (TOO-morz) are abnormal growths of body tissue that have no known cause or physiologic purpose. Tumors may or may not be cancerous.

* **cancer** is a condition characterized by abnormal overgrowth of certain cells, which may be fatal.

* **menopause** (MEN-o-pawz) is the end of menstruation.

* **hormones** are chemical substances that are produced by various glands and sent into the bloodstream carrying messages that have certain effects on other parts of the body.

Important Statistics About Uterine Cancer

The American Cancer Society published important facts and statistics about Uterine Cancer in 2008. These include:

- Cases of uterine cancer decreased steadily between 1998 and 2008.

- The odds of a woman being diagnosed with uterine cancer in her lifetime are about 1 in 41.

- The average five-year survival rate of uterine cancer is 88 percent.

* **Pap smear** is a common diagnostic test used to look for cancerous cells in the tissue of the cervix.

* **lymph nodes** (LIMF) are small, bean-shaped masses of tissue containing immune system cells that fight harmful microorganisms. Lymph nodes may swell during infections.

* **biopsy** (BI-op-see) is a test in which a small sample of skin or other body tissue is removed and examined for signs of disease.

* **chemotherapy** (KEE-mo-THER-a-pee) is the treatment of cancer with powerful drugs that kill cancer cells.

* **fallopian tubes** (fa-LO-pee-an tubes) are the two slender tubes that connect the ovaries and the uterus in females. They carry the ova, or eggs, from the ovaries to the uterus.

* **ovaries** (O-vuh-reez) are the sexual glands from which ova, or eggs, are released in women.

* **menstrual** (MEN-stroo-al) refers to menstruation (men-stroo-AY-shun), the discharging through the vagina of blood and tissue from the uterus that recurs each month in women of reproductive age.

- Early onset of menstruation/late onset of menopause
- Never having been pregnant
- Certain hormone therapies

How Is Uterine Cancer Diagnosed and Treated?

Uterine cancer is usually curable if it is found early, but unfortunately, there are no reliable routine tests for this disease (although a Pap smear* sometimes can detect early forms). Typically, it is found only after a woman experiences symptoms, such as unusual bleeding or other discharge from the vagina, pain or pressure, or weight loss.

If it is not caught early, uterine cancer can grow through the wall of the uterus and metastasize (spread) to nearby organs. The cancer cells also can enter nearby lymph nodes* and be carried to other parts of the body. Uterine cancer affects about 40,000 women each year.

If doctors suspect uterine cancer based on a woman's symptoms and a physical examination, a biopsy* is necessary to confirm the diagnosis.

The most common treatments are surgery, radiation therapy, and chemotherapy*. Surgery involves hysterectomy (the removal of the uterus and nearby reproductive organs such as the fallopian tubes* and ovaries*) and the removal of the lymph nodes near the tumor.

After the treatment is finished, most women can lead normal lives. If their uterus was removed, however, they can no longer bear children. This often is not an issue for women in their 50s and 60s, but younger women in their 20s, 30s, and 40s may find it hard to adjust to this loss.

How Can Uterine Cancer Be Prevented?

Because the causes of uterine cancer are not fully understood, prevention is not understood either. Smoking should be avoided, and it is essential that women see their doctors yearly for an examination and a Pap smear. Women who have irregular menstrual* periods, which may indicate that they have a hormonal imbalance, should be evaluated by a doctor. Hormonal treatment may reduce the risk of uterine cancer. Maintaining a healthy diet high in fruits and vegetables and low in animal fat and proper body weight seem to play some role in lowering the risk of developing this cancer.

▶ See also **Cancer: Overview** • **Cervical Cancer** • **Genital Warts**

Resources

Books and Articles

Hartmann, Lynn C., and Charles L. Loprinzi. *Mayo Clinic Guide to Women's Cancers.* New York: Mayo Clinic, 2005.

Luesley, David M., Frank Lawton, and Andrew Berchuck, eds. *Uterine Cancer.* New York: Taylor and Francis Group, 2006.

Organizations

American Cancer Society. 1599 Clifton Road NE, Atlanta, GA, 30329-4251. Toll free: 800-227-2345. Web site: http://www.cancer.org/docroot/lrn/lrn_0.asp.

National Cancer Institute. Public Inquiries Office, 6116 Executive Boulevard, Room 3036A, Bethesda, MD, 20892-8322. Toll free: 800-4-CANCER. Web site: http://www.cancer.gov/cancertopics/wyntk/uterus.

National Women's Health Information Center. 8270 Willow Oaks Corporate Drive, Fairfax, VA, 22031. Toll free: 800-994-9662. Web site: http://www.4women.gov/FAQ/uterine-cancer.cfm.

V

Vaccination (Immunization)

Vaccination (vak-sih-NAY-shun) is a way of producing immunity* to a specific disease by introducing into a person's body an inactive, altered, or weakened form of a microorganism* and thereby provoking an immune response.

Vaccination Development

Before the 19th century, a dangerous disease known as smallpox killed millions of people throughout the world. All that was soon to change as the result of an observation made by Edward Jenner (1749–1823), an English country doctor, in 1796. Jenner reported that milkmaids who milked cows infected with a disease known as cowpox did not contract smallpox. Instead, the milkmaids had a mild case of a similar rash-producing disease. Jenner concluded that cowpox must somehow protect these milkmaids against the smallpox infection.

Although Jenner is credited with being the discoverer of the principles of immunization and the developer of the first vaccine against smallpox, men and women had grasped or intuited the principles of immunization for at least several thousand years before him. There are historical accounts of successful vaccinations against contagious illnesses in Ancient Greece, India, and China. In England, approximately 75 years before Jenner's pioneering work, Lady Mary Wortley Montagu (1689–1762), wife of the British ambassador to the Ottoman Empire, vigorously promoted the practice of variolation (administering material from smallpox lesions to healthy people to produce immunity to smallpox). Montagu had observed this practice while living in what later became Turkey. She studied the method of Turkish women, who for centuries had collected in walnut shells the fluid from lesions of persons with smallpox and used lancets to press this material into the skin of healthy people to protect them from the disease. Back in England, she enthusiastically promoted this method and witnessed its many successes, albeit not without encountering a fair amount of resistance from the British medical establishment.

The milkmaids observed by Jenner who had contact with cows with cowpox had in fact become ill with cowpox themselves. (Cowpox infected humans as well as cows and in humans produces symptoms similar to those of smallpox, but cowpox in humans is a relatively benign* illness.

---

* **immunity** (ih-MYOON-uh-tee) is the condition of being protected against an infectious disease. Immunity often develops after a germ has entered the body. One type of immunity occurs when the body makes special protein molecules called antibodies to fight the disease-causing germ. The next time that germ enters the body, the antibodies quickly attack it, usually preventing the germ from causing disease.

* **microorganism** is a tiny organism that can be seen only by using a microscope. Types of microorganisms include fungi, bacteria, and viruses.

* **benign** (be-NINE) refers to a condition that is not cancerous or serious and will probably improve, go away, or not get worse.

* **poliomyelitis** (po-lee-o-my-uh-LYE-tis) is a condition caused by the polio virus that involves damage of nerve cells. It may lead to weakness and deterioration of the muscles and sometimes paralysis.

* **diphtheria** (dif-THEER-e-uh) is an infection of the lining of the upper respiratory tract (the nose and throat). It is a disease that can cause breathing difficulty and other complications, including death.

* **pertussis** (per-TUH-sis) is a bacterial infection of the respiratory tract that causes severe coughing.

* **vaccines** (vak-SEENS) are preparations of killed or weakened germs, or a part of a germ or product it produces, given to prevent or lessen the severity of the disease that can result if a person is exposed to the germ itself. Use of vaccines for this purpose is called immunization.

* **antigen** (AN-tih-jen) is a substance that is recognized as a threat by the body's immune system, which triggers the formation of specific antibodies against the substance.

* **immune system** (im-YOON SIS-tem) is the system of the body composed of specialized cells and the substances they produce that helps protect the body against disease-causing germs.

The milkmaids became ill with cowpox, but they did not get the more serious illness. Jenner concluded that having had cowpox somehow protected these milkmaids against the smallpox infection.

As an experiment, Jenner extracted material from the blister-like lesions of persons with cowpox and inoculated healthy people with the cowpox material (introduced this material into their systems). Jenner deliberately gave people the mild cowpox infection. Jenner was experimenting with vaccination. He discovered that the body's natural defense system can be stimulated to become protective against a specific illness after having been ill with a similar and more benign version of that illness. In the late 19th century, the French scientist Louis Pasteur (1822–1895) developed the concept further and named it "vaccination," a word derived from the Latin word for cow, "vacca." The first vaccine Pasteur developed was a vaccine for animals against sheep anthrax (AN-thraks).

After Jenner's time, scientists developed many effective vaccines, including ones against poliomyelitis*, measles, diphtheria*, and pertussis* (whooping cough). Overall, these vaccinations prevented disease and saved hundreds of millions of lives.

What Is Vaccination?

Vaccines*, the preparations used in vaccinations, stimulate the body's immune response by mimicking the substances that cause disease. Small amounts of antigenic* material (the vaccines themselves) are administered by oral ingestion or injection (usually intramuscular injection). Vaccines mimic a natural infection without actually causing disease. The antigenic substances promote immunologic memory, whereby specialized cells of the immune system become memory cells, that is, able to recognize and respond to any substance that bears the same antigen (if and when the actual disease-causing agent enters the body). When a person's immune system* can respond rapidly and effectively to an infection that is just beginning so that it cannot spread and cause damage within the body, that person has developed resistance to the infectious agent.

Booster vaccinations are second (or subsequent) vaccinations, separated from the first or prior vaccination by certain periods (often a span of several years) that result in an upsurge in or an extension of the effectiveness of the original vaccinations. Booster vaccinations take advantage of immunologic memory. When the white blood cells that have the ability to recognize and respond to a particular antigen are exposed to that antigen as part of a booster vaccination, those abilities are strengthened and reinforced. Some vaccinations require booster doses, whereas others do not.

Vaccinations protect more people than just the persons who receive them. They also protect unvaccinated people who live around those who have been vaccinated, a concept known as "herd immunity." A vaccination protects a person from contracting and then spreading an infection. When enough people living in an area have been immunized, the relevant

Recommended childhood and adolescent immunization schedule, United States

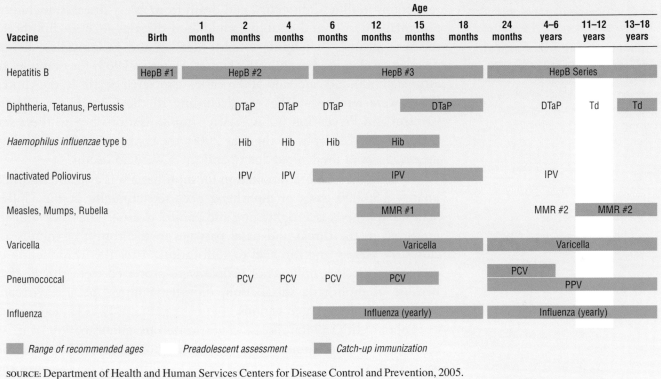

Vaccine	Birth	1 month	2 months	4 months	6 months	12 months	15 months	18 months	24 months	4–6 years	11–12 years	13–18 years
							Age					
Hepatitis B	HepB #1	HepB #2				HepB #3				HepB Series		
Diphtheria, Tetanus, Pertussis			DTaP	DTaP	DTaP		DTaP			DTaP	Td	Td
Haemophilus influenzae type b			Hib	Hib	Hib	Hib						
Inactivated Poliovirus			IPV	IPV		IPV				IPV		
Measles, Mumps, Rubella						MMR #1				MMR #2		MMR #2
Varicella							Varicella				Varicella	
Pneumococcal			PCV	PCV	PCV	PCV				PCV / PPV		
Influenza						Influenza (yearly)				Influenza (yearly)		

■ *Range of recommended ages* □ *Preadolescent assessment* ■ *Catch-up immunization*

SOURCE: Department of Health and Human Services Centers for Disease Control and Prevention, 2005.

disease-causing agent will have difficulty spreading in that area because it cannot find new human hosts*. The disease is much less likely to be passed on, even to those few people who remain unvaccinated. It is estimated that the protection of unvaccinated people in a community occurs when the proportion of persons in that community who are vaccinated reaches 95 percent.

Vaccinations boost immunity through a so-called active process, meaning that the immune system, in responding to an antigen, is reacting actively. There is also passive immunity, which is immunity acquired through the transfer of antibodies*. Infants are born with a passive immunity that protects them from some diseases. This immunity arises from the protective antibodies passed from mother to fetus and after birth from the mother's breast milk to the infant. A mother who has immunity against tetanus, a disease of the central nervous system caused by the toxin secreted by the tetanus bacterium, for example, will pass this immunity along to the developing fetus through the transfer of antibodies while she is pregnant. The offspring's immunity is only temporary, however. The infant's passive immunity disappears in the months after birth. Infants later make their own antibodies after being exposed to an infectious agent or receiving a vaccine.

Illustration by GGS Information Services, Inc. Reproduced by permission of Gale, a part of Cengage Learning.

* **hosts** are organisms that provide another organism (such as a parasite or virus) with a place to live and grow.

* **antibodies** (AN-tih-bah-deez) are protein molecules produced by the body's immune system to help fight specific infections caused by microorganisms, such as bacteria and viruses.

* **mucus** (MYOO-kus) is a thick, slippery substance that lines the insides of many body parts.

* **paralysis** (pah-RAH-luh-sis) is the loss or impairment of the ability to move some part of the body.

* **respiratory failure** is a condition in which breathing and oxygen delivery to the body are dangerously altered. This may result from infection, nerve or muscle damage, poisoning, or other causes.

How Successful Are Vaccinations?

Vaccinations are one of the great success stories of public health programs in the 20th century. Widespread use of vaccines has brought about dramatic reductions in illness, disability, and death from many diseases, including potentially deadly and disabling childhood diseases such as diphtheria, tetanus, pertussis (whooping cough), measles, and poliomyelitis. Before measles vaccination began in the United States in 1963, for example, an estimated 500,000 cases and 500 measles-associated deaths in the United States were reported each year, according to the Centers for Disease Control and Prevention (CDC). After immunizations began, these statistics dropped sharply. In the year 2000, there were only 86 confirmed measles cases in the United States, and there were no deaths.

In the 1920s, before vaccination for diphtheria was available, approximately 150,000 cases of diphtheria occurred annually in the United States. Diphtheria is a frightening and painful disease. The thick mucus* produced in the throat and nasal passages in the course of the disease closes the airway and can lead to suffocation. After the introduction of diphtheria vaccine, millions of people were protected from this disease. Because of diphtheria vaccination, diphtheria illness became virtually nonexistent in developed nations.

Poliomyelitis, a viral disease characterized by inflammation of nerve cells in the brain and spinal cord, also known as polio and infantile paralysis, was a health scourge in the United States until the 1950s. The virus can spread along nerve fiber pathways, damaging and even destroying motor neurons (especially the motor neurons that supply muscles in the legs). As a result of this damage to nerve tissue, the illness often produces muscle weakness and paralysis*. The virus may damage neurons that supply the chest wall muscles and the diaphragm, a thin sheet of muscle separating the chest from the abdomen that is essential to breathing. Paralysis of these muscles can lead to respiratory failure* and death. In 1952 there were more than 21,000 cases of paralytic (pair-uh-LIH-tik) poliomyelitis in the United States. After the introduction of polio vaccine in 1955, the incidence of this disease steadily declined, and between 1979 and 2009 there were no naturally occurring cases in the United States.

Smallpox is the only disease that has been eradicated entirely from the global population through an aggressive international immunization program. This highly contagious disease once killed as many as one out of every three infected individuals, but as of 2009, the last known naturally occurring case was reported in Somalia, Africa, in 1977. The World Health Organization declared smallpox to be eradicated in 1980.

What Vaccines Are Used in the 21st Century?

The 20th century saw both tremendous success of vaccines and advances in vaccine technology. Some earlier vaccines were improved, and new vaccines were introduced. There were four different types of vaccines available as of 2009:

■ *Live attenuated vaccines* contain virus particles that have been cultivated under conditions that considerably weaken them. Attenuated (ah-TEN-yoo-a-tid) types of vaccine contain live but weaker forms of a virus. These viruses usually do not cause disease symptoms, but they do stimulate the body to develop immunity to the virus. Attenuated vaccines include the combined vaccine for measles, mumps*, and rubella* (German measles), known as the MMR vaccine; the vaccine for varicella (var-uh-SEH-luh), or chickenpox; and the oral polio vaccine. Although these immunizations last longer than others, vaccines of this type occasionally create serious infections in people, particularly those with weakened immune systems.

■ *Killed vaccines* contain microorganisms (bacteria or viruses) that have been killed with chemicals or heat. Examples of this type of vaccine are the influenza* virus; the hepatitis A virus vaccine; the injected polio vaccine; and the cholera vaccine. Although they are not alive, the microorganisms in these vaccines cause an immune response in the body. These vaccines are considered safe for people with weakened immune systems.

■ *Toxoid (TOX-oyd) vaccines* contain a (partially inactivated) toxin (poison) produced by the infecting microorganisms (and not the microorganisms themselves). This type of vaccine is used for diseases in which the symptoms are caused principally by the toxin, rather than by the microorganism. If and when the body encounters live invading organisms that secrete the same toxin, the immune system responds. Diphtheria and tetanus vaccines are both of the toxoid type.

■ *Subunit or component vaccines* contain fragments or parts of the disease-causing microorganisms (and not the microorganisms themselves) that are able to trigger the immune response. The acellular vaccine for pertussis ("acellular," meaning it contains no whole cells) is an example of a subunit vaccine. Some subunit vaccines are semi-synthetic compounds, that is, compounds isolated from natural sources that have undergone man-made modifications. One example is the Haemophilus influenzae type B (Hib) vaccine, which contains two naturally occurring antigens combined to make a conjugate molecule.

What Vaccinations Are Recommended in the United States?

Vaccine preparations are produced by drug manufacturers and in the United States must be approved for use and licensed by the Food and Drug Administration. Vaccines are also patented, which diminishes their availabilities.

A vaccination schedule is a list of recommended vaccines that includes the recommended timings of all vaccine doses. Vaccination schedules are

* **mumps** is a contagious viral infection that causes inflammation and swelling in the glands of the mouth that produce saliva.

* **rubella** (roo-BEH-luh) is a viral infection that usually causes a rash and mild fever.

* **influenza** (in-floo-EN-zuh), also known as the flu, is a contagious viral infection that attacks the respiratory tract, including the nose, throat, and lungs.

* **cirrhosis** (sir-O-sis) is a condition that affects the liver, involving long-term inflammation and scarring, which can lead to problems with liver function.

* **meningitis** (meh-nin-JY-tis) is an inflammation of the meninges, the membranes that surround the brain and the spinal cord. Meningitis is most often caused by infection with a virus or a bacterium.

* **sepsis** is a potentially serious spreading of infection, usually bacterial, through the bloodstream and body.

compiled by the Advisory Committee on Immunization Practices (ACIP), a 15-member panel that advises the Centers for Disease Control and Prevention (CDC) and the Department of Health and Human Services. Vaccines are usually administered during early childhood, although some vaccinations may need to be given later in life.

The ACIP and the CDC recommend vaccinations. For the general population (including the general pediatric population), vaccinations are recommended but not mandated. However, in the United States all fifty states require children to be immunized against measles, diphtheria, Haemophilus influenza type B, poliomyelitis, and rubella in order to enroll in day care and/or public school.

In 2009 the CDC in its Recommended Childhood Immunization Schedule recommended the following vaccines for children six years of age or younger:

- *Hepatitis B vaccine* (HBV) protects against hepatitis B virus infection. This is the most dangerous of the hepatitis viruses, and hepatitis B (the illness) often has a severe course and can be life-threatening. People who are infected with hepatitis B are at risk for chronic liver disease, cirrhosis* of the liver, and liver cancer. Hepatitis B is one of the most common causes of cancer deaths worldwide. Hepatitis B vaccine is usually given as a series of three inoculations: one shortly after birth, another at one or two months of age, and the third at six to 18 months of age.

- *Hepatitis A vaccine* is caused by the hepatitis A virus and is the most common form of hepatitis. The illness usually follows a mild course and does not cause permanent liver damage. Hepatitis A vaccine is recommended for all children beginning at one year of age. Two separate doses are given six months apart. The CDC made this recommendation in 2006.

- *Pneumococcal conjugate vaccine* (PCV) is intended to protect infants and young children against diseases caused by the bacterium Streptococcus pneumoniae (also known as pneumococcus, or pneumococcal bacteria), including pneumonia, meningitis*, and sepsis*. The word "conjugate" refers to the conjugation (joining) of two components. PCV is given as a series of four shots, when an infant is 2 months, 4 months, 6 months, and 12 to 15 months old.

- *Diphtheria-tetanus-pertussis vaccine* (DTaP, the "aP" referring to acellular pertussis) is a mixture of three vaccines that protects against these three diseases. The acellular vaccine uses antigenic fragments of the pertussis bacterium due to the enhanced safety of this vaccine. DTaP is given as a series of five shots, usually administered to a child at the age of 2 months, 4 months, 6 months, 15 to 18 months, and 4 to 6 years (or before starting school). Five years after the last of these immunizations, generally at age 11 or 12, children receive a booster shot for diphtheria, tetanus, and pertussis known as dTap or Tdap (the lowercased "d" and "p" indicating the reduced concentrations of the diphtheria and pertussis components). Doctors recommend that people receive dTap/Tdap boosters once every 10 years after that, throughout adulthood. DTap should not be given to persons 7 years of age or older. It is licensed for children under the age of 7 years.

- *Haemophilus influenzae type b vaccine* protects against the serious disease caused by the Haemophilus influenzae bacterium, type b (Hib), which usually strikes children under the age of 5 years, once a leading cause of meningitis in children. The vaccine is given by injection to children at age 2 months, 4 months, and 6 months. A booster dose is given at age 12 to 15 months.

- *Inactivated polio vaccine* (IPV) protects again poliomyelitis infection. It is given by injection at age 2 months, 4 months, 6 to 18 months, and 4 to 6 years (or before entering school).

- *Measles-mumps-rubella vaccine* is a mixture of three live, attenuated viruses administered by injection that protects against measles, mumps, and rubella (German measles). The vaccine is administered in two doses, the first at age 12 to 15 months and the second before a child starts school, generally at age 4 to 6 years.

- *Varicella (chickenpox) vaccine* protects against varicella (caused by the varicella virus), also known as chickenpox, a common childhood viral illness. Children who have never had chickenpox are given two doses of the vaccine (via injection): at age 12 to 15 months, and at 4 to 6 years. Children who have had chickenpox do not need the vaccine. Older children and adults who have never had chickenpox can also receive the vaccine.

- *Influenza vaccine* is recommended for all children, but it is particularly recommended for children with certain conditions, including diabetes* and sickle-cell disease*, which put them at even greater risk of serious influenza infection.

- *Rotavirus vaccine* protects against rotavirus, which causes severe diarrhea in infants and young children and is the leading cause of severe diarrhea in that population. The vaccine is given orally. Vaccination is recommended for infants at age 2 months, 4 months, and 6 months.

The CDC recommends the following vaccines for adolescents between the ages of 11 and 18 years:

- DTaP (described above) is recommended for young people between the ages of 11 or 12. This booster dose of DTaP protects them against pertussis.

- *Human papillomavirus vaccine* (for girls) protects against the human papillomavirus (HPV), the most common sexually transmitted virus in the United States. This virus has many subtypes. Two of these cause about 70 percent of all cervical cancer cases.

* **diabetes** (dye-uh-BEE-teez) is a condition in which the body's pancreas does not produce enough insulin or the body cannot use the insulin it makes effectively, resulting in increased levels of sugar in the blood. This can lead to increased urination, dehydration, weight loss, weakness, and a number of other symptoms and complications related to chemical imbalances within the body.

* **sickle-cell disease** is a hereditary condition in which the red blood cells, which are usually round, take on an abnormal crescent shape and have a decreased ability to carry oxygen throughout the body.

* **tetanus** (TET-nus) is a serious bacterial infection that affects the body's central nervous system.

* **rabies** (RAY-beez) is a viral infection of the central nervous system that usually is transmitted to humans by the bite of an infected animal.

* **epidemic** (eh-pih-DEH-mik) is an outbreak of disease, especially infectious disease, in which the number of cases suddenly becomes far greater than usual. Usually epidemics are outbreaks of diseases in specific regions, whereas widespread epidemics are called pandemics.

in the United States. This vaccine prevents most cases of cervical cancer and is recommended for girls 11 and 12 years of age. It is also recommended that girls receive the vaccine prior to their first sexual contact. The vaccine is given by injection in three doses.

■ *Meningococcus vaccine* protects against meningococcal disease, which is a leading cause of bacterial meningitis in persons between the ages of 2 to 18 years in the United States. The vaccine is recommended for adolescents between the ages of 11 and 18 years. College students who live in dormitories and adolescents age 15 to 19 years are at increased risk for meningococcal disease.

In addition to children and adolescents, adults require vaccines. For example, adults generally need a tetanus booster vaccination every 10 years, and older adults or adults with some medical conditions are advised to get a flu shot every year. Adults who did not undergo immunization as children, those who have emigrated from a country where vaccines are not readily available, and those who travel to areas where there is a higher risk of certain infectious diseases also receive vaccinations.

Vaccines against tetanus* and rabies* may prevent disease if they are given immediately after exposure to the disease-causing agent. But the vaccines are effective only within a very short time period after exposure. A rabies vaccine is typically administered after a person is bitten by an animal that could have the disease or when a person plans to spend more than 30 days in a place where rabies is common.

What Are Common Fears about Vaccinations?

Vaccinations have been proven to reduce (and reduce drastically) the incidence and mortality rates of many diseases and to eradicate (eliminate) some diseases from entire populations. Still, some parents are reluctant to vaccinate their children for a variety of reasons. Some parents feel that children receive too many vaccines and that the administration of vaccines begins too early. Others worry about possible adverse reactions. Still others believe, erroneously, that with lower rates of certain diseases in the United States, regular vaccinations are no longer necessary.

A dramatic example proves otherwise. The United Kingdom, Japan, and Sweden cut back their use of pertussis vaccine in the 1970s when some medical experts in those countries believed that the risks of using the vaccine outweighed the benefits. Between 1971 and 1979, the United Kingdom experienced more than 100,000 cases of the disease and 36 pertussis-related deaths. From 1974 to 1979, Japan's vaccination coverage in the general population dropped from 80 percent to 20 percent, while the annual number of pertussis cases rose from a low of 393 in 1974, with no deaths, to a epidemic* high of 13,000 cases and 41 deaths. In Sweden, the annual incidence of pertussis per 100,000 children up to age six leaped from 700 in 1981 to 3,200 in 1985.

Another common belief is that vaccines cause the infectious diseases that they are intended to protect against. In fact, killed vaccines or those made from only a component of the infectious agent, such as a protein, cannot cause the infectious disease. In addition, continual efforts are made by the manufacturers of vaccines to minimize the possibility of contracting disease from a live vaccine. For example, in January 2000 the ACIP recommended that the polio vaccine be switched from an attenuated oral version to a killed vaccine to reduce or eliminate whatever risk there was of contracting vaccine-associated paralytic polio. Although the live oral vaccine was largely responsible for ridding the United Sates of polio, it caused polio in one of every 1.4 million people who received their first dose of the vaccine. The killed version, however, cannot cause polio.

What Are the Side Effects of Vaccination?

Although vaccinations prevent many cases of serious, and even fatal, illness, any vaccine can have side effects, and many people experience them after receiving vaccines. Potential side effects for all of the vaccines listed in this entry include low-grade fever; mild pain, tenderness, and redness at the site of the injection; rash; and irritability. Less common, but more serious, reactions include seizures*, usually as a result of fever, and allergic reactions to components of the vaccine. Reports that link childhood vaccinations to autism*, sudden infant death syndrome*, and brain damage had not been proven as of 2009 but remained hotly debated.

Why Is It Important to Vaccinate?

Vaccination provides the best protection against many well-known childhood diseases, and preventing the spread of these diseases is vital to public health. Vaccines protect the people who receive them, and they also prevent the spread of disease to people who have not been vaccinated. Modern science has produced many effective vaccines. International travel and a rapidly shrinking globe means that diseases can easily cross national and continental lines. Diseases once rarely seen in one country can be easily imported from another. This fact makes receiving vaccinations an ongoing necessity. If people somehow start to believe that they or their children do not need to get vaccinated or if they depend on others to get vaccinated, overall vaccination levels will drop. This could lead to the return of diseases that are easily prevented by vaccination.

What Vaccines May Be Developed in the Future?

In the early 21st century, medical researchers continued to work to develop vaccines for a wide range of diseases, including HIV*/AIDS*. The quest for an HIV/AIDS vaccine was complicated by the fact that HIV mutates (changes) rapidly (leading to the existence of a large number of distinct viral subspecies) and because HIV damages the very cells that are needed by the body in any response to an antigen. Malaria vaccines were also the subject of intensive research. Several drug manufacturers coninue to work on the development of vaccines that will protect against tuberculosis infection, and several clinical trials were underway as of 2009. But there was no effective tuberculosis vaccine available as of 2009. In 2006 the

* **seizures** (SEE-zhurs) are sudden bursts of disorganized electrical activity that interrupt the normal functioning of the brain, often leading to uncontrolled movements in the body and sometimes a temporary change in consciousness.

* **autism** (AW-tih-zum) is a developmental disorder in which a person has difficulty interacting and communicating with others and usually has severely limited interest in social activities.

* **sudden infant death syndrome** or SIDS, is the sudden death of an infant less than a year old that is not explained even after an autopsy or examination of the death scene. Most cases occur while the otherwise well baby is asleep on its stomach.

* **HIV** or human immunodeficiency virus (HYOO-mun ih-myoo-no-dih-FIH-shen-see), is the virus that causes AIDS (acquired immunodeficiency syndrome).

* **AIDS** or acquired immunodeficiency (ih-myoo-no-dih-FIH-shen-see) syndrome, is an infection that severely weakens the immune system; it is caused by the human immunodeficiency virus (HIV).

* **virus** (VY-rus) is a tiny infectious agent that can cause infectious diseases. A virus can only reproduce within the cells it infects.

* **herpesvirus family** (her-peez-VY-rus) is a group of viruses that can store themselves permanently in the body. The family includes varicella zoster virus, Epstein-Barr virus, and herpes simplex virus.

* **herpes** (HER-peez) is a viral infection that can produce painful, recurring skin blisters around the mouth or the genitals, and sometimes symptoms of infection elsewhere in the body.

* **vaccines** (vak-SEENS) are preparations of killed or weakened germs, or a part of a germ or product it produces, given to prevent or lessen the severity of the disease that can result if a person is exposed to the germ itself. Use of vaccines for this purpose is called immunization.

FDA approved the first vaccine for adult shingles, a painful viral disease caused by viral infection of nerve endings in skin.

In general, however, such research takes years and is costly. Because almost all vaccinations carry some risk, an important part of their development is to assess how effective they are and whether the benefits of a new vaccine outweigh the risks.

Resources

Books and Articles

Alter, Judith. *Vaccines*. Ann Arbor, MI: Cherry Lake, 2009.

Feder, Lauren. *The Parents' Concise Guide to Childhood Vaccinations: Practical Medical and Natural Ways to Protect Your Child*. Long Island City, NY: Hatherleigh, 2007.

Gray, Shirley Wimbish. *Prevention and Good Health*. Chanhassen, MN: Child's World, 2004.

Organizations

Centers for Disease Control and Prevention. 1600 Clifton Road, Atlanta, GA, 30333. Toll free: 800-311-3435. Web site: http://www.cdc.gov/vaccines.

Immunization Action Coalition. 1573 Selby Avenue, Suite 234, St. Paul, MN, 55104. Telephone: 651-647-9009. Web site: http://www.immunize.org.

Vaginal Yeast Infection *See Yeast Infection, Vaginal.*

Valley Fever *See Coccidioidomycosis.*

Varicella (Chicken Pox) and Herpes Zoster (Shingles)

Infection with the varicella zoster (var-uh-SEH-luh ZOS-ter) virus* (VZV), a member of the herpesvirus family*, causes the common childhood illness varicella or chicken pox. Reactivation of the virus later in life causes herpes* zoster, commonly known as shingles. Vaccines* are available that prevent or ameliorate (reduce) the symptoms of both diseases.

What Are Varicella and Herpes Zoster?

Varicella or chicken pox is a highly contagious* disease caused by the initial or primary infection with VZV. It is characterized by the appearance of red, itchy spots on the skin. The spots progress to blisters and eventually crust over.

Most people cannot contract varicella a second time because the body's immune system* makes protective antibodies*. However VZV remains in the nerve tissues of the body in a dormant or inactive state. Years later—most often after a person is 50 years of age—VZV can be reactivated in the form of herpes zoster or shingles. Sometimes this reactivation occurs at a time of emotional or physical stress. Shingles usually appears first as one or more local areas of intense pain, followed by a red rash or blisters. Sometimes, especially in the elderly, shingles causes nerve damage that can result in severe pain called post-herpetic neuralgia that may last for months or years.

How Common Are Varicella and Herpes Zoster?

Chicken pox was once a disease experienced by nearly every child, causing an estimated 4 million illnesses, 11,000 hospitalizations, and 100 deaths each year in the United States. After the introduction of a varicella vaccine in 1995, the incidence* of chicken pox, especially in younger children, decreased dramatically. However, in the early 2000s, chicken pox remains relatively common among unvaccinated children and adults and 10 to 15 percent of vaccinated children also contract the disease.

Nearly one in three Americans eventually develops shingles, and there are at least one million cases in the United States each year. Anyone who has ever had chicken pox or received the varicella vaccine is at risk for shingles. About half of all cases occur in people 60 years of age or older. The risk of shingles increases with age and with any condition that weakens the immune system. Susceptibility* to shingles tends to run in families.

Are Varicella and Herpes Zoster Contagious?

Most people who have never had chicken pox or been vaccinated against it will contract varicella if they come in close contact with someone who has the illness. Anyone with chicken pox is contagious from one or two days before the rash first appears until the pox blisters have crusted over. VZV is spread in the air through the coughs or sneezes of an infected person. It can also be spread by contact with the fluid in pox blisters.

Shingles itself is not contagious. However, the virus can be transmitted to someone who has never had chicken pox by direct contact with the shingles rash. That person will develop chicken pox. Only people who have had chicken pox or received the varicella vaccine can get shingles.

How Do People Know They Have Chicken Pox or Shingles?

The symptoms and signs of chicken pox usually appear within two to three weeks after exposure to the virus and typically begin with fever, headache, and fatigue. The classic chicken pox rash starts as red spots on

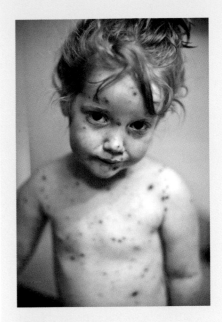

▲
The majority of children in the United States contracted chicken pox until a vaccine, which became available in 1995, dramatically reduced the rate of infection. © *Justin Leighton/Alamy.*

Chickpea pox?

The term "chicken pox" may come from *cicer,* the Latin word for "chickpea." Chickpeas or garbanzo beans, a popular ingredient in salads and spreads such as hummus (HUH-mus), are round, buff-colored, and a bit larger than green peas. Chicken pox blisters look a bit like chickpeas on the skin.

* **contagious** (kon-TAY-jus) means transmittable from one person to another, usually referring to an infection.

* **immune system** (im-YOON SIS-tem) is the system of the body composed of specialized cells and the substances they produce that helps protect the body against disease-causing germs.

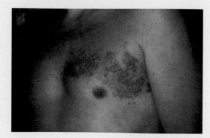

The shingles rash is a patch of small blisters filled with the herpes zoster virus. *Biophoto Associates/Photo Researchers, Inc.*

* **antibodies** (AN-tih-bah-deez) are protein molecules produced by the body's immune system to help fight specific infections caused by microorganisms, such as bacteria and viruses.

* **incidence** means rate of occurrence.

* **susceptibility** (su-sep-ti-BIL-i-tee) means having less resistance to and higher risk for infection or disease.

* **nausea** (NAW-zha) refers to a feeling of being sick to one's stomach or needing to vomit.

* **diarrhea** (di-ah-RE-a) refers to frequent, watery stools (bowel movements).

* **antihistamines** (an-tie-HIS-tuh-meens) are drugs used to combat allergic reactions and relieve itching.

* **Reye's syndrome** (RYES SIN-drome) is a rare condition that involves inflammation of the liver and brain, and sometimes appears after illnesses such as chicken pox or influenza. It has also been associated with taking aspirin during certain viral infections.

* **acetaminophen** (uh-see-teh-MIH-noh-fen) is a medication commonly used to reduce fever and relieve pain.

the face, chest, back, buttocks, and, less commonly, arms and legs. The spots quickly turn into blisters that break, ooze fluid, and then crust over. The pox often pop up in groups over a period of four or five days. The number of blisters varies from very few to hundreds. The rash ranges from mildly to severely itchy.

The first symptoms of shingles are local areas of intense tingling, burning, itching, or severe pain, usually on one side of the face or body (people suffering from impairment of the immune system may developed more generalized shingles covering larger areas of the body). A rash or fluid-filled blisters on reddened skin appears next. The rash follows the path of the inflamed nerve tissue and looks like a streak or a band. Before the rash develops the pain of shingles is easily confused with other conditions. The rash can last two to three weeks before healing and scabbing over. Shingles pain usually subsides when the rash disappears, but it may last much longer, with one in five people developing post-herpetic neuralgia.

Uncommon symptoms of shingles include:

- Chills
- Fever
- Headache
- Nausea*
- Stomach pain
- Diarrhea*

How Do Doctors Diagnosis and Treat Chicken Pox and Shingles?

Diagnosis Doctors usually recognize chicken pox or shingles by their distinctive rashes. Laboratory tests on the fluid in blisters from either disease can diagnose VZV infection. Blood tests for antibodies against VZV can determine whether a person is immune to chicken pox.

Treatment In general, the goal of chicken-pox treatment is to ease the discomfort caused by itchy blisters. Cool compresses or lukewarm baths in water sprinkled with uncooked oatmeal or baking soda can soothe the skin and relieve itching. Over-the-counter antihistamines* can also help control itching. Children with chicken pox should not be given aspirin for fever due to the risk of Reye's syndrome*. A non-aspirin fever reducer such as acetaminophen* is recommended instead. A child's fingernails should be cut short, because scratching the blisters can lead to secondary skin infections caused by bacteria*. Children usually recover from chicken pox within one to two weeks. Adults may take longer to recover. Adults and those with weakened immune systems are at greater risk for complications of chicken pox and may be treated with antiviral medications for a few days to control the infection.

If shingles is recognized soon after the rash first appears, it can be treated with oral* antiviral medication, which may shorten the course of the disease and minimize pain. Blisters from shingles typically clear up after two to three weeks, but the nerve pain can linger for weeks or months, sometimes even years.

Complications   The most common complication of chicken pox is cellulitis*, a skin infection caused by bacteria such as streptococci (strep-tuh-KAH-kye) and staphylococci (stah-fih-lo-KAH-kye), which can invade the skin through repeated scratching of pox sores.

If a woman becomes infected with chicken pox during the first 20 weeks of pregnancy, there is a 2 percent risk that her baby will be born with congenital* varicella syndrome*, including multiple birth defects. Maternal infection during the final stages of pregnancy, before the mother has developed antibodies, can cause life-threatening varicella infection in her baby.

People with weakened immune systems, such as those with HIV*/AIDS* or cancer* or who are undergoing chemotherapy* are at particular risk for widespread infection from either chicken pox or shingles. Varicella infection can spread to the lungs causing pneumonia*. Even in healthy people pneumonia from varicella can be dangerous and potentially fatal. Newborn babies, teens, and adults are at greater risk than children. Adults are also more at risk for other serious—but rare—complications, including liver* and kidney* disease and encephalitis*.

Untreated shingles rash on the face can spread to the eye. Involvement of the cornea* can lead to temporary or permanent blindness. Rarely shingles can cause hearing loss or death.

Can Chicken Pox and Shingles Be Prevented?

The American Academy of Pediatrics recommends that all children be vaccinated against chicken pox before two years of age. Older children and teens who have not had chicken pox are usually vaccinated as part of routine health care. Women who have not had chicken pox or been previously vaccinated should be vaccinated before they become pregnant. Pregnant women cannot be vaccinated because the vaccine contains live virus that could harm the fetus*. However, vaccinations* for family members and others in close contact with a pregnant woman can help protect her from infection. People who become infected with varicella despite vaccination usually have a milder case of chicken pox.

A single dose of varicella zoster immune globulin* (VZIG) can be administered intravenously* to protect a person with a weakened immune system who comes into contact with the virus. VZIG contains antibodies against VZV and, if it is given within three to four days of exposure, offers temporary protection. Exposure to varicella by a non-immune pregnant woman can also be treated with VZIG to reduce the risk of transmitting the virus to her fetus.

People with shingles should avoid contact with anyone who has not had chicken pox or been vaccinated, particularly pregnant women, newborns, and those with weakened immune systems.

* **bacteria** (bak-TEER-ee-a) are single-celled microorganisms, which typically reproduce by cell division. Some, but not all, types of bacteria can cause disease in humans. Many types can live in the body without causing harm.

* **oral** means by mouth or referring to the mouth.

* **cellulitis** (sel-yoo-LYE-tis) is an infection of the skin and the tissues beneath it.

* **congenital** (kon-JEH-nih-tul) means present at birth.

* **syndrome** is a group or pattern of symptoms or signs that occur together.

* **HIV** or human immunodeficiency virus (HYOO-mun ih-myoo-no-dih-FIH-shen-see), is the virus that causes AIDS (acquired immunodeficiency syndrome).

* **AIDS** or acquired immunodeficiency (ih-myoo-no-dih-FIH-shen-see) syndrome, is an infection that severely weakens the immune system; it is caused by the human immunodeficiency virus (HIV).

* **cancer** is a condition characterized by abnormal overgrowth of certain cells, which may be fatal.

* **chemotherapy** (KEE-mo-THER-a-pee) is the treatment of cancer with powerful drugs that kill cancer cells.

* **pneumonia** (nu-MO-nyah) is inflammation of the lungs.

* **liver** is a large organ located beneath the ribs on the right side of the body. The liver performs numerous digestive and chemical functions essential for health.

* **kidney** is one of the pair of organs that filter blood and remove waste products and excess water from the body in the form of urine.

* **encephalitis** (en-seh-fuh-LYE-tis) is an inflammation of the brain, usually caused by a viral infection.

* **cornea** (KOR-nee-uh) is the transparent circular layer of cells over the central colored part of the eyeball (the iris) through which light enters the eye.

* **fetus** (FEE-tus) is the term for an unborn human after it is an embryo, from 9 weeks after fertilization until childbirth.

* **vaccinations** (vak-sih-NAY-shunz), also called immunizations, are the giving of doses of vaccines, which are preparations of killed or weakened germs, or a part of a germ or product it produces, to prevent or lessen the severity of the disease that can result if a person is exposed to the germ itself.

* **immune globulin** (ih-MYOON GLAH-byoo-lin), also called gamma globulin, is the protein material that contains antibodies.

* **intravenous** (in-tra-VEE-nus) or IV, means within or through a vein. For example, medications, fluid, or other substances can be given through a needle or soft tube inserted through the skin's surface directly into a vein.

* **tuberculosis** (too-ber-kyoo-LO-sis) is a bacterial infection that primarily attacks the lungs but can spread to other parts of the body.

A single-dose vaccine against shingles became available in 2006 and was recommended for most people 60 years of age and older. It appeared to prevent shingles in about 50 percent of vaccinated people and reduces the pain associated with shingles in others. It was believed to help prevent post-herpetic neuralgia. People should not receive the shingles vaccine if any of the following conditions apply to them:

- Have a weakened immune system
- Have active, untreated tuberculosis*
- Are pregnant or could become pregnant within three months of being vaccinated
- Have a moderate or severe illness or fever

▶ *See also* **Congenital Infections • Encephalitis • Herpes Simplex Virus Infections • Immune Deficiencies • Mononucleosis, Infectious • Skin and Soft Tissue Infections • Staphylococcal Infections • Streptococcal Infections**

Resources

Books and Articles

Glaser, Jason. *Chicken Pox.* Mankato, MN: Capstone Press, 2006.

Gupta, Sanjay. "Rash Redux." *Time* 172, no. 4 (July 28, 2008): 53.

Heininger, Ulrich, and Jane F. Seward. "Varicella." *Lancet* 368, no. 9544 (October 14–20, 2006): 1365–1376.

Siegel, Mary-Ellen, and Gray Williams. *Shingles: New Hope for an Old Disease,* updated ed. Lanham, MD: M. Evans, 2008.

Organizations

American Academy of Pediatrics. 141 Northwest Point Boulevard, Elk Grove Village, IL, 60007-1098. Telephone: 847-434-4000. Web site: http://www.aap.org.

Centers for Disease Control and Prevention. 1600 Clifton Road, Atlanta, GA, 30333. Toll free: 800-311-3435. Web site: http://www.cdc.gov.

Varicose Veins

Varicose veins are damaged superficial veins that have become stretched, enlarged, and/or twisted. They can develop virtually anywhere in the body, but they develop most commonly in the legs. They can often be seen on the legs, just below the surface of the skin, and they may give affected areas a lumpy appearance.

What Are Veins and Arteries?

The circulatory system has two main types of vessels for carrying blood to and from all of the body's cells, tissues, and organs. Arteries carry oxygen-rich blood from the heart to the organs, and veins return oxygen-poor blood to the heart. Both arteries and veins are vessels or tubes through which blood flows, but they are dissimilar in many ways. Arteries have much thicker walls than veins of comparable size. Both arteries and veins have rings of smooth muscle surrounding them, but arteries have thicker rings. Arteries have many more elastic fibers than veins and have the property of elasticity. Veins are relatively inelastic. In addition, blood pressure in the veins is much lower than it is in the arteries. Veins do have valves, which help to keep blood from pooling in the veins. When these valves start to break down, as often happens in older or inactive people, the veins sometimes dilate* or collapse and become varix, varices, varicose*. The result is varicose veins. Although varicose veins can be painful, most varicose veins are relatively benign*.

Where Do Varicose Veins Occur?

Varicose veins very often in the area behind the knee joint and in the calf area. The veins look bluish and may become swollen, which may give the affected area a lumpy appearance. About 15 percent of adults in the United States have varicose veins. Women have varicose veins more often than men do and are particularly prone to developing them during pregnancy. In addition, varicose veins tend to run in families.

What Is the Treatment for Varicose Veins?

Many people with varicose veins have no symptoms, but some people feel pain in their legs, especially when they stand for long periods of time. People with varicose veins will sometimes seek treatment for cosmetic reasons.

Conservative treatment   In mild cases, doctors usually suggest that their patients exercise to improve circulation and that they wear support hose or stockings to promote circulation in the legs and the return of blood to the heart. Doctors also typically tell people with varicose veins to sit with their feet up as often as possible and to avoid standing for prolonged periods of time.

Interventional treatment   Medical intervention can be divided into two classes: surgical and non-surgical. Varicose veins can be removed surgically via a process know as vein stripping. This process takes about 30 minutes and is often quite successful. Vein stripping is commonly used to improve the appearance of the legs. There are also less invasive treatments include sclerotherapy, endovenous laser therapy ablation, and radiofrequency ablation.

Sclerotherapy is the injection of a chemical irritant into a vein to "sclerose" or harden it. The chemical substance irritates the lining of the vein, causing it to swell and the blood to clot. The vein loses its function

* **dilate** (DY-late) means to become enlarged or stretched beyond the usual boundaries.

* **varix, varices, varicose** are the Latin words that describe veins, arteries, or lymph vessels that have become stretched or enlarged.

* **benign** (be-NINE) refers to a condition that is not cancerous or serious and will probably improve, go away, or not get worse.

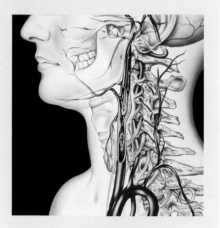

A blood clot (lower center) approaches a junction (center) of the left carotid artery that has been narrowed by atherosclerotic plaques (yellow). These fatty deposits of cholesterol on the artery walls have caused stenosis (narrowing) of the artery. If the blood clot lodges (an embolism), then the oxygenated blood supply to the head and brain will be interrupted. This will cause an ischemic stroke, where the brain is damaged due to hypoxia (lack of oxygen). The blood clot (thrombus) may have detached from a site of deep vein thrombosis. The backbone, its nerves (yellow), and skull bones and throat structures are also seen. *John Bavosi/Photo Researchers, Inc.*

* **cholesterol** (ko-LES-ter-ol) is a fatlike substance found in the blood and body tissues.

* **plaque** (PLAK) is a raised patch or swelling on a body surface. Arterial plaque occurs on the inner surface of an artery and is produced by fatty deposits.

* **blood clot** is a thickening of the blood into a jelly-like substance that helps stop bleeding. Clotting of the blood within a blood vessel can lead to blockage of blood flow.

* **heart attack** is a general term that usually refers to a sudden, intense episode of heart injury. It is usually caused by a blockage of a coronary artery, which stops blood from supplying the heart muscle with oxygen.

entirely. Most of the vein tissue turns into scar tissue. Blood flow shifts to nearby healthy veins. Endovenous laser ablation therapy is a treatment for varicose veins in which a laser source is inserted into the vein to be treated, and laser light is emitted that strikes the interior of the vein. This causes the vein to contract, and the laser source is then withdrawn. An alternative treatment is radiofrequency ablation, which is similar to endogenous laser therapy, but uses electromagnetic radiation of the radio-frequency range instead of laser light to close the vein.

Resources

Organization

National Heart, Lung, and Blood Institute. P.O. Box 30105, Bethesda, MD, 20824-0105. Telephone: 301-592-8573. Web site: http://www.nhlbi.nih.gov/health/dci/Diseases/vv/vv_whatis.html.

Vascular Diseases

Vascular diseases include a group of conditions that affect blood vessels. These conditions are common, affecting about 20 to 30 million Americans yearly. Major types are heart disease, including diseases that affect the peripheral arteries (arteries other than the coronary arteries, such as those that carry blood to the limbs, the carotid arteries that carry blood to the brain, or the renal arteries that carry blood to the kidneys); aneurysms; Raynaud's phenomenon; Buerger's disease, varicose veins; blood clotting disorders; and lymphedema. Each of these has its own underlying causes, symptoms, diagnostic requirements, and treatments.

What Are Some Types of Vascular Disease?

Heart disease and stroke Heart disease (also called coronary artery disease) occurs when the arteries that supply blood to the heart muscle narrow and harden. This condition is due to a process called atherosclerosis, in which cholesterol* combines with other substances to form plaque* that attaches in patches to arterial walls. As these patches expand in size, they may block blood flow to the heart muscle. Over time, this blockage can become complete enough to deprive the heart muscle of oxygen, damaging or destroying that area of heart muscle. Sometimes a blood clot* forms on top of the plaque, which can result in complete blockage of blood flow, leading to heart attack*. Other times, the blood clot may break away from the plaque, travel through the bloodstream, and cause a blockage in another location. If the blood clot stays within the circulation of the heart, a heart attack occurs; if the blood clot travels to the brain, a stroke* may occur.

Coronary artery disease is more common in people who have high concentrations of cholesterol in their blood, high blood pressure, diabetes*, family history of coronary artery disease, or who are smokers, obese*, or sedentary. Symptoms of coronary artery disease include bouts of angina (chest pain), frank heart attack (symptoms being pain in the jaw, neck, or back; chest pain; dizziness/faintness; pain in the arms or shoulders; shortness of breath), or signs of stroke (symptoms being sudden weakness or numbness in limbs or face; sudden confusion, difficulty speaking, or understanding others; sudden visual problems in one or both eyes; and sudden problems walking or maintaining balance).

Heart disease is diagnosed by correlating the results of a number of tests, including:

- Blood tests to look at cholesterol levels and the presence and levels of substances that indicate heart muscle damage

- Imaging studies that allow the coronary arteries to be visualized and demonstrate the presence of narrowing and plaque (such as cardiac catheterization, CT scans*, and MRIs*

- Tests of the heart's electrical system (electrocardiogram*)

- Ultrasound* to observe the movements of the heart and any obstruction

- Tests that demonstrate the heart's functioning (echocardiogram*)

- Stress tests* to evaluate how well the heart performs during periods of exercise

Treating coronary artery disease is determined by the severity of the disease. In people who have more mild disease, lifestyle changes (e.g., weight loss, smoking cessation, increased exercise, learning to deal with stress, and eating a healthier diet) may be sufficient. In more complicated cases, blood cholesterol and high blood pressure may need to be lowered with medications. Other medications may also be used, including blood thinners (anticoagulants), beta blockers, calcium channel blockers, and nitroglycerin (to treat chest pain from angina).

When blockages are more severe, one of two surgical operations may be required. Angioplasty involves slipping a small balloon into an obstructed artery and inflating the balloon to widen the narrowed artery, a procedure that may be combined with stent placement, in which an artificial tube is permanently positioned inside the artery to keep it open. Coronary artery bypass grafting involves open-heart surgery. The obstructed sections of the coronary arteries are removed and replaced with grafts* made from arteries or veins that are harvested (taken) from elsewhere in the body, often times from a leg.

While coronary artery disease often runs in families, an individual's risk can be lowered by adhering to basic preventive measures, including maintaining a healthy weight, eating a low-fat/low-cholesterol diet, never smoking, drinking only moderate quantities of alcohol, exercising regularly, learning and practicing stress reduction, and following all prescriptions to maintain normal blood cholesterol and blood pressure.

* **stroke** is a brain-damaging event usually caused by interference with blood flow to the brain. A stroke may occur when a blood vessel supplying the brain becomes clogged or bursts, depriving brain tissue of oxygen. As a result, nerve cells in the affected area of the brain, and the specific body parts they control, do not properly function.

* **diabetes** (dye-uh-BEE-teez) is a condition in which the body's pancreas does not produce enough insulin or the body cannot use the insulin it makes effectively, resulting in increased levels of sugar in the blood. This can lead to increased urination, dehydration, weight loss, weakness, and a number of other symptoms and complications related to chemical imbalances within the body.

* **obesity** (o-BEE-si-tee) is an excess of body fat. People are considered obese if they weigh more than 30 percent above what is healthy for their height.

* **CT scans** or CAT scans are the shortened name for computerized axial tomography (to-MOG-ra-fee), which uses computers to view structures inside the body.

* **MRI** which is short for magnetic resonance imaging, produces computerized images of internal body tissues based on the magnetic properties of atoms within the body.

* **electrocardiogram** (e-lek-tro-KAR-dee-o-gram), also known as an EKG, is a test that records and displays the electrical activity of the heart.

* **ultrasound** also called a sonogram, is a diagnostic test in which sound waves passing through the body create images on a computer screen.

* **echocardiogram** (eh-ko-KAR-dee-uh-gram) is a diagnostic test that uses sound waves to produce images of the heart's chambers and valves and blood flow through the heart

* **stress test** measures the health of a person's heart while the heart is intentionally stressed by exercise or medication.

* **grafts** are tissue or organ transplants.

* **gangrene** (GANG-green) is the decay or death of living tissue caused by a lack of oxygen supply to the tissue and/or bacterial infection of the tissue.

* **aorta** (ay-OR-ta) is the major large artery that carries blood from the heart to the rest of the body.

* **aortic aneurysm** (ay-OR-tik AN-yoo-rizm) is a weak spot in the aorta, the body's largest blood vessel. The weak spot can rupture or break, causing massive internal bleeding.

Peripheral artery disease Peripheral artery disease develops when the arteries outside the heart narrow and harden. Like coronary artery disease, this condition develops because plaque obstructs blood flow. Peripheral artery disease has many of the same risk factors as coronary artery disease, including aging, family history, smoking, diabetes, high blood pressure, high cholesterol, and obesity, as well as high blood levels of a particular amino acid (homocysteine). Blockage in the carotid arteries, which carry blood through the neck to the brain) can lead to a transient ischemic attack, or stroke. Blockage in the arteries that carry blood to the legs can result in poor blood circulation in the legs, leading to leg pain and cramps with activity (called intermittent claudication), delayed healing, open ulcers, and even gangrene*. Initially, pain only occurs with activity, but over time it may also occur at rest. Blockage in the renal (kidney) arteries can result in high blood pressure, congestive heart failure, and, over time, kidney failure.

Peripheral artery disease is diagnosed by using a stethoscope to listen for abnormal sounds over the carotid arteries, comparing the blood pressure in the patient's arms and legs (called the ankle-brachial index), testing for high blood cholesterol and homocysteine, and demonstrating poor blood flow through the arteries of concern via ultrasound tests, MRI or CT scans, or angiography (during which dye is injected into the blood vessels to highlight areas of obstruction).

Treatment of peripheral artery disease can include the same types of lifestyle changes used to treat coronary artery disease (weight loss, smoking cessation, increased exercise, learning to deal with stress, and eating a healthier diet). Medications may be used to lower high cholesterol and high blood pressure; to avoid blood clots with blood thinners (anticoagulants), aspirin, or clopidogrel; and to improve the ability to walk distances pain-free with cilostazol. More severe arterial obstructions may require surgery. As with coronary arteries, both angioplasty and bypass grafting can be used to treat peripheral artery disease. Additionally, the carotid arteries may require endarterectomy, a surgical procedure which cleans out the plaque within the carotid arteries and places a permanent artificial tube or stent inside the artery to keep it open.

While peripheral artery disease is a common problem of aging and often runs in families, an individual's risk can be lowered by adhering to basic preventive measures, including maintaining a healthy weight, eating a low-fat/low-cholesterol diet, never smoking, drinking only moderate quantities of alcohol, exercising regularly, learning and practicing stress reduction, and following directions for taking all prescriptions to maintain normal blood cholesterol and blood pressure and treat diabetes.

Aneurysms Aneurysms are abnormal bulges in the wall of an artery. Any artery can develop an aneurysm, although aneurysms are simultaneously most common and most dangerous when they occur within the largest artery of the body, the aorta* (called an abdominal aortic aneurysm* or thoracic aortic aneurysm, depending on its specific location), and when they occur within arteries of the brain (called intracerebral aneurysms). An aneurysm may be present at birth (congenital) or may occur over time.

Some of the same factors that cause the atherosclerosis responsible for coronary artery disease and peripheral artery disease can also increase an individual's risk for developing an aneurysm. Risk factors for aneurysm include being a male over age 60, having a family history of aneurysm, high blood pressure, smoking, high cholesterol, and excess alcohol intake. Additionally, aneurysms may occur in conjunction with a number of other medical conditions, such as Kawasaki syndrome, Marfan syndrome, presence of an abnormal bicuspid aortic valve, giant cell arteritis, polycystic kidney disease, systemic lupus erythematosus, and Ehler-Danlos syndrome. Initially, an aneurysm does not usually cause symptoms, but it will continue to expand over time very gradually. Clots may form over the area of an aneurysm, risking obstruction of the blood vessel. The clot may also break off of the site, travel through the blood circulation, and obstruct a vessel at a distance, causing death or disability. Alternatively, the aneurysm may eventually reach a size at which it presses on other structures, organs, or nerves in the vicinity, causing pain or disability. Most dangerous, as an aneurysm grows, the adjacent area of artery wall becomes thinner and more fragile. Eventually, the aneurysm may rupture (burst) and cause life-threatening hemorrhage* (bleeding).

Rupture of an aneurysm is a serious emergency. Symptoms of a ruptured aneurysm depend on its location. Rupture of an aortic aneurysm leads to severe abdominal and back pain, low blood pressure, dizziness, lightheadedness, and ultimately unconsciousness. Rupture of a brain aneurysm leads to stroke symptoms, such as severe headache, confusion, facial drooping, visual problems, problems speaking or understanding speech, difficulty walking, weakness or paralysis of the muscles on one side of the body. An aneurysm may be suspected when a physician discovers a pulsing abdominal mass during a physical examination, although aneurysms are often discovered incidentally during tests for other conditions. Tests to confirm the presence of an aneurysm include ultrasound, CT scan, and angiography.

Smaller aneurysms can be monitored over time, without specific treatment. Some aneurysms can be repaired and reinforced by permanently placing a graft made of artificial material into the area of artery where the aneurysm is located. A large aneurysm may call for surgery to remove the aneurysm and replace that area with a graft. A ruptured aneurysms requires immediate, emergency surgery. While coronary artery disease often runs in families, an individual's risk can be lowered by adhering to basic preventive measures, including maintaining a healthy weight, eating a low-fat/low-cholesterol diet, never smoking, drinking only moderate quantities of alcohol, exercising regularly, learning and practicing stress reduction, and following all directions for taking prescription medications to maintain normal blood cholesterol and blood pressure. Prevention of aneurysms requires practice of the same measures.

Raynaud's disease Raynaud's disease is an abnormality of the small arteries that bring blood to the fingers and toes. In this disease,

* **hemorrhage** (HEH-muh-rij) is uncontrolled or abnormal bleeding.

* **chemotherapy** (KEE-mo-THER-a-pee) is the treatment of cancer with powerful drugs that kill cancer cells.

* **ulcers** are open sores on the skin or the lining of a hollow body organ, such as the stomach or intestine. They may or may not be painful.

certain factors (exposure to cold temperatures or stressful and emotional situations) cause these arteries to spasm, preventing normal blood flow. About 75 percent of all Raynaud's sufferers are women between the ages of 15 and 40.

Risk factors for Raynaud's disease include repetitive stress injuries, exposure to certain chemicals, nicotine, caffeine, certain medicines (including chemotherapy* agents, drugs used to treat migraine headache or high blood pressure, nonprescription cold and allergy medicines, oral contraceptives); previous injury due to frostbite or other extreme cold exposure/hypothermia); and other diseases such as rheumatoid arthritis, Sjogren's syndrome, Buerger's disease, scleroderma, systemic lupus erythematosus, dermatomyositis, polymyositis, and atherosclerotic disease.

Symptoms of Raynaud's disease occur when the small arteries spasm, preventing blood and oxygen from reaching the tissues. The skin turns white or blue, very cold, numb, tingly, and painful. In severe cases, Raynaud's disease can result in poorly healing ulcers* and even gangrene and tissue death. Bouts may occur several times daily and may last between 15 minutes and several hours.

Raynaud's disease is often provisionally diagnosed based on the very characteristic symptoms that are reported. Testing can be done to confirm the condition, including a cold simulation test that uses temperature sensors affixed to the fingers to measure the response to cold exposure. Nailfold capillaroscopy involves placing a drop of oil on the skin at the base of fingernail, and then examining the area with a microscope, which may reveal the presence of abnormal blood vessels. A variety of blood tests may be done to evaluate for the presence of one of the conditions that are strongly associated with Raynaud's disease.

Raynaud's disease is treated by encouraging sensible lifestyle changes, such as avoidance of cold temperatures and use of gloves and mittens when they cannot be avoided. Known precipitants (factors that bring on attacks), such as medications, chemicals, activities, or stress should be avoided. A variety of medications may be used to improve dilatation of blood vessels. Aspirin and heparin may be used to prevent blood clotting. Very severe cases may require surgery to cut the nerve responsible for the spasms in small arteries or to perform a bypass to replace the length of malfunctioning blood vessel with a graft.

Buerger's disease Buerger's disease, also called thromboangiitis obliterans, occurs when small- and medium-sized arteries and veins develop severe inflammation. Although this rare condition is not due to the presence of atherosclerotic plaque, it can result in similar problems, because the inflamed arteries and veins become narrowed and significantly decrease blood flow. Organs and tissues are deprived of oxygen and nutrients. Blood clots may form within the inflamed blood vessels, resulting in further obstruction. Arms and legs are most frequently affected. Buerger's disease usually begins prior to the age of 40 and is more common in men, smokers, and people who live in Asia, the Far East, and the Middle East.

Symptoms of Buerger's disease include pain with activity and at rest, decreased sensation in the affected limb, poor healing, and open ulcers and sores. Over time, gangrene may develop, with the necessity of amputation (surgical removal of a body part). There is no one test that can definitely diagnose Buerger's disease. Blood tests and an echocardiogram may be done in order to rule out other disease. Angiography involves taking x-rays, CT scans, or MRI scans, after the injection of dye into blood vessels. This test allows any obstructions to be visualized.

The first step of treatment in Buerger's disease is smoking cessation. Very severe cases may require surgery to cut the nerve responsible for the spasm or to perform a bypass to replace the length of malfunctioning blood vessel with a graft. If gangrene develops, amputation may be necessary and life-saving. Although imperfect, avoiding smoking is the only potential form of prevention.

Varicose veins   Varicose veins are enlarged, twisted veins. Milder cases are simply a cosmetic annoyance; more severe cases can cause pain and disability. Varicose veins happen when there is increased back-pressure on the veins that are attempting to carry blood to the heart (for example, during pregnancy). Veins become less elastic, more extended, and unable to prevent the backflow of blood, due to weakening of the valves within the veins that normally keep blood flowing toward the heart. When blood accumulates within the veins, the veins stretch even more, become more enlarged, and begin to take on a gnarled, twisted appearance. Because the blood within the veins has already delivered oxygen to the tissues, it is bluer in color, which causes the varicose veins to appear very blue and more obvious under the skin.

About 15 percent of all men and 25 percent of all women in the United States have varicose veins. The tendency seems to run in families and increases with increasing age. Predisposing conditions include pregnancy, obesity, history of long periods of standing, and use of oral contraceptives or estrogen replacement therapy. Symptoms of varicose veins include their characteristic appearance of thick, winding, blue cords visible beneath the skin. Other symptoms may include a heavy, aching in the legs; itchiness in the area around visible veins; poorly healing sores; and the emergence of ulcers in the skin around the ankles.

Diagnosis is usually straightforward, because varicose veins are so visible. An ultrasound test of the affected veins may be performed to evaluate whether the valves are working, how hampered the blood flow is, and whether any blood clots are forming within the veins. Treatment usually begins with basic steps, such as maintaining a normal weight, exercising, avoiding tight clothing, avoiding prolonged sitting (with legs dangling) or standing, and keeping feet and legs elevated when possible. For more severe and symptomatic varicose veins, a number of procedures are available:

- Sclerotherapy (in which a caustic chemical solution is injected into affected veins, thus scarring them closed)
- Laser surgery (which uses light to get rid of the affected vein)

- Catheter-assisted procedures (in which a narrow, flexible tube is placed into a varicose vein; the tube heats the vein, causing it to seal closed)
- Vein stripping (the removal of veins through tiny incisions in the leg)
- Endoscopic vein surgery (which also removes the veins through tiny incisions, but requires the insertion of a tiny camera in order to visualize, close, and remove the affected vein)

Clotting disorders   Clotting disorders include both conditions that prevent normal blood clotting and those that promote abnormal blood clotting.

BLEEDING DISORDERS   Bleeding disorders are diseases that interfere with the blood's ability to form a clot. Twenty different clotting factors are involved in the ability of the blood to clot normally; absence or deficiency in any of these factors can result in a tendency to bleed. Types of bleeding disorders include von Willebrand's disease and various forms of hereditary hemophilia, such as hemophilia A (also called classic hemophilia or factor VIII deficiency), hemophilia B (also called Christmas disease or factor IX deficiency), and hemophilia C (also called factor XI deficiency). People with bleeding disorders are at risk of severe bleeding and hemorrhage from seemingly minor cuts or trauma. Severe hemophiliacs can begin to bleed spontaneously, resulting in unexpected gushing nosebleeds, severe bruising, bleeding into the joints, or bleeding from the gastrointestinal or urinary tract.

Hemophilia is an inherited disorder, often affecting many members of a family. Some types of hemophilia only affect males; other types can strike either males or females. Hemophilia is often suspected due to a family history of the disorder, although some mild cases are only diagnosed after an injury or surgical procedure results in excess bleeding. Blood tests may reveal a lack of specific clotting factors associated with hemophilia or decreased levels of the specific protein (von Willebrand factor) deficient in von Willebrand's disease. Treatment of hemophilia may require infusions of fresh frozen plasma (fluid part of blood) or specific clotting factors to help stop or prevent bleeding.

HYPERCOAGULATION DISORDERS   The opposite of hemophilia occurs when the blood has a tendency to clot too easily, resulting in the formation of thromboses (blood clots) that can obstruct the blood circulation, causing ischemia (oxygen deprivation) in tissues or organs that are unable to receive normal blood flow. One form of this condition is called deep-vein thrombosis or DVT, in which clots form spontaneously in the deep veins of the legs. A DVT will cause swelling in the affected leg, as well as warmth, redness, and pain in the area of the clot. This condition is particularly dangerous, because pieces of the clot (or the entire clot) can break loose, travel through the bloodstream, and obstruct blood vessels. The blood clot can lodge in the heart, resulting in heart attack; the lungs (pulmonary embolism), resulting in extreme difficulty breathing or even respiratory arrest; or brain (resulting in stroke).

Hypercoagulation (excessive clotting) may be hereditary (as in protein S deficiency) or acquired. People at risk of developing thromboses include women who are using oral contraceptives, estrogen replacement therapy, or who are pregnant; smokers; cancer patients; people who have recently had surgery or suffered trauma; hospitalized or debilitated patients; and individuals who are obese and/or sedentary. Diagnosis of hypercoagulation disorders usually involves demonstrating the presence of a DVT, via ultrasound, CT, MRI or venography (in which dye is injected into the vein and images are taken that can reveal the presence of a blood clot). Blood tests may reveal an elevation of a substance called D dimmer. Treatment of hypercoagulation requires anticoagulation via blood thinner medications such as heparin and warfarin.

Lymphedema Lymphedema occurs when there is an obstruction in the lymphatic system*, reducing the normal flow of lymph (clear fluid that contains white blood cells) through the lymph vessels. As lymph fluid backs up, the vessels become leaky, allowing the fluid to seep out into the surrounding tissues and causing swelling in the affected arm or leg or other part of the body.

Lymphedema can occur due to congenital (present at birth) malformation of the lymph vessels, as occurs in a number of diseases, including Milroy disease (congenital lymphedema); Meige disease (lymphedema praecox); and lymphedema tarda (late-onset lymphedema). Lymphedema can also occur in the following situations:

- After injury or disease damages the lymph vessels, such as after surgery that involves removal of lymph nodes or vessels (for example, due to a lymph node dissection during a mastectomy*)

- Due to scarring from radiation treatment

- Due to obstruction of lymph vessels by cancer cells or pressure from a nearby expanding tumor*

- After traumatic injury involving lymph vessels

- Due to parasitic infection that blocks the lymph vessels (such as filiariasis, also known as elephantiasis)

The diagnosis may be quite obvious, depending on the individual's history, but further visualization of the area may be obtained through ultrasound, MRI or CT scans, or lymphoscintigraphy, during which radioactive dye is injected into the lymph vessels. Subsequent imaging of the dye flow can reveal the location of a lymphatic obstruction.

Treatment of lymphedema includes special exercises or massage to encourage better lymph flow; the wearing of elastic pressure bandages and special compression garments (such as a sleeve, stockings, or glove) to improve lymph flow back towards the heart; or the application of a pneumatic pressure device to "milk" the lymph fluid back into circulation. Prevention focuses on those individuals at particularly high risk of

* **lymphatic system** (lim-FAH-tik) is a system that contains lymph nodes and a network of channels that carry fluid and cells of the immune system through the body.

* **mastectomy** (mas-TEK-to-mee) is the surgical removal of the breast.

* **tumor** (TOO-mor) is an abnormal growth of body tissue that has no known cause or physiologic purpose. A tumor may or may not be cancerous.

developing lymphedema, such as women who have undergone mastectomy with lymph node dissection. These individuals should treat their at-risk limb with particular care, keeping it scrupulously clean; avoiding injury; carefully treating even small scratches, cuts or punctures; keeping it elevated above heart-level; avoiding application of heat; and making sure that clothing is not overly constricting.

▶ *See also* **Aneurysm**

Resources

Books and Articles

Ferri, Fred, ed. *Ferri's Clinical Advisor 2008.* Philadelphia, PA: Mosby Elsevier, 2008.

Sutton, Amy L., ed. *Blood and Circulatory Disorders Sourcebook,* 2nd ed. Detroit, MI: Omnigraphics, 2005.

Organizations

American Heart Association. 7272 Greenville Avenue, Dallas, TX, 75231-4596. Toll free: 800-AHA-USA1. Web site: http://www.americanheart.org/presenter.jhtml?identifier=1200000.

National Heart, Lung, and Blood Institute. P.O. Box 30105, Bethesda, MD, 20824-0105. Telephone: 301-592-8573. Web site: http://www.nhlbi.nih.gov/index.htm.

National Hemophilia Foundation. 116 West 32nd Street, 11th Floor, New York, NY, 10001. Telephone: 212-0328-3700. Web site: http://www.hemophilia.org.

Vascular Disease Foundation. 1075 S. Yukon, Suite 320, Lakewood, CO, 80226. Telephone: 303-989-0500. Web site: http://www.aad.org.

Venous Thrombosis *See Phlebitis and Venous Thrombosis.*

Vertigo

Vertigo (VER-ti-go) is dizziness which causes people to feel that they or their surroundings are moving, often causing loss of balance.

What Is Vertigo?

Vertigo is different from other forms of dizziness because it is caused by disturbances in the structures that control the sense of balance. These structures include the vestibule and semicircular canals in the ear, the vestibular (ves-TIB-u-lar) nuclei in the brain stem*, and the eyes. There are many different kinds of vertigo.

Benign paroxysmal vertigo of childhood Benign* paroxysmal (par-ok-SIZ-mal) vertigo is a condition that sometimes affects toddlers, who may suddenly lose their balance, roll their eyes, and become pale, dizzy, or nauseated for a few minutes. They usually recover quickly and often outgrow this form of vertigo.

Positional vertigo Positional vertigo may occur following changes in head position, especially when lying on one ear or when tipping back the head to look up. The symptoms tend to appear in clusters that last for several days. The vertigo begins several seconds after head movement and usually stops in under a minute. Some of the causes of positional vertigo are trauma to the ear, an ear infection, ear surgery, or degeneration due to aging inner ear organs that are involved in balance. Surgery can sometimes correct positional vertigo.

Ménière's disease Sometimes called Ménière's syndrome or recurrent aural vertigo, Ménière's disease is caused by damage to the balance organs in the ears, although doctors often do not know the cause of the damage. In addition to vertigo, symptoms are likely to include tinnitus (ti-NY-tis), which is a ringing, buzzing, or roaring in the ears. It may also cause gradual deafness in the affected ear. Ménière's disease can be controlled with medication, but it cannot be cured.

Labyrinthitis Labyrinthitis (lab-i-rin-THY-tis) is an inflammation of the labyrinth in the inner ear, possibly as a result of viral infection in the upper respiratory tract. The labyrinth is a group of canals in the inner ear that is important for balance. Symptoms of labyrinthitis are sudden onset of severe vertigo lasting for several days, hearing loss, and tinnitus in the affected ear. During the recovery period, which may last several weeks, rapid head movement causes temporary vertigo.

Vestibular neuronitis Vestibular neuronitis (noo-ro-NY-tis) is sometimes called epidemic vertigo and is thought to be the result of a virus that causes inflammation of the vestibular nerve cells. Vestibular neuronitis usually causes a single attack of severe vertigo with nausea and vomiting that lasts for a few days. There is no hearing loss or tinnitus, and doctors often prescribe medication to help with the dizziness and nausea.

Traumatic vertigo Traumatic vertigo is one of the most common types of vertigo. It usually follows a head injury. The symptoms generally start to improve within several days but may last for weeks. Deafness

* **brain stem** is the part of the brain that connects to the spinal cord. The brain stem controls the basic functions of life, such as breathing and blood pressure.

* **benign** (be-NINE) means a condition is not cancerous or serious and will probably improve, go away, or not get worse.

often accompanies the vertigo on the side of the head that received the trauma. In some cases, surgery may be required to correct damage to the ear structures.

Acoustic neuromas Acoustic neuromas are benign tumors that form in the vestibular nerve, affecting nerve signals for balance and hearing from the ear to the brain. Symptoms are hearing loss, tinnitus, dizziness, and unsteadiness. Surgery to remove the tumor improves the vertigo.

How Do Doctors Treat Vertigo?

Doctors often prescribe medication to reduce the dizziness, nausea, and sense of motion of vertigo. Other treatments vary according to the cause of the vertigo.

▶ *See also* **Deafness and Hearing Loss • Motion Sickness • Otitis (Ear Infections) • Tinnitus**

Resources

Books and Articles

Poe, Dennis, ed. *The Consumer Handbook on Dizziness and Vertigo.* Sedona, AZ: Auricle Ink, 2005.

Organizations

National Institute on Deafness and Other Communication Disorders, National Institutes of Health. 31 Center Drive, MSC 2320, Bethesda, MD, 20892-2320. Toll free: 800-241-1044. Web site: http://www.nidcd.nih.gov.

National Library of Medicine. 8600 Rockville Pike, Bethesda, MD, 20894, Web site: http://www.nlm.nih.gov/medlineplus/dizzinessandvertigo.html.

Vestibular Disorders Association. P.O. Box 13305, Portland, OR, 97213-0305, Web site: http://www.vestibular.org.

Violence

Violence is the use of physical force to injure people or property. Violence may cause physical pain to those who experience it directly, as well as emotional distress to those who either experience or witness it. Individuals, families, schools, workplaces, communities, national societies, and local and global environments all are harmed by violence.

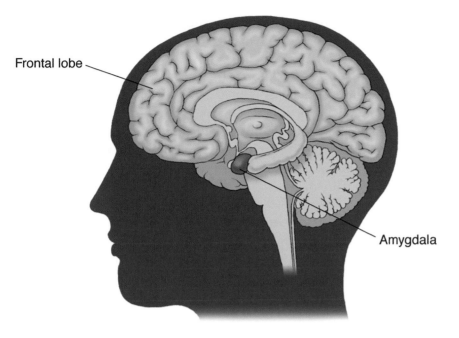

Frontal lobe

Amygdala

The frontal lobe and amygdala are the parts of the human brain affected by anger and violence. *Illustration by Frank Forney. Reproduced by permission of Gale, a part of Cengage Learning.*

What Is Violence?

Violence is a social and health problem for all who experience and witness it. Violence takes many forms, including:

- Family violence, often referred to as domestic abuse, child abuse, child maltreatment, spouse abuse, and wife battering
- Peer group violence, which includes workplace violence, school violence, gang violence, and bullying*
- Sexual violence, which includes rape*, date rape, marital rape, intimate partner abuse, and child sexual abuse
- Abuse of power, which includes mistreatment of children, students, elders, people with disabilities, and others who are smaller or less powerful than the abuser
- Community violence, which includes assaults, fights, shootings, homicides, and most forms of peer violence
- Hate crimes and hate speech, which target victims based on gender, age, race, ethnicity, religious belief, or sexual orientation
- Media violence, shown on television, in film, and in video games.

Why Do People Behave Violently?

Research indicates that violent behavior may have many different causes, some of which are inborn but most of which are learned from experiencing or witnessing violent behavior by others, particularly those who are role models.

Genetics   Chromosomes carry genetic messages from parents to offspring, and there is some research that suggests that, in some cases, aggressiveness may be inherited.

* **bullying** is when a person repeatedly intimidates or acts aggressively toward those with less power or ability to defend themselves.

* **rape** is when a person forces another person to have sexual intercourse, or engage in other unwanted sexual activities.

What Is Wrong with Media Violence?

Research indicates that media violence can lead to real violence in multiple ways. The surgeon general and the National Institute of Mental Health have both reported that watching violence depicted on television is an important predictor of aggressive behavior. Children's cartoons and music videos in particular often portray violence. American children see about 16,000 simulated murders and 200,000 acts of violence on television by age 18. In nearly 75 percent of those cases, punishment is not shown to be a consequence of violent behavior.

Perhaps even more serious is the link between violence and some interactive video games. During violent video games, the player identifies with the point of view of the aggressor and imitates or enacts violent thoughts, feelings, and simulated actions. For some people, with enough reinforcement, violent behaviors can become accessible or even automatic if and when the player later encounters conflict in real life.

Brain injury   Injury to the front parts of the brain may remove some personal control over anger and aggression.

Antisocial personality disorder   People with antisocial personality disorder often behave violently even as children. They may disregard their own safety and the safety of others. People with this disorder do not seem to understand that violence harms other people, and they do not seem to have a conscience that distinguishes between right and wrong. The terms sociopath and psychopath sometimes are used to describe people with antisocial personality disorder.

Alcohol and substance abuse   Drinking and drugs often play a role in violence. For some, these substances interfere with otherwise good judgment or behavior. Some people try to use alcohol or drugs to treat their feelings of anger or depression, but instead feel worse. Violence toward others—or towards themselves—can result.

Desensitization   Constantly viewing violence at home, in communities, or on television can lead people to believe that violence is a normal part of life. People who are surrounded by violence may reach a point at which they no longer notice violent events or remember that peaceful behavior is a possibility.

Learned helplessness   People who accept the belief that violence is an inevitable part of their lives may give up trying to avoid or escape that violence. They may become passive and unable to create safety for themselves or their families. Battered wives who remain at home with battering husbands, for example, may believe that that they are unable to escape violence. This resignation to violence exposes them to more of it.

Social modeling   Children learn by observation and by imitation. Children who observe their home, school, or media role models behaving in violent ways may come to believe that turning angry feelings into angry actions is acceptable behavior or even the most effective way to solve problems. Such children may never learn peaceful behaviors or cooperative ways to solve problems.

Parents who model abusive behavior at home can create a cycle of violence, teaching children to grow up to be abusive adults. The importance of positive role models and the dangers of negative role models should not be underestimated.

Learning the boundaries between anger (emotion) and violence (physical force) is an important developmental task for all people and all cultures. It is possible to have angry feelings without turning those feelings into angry actions or violent behaviors. Expressing anger in a nonviolent way can be healthy. However, parents, adult mentors, media, and community leaders first must model nonviolent conflict-resolution skills for young people to learn them.

SOCIAL MODELING AND SELF-REGULATION

Social psychologist Albert Bandura (b. 1925) began studying social modeling, observational learning, aggression, and self-regulation in the 1970s. Bandura's theories suggest that role models (social modeling) can influence people toward creativity or toward violence. If children observe violent behavior at home, in school, or on television, they may come to believe that turning angry feelings into angry actions is acceptable behavior. When these children become angry themselves, they may display the behaviors they have observed, and they even may create new angry behaviors that go beyond what they have learned from their models.

Another important aspect of Bandura's research focused on self-direction and self-efficacy or people's beliefs about their own abilities to influence and affect the world around them. If children observe adults failing to control their own angry feelings or violent behaviors or if they observe violent behavior going unpunished, they may come to believe that peaceful behaviors cannot succeed or are not worthwhile activities. They may lose their motivation to learn cooperative problem-solving skills, or they may quit before they achieve success in using these skills.

* **post-traumatic stress disorder** (post-traw-MAT-ik STRES dis-OR-der) is a mental disorder that interferes with everyday living and occurs in people who survive a terrifying event, such as school violence, military combat, or a natural disaster.

How Is Violence Treated and Prevented?

People who experience or witness violence should react immediately. Police and violence hotlines should be called in an emergency. People who have been injured should be taken to a clinic or hospital emergency room for treatment. When an immediate crisis has ended, a family doctor or school counselor or member of the clergy should be contacted for counseling and referrals. Shelters and child protection agencies can help battered women and children. Counseling can help batterers and their families to learn better behaviors for managing stress, conflict, and anger. Therapists can help people with post-traumatic stress disorder* achieve emotional recovery from the aftermath of violence.

Those who commit violent acts or have violent or angry feelings need to receive treatment. Emotional problems, drug and alcohol abuse, and other conditions which make a person more prone to violence need to be handled. The social forces that prevent violence—family, friends, and the community—need to take positive steps to make violence less likely and to increase safety.

Physical violence is never an acceptable form of behavior. Everyone has choices. Becoming aware of the problems, deciding not to follow violent patterns, and making a commitment to learn new ways of relating are the keys to change and increased wellness. It is never too late to change the pattern of violence in families, communities, or society.

▶ *See also* **Antisocial Personality Disorder • Conduct Disorder • Oppositional Defiant Disorder • Personality and Personality Disorders • Post-Traumatic Stress Disorder • Rape**

Resources

Books and Articles

Armitage, Ronda. *Violence in Society: The Impact on Our Lives.* Chicago: Raintree, 2004.

Jones-Smith, Elsie. *Nurturing Nonviolent Children: A Guide for Parents, Educators, and Counselors.* Westport, CT: Praeger, 2008.

Monteverde, Matthew. *Making Smart Choices about Violence, Gangs, and Bullying.* New York: Rosen Publishings Rosen Central, 2008.

Organizations

Center for the Prevention of School Violence. 313 Chapanoke Road, Suite 140, Raleigh, NC, 27603. Toll free: 800-299-6054. Web site: http://www.ncsu.edu/cpsv.

Centers for Disease Control and Prevention. 1600 Clifton Road, Atlanta, GA, 30333. Toll free: 800-311-3435. Web site: http://www.cdc.gov.

National Institute of Mental Health. Science Writing, Press, and Dissemination Branch, 6001 Executive Boulevard, Room 8184, MSC 9663, Bethesda, MD, 20892-9663. Toll free: 866-615-6464. Web site: http://www.nimh.nih.gov/health/topics/child-and-adolescent-mental-health/children-and-violence.shtml.

Viral Infections

Viral infections occur when viruses enter cells in the body and begin reproducing, often causing illness. Viruses are tiny germs that can reproduce only by invading a living cell.

How Are Viruses Different from Bacteria?

Viruses are far smaller than bacteria. They are so small that they could not be seen until the electron microscope was invented in the 1940s. Unlike most bacteria, viruses are not complete cells that can function on their own. They cannot convert carbohydrates to energy, the way that bacteria and other living cells do. Viruses depend on other organisms for energy.

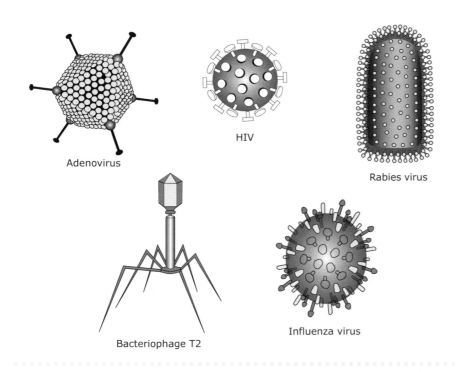

Adenovirus

HIV

Rabies virus

Bacteriophage T2

Influenza virus

There are thousands of kinds of viruses. Most consist only of tiny particles of genetic material surrounded by a coat of protein and sometimes an outer envelope. Specific viruses attach themselves to the outsides of specific host cells, and then work their way inside through the host's outer membranes. Once inside their host cells, the viruses reproduce. The new viruses can destroy their host cells and then move on to attack new host cells. *Illustration by Frank Forney. Reproduced by permission of Gale, a part of Cengage Learning.*

◀

Moreover, viruses cannot reproduce unless they get inside a living cell. Most viruses consist only of tiny particles of nucleic acid (the material that makes up genes) surrounded by a coat of protein. Some have an outer envelope as well.

Thousands of viruses There are thousands of viruses, and in humans they cause a wide range of diseases. For instance, rhinoviruses cause colds, influenza viruses cause flu, adenoviruses* cause various respiratory problems, and rotaviruses cause gastroenteritis. Polioviruses can make their way to the spinal cord and cause paralysis, whereas coxsackieviruses (sometimes written as Coxsackie viruses) and echoviruses* sometimes infect the heart or the membranes surrounding the spinal cord or lungs. Herpesviruses cause cold sores, chickenpox, and genital herpes, which is a sexually transmitted disease. Other viruses cause a variety of conditions from measles and mumps to AIDS.

The body's defense system Most viruses do not cause serious diseases and are killed by the body's immune system*—its network of natural defenses. In many cases, people never even know they have been infected. But unlike bacteria, which can be killed by antibiotics, most viruses are not affected by existing medicines. Fortunately, scientists have been able to make vaccines, which help the body develop natural defenses to prevent many viral infections.

How Do Viruses Infect the Body?

Viruses can enter the human body through any of its openings, but most often they use the nose and mouth. Once inside, the virus attaches itself to the outside of the kind of cell it attacks, called a host cell. For example,

Are Viruses Alive?

It would seem to be a simple matter to determine if something is alive. But biologists disagree on whether viruses are a form of life.

Viruses lack certain features that other forms of life have. They cannot convert carbohydrates, proteins, or fats into energy, a process called metabolism. They cannot reproduce on their own but must enter a living cell and use the host cell's energy. Yet, like all life forms, viruses do have genes made of nucleic acid that contain the information they need to reproduce.

Biologists have an elaborate way of classifying every form of life. Each is grouped into a kingdom (such as the animal kingdom) and smaller subcategories called the phylum, class, genus, and species.

Bacteria and fungi each have a kingdom of their own, but viruses are left out of this system. Many biologists think that, unlike the forms of life grouped into kingdoms, viruses did not evolve (develop) as a group. Instead, viruses may have developed individually from the kind of cells they now infect—animal cells, plant cells, or bacteria.

The replication of a virus. *Chart by Hans & Cassidy. Reproduced by permission of Gale, a part of Cengage Learning.*

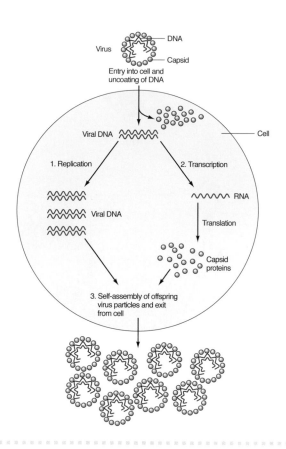

---

* **adenoviruses** (ah-deh-no-VY-ruh-sez) are a type of viruses that can produce a variety of symptoms, including upper respiratory disease, when they infect humans.

* **echoviruses** a group of viruses found in the intestinal tract. The word echo in the name is acronym for enteric cytopathic human orphan viruses. When these viruses were named, they were not associated with any disease, hence the use of the word orphan. However, later these viruses were associated with various diseases, including meningitis and encephalitis.

* **immune system** (im-YOON SIS-tem) is the system of the body composed of specialized cells and the substances they produce that helps protect the body against disease-causing germs.

a rhinovirus attacks cells in the nose, whereas an enterovirus binds to cells in the stomach and intestines. Then the virus works its way through the host cell's outer membrane.

After entering the cell, the virus begins making identical viruses from the host cell's protein. These new viruses may make their way back out through the host cell's membrane, sometimes destroying the cell, and then attacking new host cells. This process continues until the body develops enough antibodies* and other defenses to defeat the viral invaders.

Not all viruses attack only one part of the body, causing what is called a localized infection. Some viruses spread through the bloodstream or the nerves, attacking cells throughout the body. For instance, HIV*, the human immunodeficiency virus that causes AIDS*, attacks certain cells of the immune system that are located throughout the body.

How Long Do Viral Infections Last?

In most types of viral infection, the immune system clears the virus from the body within days to a few weeks. But some viruses cause persistent or latent* infections, which can last for years. In these cases, a person may get infected and seem to recover or may not be aware of being infected at all. Then years later, the illness occurs again, or symptoms start for the first time. Viruses that can cause latent infections include herpesviruses, Hepatitis B and C viruses, and HIV.

How Do Viruses Cause Illness?

Viruses can cause illness by destroying or interfering with the functioning of large numbers of important cells. Sometimes, as mentioned earlier, the cell is destroyed when the newly created viruses leave it. Sometimes the virus keeps the cell from producing the energy it needs to live, or the virus upsets the cell's chemical balance in some other way. Sometimes the virus seems to trigger a mysterious process called "programmed cell death" or apoptosis (ap-op-TO-sis) that kills the cell.

Some persistent or latent viral infections seem to transform cells into a cancerous state that makes them grow out of control. It has been estimated that 10 to 20 percent of cancers are caused by viral infections. The most common are liver cancer caused by persistent infection with hepatitis B or hepatitis C virus and cancer of the cervix (the bottom of a woman's uterus or womb), both of which are linked to certain strains of the human papillomavirus.

Sometimes a viral illness is caused not by the virus itself, but by the body's reaction to it. The immune system may kill cells in order to get rid of the virus that is inside them. This process can cause serious illness if the cells being killed are very important to the body's functioning, such as those in the lungs or central nervous system, or if the cells cannot reproduce quickly enough to replace the ones being destroyed.

How Are Viral Infections Diagnosed and Treated?

Symptoms   Symptoms vary widely, depending on the virus and the organs involved. Many viruses, like many bacteria, cause fever, and either respiratory symptoms (coughing and sneezing) or intestinal symptoms (nausea, vomiting, diarrhea). Viral illnesses often cause high fevers in young children, even when the illnesses are not dangerous.

Diagnosis   Some viral infections, such as influenza, the common cold, and chickenpox, are easily recognized by their symptoms and no lab tests are needed. For many others, such as viral hepatitis, AIDS, and mononucleosis, a blood sample is analyzed for the presence of specific antibodies to the virus. If present, these antibodies help confirm the diagnosis. In some cases, a virus may be grown in the laboratory, using a technique called tissue culture*, or identified by its nucleic acid, using a technique called polymerase chain reaction (PCR). Tests such as tissue culture or PCR are used when antibody tests are not precise enough or when the actual amount of a virus in the body must be determined.

Treatment   Viruses cannot be treated with the antibiotics that kill bacteria. Fortunately, a few drugs, such as ribavirin and acyclovir, can control the spread of viral invaders without destroying host cells. Intense research to find better treatments for AIDS led to development of many drugs

* **antibodies** (AN-tih-bah-deez) are protein molecules produced by the body's immune system to help fight specific infections caused by microorganisms, such as bacteria and viruses.

* **HIV** or human immunodeficiency virus (HYOO-mun ih-myoo-no-dih-FIH-shen-see), is the virus that causes AIDS (acquired immunodeficiency syndrome).

* **AIDS** or acquired immunodeficiency (ih-myoo-no-dih-FIH-shen-see) syndrome, is an infection that severely weakens the immune system; it is caused by the human immunodeficiency virus (HIV).

* **latent** infections are dormant or hidden illnesses that do not show the signs and symptoms of active diseases.

* **culture** (KUL-chur) is a test in which a sample of fluid or tissue from the body is placed in a dish containing material that supports the growth of certain organisms. Typically, within days the organisms will grow and can be identified.

What Is a 24-Hour Virus?

When people have a mild illness—perhaps fever and an upset stomach, perhaps nausea and diarrhea—they often say they have a "24-hour virus" or a "stomach virus." Many viruses can cause these kinds of symptoms, but there are many other possible causes as well, including bacterial infection or bacterial food poisoning. People usually recover from these brief or mild illnesses before doctors can do the tests that determine the causes. So a "stomach virus" may or may not be a virus at all.

that help fight the virus. Unfortunately, as of 2009, none of these drugs was able to treat viral infections as effectively as antibiotics treat bacterial infections.

How Are Viral Infections Prevented?

Hygiene and sanitation   The first step in preventing the spread of viral infections is simply to practice good hygiene. Doing so involves washing the hands often, and eating only food that has been prepared properly. It also involves building and maintaining facilities for getting rid of sewage safely and for providing clean drinking water.

Vaccination   Another important preventive measure is immunizing people against viruses. Immunization involves giving people vaccines that stimulate the immune system to make antibodies, proteins that target a specific germ. Vaccines to prevent hepatitis B, polio, mumps, measles, rubella (German measles), and chickenpox are usually given to babies and young children in the United States. Vaccines also can prevent influenza and hepatitis A.

Vaccines are useful only against certain kinds of viruses. For example, the polioviruses that cause poliomyelitis (polio), a great crippler of children in the past, are few in number and relatively stable. So it was possible in the 1950s to make a vaccine that protects children from getting polio (although the illness still occurs in the developing world where fewer children are vaccinated). By contrast, influenza viruses change in minor ways every few years and in a major way about every ten years, so a flu vaccine is useful for only a year or two.

One reason a vaccine for the common cold has never been developed is that there are at least a hundred different rhinoviruses that cause colds, and as of 2009 it had not been possible to make a vaccine that works against all of them. A similar problem with HIV, which has many different and fast-changing strains (variations), is one of several reasons why progress toward an AIDS vaccine was slow.

Resources

Books and Articles

Shors, Teri. *Understanding Viruses.* Sudbury, MA: Jones and Bartlett, 2009.

Sonenklar, Carol. *Virus Hunters.* Brookfield, CT: Twenty-First Century Books, 2003.

Organizations

American Society for Microbiology. 1752 N Street, NW, Washington, DC, 20036-2904. Telephone: 202-737-3600. Web site: http://www.microbeworld.org/microbes/virus.

HealthInsite. Editorial Team Service Access Programs Branch, Department of Health and Ageing, MDP 2, GPO Box 9848, Canberra, ACT, 2601, Australia. Telephone: 02 6289 8488. Web site: http://www.healthinsite.gov.au/topics/Viral_Infections.

Karolinska Institutet. SE-171 77, Stockholm, Sweden. Telephone: +46 8 524 800 00. Web site: http://www.mic.ki.se/Diseases/C02.html.

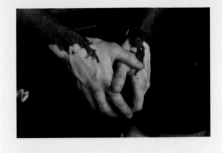

The hands of a person with vitiligo.
© *Bruce Coleman Inc./Alamy.*

> **Vitamin Deficiencies** *See Dietary Deficiencies.*

* **pigment** (PIG-ment) is a substance that imparts color to another substance.

* **immune system** (im-YOON SIS-tem) is the system of the body composed of specialized cells and the substances they produce that helps protect the body against disease-causing germs.

Vitiligo

Vitiligo is a condition that causes white patches of skin due to a loss of pigment in the cells and tissues of the body.

What Is Vitiligo?

Melanocytes (MEL-a-no-sites) are special skin cells that make the pigment* that colors the skin, hair, eyes, and body linings. If these cells die or cannot make pigment, the affected skin gets lighter or completely white, causing vitiligo (vit-i-LY-go). The hair in affected areas also may turn white, and people with dark skin may notice a loss of color inside their mouths. No one knows for sure what makes melanocytes die or stop working in vitiligo.

Who Gets Vitiligo?

Vitiligo affects people of all races and both sexes equally. It affects one or two out of every 100 people. About half of all people who have vitiligo begin to lose pigment before they are 20 years of age.

Vitiligo is common in people with certain immune system* diseases and in children with parents who have the condition. However, most people with vitiligo have no immune system disease, and most children will not get vitiligo even if a parent has it. In fact, most people with vitiligo are in good general health and do not have a family history of the condition.

Vitiligo is more obvious in people with dark skin. Light-skinned people may notice the contrast between patches of vitiligo and areas of suntanned skin in the summer. The amount of pigment that is lost varies from person to person. The first white patches often occur on the hands, feet, arms, face, or lips. Other common areas for patches to appear are the

* **ultraviolet** light is a wavelength of light beyond visible light; on the spectrum of light, it falls between the violet end of visible light and x-rays.

armpits, the groin (the area where the inner thighs join the trunk), and around the navel (belly button) and genitals.

There is no way to know if vitiligo will spread to other parts of the body, but it usually does spread over time. For some people, this spread occurs rapidly, but for other people, it takes place over many years. Both sides of the body usually are affected in a similar way. There may be a few patches or there may be many.

How Is Vitiligo Diagnosed and Treated?

Diagnosis To diagnose vitiligo, the doctor may ask about the person's symptoms, whether the person has an immune system disorder, and whether vitiligo runs in the person's family. The doctor also may suggest various tests to rule out other medical problems that can cause light skin patches.

Treatment Vitiligo does not always need treatment. For some people with light skin, simply avoiding a suntan on areas of normal skin is enough to make the patches of vitiligo almost unnoticeable. Other people use makeup, skin dyes, or self-tanning products to cover up the vitiligo. Self-tanning products are creams that give the skin a tan color, but not a true tan. The color tends to wear off after a few days. These strategies do not change the condition, but they can make the vitiligo less noticeable. In children, vitiligo usually is just covered up.

In adults, if covering up the vitiligo is not enough, a medical treatment may be tried, although results often cannot be seen for 6 to 18 months. The choice of treatment depends on the person's wishes, how many white patches the person has, and how widespread the patches are. Not every treatment works for every person. There are several choices:

- Corticosteroid (kor-ti-ko-STEER-oid) creams can be applied to the skin and sometimes can return color to small areas of vitiligo.

- Psoralen (SOR-a-len) and ultraviolet* therapy entails taking medication by mouth or applied to the skin and then exposing the light patches of skin to ultraviolet A light from a special lamp. Ultraviolet A is the part of sunlight that can cause the skin to tan, and psoralens are substances that react with ultraviolet light to darken the skin.

- Skin grafting is an operation that involves moving skin from normal areas to white patches. It is useful only for a small number of people with vitiligo.

- Depigmentation therapy involves using medication to fade the normal skin to match the whitened areas of vitiligo.

Living with Vitiligo

The white patches of vitiligo have no natural protection from the sun and are very easily sunburned. People with vitiligo should be careful to avoid exposure to midday sun, to cover up with clothing and a hat, and to use a sunscreen with a high SPF (sun protection factor) rating.

▶ *See also* **Immune Deficiencies • Skin Conditions**

Resources

Books and Articles

Thomas, Lee. *Turning White: A Memoir of Change.* Troy, MI: Momentum Books, 2007.

Organizations

American Academy of Dermatology. P.O. Box 4014, Schaumburg, IL, 60168-4014. Toll free: 866-503-SKIN. Web site: http://www.aad.org/public/publications/pamphlets/common_vitilgo.html.

National Institute of Arthritis and Musculoskeletal and Skin Diseases. 1 AMS Circle, Bethesda, MD, 20892-3675. Toll free: 877-226-4267. Web site: http://www.niams.nih.gov/health_info/Vitiligo/default.asp.

National Vitiligo Foundation. P.O. Box 23226, Cincinnati, OH, 45223. Telephone: 513-541-3903. Web site: http://nvfi.org.

W

Wall Eyes *See Strabismus.*

Warts

Warts are small growths on the skin or inner linings of the body that are caused by a type of virus.

What Are Warts?

Warts are small areas of hardened skin that can grow on almost any part of the body. Human papilloma (pah-pih-LO-mah) viruses, or HPV, causes warts. More than 100 different kinds, or strains, of HPV exist. Warts are usually skin-colored and bumpy or rough, but sometimes they are dark and smooth. The way a wart looks depends on where it is growing, and different kinds of warts appear on different parts of the body.

Common warts usually grow on fingers and hands, especially around fingernails. These warts usually have a rough, bumpy surface with tiny black dots, which are the blood vessels that feed the wart and allow it to grow. Flat warts are much smaller than common warts and are very smooth. This type of wart typically grows in little bunches on the face and legs; as many as 100 flat warts may grow together in one place. Common warts and flat warts generally are not painful except under certain circumstances, such as when the pressure of a pencil pushes against a wart on the finger while writing. Plantar warts, which grow on the soles of the feet, can be quite painful as a person walks on them, flattening them and pushing them back into the skin. Like a common wart, a plantar wart is covered with black dots marking the place of blood vessels.

Genital warts are small and pink, and they can grow one at a time or in bunches that make them look a bit like cauliflower. This type of wart can grow on the genitals*, the skin around the genitals, the rectum*, the buttocks, or in the vagina* or cervix*. Although most warts do not cause major health problems, genital warts may itch or bleed, and the ones caused by some strains of HPV are known to increase a woman's chances of developing cancer of the cervix without causing a wart.

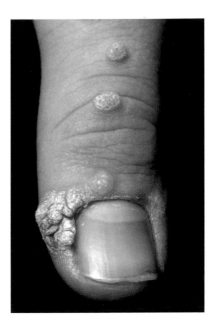

▲

Warts commonly appear on the fingertips, where skin is more likely to be broken and susceptible to HPV infection. *Medical-on-Line/Alamy.*

* **genitals** (JEH-nih-tuls) are the external sexual organs.

* **rectum** is the final portion of the large intestine, connecting the colon to the outside opening of the anus.

* **vagina** (vah-JY-nah) is the canal, or passageway, in a woman that leads from the uterus to the outside of the body.

* **cervix** (SIR-viks) is the lower, narrow end of the uterus that opens into the vagina.

* **immune system** (im-YOON SIS-tem) is the system of the body composed of specialized cells and the substances they produce that helps protect the body against disease-causing germs.

* **chronic** (KRAH-nik) lasting a long time or recurring frequently.

* **pelvic exam** is an internal examination of a woman's reproductive organs.

* **Pap smear** is a common diagnostic test used to look for cancerous cells in the tissue of the cervix.

WARTS MYTHS

Warts have a long history in folklore, and the myths about them abound. Touching a frog, for example, has been thought both to cause and to cure warts. Other unconventional treatments have become popular. Among the many wart so-called remedies, none of which has been proven to work, are the following:

■ Put pebbles in a bag with a silver coin. Then tie up the bag and throw it in the street. The person who finds the money and keeps it will also keep the warts.

■ Rub a dirty washcloth on the warts. Next, bury the washcloth by the light of the full moon.

■ Make the wart bleed. Put one drop of blood on seven grains of corn and feed it to a black hen.

■ Apply a piece of raw meat to the warts and then bury the meat. As it decays underground, the warts will disappear.

■ Mix brown soap with saliva and make a paste. Apply it to the warts and leave it there for 24 hours.

■ Write a wish for your warts to disappear on a piece of paper, take it to the intersection of two roads, tear it up, and cast it to the winds.

Who Has Warts and Why?

About one in four people have common, flat, or plantar warts at some time in their lives. Children tend to have warts more often than adults do, and people who bite their fingernails or pick at hangnails may be more likely to have warts because tiny openings in the skin provide a way for HPV to enter the body. Someone with a weakened immune system*, due to a chronic* illness or an infection, for example, also may be more likely to have warts. Warts are very contagious because HPV can pass easily from one person to another by contact. Genital warts spread through sexual intercourse. In fact, they are the most common cause of sexually transmitted disease in the United States. In rare cases, a mother with genital warts can pass HPV to her baby during birth. The virus can cause growths on the baby's vocal cords or elsewhere in the infant's respiratory tract.

How Are Warts Diagnosed and Treated?

Healthcare providers can diagnose a wart by its appearance. If individuals have a wart, they should see a professional who can examine the wart, determine exactly what is growing on the skin, and recommend the best treatment. In the case of genital warts, a doctor may also screen a woman for cervical cancer by performing a pelvic exam*, including a Pap smear*. In some cases, warts eventually disappear without any treatment. However, if a person has several warts or if the warts are painful or seem to be spreading, several possible treatments exist.

Over-the-counter medicines containing salicylic (sah-lih-SIH-lik) acid can remove common warts. Depending on the particular brand of medicine, the person may be able to paint it on or may be able to use a stick-on patch that attaches directly to the wart. These over-the-counter medicines can take longer than other treatments do, but they are painless. People who have diabetes* or other conditions that affect the circulatory system should first consult with a doctor before using these over-the-counter medicines.

Another typical treatment for common warts and also for plantar warts is cryotherapy, or freezing. In cryotherapy, a medical professional freezes the wart with a special chemical. Afterward, a scab develops as the skin heals. Plantar warts can be difficult to treat, however, because most of the wart is located beneath the surface of the skin. Medical professionals may use electrosurgery to burn plantar warts—and also sometimes common warts—with a tool that uses an electric current. Sometimes, a doctor will recommend an acid-containing chemical peel to treat flat warts, which grow in such large bunches that the other types of treatments usually are not efficient. These chemicals, which are applied to the skin, eventually peel away the warts. Doctors also may use laser treatment to destroy any type of wart that proves difficult to remove. In some cases, doctors may use a cream called imiquimod, which is applied to the site of the wart and stimulates the body's immune system to fight the HPV.

Genital warts require treatment from a doctor. To remove them, doctors may use cryotherapy, lasers, medicines that can be applied directly to the warts, or surgery. If a woman has had genital warts, doctors may advise her to have Pap smears more often. In some cases, certain types of HPV infection can lead to cancer of the cervix, and a Pap smear allows the doctor to find and treat the disease in its early stages.

Can Warts Be Prevented?

It can be very difficult for people to protect themselves from common, flat, and plantar warts, because they are so common, and the virus spreads so easily. In addition, individuals can come into contact with HPV many months or even a year before a wart grows big enough to see, so it is often impossible to know for sure where and how they got the virus. If people have a wart, it is best for other people not to touch it. It is also advisable to avoid sharing towels and washcloths with someone who has a wart and to wear sandals at public showers or pools or in locker rooms, to avoid infection. The prevention of genital warts can be difficult, because skin-to-skin contact spreads them. Condoms may limit the spread of genital warts, but because some warts grow on the skin around the genitals and on the buttocks, a condom may not cover every one of them, making it still possible for the HPV to pass between sexual partners. Abstaining from sex with a person who has genital warts is the safest choice.

In 2006, the Food and Drug Administration licensed a vaccine to fight HPV infection. Medical professionals recommend the vaccine,

* **diabetes** (dye-uh-BEE-teez) is a condition in which the body's pancreas does not produce enough insulin or the body cannot use the insulin it makes effectively, resulting in increased levels of sugar in the blood. This can lead to increased urination, dehydration, weight loss, weakness, and a number of other symptoms and complications related to chemical imbalances within the body.

* **flavivirus family** (FLAY-vih-vy-rus) is a group of viruses that includes those that cause dengue fever and yellow fever.

* **hosts** are organisms that provide another organism (such as a parasite or virus) with a place to live and grow.

determine if it can also protect others groups of people, including boys and men, from HPV infections.

▶ *See also* **Skin and Soft Tissue Infections**

Resources

Books and Articles

Royston, Angela. *Warts.* Chicago: Heinemann Library, 2002.

Organizations

American Academy of Dermatology. PO Box 4014, Schaumburg, IL, 60168-4014. Toll free: 866-503-SKIN. Web site: http://www.aad.org/public/publications/pamphlets/common_warts.html.

American Academy of Family Physicians. P.O. Box 11210, Shawnee Mission, KS, 66207-1210. Toll free: 800-274-2237. Web site: http://familydoctor.org/online/famdocen/home/common/skin/disorders/209.html.

West Nile Fever

West Nile fever is a viral infection that can result in inflammation of the brain, called encephalitis (en-seh-fuh-LYE-tis). The virus that causes it spreads to humans by way of infected mosquitoes.

What Is West Nile Fever?

West Nile fever (WNF) is caused by West Nile virus (WNV), which is part of the flavivirus family*. First discovered in Africa, WNV can infect animals and humans, although animals (mainly birds, but also horses, cats, and bats) are the primary hosts* for the virus.

Most of the time, people with WNF become only mildly ill. In some cases, however, WNF can develop into a life-threatening disease. If the virus passes into the brain, the infection can cause serious inflammation and complications affecting the nervous system. Of those infected, people 50 years of age or older have the greatest risk of developing severe disease.

Do Many People Contract West Nile Fever?

WNF is found most frequently in Africa, the Middle East, Western Europe, and Asia. It was not found in the Western Hemisphere until 1999, when the first case appeared in the United States. Between 1999 and 2008, presence of the virus was documented in 39 states and the

District of Columbia. In 2007, the Centers for Disease Control (CDC) reported a total of 3,630 WNF cases in the United States. WNF tends to occur more often in the summer and early fall, but the vast majority of cases likely go unreported because they cause only mild illness, if any. Of the 3,630 total in 2007, 124 (3 percent) resulted in death from the disease. Those numbers represented a decrease compared with 2006, when the CDC reported 4,269 cases and 177 deaths. Some experts believed that the U.S. population was starting to develop immunity to the virus.

Is West Nile fever Contagious?

Generally, a person cannot contract WNF from another infected person or from an infected animal, although transmission of the virus through a blood transfusion* has been confirmed in some cases. Likewise, infected people cannot spread the virus to animals. Scientists think that the virus is transmitted almost exclusively by the bite of an infected mosquito. The chances of becoming ill with WNF actually are very small. Of all the mosquitoes in any area where infected mosquitoes have been found, less than 1 percent carry the virus.

The transmission cycle begins when a mosquito bites an infected bird and takes in blood that contains WNV. If the mosquito then bites a human, it can transmit the virus to that person. Scientists have found no evidence that humans can contract the disease by handling live or dead birds or any other animal that has been infected with the virus. Still, experts recommend that people never handle a dead animal with bare hands, instead always using disposable gloves and placing the dead animal in a plastic bag when discarding it.

How Do People Know They Have West Nile Fever?

The first symptoms of WNV infection are usually fever, headache, and body aches, sometimes accompanied by a rash and swollen lymph nodes*. Serious cases of the disease may cause more severe symptoms, including high fever, stiff neck, muscle weakness, convulsions*, confusion, paralysis*, and coma*. Very severe cases can result in death, but this is rare. Symptoms usually begin 3 to 15 days after infection.

How Is West Nile fever Diagnosed and Treated?

If WNF is suspected, the first step for the physician is take a history, which means asking a person about prior health, when symptoms began, and recent travels and activities. This may help determine if the person might have been exposed to an infected mosquito. A blood test can confirm the presence of the virus.

For mild cases of WNF, no specific treatment exists. A doctor usually recommends rest and over-the-counter medications, such as acetaminophen*, to ease fever and aches. Severe cases of WNF may require hospitalization and more specialized care, such as intravenous (in-tra-VEE-nus) fluids (fluids given directly into a vein) to prevent dehydra-

* **blood transfusion** is the process of giving blood (or certain cells or chemicals found in the blood) to a person who needs it due to illness or blood loss.

* **lymph nodes** (LIMF) are small, bean-shaped masses of tissue containing immune system cells that fight harmful microorganisms. Lymph nodes may swell during infections.

* **convulsions** (kon-VUL-shuns), also called seizures, are involuntary muscle contractions caused by electrical discharges within the brain and are usually accompanied by changes in consciousness.

* **paralysis** (pah-RAH-luh-sis) is the loss or impairment of the ability to move some part of the body.

* **coma** (KO-ma) is an unconscious state, like a very deep sleep. A person in a coma cannot be awakened, and cannot move, see, speak, or hear.

* **acetaminophen** (uh-see-teh-MIH-noh-fen) is a medication commonly used to reduce fever and relieve pain.

* **dehydration** (dee-hi-DRAY-shun) is a condition in which the body is depleted of water, usually caused by excessive and unreplaced loss of body fluids, such as through sweating, vomiting, or diarrhea.

* **ventilator** (VEN-tuh-lay-ter) is a machine used to support or control a person's breathing.

WEST NILE INVADES NEW YORK

In the summer of 1999, dead birds began appearing all over the New York City metropolitan area. Public health officials were called in to find out why. They soon learned that the deaths were linked to the virus that causes West Nile fever, an infection that is spread by mosquitoes. Before 1999, West Nile fever had never been seen in the Western Hemisphere.

---

dehydration* in someone who is too sick to drink or who is vomiting. A person who is having trouble breathing may be put on a ventilator*.

How long WNV illness lasts depends on the severity of the infection. If a person has a mild infection, symptoms often go away in about a week. Recovery from serious infection may take several weeks to months. Most people who are infected with WNV do not become very sick. Only about 1 percent of all infected people become severely ill. Of these severe cases, up to 15 percent are fatal. Elderly people have the highest risk of developing serious complications from the disease.

Can West Nile Fever Be Prevented?

No vaccine is available for WNF, so the best way to prevent the spread of the virus is to prevent mosquito bites. To do so, experts recommend that people avoid being outside at times when mosquitoes are most active (dawn, dusk, and early evening), that they wear long sleeves and long pants, and that they use insect repellent when outside. When using repellent, everyone, especially children, should carefully follow the instructions on the package.

In the United States, health officials have often traced WNV to areas where dead birds have been found. By tracking the disease and looking for patterns of infection, public health officials are better able to prevent future outbreaks. Experts advise people to contact the local or state health department if a dead bird is found in an area where WNV has been reported; a representative will collect the bird for testing.

▶ *See also* **Encephalitis** • **Zoonoses**

Resources

Books and Articles

Lew, Kristi. *Mosquito-borne Illnesses.* New York: Marshall Cavendish Benchmark, 2010.

Sfakianos, Jeffrey N. *West Nile Virus.* Philadelphia, PA: Chelsea House, 2005.

Organizations

Centers for Disease Control and Prevention. 1600 Clifton Road, Atlanta, GA, 30333. Toll free: 800-311-3435. Web site: http://www.cdc.gov/ncidod/dvbid/westnile.

National Biological Information Infrastructure, USGS Biological Informatics Office. 302 National Center, Reston, VA, 20192. Telephone: 703-648-4216. Web site: http://westnilevirus.nbii.gov.

Whiteheads *See Acne.*

Whooping Cough *See Pertussis (Whooping Cough).*

Williams Syndrome *See Intellectual Disability.*

Wisdom Teeth *See Impacted Teeth.*

Worms

Disease-causing worms are parasitic organisms that must live on or inside another organism to survive.

What Are Worms?

Worms that cause human disease are parasitic organisms that must live on or inside another organism to survive. An animal or human harboring a worm is called its host. Worms live at the expense of the host and may cause illness. Worms live part of their life cycle within the gastrointestinal* tract and the organs of the digestive system. Worms may cause diarrhea or malnutrition despite a healthy diet.

What Are Types of Worms?

In humans, there are three major types of worm parasites: flukes (trematodes), tapeworms (cestodes), and roundworms (nematodes). While worms complete a part of their life cycle within the gastrointestinal tract, some may also travel to other parts of the body and invade other organs. Worms enter the body through different routes and at various life cycle stages. For example, tapeworms may enter the human body through ingestion of food

* **gastrointestinal** (gas-tro-in-TES-tih-nuhl) means having to do with the organs of the digestive system, the system that processes food. It includes the mouth, esophagus, stomach, intestines, colon, and rectum and other organs involved in digestion, including the liver and pancreas.

* **endemic** (en-DEH-mik) describes a disease or condition that is present in a population or geographic area at all times.

the egg and larval forms. There are some types of worm parasites that can enter the body directly through the skin.

While typically worm infestation is not fatal, it is still a serious health and economic problem. Parasitic worms create a lot of sickness in the tropics and subtropics, especially among rural, poor people. They are a common problem in areas with poor sanitation. Worms may interfere with the normal growth and development of children and cause chronic illness in adults. In the United States, cases of worms occur among people who were infected during travels to endemic* countries.

Flukes (Trematodes)   After malaria, the most prevalent tropical disease in the world is schistosomiasis, which is caused by a fluke of the genus *Schistosoma*. The fluke that causes schistosomiasis lives on a type of freshwater snail. Humans may be infected by contaminated water carrying the fluke. Schistosomiasis affects large populations in developing countries, especially among children who become infested while playing in water containing the snail host. Although it is usually not fatal, schistosomiasis causes chronic illness that may damage internal organs and impair both physical and mental development. One form of schistosomiasis involves a type of fluke that enters the urinary tract and is associated with increased risk for bladder cancer in adults. Individuals from the United States traveling to tropical areas may become infested while abroad.

Tapeworms (Cestodes)   Human tapeworm infestations usually are caused by eating meat or fish contaminated with worm larvae, but it may also be caused by eating soil or water contaminated with human fecal matter containing the eggs. Meat contaminated with tapeworm larvae has larvae enclosed in cyst form within the meat. Like other types of worms, tapeworms frequently cause infestations in areas with poor sanitation, where livestock animals are exposed to contaminated soil or fish to contaminated water, and these have parasites in their body tissues. After humans ingest contaminated tapeworm encysted meat or fish, the larvae travel to the intestines, where they latch onto the lining of the intestines and gradually grow into adults. The worms shed their eggs into the feces, from which they contaminate soil and water, are ingested by animals or fish, and reenter the cycle. Tapeworms cause the most health problems in areas of Latin America and Asia. Tapeworm infestation is rare in the United States. Fish tapeworm infestations in the United States tend to occur among Eskimos of western Alaska and in individuals from the west coast.

Ascariasis (Nematode)   Ascariasis is caused by *Ascaris lumbricoides*, an intestinal roundworm. It is one of the most common intestinal parasites in areas with poor sanitation, affecting people in all parts of the world. In the United States, ascariasis is extremely common in rural parts of the Southeast. Exposure to pigs and pig manure increases the risk of infestation. An estimated 4 million individuals may be infected in the United States. Approximately 1.4 billion people may be infected worldwide. Indonesia has an especially high rate of infestation with Ascariasis, with 90 percent of the people in some regions being affected. The life cycle of this worm begins when an adult worm lays its eggs in the intestines of an infected person. The eggs leave the body through the feces and can live in soil for up to two years. When people eat raw food containing this contaminated soil, they may ingest the eggs, which hatch in the stomach as larvae. Part of the life cycle of the larvae is to migrate outside the gastrointestinal tract. The larvae invade the walls of the gastrointestinal tract, migrate through the blood to the lungs and then to the throat, where they are swallowed. Eventually, they pass into the intestines, where adult worms form and begin the cycle again.

Strongyloidiasis/Threadworm (Nematode) Strongyloidiasis is caused by a type of roundworm commonly referred to as the threadworm, *Strongyloides stercoralis*. Strongyloidiasis is common in the tropics and is especially prevalent in West Africa, the Caribbean, and Southeast Asia. Strongyloidiasis is rare in the United States, except in some areas of the Southeast and Appalachia. It is more common among military veterans who served in Southeast Asia. Worldwide approximately 35 million cases occurred in 2008. Although the route of infestation can be fecal-oral, this infestation most commonly comes from contact with contaminated soil where the larvae of the parasite can burrow directly through the skin. The larvae travel to the lungs, are coughed up into the mouth, swallowed, and enter the intestines. In the intestines the worm matures to adulthood and begins laying eggs. The eggs can hatch inside the intestines and the worm can continue to cycle through many generations without leaving the body. Such an infestation can last for decades. Some larvae may invade the lungs and other organs. This infestation can be fatal.

Hookworm (Nematode) Hookworms are a type of roundworm and a common intestinal parasite. The Centers for Disease Control and Prevention (CDC) estimates that one-fourth of the population worldwide has hookworm infestations, although improved sanitation has reduced the number of cases in the United States. Two species can infest humans. The hookworm eggs hatch into larvae in the soil. Hookworms can directly penetrate human skin. Humans may be infested by walking barefoot in or touching contaminated soil, as well as ingesting food with contaminated soil on it. The hookworm larvae travel to the lungs via the bloodstream. The larvae then travel to the throat and are swallowed, in a similar fashion to the ascaris worm. When they reach the small intestine, the larvae latch onto the intestinal walls and suck blood. There they mature and eventually lay eggs, which pass out of the body in the feces. Hookworms can live for one to two years in the human body.

Enterobiasis/Pinworm (Nematode) Enterobiasis, also known as pinworm infestation, is caused by a staple-size worm known as *Enterobius vermicularis*. Pinworm tends to occur in temperate regions, rather than

* **antibodies** (AN-tih-bah-deez) are protein molecules produced by the body's immune system to help fight specific infections caused by microorganisms, such as bacteria and viruses.

* **endoscope** (EN-doh-skope) is a tool for looking inside parts of the body. It consists of a lighted tube and optical fibers and/or lenses.

the tropics. It is the most common worm infestation in the United States and is found primarily in children. Crowded living conditions are often associated with pinworm infestation. Outbreaks of pinworm often occur among individuals who are grouped together in institutions, such as schools and daycare centers. From there, infested children may spread the worms to their family members. In the United States, in some small regions pinworm infestation has affected 12 percent of the population. School-aged children and adults from 30 to 39 years of age who have children are most commonly infested.

Trichinosis (Nematode)   Trichinosis arises from several varieties of roundworms of the genus *Trichinella.* Although once very common, trichinosis was as of 2009 relatively rare in the United States, with the CDC reporting an average of just 38 cases per year. Trichinosis is more common in developing countries. Trichinella larvae live encysted in the tissues of pigs and wild animals. When people eat their meat raw or undercooked, the larval cysts travel to the stomach, where acid dissolves the walls of the cysts and releases the immature, larval worms. These migrate to the small intestine, mature to adults, and lay eggs. Once the eggs hatch, the worms travel through the bloodstream to muscles, where they burrow in, forming new cysts. This ends the cycle in humans.

How Is Worm Infestation Diagnosed?

Physicians may use fecal samples, sometimes taken a day or two apart, to diagnose intestinal parasitic diseases. The feces are examined for evidence of parasites, such as eggs, larvae, or adult forms. Blood samples may also be taken to check for antibodies* made by the body against specific parasites. Physicians may also use an endoscope* that allows them to view the internal structures of the gastrointestinal tract and to examine the intestines for infection. To detect pinworms, physicians often request that patients take a "tape test". For this test, patients briefly apply a piece of transparent tape to the skin around the anus in the early morning, the time right after the worm has laid its eggs. The tape is removed and examined at the doctor's office for any eggs that might be sticking to it.

How Is Worm Infestation Treated?

Some cases of intestinal parasites require little or no treatment, and the parasites eventually disappear on their own. Other cases require antibiotics or anthelmintics, a type of drug used to fight worm infections. Different types of infestation are treated with different medicines. It is critical that the type of worm be identified so that the correct medication can be prescribed. Some anthelmintics work by inhibiting the development of the worm from egg to larvae. Others may inhibit an enzyme specific to worms, not present in human cells, and necessary for worm bodily function. Anthelmintics can also paralyze the worm so that it can no longer remain attached to the human body and is either digested or simply expelled. Anthelmintics may kill the worm by preventing its absorption of nutrients.

In most cases, patients can remain at home and maintain a normal schedule. However, many side effects are associated with anthelmintics for the duration of treatment, including nausea, vomiting, abdominal pain, dizziness, and headache. Patients experiencing diarrhea are usually advised to drink plenty of fluids to avoid dehydration*. Infants and young children are particularly vulnerable to dehydration and nutrition problems when they become infested. Antidiarrheal medicine is usually not recommended because it may keep the parasites in the body longer. More severe cases of infestations may require treatment in the hospital.

Prevention of Worm Infestation

Intestinal parasite infestation is best prevented through careful personal hygiene, which includes frequent and thorough hand washing, especially after changing diapers, after going to the bathroom, and before handling food. In areas known for parasites that live in the soil and burrow directly through the skin, wearing shoes may prevent parasites from entering the body. Individuals who travel to foreign countries known to have parasite problems should drink bottled water only and brush their teeth with bottled water. They should avoid eating raw fruits and vegetables, food from street vendors, and unpasteurized dairy products. In addition, cooking all food until it is steaming hot kills parasites. Avoiding swimming in bodies of fresh water such as ponds, rivers, and lakes in these areas can reduce possible exposure to contaminated water.

▶ *See also* **Ascariasis • Hookworm • Parasitic Diseases: Overview • Pinworm Infestation • Tapeworm • Trichinosis**

Resources

Books and Articles

Tilden, Thomasine E. Lewis. *Belly-Busting Worm Invasions! Parasites That Love Your Insides!* New York: Franklin Watts, 2008.

Organizations

Centers for Disease Control and Prevention. 1600 Clifton Road, Atlanta, GA, 30333. Toll free: 800-311-3435. Web site: http://www.cdc.gov.

Food and Drug Administration, Center for Food Safety and Applied Nutrition. 5100 Paint Branch Parkway, College Park, MD, 20740. Toll free: 888-SAFEFOOD. Web site: http://www.cfsan.fda.gov.

* **dehydration** (dee-hi-DRAY-shun) is a condition in which the body is depleted of water, usually caused by excessive and unreplaced loss of body fluids, such as through sweating, vomiting, or diarrhea.

Y-Z

Yeast Infection, Vaginal

The vaginal yeast infection candidiasis (kan-di-DY-a-sis) results from an overabundance of a certain kind of fungus* in the genital area. Its symptoms include an itching or burning sensation in the genital area and often a white discharge from the vagina. Genital candidiasis occurs much more frequently in women, but it also occurs in men.

What Is Candidiasis?

The fungus that causes most vaginal yeast* infection is usually *Candida albicans* (KAN-di-da AL-bi-kanz). It is naturally present in the vagina (va-JY-na), the gastrointestinal* tract, and the mouth. It is part of the vaginal and gastrointestinal flora. In the vagina and in the gastrointestinal tract, the Candida organisms usually remains in balance with various bacteria* that are also found in these naturally moist areas (meaning that the presence of bacteria and other components of the flora helps to keep Candida growth in check). All of these microorganisms are competitors for the same resources, and a reduction in the level of one becomes an opportunity for another to flourish. When this ecological balance is disrupted, Candida growth may become Candida overgrowth (candidiasis). Vaginal candidiasis will develop quickly when this excessive growth occurs in the vaginal area. (When *Candida* infection involves the mouth, it is called thrush. When it involves babies' diaper area, it is called candidal diaper rash.)

Candida fungus cells can multiply too much when a person is taking an antibiotic*, which may destroy too many of the bacteria that usually keep the fungus in check. Other situations that may cause the fungus to grow out of control are the use of birth control pills, pregnancy, and the use of drugs that suppress the immune system*. When a woman becomes immunocompromised (has an immunodeficiency disease such as AIDS, or is taking an immunosuppressant medication—for example, in preparation for organ transplantation) she will also be more likely to develop a vaginal yeast infection. Sugar causes yeasts to multiply. Women with diabetes have higher blood sugar levels, and their vaginal secretions contain more glucose. Thus, a woman with diabetes is more likely to develop a vaginal yeast infection.

Estimates indicate that about 75 percent of women have a yeast infection at least once in their lifetime. Half of them have the infection more than once

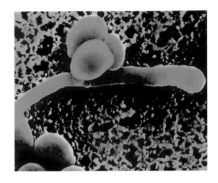

▲

Candida albicans magnified 3000 times.
© *PHOTOTAKE Inc./Alamy.*

* **fungus** (FUN-gus) is any organism belonging to the kingdom Fungi (FUN-ji), which includes mushrooms, yeasts, and molds.

* **yeast** (YEEST) is a general term describing single-celled fungi that reproduce by budding.

* **gastrointestinal** (gas-tro-in-TES-tih-nuhl) means having to do with the organs of the digestive system, the system that processes food. It includes the mouth, esophagus, stomach, intestines, colon, and rectum and other organs involved in digestion, including the liver and pancreas.

* **bacteria** (bak-TEER-ee-a) are single-celled microorganisms, which typically reproduce by cell division. Some, but not all, types of bacteria can cause disease in humans. Many types can live in the body without causing harm.

* **antibiotics** (an-tie-by-AH-tiks) are drugs that kill or slow the growth of bacteria.

1803

Antibiotics and Yogurt

Antibiotics prescribed to treat bacterial infections also kill beneficial bacteria. When the beneficial bacteria found normally in the mucous membranes of the vagina and other mucous membranes die, yeast cells can grow unchecked, which leads lead to a yeast infection.

Eating active-culture yogurt daily while taking an antibiotic may help replenish the supply of beneficial bacteria. Besides yogurt, most pharmacies and health stores carry a capsule or powder form of the same beneficial bacteria that are in active-culture yogurt. These beneficial bacteria, also known as probiotics, include *Lactobacillus acidophilus* and *Lactobacillus bifidus* species. Another probiotic that shows promise in treatment and prevention of yeast infections is a beneficial yeast called *Saccharomyces boulardii*, which is marketed in the United States as Florastor.

* **immune system** (im-YOON SIS-tem) is the system of the body composed of specialized cells and the substances they produce that helps protect the body against disease-causing germs.

* **antifungal drugs** (an-ty-FUNG-al drugs) are medications that kill fungi.

What Are the Symptoms of Candidiasis?

The most common symptom of vaginal yeast infection is an itching sensation in and around the vagina and/or vulva. The itching may be accompanied by a burning sensation and sharp, or even severe, pain. A vaginal discharge is not always present, but when it occurs it typically has a whitish appearance and a texture like that of cottage cheese. The area around the vagina also may itch or feel irritated. In yeast infections in men, the head of the penis becomes inflamed or shows a rash.

How Is Candidiasis Diagnosed and Treated?

The diagnosis of vaginal yeast infection is usually a simple matter of microscopic examination. A scraping or swab of the infected area, or a small sample of the vaginal discharge, is placed on a microscope slide. The treatment is antifungal drugs* that are applied to the affected area or taken by mouth.

An individual who notices a vaginal yeast infection for the first time should see her doctor, who can then diagnose it properly before she begins treatment. Health professionals recommend that anyone with a vaginal yeast infection should also have her partner examined for infection. Women who have had previous vaginal yeast infections are often familiar enough with the infection to diagnose it themselves and begin treatment with over-the-counter creams.

How Can Candidiasis Be Prevented?

The following measures can help prevent a vaginal yeast infection:

- Wearing cotton underwear
- Avoiding tight-fitting underwear made of synthetic fiber such as nylon
- Avoiding the daily use of panty hose
- Using white, non-perfumed toilet paper
- Keeping the genital area clean
- Using a towel (not a blow dryer) to dry the genital area
- Removing a wet bathing suit as soon as possible after swimming
- Avoiding douches and feminine hygiene sprays
- Using sanitary pads or tampons that are free of perfume

▶ *See also* **Fungal Infections • Sexually Transmitted Diseases (STDs) • Thrush**

Resources

Organizations

Centers for Disease Control and Prevention. 1600 Clifton Road, Atlanta, GA, 30333. Toll free: 800-232-4636. Web site:http://www.cdc.gov/nczved/dfbmd/disease_listing/candidiasis_gi.html.

Mayo Clinic. 200 First Street SW, Rochester, MN, 55905. Web site: http://www.mayoclinic.com/health/male-yeast-infection/HO00172.

National Women's Health Information Center. 8270 Willow Oaks Corporate Drive, Fairfax, VA, 22031. Toll free: 800-994-9662. Web site:http://www.4woman.gov/faq/vaginal-yeast-infections.cfm.

Yellow Fever

Yellow fever is an infectious disease caused by a virus that is transmitted to humans by mosquitoes.

What Is Yellow Fever?

Yellow fever is a disease caused by yellow fever virus, a member of the flavivirus (FLAY-vih-vy-rus) group of viruses. The disease gets its name because it often causes jaundice*, which tints the skin yellow, and a high fever. Yellow fever also can cause kidney failure and uncontrolled bleeding, or hemorrhaging (HEM-rij-ing). Many cases produce only mild illness, but severe cases of yellow fever can be fatal. Once someone has survived the disease, the person has lifetime immunity* against it.

Yellow fever afflicts both humans and monkeys and has been known since at least the 1600s. The disease is not spread by person-to-person contact. It is transmitted by several different species of mosquitoes; a person can contract yellow fever only from the bite of a mosquito that has bitten an infected person or monkey.

The disease once caused epidemics* in the Americas, Europe, and the Caribbean, but at the beginning of the 21st century the disease occurred almost exclusively in South America and Africa. Each year, outbreaks lead to an estimated 200,000 cases and 30,000 deaths worldwide. Vaccines against the virus were developed in 1928 and 1937, and mosquito-eradication programs made great progress in controlling the disease. The last recorded outbreak of yellow fever in the United States was in New Orleans in 1905. However, lapses in prevention programs in Africa and South America allowed yellow fever to once again become a serious public health issue on those continents.

Are There Different Kinds of Yellow Fever?

Yellow fever occurs as three subtypes: epidemic (urban), intermediate, and jungle-acquired. Epidemic yellow fever spreads in densely populated areas of Africa and South America via the bite of Aedes aegypti (a-E-deez eh-JIP-tie) mosquitoes. Intermediate yellow fever occurs in Africa as the result of

* **jaundice** (JON-dis) is a yellowing of the skin, and sometimes the whites of the eyes, caused by a buildup in the body of bilirubin, a chemical produced in and released by the liver. An increase in bilirubin may indicate disease of the liver or certain blood disorders.

* **immunity** (ih-MYOON-uh-tee) is the condition of being protected against an infectious disease. Immunity often develops after a germ has entered the body. One type of immunity occurs when the body makes special protein molecules called antibodies to fight the disease-causing germ. The next time that germ enters the body, the antibodies quickly attack it, usually preventing the germ from causing disease.

* **epidemics** (eh-pih-DEH-miks) are outbreaks of diseases, especially infectious diseases, in which the number of cases suddenly becomes far greater than usual. Usually, epidemics that involve worldwide outbreaks are called pandemics.

WALTER REED AND THE U.S. YELLOW FEVER COMMISSION

Walter Reed (1851–1902), American military surgeon and head of the U.S. Army Yellow Fever Commission, is widely known as the man who conquered yellow fever by tracing its origin to a particular mosquito species.

Walter Reed was born on in Belroi, Virginia, the son of a Methodist minister. After attending private schools, Reed entered the University of Virginia, where he received his medical degree in 1869, after completing only two years. He then went to New York, where he received a second medical degree from the Bellevue Hospital Medical College in 1870. In June 1875, after working for the Board of Health of New York and Brooklyn, Reed was commissioned an assistant surgeon in the U.S. Army with the rank of first lieutenant. Then followed 11 years of frontier garrison duty, further study at Johns Hopkins Hospital while on duty in Baltimore, and an assignment as professor of bacteriology and clinical microscopy at the newly organized Army Medical School in Washington in 1893.

When yellow fever made its appearance among U.S. troops in Havana, Cuba, in 1900, Reed was appointed head of the commission of Army medical officers to investigate the cause and mode of transmission. After some months of fruitless work in searching for the cause of the disease, Reed and his associates decided to concentrate upon determining the mode of transmission. Carlos Juan Finlay first advanced the theory that yellow fever was transmitted by mosquitoes (he blamed it on the *Stegomyia fasciata*, later known as the *Aedes aegypti*) and proved it by experiments, but physicians generally did not credit the possibility. Walter Reed confirmed Finlay's findings by using human subjects. Reed and his associates argued that there was no alternative to experimentation with humans and that their results would justify the practice. Mosquitoes that had been fed on yellow fever-infected blood were applied to several of Reed's associates, including Dr. James Carroll, who developed the first experimental case of the disease.

There followed a series of controlled experiments with soldier volunteers. In all, 22 cases of experimental yellow fever were produced: 14 by mosquito bites, 6 by injections of blood, and 2 by injections of filtered blood serum. At the same time, in order to disprove the theory that the disease could be transmitted by mere physical contact, Dr. Robert P. Cook and a group of soldiers slept in a detached building with the clothing and bedding of yellow fever patients from the camp hospital. No cases of the illness resulted, the theory was conclusively falsified.

The value of the commission's work quickly became evident. In 1900 there had been 1,400 cases of yellow fever in Havana; by 1902, after more than a year of mosquito eradication prompted by the Reed Commission's report, there was not a single case. Once its mode of transmission was known, there was no danger of yellow fever in any country with adequate control facilities.

---

* **incubation** (ing-kyoo-BAY-shun) is the period of time between infection by a germ and when symptoms first appear. Depending on the germ, this period can be from hours to months.

mosquitoes breeding in humid flat grasslands (savannahs) during rainy seasons, then infecting both monkeys and humans. In dry seasons, the virus can remain alive in unhatched mosquito eggs that are resistant to the heat.

Jungle-acquired yellow fever occurs mainly in South America when mosquitoes pick up the virus from infected forest monkeys and then transmit the disease to humans in jungles and rainforests. People who are regional settlers, soldiers, or agricultural or forestry workers are at greater risk for this less common form of the disease.

How Do People Know They Have Yellow Fever?

After an incubation* period of three to six days, the yellow fever virus begins to produce symptoms. An early phase of disease occurs, which includes fever, headache, muscle aches, and vomiting. The infected person may have a slower heartbeat than that expected with a high fever. After a few days, most of the symptoms disappear. Many people recover from yellow fever at this point without complications. However, about 15 percent of patients develop a second, toxic phase of the disease, in which fever reappears and the disease becomes more severe. Inflammation* of the liver occurs, along with jaundice, stomach pains, and vomiting. The mouth, nose, eyes, and stomach can bleed uncontrollably, with blood present in vomited material and bowel movements. The kidneys may begin to fail, and patients may go into a coma (an unconscious state in which a person cannot be awakened).

How Do Doctors Diagnose and Treat Yellow Fever?

Early stages of yellow fever can be easily confused with other diseases such as malaria*, typhoid fever*, and other hemorrhagic (heh-muh-RAH-jik) fevers and types of viral hepatitis*. Blood tests can detect whether a patient's body has produced yellow fever antibodies* to fight the infection. Doctors also will take a travel history to see if a patient recently has visited a country where yellow fever occurs.

No specific treatment exists for yellow fever. Care is geared toward treating complications of the disease. In serious cases, intensive care in the hospital usually is needed. Patients may be given fluids to prevent dehydration*, and blood transfusions* may be necessary if bleeding is severe.

Most people who contract yellow fever recover from the early phase of the disease within a week; those who progress to the toxic phase may take several weeks or longer to recover. About half of those who develop toxic phase symptoms die within two weeks; the other half may recover without significant long-term problems.

How Can Yellow Fever Be Prevented?

Vaccination* against yellow fever is the single most important prevention measure, and it is a must for people traveling to countries where the disease is common. Most countries in which yellow fever occurs require a certificate proving that travelers have been vaccinated before they are allowed into the country. One dose of vaccine provides at least 10 years of immunity.

Doctors recommend that infants under six months of age, pregnant women, people allergic to eggs (eggs are used in producing the vaccine), and people with a weakened immune system* (such as people who have AIDS* or certain cancers) not receive the vaccine; these people are advised to delay visits to countries where yellow fever is endemic*.

Avoiding mosquito bites when traveling abroad reduces the risk of contracting yellow fever. To help prevent infection, experts suggest that travelers do the following:

- Wear long sleeves and pants
- Avoid going outside when mosquitoes are active—at dawn, dusk, and early evening
- Use mosquito repellent
- Sleep beneath a mosquito net

* **inflammation** (in-fla-MAY-shun) is the body's reaction to irritation, infection, or injury that often involves swelling, pain, redness, and warmth.

* **malaria** (mah-LAIR-e-uh) is a disease spread to humans by the bite of an infected mosquito.

* **typhoid fever** (TIE-foyd FEE-ver) is an infection with the bacterium Salmonella typhi that causes fever, headache, confusion, and muscle aches.

* **hepatitis** (heh-puh-TIE-tis) is an inflammation of the liver. Hepatitis can be caused by viruses, bacteria, and a number of other noninfectious medical conditions.

* **antibodies** (AN-tih-bah-deez) are protein molecules produced by the body's immune system to help fight specific infections caused by microorganisms, such as bacteria and viruses.

* **dehydration** (dee-hi-DRAY-shun) is a condition in which the body is depleted of water, usually caused by excessive and unreplaced loss of body fluids, such as through sweating, vomiting, or diarrhea.

* **transfusions** (trans-FYOO-zhunz) are procedures in which blood or certain parts of blood, such as specific cells, are given to a person who needs them due to illness or blood loss.

* **vaccination** (vak-sih-NAY-shun), also called immunization, is giving, usually by an injection, a preparation of killed or weakened germs, or a part of a germ or product it produces, to prevent or lessen the severity of the disease caused by that germ.

* **immune system** (im-YOON SIS-tem) is the system of the body composed of specialized cells and the substances they produce that helps protect the body against disease-causing germs.

* **AIDS** or acquired immunodeficiency (ih-myoo-no-dih-FIH-shen-see) syndrome, is an infection that severely weakens the immune system; it is caused by the human immunodeficiency virus (HIV).

* **endemic** (en-DEH-mik) describes a disease or condition that is present in a population or geographic area at all times.

* **parasites** (PAIR-uh-sites) are organisms such as protozoa (one-celled animals), worms, or insects that must live on or inside a human or other organism to survive. An animal or plant harboring a parasite is called its host. Parasites live at the expense of the host and may cause illness.

* **bacteria** (bak-TEER-ee-a) are single-celled microorganisms, which typically reproduce by cell division. Some, but not all, types of bacteria can cause disease in humans. Many types can live in the body without causing harm.

* **viruses** (VY-rus-sez) are tiny infectious agents that can cause infectious diseases. Viruses can only reproduce within the cells they infect.

▶ *See also* **Dengue Fever** • **Hepatitis** • **Malaria** • **West Nile Fever**

Resources

Books and Articles

Dickerson, James L. *Yellow Fever: A Deadly Disease Poised to Kill Again.* Amherst, NY: Prometheus Books, 2006.

Pierce, John R., and Jim Writer. *Yellow Jack: How Yellow Fever Ravaged America and Walter Reed Discovered Its Deadly Secrets.* Hoboken, NJ: Wiley, 2005.

Organizations

Centers for Disease Control and Prevention. 1600 Clifton Road, Atlanta, GA, 30333. Toll free: 800-311-3435. Web site:http://www.cdc.gov/ncidod/dvbid/YellowFever/index.html.

World Health Organization. Avenue Appia 20, CH - 1211 Geneva 27, Switzerland. Telephone: +41 22 791 2111. Web site:http://www.who.int/mediacentre/factsheets/fs100/en.

Yersinia *See Plague.*

Zoonoses

Zoonoses (zoh-ah-NO-seez) are infections that humans contract from animals.

What Are Zoonoses?

Zoonoses are infections caused by parasites*, bacteria*, or viruses* that pass from animals to humans. Most people contract zoonotic (zoh-uh-NAH-tik) infections from pets, farm animals, and animals with which they are in contact. Alternatively, there may be an intermediate between the animal and the human, such as food or water. Wild animals and insects can be the source of disease, too, particularly for diseases spread by the bite of a tick, mosquito, or fly. Animals such as wild rodents, raccoons, and bats also can carry diseases that may be harmful to humans.

Zoonoses can either cause minor or serious illness. In some cases, the organisms involved infected humans, but the people do not become ill.

Disease-causing Organism	Animal or Insect Carrier	Human Disease
Bartonella hensalae bacteria	Cats	Cat scratch disease
Chlamydia psittaci bacteria	Birds	Psittacosis
Mononegavirales virus	Mammals, including bats, raccoons, skunks, foxes, and coyotes	Rabies
Yersinia pestis bacteria	Fleas and rodents, including rats, chipmunks, prairie dogs, ground squirrels, and mice	Plague
Hantavirus	Rodents, including rats and mice	Hantavirus pulmonary syndrome
Borrelia burgdorferi bacteria	Ticks, deer, and mice	Lyme disease
Toxoplasma gondii bacteria	Cats and farm animals	Toxoplasmosis
Trichinella larvae	Bears, foxes, and other wild game; pigs and horses	Trichinosis

Other zoonoses can be very dangerous to people, some of which to especially anyone with an immune system weakened by age or illness.

Are Zoonoses Contagious?

Most of these infections do not spread from person to person or do so only in rare instances. Usually they spread from animals to humans in the following ways:

- Bite of an infected insect
- Contact with an animal's feces* or urine, either through the mouth (perhaps by touching a contaminated object and then touching the mouth) or by breathing in dust from dried feces
- Bite or scratch of an infected animal
- Consumption of the meat of an infected animal

▲

A sampling of infections contracted from animals. *Illustration by Frank Forney. Reproduced by permission of Gale, a part of Cengage Learning.*

* **feces** (FEE-seez) is the excreted waste from the gastrointestinal tract.

* **lymph nodes** (LIMF) are small, bean-shaped masses of tissue containing immune system cells that fight harmful microorganisms. Lymph nodes may swell during infections.

* **delirium** (dih-LEER-e-um) is a condition in which a person is confused, is unable to think clearly, and has a reduced level of consciousness.

* **seizures** (SEE-zhurs) are sudden bursts of disorganized electrical activity that interrupt the normal functioning of the brain, often leading to uncontrolled movements in the body and sometimes a temporary change in consciousness.

* **coma** (KO-ma) is an unconscious state, like a very deep sleep. A person in a coma cannot be awakened, and cannot move, see, speak, or hear.

* **vaccinations** (vak-sih-NAY-shunz), also called immunizations, are the giving of doses of vaccines, which are preparations of killed or weakened germs, or a part of a germ or product it produces, to prevent or lessen the severity of the disease that can result if a person is exposed to the germ itself.

* **epidemics** (eh-pih-DEH-miks) are outbreaks of diseases, especially infectious diseases, in which the number of cases suddenly becomes far greater than usual. Usually, epidemics that involve worldwide outbreaks are called pandemics.

What Are Examples of Zoonoses?

Cat scratch disease   A cat carrying *Bartonella henselae* (bar-tuh-NEH-luh HEN-suh-lay), the bacterium responsible for cat scratch disease, usually does not have symptoms, but if the bacteria are passed to a human through a scratch or bite, the person may experience skin sores, swollen and sore lymph nodes*, extreme tiredness, headaches, and fever. Doctors may prescribe antibiotics to treat the infection.

Psittacosis   People who have contact with birds may be at risk for psittacosis (sih-tuh-KO-sis), also known as parrot fever. If a person inhales bird feces or urine particles while cleaning a bird's cage, the person may develop symptoms of pneumonia (nu-MO-nyah, inflammation of the lung), such as fever, coughing, or chest pain. Medical professionals use antibiotics to treat psittacosis.

Rabies   A virus that is carried in the saliva of infected animals can cause rabies when transmitted through a bite or, less commonly, through contact with saliva. Rabies in the United States is most often associated with raccoons, followed by bats and skunks, but any bite produced by an animal, whether domestic, stray, or wild, should be reported immediately to a local animal control agency. Symptoms include fever, difficulty swallowing, delirium*, seizures*, and coma*. If treatment does not begin very soon after the bite, death can result. Treatment includes intensive care in a hospital. A series of vaccinations* started at the time of a bite from a possibly infected animal can prevent the person from developing the disease.

In 2006, the Centers for Disease Control and Prevention (CDC) reported that tests of more than 113,000 animals in 49 states, the District of Columbia, and Puerto Rico resulted in 6,940 cases of rabies in animals and three human cases. Only one state, Hawaii, was free of rabies. Rabies is much more common in many other countries, especially developing ones.

Plague   Plague (PLAYG) is a bacterial infection caused by *Yersinia pestis* (yer-SIN-e-uh PES-tis). People can contract plague through the bite of a flea that has become infected through contact with an infected rodent, such as a rat. The disease causes such symptoms as fever and swollen lymph nodes. In some cases the infection spreads through the blood and can infect the lungs. If this happens, plague can spread from person to person through coughing or sneezing. Plague was the cause of epidemics* in Europe and Asia during the Middle Ages, and it is still seen in the 21st century in many developing countries. It occurs in many developed countries too, including the United States, although not as many cases occur. The disease can be fatal if it is not treated with antibiotics.

Hantavirus   Rodents, such as mice and rats, may carry hantavirus (HAN-tuh-vy-rus), which can spread to humans when they inhale particles from rodent feces, saliva, or urine. People infected with hantavirus can develop hantavirus pulmonary (PUL-mo-nar-ee) syndrome (HPS), which causes such symptoms as fever, headaches, muscle aches, nausea (NAW-zee-uh), vomiting, diarrhea (dye-uh-REE-uh), abdominal* pain, and chills. In severe cases a person may experience shortness of breath and the lungs may fill with fluid. No cure is available for hantavirus infection, but people who have HPS typically are hospitalized in an intensive care unit, where they receive oxygen and other types of supportive care.

Lyme disease   *Borrelia burgdorferi* (buh-REEL-e-uh burg-DOR-fe-ree) bacteria inside an infected tick can cause Lyme (LIME) disease in humans after a tick attaches to the skin and feeds on a person's blood. Ticks pick up the bacterium by feeding on the blood of infected deer and mice, which serve as reservoirs for the organism. Lyme disease can produce a number of symptoms, such as extreme tiredness, muscle aches, and swollen painful joints. Patients often describe the symptoms as being flu-like and pay a visit to the doctor's office because no one else they know has the flu. At the site of the tick bite, some (but not all) people develop a bull's-eye rash, a red rash surrounded by rings that resembles a bull's-eye target. A person with Lyme disease usually is treated with antibiotics.

Toxoplasmosis   Eating contaminated meat or having contact with the feces of an infected cat can put a person at risk for toxoplasmosis (tox-o-plaz-MO-sis). This zoonosis is caused by a parasite and can produce such symptoms as swollen lymph nodes, muscle aches, headaches, and sore throat in a healthy person, and life-threatening brain infections in people with weakened immune systems, especially those who have HIV*/AIDS*. If a pregnant woman becomes infected with the parasite, she can transmit the infection to her unborn baby, which can lead to a number of health problems in the child. Doctors treat those people who have severe forms of the disease, as well as pregnant women, with antibiotics.

Trichinosis   If people eat meat (especially pork products, such as sausage or ham, or the meat of wild carnivorous animals) infected with the eggs of *Trichinella* (trih-kih-NEH-luh) worms, the people can contract trichinosis (trih-kih-NO-sis), also known as trichinellosis. Trichinosis is a disease that produces such symptoms as diarrhea, vomiting, and abdominal pain. It can cause nerve and muscle damage and heart and lung problems. Medication treats this condition.

How Are Zoonoses Treated?

The treatment of a zoonotic infection depends on the specific disease, but many are treated with prescription medications, such as antibiotics.

How Are Zoonoses Prevented?

Because household pets may carry zoonotic organisms, pet owners should keep their animals healthy and vaccinated to avoid infection. Some other ways people can protect against zoonoses include the following:

* **abdominal** (ab-DAH-mih-nul) refers to the area of the body below the ribs and above the hips that contains the stomach, intestines, and other organs.

* **HIV** or human immunodeficiency virus (HYOO-mun ih-myoo-no-dih-FIH-shen-see), is the virus that causes AIDS (acquired immunodeficiency syndrome).

* **AIDS** or acquired immunodeficiency (ih-myoo-no-dih-FIH-shen-see) syndrome, is an infection that severely weakens the immune system; it is caused by the human immunodeficiency virus (HIV).

- Have pets regularly examined by a veterinarian
- Avoid contact with stray, unfamiliar, or wild animals
- Clean litter boxes daily and animal cages frequently to prevent the growth of bacteria and parasites
- Have someone who does not have a weakened immune system and is not pregnant empty pet litter boxes, bathe pets, clean pet cages, and pick up pet feces
- Cook meat until it is no longer pink inside and the juices run clear
- Wash hands with soap and warm water after handling animals and before eating
- Clear brush and other areas around the house where rodents might live
- Avoid storing food or trash in an area where it could attract animals
- Wear long sleeves and long pants when outdoors, especially in wooded areas, to discourage tick and mosquito bites
- Use insect and mosquito repellent
- Examine the body and pets for ticks after spending time outside in areas where ticks are found

▶ *See also* **Cat Scratch Disease • Chlamydial Infections • Hantavirus Pulmonary Syndrome • Lyme Disease • Plague • Rabies • Toxoplasmosis • Trichinosis**

Resources

Books and Articles

Brownlee, Christen. *Cute, Furry, and Deadly: Diseases You Can Catch from Your Pet!* New York: Franklin Watts, 2008.

DiConsiglio, John. *When Birds Get Flu and Cows Go Mad! How Safe Are We?* New York: Franklin Watts, 2008.

Torrey, E. Fuller, and Robert H. Yolken. *Beasts of the Earth: Animals, Humans, and Disease.* New Brunswick, NJ: Rutgers University Press, 2005.

Organizations

Centers for Disease Control and Prevention. 1600 Clifton Road, Atlanta, GA, 30333. Toll free: 800-232-4636. Web site:http://www.cdc.gov/ncidod/dpd/animals.htm.

New York State Department of Health. Corning Tower, Empire State Plaza, Albany, NY, 12237. Web site: http://www.health.state.ny.us/diseases/communicable/botulism/fact_sheet.htm.

Bibliography

The following is an alphabetical compilation of books and articles listed in the ***Resources*** section of the main body entries. Although the list is comprehensive, it is by no means exhaustive and is intended to serve as a starting point for further research. Cengage Learning is not responsible for the content of the materials.

Abbruzzese, James L., and Ben Ebrahimi. *Myths & Facts About Pancreatic Cancer: What You Need to Know.* Melville, NY: PRR, 2002.

Abeloff, Martin D., James O. Armitage, John E. Niederhuber, et al. *Abeloff's Clinical Oncology,* 4th ed. Philadelphia, PA: Elsevier, 2008.

Abraham, Kimberly, Marney Studaker-Cordner, with Kathryn O'Dea. *The Whipped Parent: Hope for Parents Raising an Out-of-Control Teen.* Highland City, FL: Rainbow Books, 2003.

Abraham, Suzanne. *Eating Disorders: The Facts,* 6th ed. New York: Oxford University Press, 2008.

Abraham, Thomas. *Twenty-first Century Plague: The Story of SARS.* Baltimore, MD: Johns Hopkins University Press, 2005.

Abramovitz, Melissa. *Muscular Dystrophy.* Detroit, MI: Lucent Books, 2008.

Adams, Francis V. *The Asthma Sourcebook (Sourcebooks),* 3rd ed. New York: McGraw-Hill, 2006.

Alcott, Louisa May. *Little Women, or, Meg, Jo, Beth, and Amy.* Boston: Roberts Brothers, 1868.

This beloved children's book contains a description of scarlet fever in the 1800s.

Aleman, Andre, and Frank Laroi. *Hallucinations: The Science of Idiosyncratic Perception.* Washington, DC: American Psychological Association, 2008.

Alexander, Ivy L. *AIDS Sourcebook,* 4th ed. Detroit, MI: Omnigraphics, 2008.

Alexander-Roberts, Colleen. *The AD/HD Parenting Handbook: Practical Advice for Parents from Parents,* 2nd ed. Lanham, MD: Taylor Trade, 2006.

Ali, Rasheda. *I'll Hold Your Hand So You Won't Fall: A Child's Guide to Parkinson's Disease.* West Palm Beach, FL: Merit Publishing International, 2005.

Allman, Toney. *Parasites! Tapeworms.* San Diego, CA: KidHaven Press, 2003.

Alschuler, Lise, and Karolyn, A. Gazella, eds. *Alternative Medicine Magazine's Definitive Guide to Cancer: An Integrative Approach to Prevention, Treatment, and Healing (Alternative Medicine).* Berkeley, CA: Celestial Arts, 2007.

This book offers a comprehensive guide to cancer to help patients and their caregivers evaluate alternative treatments, providing discussions on twenty specific cancers.

Alter, Judith. *Vaccines.* Ann Arbor, MI: Cherry Lake, 2009.

Amato, Anthony, and James Russell. *Neuromuscular Disorders.* New York: McGraw-Hill Professional, 2008.

American Academy of Pediatrics. *Your Baby's First Year,* 2nd ed. New York: Bantam Dell, 2005.

American Cancer Society. *Lymphedema: Understanding and Managing Lymphedema After Cancer Treatment.* Atlanta, GA: American Cancer Society, 2006.

American Diabetes Association. *American Diabetes Association Complete Guide to Diabetes,* 4th ed. New York: Bantam, 2006.

American Diabetes Association. *Gestational Diabetes: What To Expect,* 5th ed. Alexandria, VA: Author, 2005.

American Medical Association, Kate Gruenwald Pfeifer, and Amy B. Middleman. *American Medical Association Boys' Guide to Becoming a Teen.* San Francisco, CA: Jossey-Bass, 2006.

Subjects addressed include healthy eating, exercise, skin care, personal feelings, relationships, and sex.

American Medical Association Guide to Preventing and Treating Heart Disease: Essential Information You and Your Family Need to Know About Having

Bibliography

Dahlman, David. *Why Doesn't My Doctor Know This? Conquering Irritable Bowel Syndrome, Inflammatory Bowel Disease, Crohn's Disease and Colitis.* Garden City, NY: Madeeasy Pub., 2008.

Dalebout, Susan. *The Praeger Guide to Hearing and Hearing Loss: Assessment, Treatment, and Prevention.* Westport, CT: Praeger, 2008.

Dann, Patty. *The Goldfish Went on Vacation: A Memoir of Loss (and Learning to Tell the Truth About it).* Boston: Trumpeter, 2007.

Darvill, Wendy, and Kelsey Powell. *In Your Jeans: A Pocket Guide to Your Changing Body.* Berkeley, CA: Ulysses Press, 2006.

Davis, Deborah L., and Mara Tesler Stein. *Parenting Your Premature Baby and Child: The Emotional Journey.* Golden, CO: Fulcrum, 2004.

Davis, Devra. *The Secret History of the War on Cancer.* New York: Basic Books, 2007.

This book describes how medical science set out to find, treat, and cure cancer but left untouched many of the factors known to cause cancer, including tobacco, the workplace, radiation, or the global environment; the book explains how and why these factors were either overlooked or suppressed.

Davis, Melanie, Caroline Overton, and Lisa Webber. *Infertility: The Facts.* New York: Oxford University Press, 2008.

Day, Doris J. *100 Questions & Answers About Acne.* Sudbury, MA: Jones and Bartlett, 2005.

Day, Jeff. *Don't Touch That! The Book of Gross, Poisonous, and Downright Icky Plants and Critters.* Chicago: Chicago Review Press, 2008.

De Geus, Eelco. *Sometimes I Just Stutter.* Memphis, TN: Stuttering Foundation of America, 1999.

This book tells young people about the causes of stuttering and discusses the fears and embarrassment of people who stutter. It is available to buy or to read at the foundation's web site: http://www.stuttersfa.org.

De Pree, Julia K. *Body Story.* Athens, OH: Swallow Press/Ohio University Press, 2004.

This book describes the troubling journey of poet Julia De Pree from adolescence to adulthood and from anorexia to health.

DeLisi, Lynn E. *100 Questions and Answers About Schizophrenia: Painful Minds.* Sudbury, MA: Jones and Bartlett, 2006.

Deboo, Ana. *Alcohol.* Chicago: Heinemann Library, 2008.

Decker, Janet, and Alan Hecht. *Mononucleosis.* Philadelphia, PA: Chelsea House, 2009.

Del Rio, Iris Quintero. *Lupus: A Patient's Guide to Diagnosis, Treatment, and Lifestyle,* 2nd ed. Roscoe, IL: Hilton, 2007.

Delpeuch, Francis et al. *Globesity: A Planet Out of Control?* London: Earthscan, 2009.

Delta Gamma Center for Children with Visual Impairments. *A Look Into Our "I's": A Compilation of Introspective Writings From a Group of Extraordinary Young People With Visual Impairments.* [St. Louis, MO]: Delta Gamma Center, 2006.

Dempsey, Sharon. *My Brain Tumour Adventures: The Story of a Little Boy Coping with a Brain Tumour.* London: Jessica Kingsley, 2003.

Deraco, M., D. Bartlett, S. Kusamura, et al. "Consensus Statement on Peritoneal Mesothelioma." *Journal of Surgical Oncology* 98, no. 4 (September 15, 2008): 268–272.

Derickson, Alan. *Black Lung: Anatomy of a Public Health Disaster.* Ithaca, NY: Cornell University Press, 1998.

This book provides historical information on black lung disease.

Deyssig, R., H. Frisch, W. F. Blum, et al. "Effect of Growth Hormone Treatment on Hormonal Parameters, Body Composition, and Strength in Athletes." *Acta Endocrinology* (Copenhagen) 128, no. 4 (April 1993):313–318.

DiConsiglio, John. *When Birds Get Flu and Cows Go Mad! How Safe Are We?* New York: Franklin Watts, 2008.

Dicker, Katie. *Explaining Deafness.* London: Franklin Watts, 2009.

Dickerson, James L. *Yellow Fever: A Deadly Disease Poised to Kill Again.* Amherst, NY: Prometheus Books, 2006.

Dizon, Don S. *100 Questions & Answers About Cervical Cancer.* Sudbury, MA: Jones and Bartlett, 2009.

Dizon, Don S. *100 Questions & Answers About Ovarian Cancer,* 2nd ed. Sudbury, MA: Jones and Bartlett, 2006.

This book provides authoritative, practical answers to questions about treatment options, post-treatment quality of life, sources of support, and much more.

Dobbert, Duane L. *Understanding Personality Disorders: An Introduction.* Westport, CT: Praeger, 2007.

Dobler, Merri Lou. *Lactose Intolerance Nutrition Guide.* Chicago: American Dietetic Association, 2003.

Domitrz, Michael J., ed. *Voices of Courage: Inspiration from Survivors of Sexual Assault.* Greenfield, WI: Awareness Publications, 2005.

Donovan, Sandy. *Keep Your Cool! What You Should Know About Stress.* Minneapolis, MN: Lerner, 2009.

Donovan, Sandy, and Jack Desrocher. *Stay Clear! What You Should Know About Skin Care.* Minneapolis, MN: Lerner, 2009.

This book is written for young people, and its discussion is enlivened by anecdotes and cartoons.

Dorris, Michael. *The Broken Cord.* New York: HarperCollins, 1989.

Dorris relates the true story about parents who adopt a boy with fetal alcohol syndrome.

Downs, Alan. *The Velvet Rage: The Pain of Growing Up Gay in a Straight Man's World.* Cambridge, MA: De Capo Press, 2006.

This book describes ways in which early childhood experiences mold the adult lives of gay men.

Drake, Kendis Moore. *Preparing for a Healthy Baby: A Pregnancy Book.* Phoenix: Trimester, 2008.

Dreger, Alice Domurat. *One of Us: Conjoined Twins and the Future of Normal.* Cambridge, MA; Harvard University Press, 2004.

Dreyer, ZoAnn. *Living with Cancer.* New York: Facts On File, 2008.

Drummond, Roger. *Ticks and What You Can Do About Them.* Berkeley, CA: Wilderness Press, 2004.

Durant, Penny. *Sniffles, Sneezes, Hiccups, and Coughs.* New York: Dorling Kindersley (DK), 2005.

Dutton, Mark. *Orthopaedic Examination, Evaluation, and Intervention.* New York: McGraw-Hill Medical, 2008.

Dvorchak, George E., Jr. *The Pocket First-Aid Field Guide: Treatment and Prevention of Outdoor Emergencies.* Accokeek, MD: Stoeger, 2007.

Ehrlich, Paul M., with Elizabeth Shimer. *Living with Allergies.* New York: Facts On File, 2007.

Eig, Jonathan. *Luckiest Man: The Life and Death of Lou Gehrig.* New York: Simon & Schuster, 2005.

A biography of Lou Gehrig, containing information about his struggle with ALS.

Ellsworth, Pamela. *100 Questions & Answers About Prostate Cancer,* 2nd ed. Sudbury, MA: Jones and Bartlett, 2009.

Ellsworth, Pamela. *100 Questions & Answers About Erectile Dysfunction,* 2nd ed. Sudbury, MA: Jones and Bartlett, 2008.

Ellsworth, Pamela, and Brett Carswell. *100 Questions & Answers About Bladder Cancer.* Sudbury, MA: Jones and Bartlett Publishers, 2006.

Ellsworth, Pamela, and David A. Gordon. *100 Questions & Answers About Overactive Bladder and Urinary Incontinence.* Sudbury, MA: Jones and Bartlett, 2006.

Emery, Alan E. M. *Muscular Dystrophy,* 3rd ed. New York: Oxford University Press, 2008.

Emmeluth, Don. *Botulism.* Philadelphia, PA: Chelsea House, 2006.

Emmeluth, Donald. *Plague.* Philadelphia, PA: Chelsea House, 2005.

Emmeluth, Donald. *Typhoid Fever.* Philadelphia, PA: Chelsea House, 2004.

Emmerson, Bryan. *Getting Rid of Gout,* 2nd ed. New York: Oxford University Press, 2003.

Epstein, Lawrence J., with Steven Mardon. *The Harvard Medical School Guide to a Good Night's Sleep.* New York: McGraw-Hill, 2007.

Esherick, Joan. *The Silent Cry: A Teen's Guide to Escaping Self-Injury and Suicide.* Philadelphia, PA: Mason Crest, 2005.

Espeland, Pamela, and Elizabeth Verdick. *Loving to Learn: The Commitment to Learning Assets.* Minneapolis, MN: Free Spirit, 2005.

Evans, Arlene. *Color Is in the Eye of the Beholder: A Guide to Color Vision Deficiency and Colorblindness.* Auburn, CA: CVD, 2003.

Evans, Dwight L., and Linda Wasmer Andrews. *If Your Adolescent Has Depression or Bipolar Disorder: An Essential Resource for Parents.* New York: Oxford University Press, 2005.

Everson, Gregory, and Hedy Weinberg. *Living with Hepatitis C: A Survivor's Guide,* 6th ed. New York: Hatherleigh Press, 2006.

Eynikel, Hilde. *Molokai: The Story of Father Damien.* Translated by Lesley Gilbert. New York: Alba House, 1999.

This is the story of the Belgian priest who cared for thousands of people with leprosy who were banished to the remote island of Molokai in the Hawaiian Islands. The book was made into a movie by the same name that is available on DVD.

Fagan, Peter J. *Sexual Disorders: Perspectives on Diagnosis and Treatment.* Baltimore, MD: Johns Hopkins University Press, 2004.

Falvo, Donna R. *Medical and Psychosocial Aspects of Chronic Illness and Disability.* Sudbury, MA: Jones and Bartlett, 2008.

This book offers both medical and psychological information about issues and concerns that those with disability and chronic illness may encounter.

"FDA Approves First U.S. Vaccine for Humans Against the Avian Influenza Virus H5N1." Press release from the U.S. Food and Drug Administration, April 17, 2007, available online at www.fda.gov/bbs/topics/NEWS/2007/NEW01611.html.

Feder, Lauren. *The Parents' Concise Guide to Childhood Vaccinations: Practical Medical and Natural Ways to Protect Your Child.* Long Island City, NY: Hatherleigh, 2007.

Feehally, John, Jurgen Floege, and Richard J. Johnson, eds. *Comprehensive Clinical Nephrology.* Philadelphia, PA: Mosby/Elsevier, 2007.

Feit, Debbie, with Heidi M. Feldman. *The Parent's Guide to Speech and Language Problems.* New York: McGraw-Hill, 2007.

Fekrat, Sharon, and Jennifer S. Weizer, eds. *All About Your Eyes.* Durham, NC: Duke University Press, 2006.

Feldman, Marc D. *Playing Sick? Untangling the Web of Munchausen Syndrome, Munchausen by Proxy, Malingering, and Factitious Disorder.* New York: Brunner-Routledge, 2004.

Feldman, Mark, Lawrence S. Friedman, Marvin H. Sleisenger, et al. *Sleisenger and Fordtran's Gastrointestinal and Liver Disease,* 8th ed. Lanham, MD: Saunders, 2006.

Felner, Kevin, and Meg Schneider. *COPD for Dummies.* Waterville, ME: Thorndike Press, 2008.

Ferreiro, Carmen. *Mad Cow Disease (Bovine Spongiform Encephalopathy).* Philadelphia, PA: Chelsea House, 2005.

Ferri, Fred, ed. *Ferri's Clinical Advisor 2008.* Philadelphia, PA: Mosby Elsevier, 2008.

Fields, Denise, and Ari Brown. *Toddler 411: Clear Answers & Smart Advice for your Toddler.* Boulder, CO: Windsor Peak Press, 2006.

A pediatrician and mother offers practical advice and information on a variety of different subjects.

Filip, David, and Sharon Filip. *Valley Fever Epidemic.* [United States]: Golden Phoenix, 2008.

Finer, Kim R. *Smallpox.* Philadelphia, PA: Chelsea House, 2004.

Firestein, Gary S., Ralph C. Budd, Edward D. Harris, et al. *Kelley's Textbook of Rheumatology,* 8th ed. Philadelphia, PA: Saunders, 2008.

Fishman, Loren, and Carol Ardman. *Sciatica Solutions: Diagnosis, Treatment, and Cure of Spinal and Piriformis Problems.* New York: Norton, 2007.

This book offers information about sciatica and various treatment options for those suffering with pain in the lower back, buttocks, and legs.

Flammer, Josef. *Glaucoma: Guide for Patients, an Introduction for Care-Providers, a Quick Reference,* 3rd rev. ed. Cambridge, MA: Hogrefe, 2006.

Flegg, Anita. *Hypoglycemia: The Other Sugar Disease.* Ottawa: Book Coach Press, 2006.

The book discusses what hypoglycemia is, its symptoms, and diagnosis, testing and interpretation. It also contains practical advice on the use of supplements.

Fleming, Shawna L. *Helicobacter Pylori.* New York: Chelsea House, 2007.

Foltz-Gray, Dorothy. *The Arthritis Foundation's Guide to Good Living with Rheumatoid Arthritis,* 3rd ed. Atlanta, GA: Arthritis Foundation, 2006.

From the Arthritis Foundation, this book discusses medications and other treatment options and research.

Fonda, Jane. *My Life So Far.* New York: Random House, 2006.

In this autobiography, Fonda admits to 30 years of bulimia and anorexia and describes her quest for self-discovery.

Ford, Melissa. *Navigating the Land of IF: Understanding Infertility and Exploring Your Options.* Emeryville, CA: Seal Press, 2009.

Fowler, Mary. *20 Questions to Ask If Your Child Has ADHD.* Franklin Lakes, NJ: Career Press, 2006.

Francis, Suzanne, with Jim Breheny. *Dangerous and Deadly Toxic Animals.* New York: Scholastic, 2007.

Fredericks, Carrie. *Obesity.* San Diego, CA: ReferencePoint, 2008.

Freedman, Jeri. *Brain Cancer: Current and Emerging Trends in Detection and Treatment.* New York: Rosen, 2008.

Freeman, Daniel, and Jason Freeman. *Paranoia: The Twenty-First Century Fear.* Oxford, UK: Oxford University Press, 2008.

Freimuth, Marilyn. *Addicted? Recognizing Destructive Behavior Before It's Too Late.* Lanham, MD: Rowman and Littlefield, 2008.

Fried, Richard G. *Healing Adult Acne: Your Guide to Clear Skin & Self-Confidence.* Oakland, CA: New Harbinger, 2005.

Friend, Milton. *Tularemia.* Reston, VA: Department of the Interior, Geological Survey, 2006.

Furgang, Kathy. *Frequently Asked Questions About Sports Injuries.* New York: Rosen, 2008.

Gallant, Joel. *100 Questions & Answers About HIV and AIDS.* Sudbury, MA: Jones and Bartlett, 2009.

Galvin, Matthew. *Clouds and Clocks: A Story for Children Who Soil,* 2nd ed. Washington, DC: Magination Press, 2007.

Gardner, James. *Phobias and How to Overcome Them.* Franklin Lakes, NJ: New Page Books, 2005.

Garie, Gretchen, and Michael J. Church, with Winifred Conkling. *Living Well with Parkinson's Disease: What Your Doctor Doesn't Tell You—That You Need to Know.* New York: Collins, 2007.

Garrison, Cheryl, and Richard A. Passwater. *The Hemochromatosis Cookbook: Recipes and Meals for Reducing the Absorption of Iron in Your Diet.* Nashville, TN: Cumberland House, 2008.

Gavigan, Christopher. *Healthy Child, Healthy World: Creating a Cleaner, Greener, Safer Home.* New York: Dutton Adult, 2008.

The author discusses ways to keep babies healthy and safe inside and outside of the home.

Geffen, Jeremy R. *The Journey Through Cancer: Healing and Transforming the Whole Person.* New York: Three Rivers Press, 2006.

This book offers suggestions for the unique challenges encountered by people living with cancer.

Gerber, Max. *My Heart vs. the Real World: Children with Heart Disease, in Photographs and Interviews.* Woodbury, NY: Cold Spring Harbor Laboratory Press, 2008.

A photo documentary volume that explores the lives of children with congenital heart disease through striking black and white photographs and interviews with subjects and their families.

Gerdes, Louise I., ed. *The Homeless.* Detroit, MI: Greenhaven Press, 2007.

Giddens, Sandra. *Frequently Asked Questions About Suicide.* New York: Rosen, 2009.

Giddens, Sandra. *Obsessive-Compulsive Disorder.* New York: Rosen, 2009.

Gipson, Fred. *Old Yeller.* New York: Harper 1956.

This classic children's coming-of-age story concerns a dog that develops rabies.

Gislason, Stephen J. *The Book of Brain,* 2nd ed. Sechelt, BC, Canada: Environmed Research, 2006.

Gittleman, Ann Louise. *Guess What Came to Dinner? Parasites and Your Health,* 2nd ed. New York: Avery, 2001.

Gizel, Kayli. *All About Me: Growing Up with Turner Syndrome and Nonverbal Learning Disabilities.* Wallingford, VT: Maple Leaf Center, 2004.

Glaser, Jason. *Chicken Pox.* Mankato, MN: Capstone Press, 2006.

Glaser, Jason. *Ear Infections.* Mankato, MN: Capstone Press, 2007.

Glaser, Jason. *Flu.* Mankato, MN: Capstone Press, 2006.

Glaser, Jason. *Pink Eye.* Mankato, MN: Capstone Press, 2006.

Glaser, Jason. *Strep Throat.* Mankato, MN: Capstone Press, 2007.

Goetz, C. G. *Goetz's Textbook of Clinical Neurology,* 3rd ed. Philadelphia, PA: Saunders, 2007.

Gogerly, Liz. *Eating Well.* New York: Crabtree, 2009.

Golden, Janet. *Message in a Bottle: The Making of Fetal Alcohol Syndrome.* Cambridge, MA: Harvard University Press, 2005.

Goldman, Lee, and Dennis Ausiello, eds. *Cecil Textbook of Internal Medicine,* 23rd ed. Philadelphia, PA: Saunders, 2008.

Goldsmith, Connie. *Meningitis.* Minneapolis, MN: Twenty-First Century Books, 2008.

Goldsmith, Connie. *Superbugs Strike Back: When Antibiotics Fail.* Minneapolis, MN: Twenty-First Century Books, 2007.

Goldstein, Andrew, Caroline Pukall, Irwin Goldstein. *Female Sexual Pain Disorders: Evaluation and Management.* Hoboken, NJ: Wiley, 2009.

Golomb, Ruth Goldfinger, and Sherrie Mansfield Vavrichek. *The Hair Pulling "Habit" and You: How to Solve the Trichotillomania Puzzle.* Silver Spring, MD: Writers' Cooperative of Greater Washington, 2000.

This workbook and guide for kids and teens, parents, and therapists presents useful strategies and tools for conquering trichotillomania.

Goodheart, Herbert P. *Acne for Dummies.* Indianapolis, IN: Wiley, 2006.

Gootman, Marilyn. *When A Friend Dies: A Book for Teens About Grieving and Healing,* rev. and updated ed. Minneapolis, MN: Free Spirit, 2005.

This book seeks to help teens cope with the death of a friend, for readers over the age of 11.

Gould, Harry J., III. *Understanding Pain: What It Is, Why It Happens, and How It's Managed.* St. Paul, MN: American Academy of Neurology Press, 2007.

Gravelle, Karen. *The Period Book: Everything You Don't Want to Ask (but Need to Know).* New York: Walker, 2006.

Gray, Shirley Wimbish. *Prevention and Good Health.* Chanhassen, MN: Child's World, 2004.

Graziano, Anthony M. *Developmental Disabilities: Introduction to a Diverse Field.* Needham, MA: Allyn and Bacon, 2001.

Green, Peter H. R. *Celiac Disease: A Hidden Epidemic.* New York: Collins, 2006.

Greenberg, Jerrold S. *Comprehensive Stress Management.* New York: McGraw-Hill, 2008.

This book discusses the physical, psychological, sociological, and spiritual components and features of stress and offers insight into various stress management and coping skills.

Greenfeld, Karl Taro. *China Syndrome: The True Story of the 21st Century's First Great Epidemic.* New York: HarperCollins, 2006.

Greenstein, Ben, and Diana F. Wood. *The Endocrine System at a Glance,* 2nd ed. Malden, MA: Blackwell, 2006.

Gregory, Robert J. *Psychological Testing: History, Principles, and Applications,* 5th ed. Boston: Pearson/Allyn and Bacon, 2007.

Grubb, Blair P. *The Fainting Phenomenon: Understanding Why People Faint and What to Do About It,* 2nd ed. Malden, MA: Blackwell, 2007.

Gruman-Trinkner, Carrie, and Blaise Winter. *Your Cleft-Affected Child: The Complete Book of Information, Resources, and Hope.* Alameda, CA: Hunter House, 2001.

Guilfoile, Patrick. *Antibiotic-Resistant Bacteria.* New York: Chelsea House, 2007.

Guilfoile, Patrick. *Diphtheria.* New York: Chelsea House, 2009.

Guilfoile, Patrick. *Tetanus.* New York: Chelsea House, 2008.

Gunther, John. *Death Be Not Proud: A Memoir.* New York: HarperPerennial Library, 1998.

First published in 1949 and made into a movie in 1975, this memoir presents a father's description of the ordeals experienced by his son who had a brain tumor and by his family.

Gupta, Sanjay. "Battling Brain Cancer." *Time* 171, no. 22 (June 2, 2008): 52.

Gupta, Sanjay. "Rash Redux." *Time* 172, no. 4 (July 28, 2008): 53.

Guthrie, Woody. *Bound for Glory.* New York: E.P. Dutton, 1943.

An autobiography by the folk singer who was later afflicted with Huntington's disease.

Hall, Ian R., Steven L. Stephenson, Peter K. Buchanan, et al. *Edible and Poisonous Mushrooms of the World.* Portland, OR: Timber Press, 2003.

Halpern, Sue. *Can't Remember What I Forgot: The Good News from the Front Lines of Memory Research.* New York: Harmony Books, 2008.

Halse, Christine, Anne Honey, and Desiree Boughtwood. *Inside Anorexia: The Experiences of Girls and Their Families.* London: Jessica Kingsley, 2008.

The Hangover Companion: A Guide to the Morning After. London: Michael O'Mara Books, 2006.

A humorous approach to the morning after full of facts and other hangover related information.

Hardman, Lizabeth. *Dementia.* Detroit, MI: Lucent Books, 2009.

Hart, Carl, Charles Ksir, and Oakley Ray. *Drugs, Society, and Human Behavior*, 13th ed. New York: McGraw-Hill, 2009.

Hartley, Karen, Chris Macro, and Philip Taylor. *Head Louse,* new ed. Chicago: Heinemann Library, 2006.

Hartmann, Lynn C., and Charles L. Loprinzi. *Mayo Clinic Guide to Women's Cancers.* New York: Mayo Clinic, 2005

Hawkins, W. Rex. *Eat Right—Electrolyte: A Nutritional Guide to Minerals in Our Daily Diet.* Amherst, NY: Prometheus Books, 2006.

Hayden, Deborah. *Pox: Genius, Madness, and the Mysteries of Syphilis.* New York: Basic Books, 2003.

Healy, Bernadine. *Living Time: Faith and Facts to Guide Your Cancer Journey.* New York: Bantam Dell, 2008.

Heaton, Jeanne A., and Claudia J. Strauss. *Talking to Eating Disorders: Simple Ways to Support Someone Who Has Anorexia, Bulimia, Binge Eating or Body Image Issues.* New York: New American Library, 2005.

This book discusses ways to deal with issues of negative body image, the images promoted in the popular media, problems with physical touching, diets, and exercise. The book includes a section on talking about these issues with children.

Hedges, Dawson, and Colin Burchfield. *Mind, Brain, and Drug: An Introduction to Psychopharmacology.* Boston: Pearson/Allyn and Bacon, 2006.

Heininger, Ulrich, and Jane F. Seward. "Varicella." *Lancet* 368, no. 9544 (October 14–20, 2006): 1365–1376.

Hempel, Sandra. *The Strange Case of the Broad Street Pump: John Snow and the Mystery of Cholera.* Berkeley: University of California Press, 2007.

Herrick, Charles, and Charlotte A. Herrick. *100 Questions & Answers About Alcoholism.* Sudbury, MA: Jones and Bartlett, 2007.

Herrin, Marcia, and Nancy Matsumoto. *The Parent's Guide to Eating Disorders: Supporting Self-Esteem, Healthy Eating, and Positive Body Image at Home.* Carlsbad, CA: Gurze Books, 2007.

The authors argue that eating disorders can be resolved at home with the effective use of time, effort, and love.

Hinds, Maurene J. *Fighting the AIDS and HIV Epidemic: A Global Battle.* Berkeley Heights, NJ: Enslow, 2008.

Hirsch, Alan R. *What Your Doctor May Not Tell You About Sinusitis: Relieve Your Symptoms and Identify the Real Source of Your Pain.* New York: Warner Books, 2004

Hirschmann, Kris. *Lice.* Farmington Hills, MI: Kidhaven Press, 2004.

Hirschmann, Kris. *Reflections of Me: Girls and Body Image.* Mankato, MN: Compass Point Books, 2009.

Hirschmann, Kris. *Salmonella.* San Diego, CA: Kidhaven Press, 2004.

Hirschmann, Kris. *The Ebola Virus.* Detroit, MI: Lucent Books, 2007.

Hoffman, John, and Susan Froemke, eds. *Addiction: Why Can't They Just Stop?* New York: Rodale Books, 2007.

Hollander, Eric, and Nicholas Bakalar. *Coping with Social Anxiety: The Definitive Guide to Effective Treatment Options.* New York: Holt, 2005.

Hollenbeck, Peter. *Treating Tourette Syndrome and Tic Disorders: A Guide for Practitioners.* New York: Guilford Press, 2007.

Holler, Teresa. *Cardiology Essentials.* Sudbury, MA: Jones and Bartlett, 2007.

Holmes, King. *Sexually Transmitted Diseases,* 4th ed. New York: McGraw Hill, 2007.

Horchler, Joani. *SIDS and Infant Death Survival Guide: Information and Comfort for Grieving Family and Friends and Professionals Who Seek to Help Them,* 3rd ed. Hyattsville, MD: SIDS Educational Services, 2003.

Horsley, Heidi, and Gloria Horsley. *Teen Grief Relief.* Highland City, FL: Rainbow Books, 2007.

This guide answers questions and helps teenagers understand a range of situations connected to dying and death.

How to Study for Success. Hoboken, NJ: Wiley, 2004.

Hreib, Kinan K. *100 Questions and Answers About Stroke: A Lahey Clinic Guide.* Sudbury, MA: Jones and Bartlett, 2008.

Huebner, Dawn. *What to Do When Your Brain Gets Stuck: A Kid's Guide to Overcoming OCD.* Washington, DC: Magination Press, 2007.

Hulit, Lloyd M. *Straight Talk on Stuttering: Information, Encouragement, and Counsel for Stutterers, Caregivers, and Speech-language Clinicians,* 2nd ed. Springfield, IL: Charles C. Thomas, 2004.

Hultquist, Alan M. *What Is Dyslexia? A Book Explaining Dyslexia for Kids and Adults to Use Together.* London: Jessica Kingsley, 2008.

The Human Body & the Environment: How Our Surroundings Affect Our Health. Westport, CT: Greenwood Press, 2003.

Hunter, Kathy. *Raindrops and Sunshine: Tales of Triumph and Laughter.* Clinton, MD: IRSA, 2007.

Hunter, Miranda, and William Hunter. *Staying Safe: A Teen's Guide to Sexually Transmitted Diseases.* Philadelphia, PA: Mason Crest, 2005.

Hyman, Bruce M., and Cherry Pedrick. *Anxiety Disorders.* Minneapolis, MN: Twenty-First Century Books, 2006.

Icon Health Publications. *Ataxia: A Medical Dictionary, Bibliography, and Annotated Research Guide to Internet References.* San Diego, CA: Author, 2004.

Imboden, John. *Current Diagnosis and Treatment in Rheumatology,* 2nd ed. New York: McGraw Hill, 2006.

Isaacs, Scott, and Fred Vagnini. *Overcoming Metabolic Syndrome.* Omaha, NE: Addicus Books, 2006.

Ishimure, Michiko. *Paradise in the Sea of Sorrow: Our Minamata Disease.* Translated by Livia Monnet. Ann Arbor: University of Michigan Center for Japanese Studies, 2003.

The author, a housewife and poet, visited the families affected by Minamata disease and wrote a documentary about it. She also organized a movement to obtain financial help for the victims.

Izzo, Joseph. *Hypertension Primer: The Essentals of High Blood Pressure,* 4th ed. Philadelphia, PA: Lippincott Williams & Wilkins, 2007.

Jacobs, Gregg D. *Say Good Night to Insomnia.* New York: Holt, 2009.

Jacobson, John W., James A. Mulick, and Johannes Rojahn, eds. *Handbook of Intellectual and Developmental Disabilities* New York: Springer, 2007.

James, Andra H., Thomas L. Ortel, and Victor F. Tapson. *100 Questions & Answers About Deep Vein Thrombosis and Pulmonary Embolism.* Sudbury, MA: Jones and Bartlett, 2008.

Janowitz, Henry D. *Your Gut Feelings.* New York: Oxford University Press, 1994.

Jarrow, Gail. *Hookworms.* San Diego. CA: Kidhaven Press, 2004.

Jennings, Kathryn Tracey. "Female Sexual Abuse of Children: An Exploratory Study." Ph.D. diss., University of Toronto (Canada), 1998.

Jensen, Dean. *The Lives and Loves of Daisy and Violet Hilton: A True Story of Conjoined Twins.* Berkeley, CA: Ten Speed Press, 2006.

Johanson, Paula. *Frequently Asked Questions About Testicular Cancer.* New York: Rosen, 2008.

Johanson, Paula. *Muscular Dystrophy.* New York: Rosen, 2008.

Johns Hopkins Complete Guide to Medical Tests: Everything You Need to Know About 170 Common Tests. Pleasantville, NY: Reader's Digest Association, 2002.

Johnson, David, and David Sandmire, with Daniel Klein. *Medical Tests That Can Save Your Life: 21 Tests Your Doctor Won't Order—Unless You Know to Ask.* Emmaus, PA: Rodale, 2004.

Johnson, Rebecca L. *Daring Cell Defenders.* Minneapolis, MN: Millbrook Press, 2008.

Johnson, Stephen. *The Ghost Map: The Story of London's Most Terrifying Epidemic.* New York: Riverhead Books, 2006.

Jones, J. Stephen. *The Complete Prostate Book: What Every Man Needs to Know.* Amherst, NY: Prometheus Books, 2005.

Jones, James Earl, and Penelope Niven. *Voices and Silences: with a New Epilogue.* New York: Limelight Editions, 2002.

Jones, Marcia L., Theresa Eichenwald, and Nancy W. Hall. *Menopause for Dummies,* 2nd ed. Hoboken, NJ: Wiley, 2007.

Jones, Paul E., with Andrea Thompson. *The Up and Down Life: the Truth About Bipolar Disorder—The Good, the Bad, and the Funny.* New York: Perigee Book, 2008.
Comedian Paul Jones describes his own struggle with bipolar disorder.

Jones, Phill. *Sickle Cell Disease.* New York: Chelsea House, 2008.

Jones-Smith, Elsie. *Nurturing Nonviolent Children: A Guide for Parents, Educators, and Counselors.* Westport, CT: Praeger, 2008.

Jong, Elaine. *The Travel and Tropical Medicine Manual,* 4th ed. Philadelphia, PA: Saunders, 2008.

Judd, Sandra J., ed. *Autism and Pervasive Developmental Disorders Sourcebook.* Detroit, MI: Omnigraphics, 2007.

Juettner, Bonnie. *Skin Cancer.* Detroit, MI: Lucent Books, 2008.

Jupiter, Jesse, Alan Levine, and Peter Trafton. *Skeletal Trauma: Basic Science, Management, and Reconstruction,* 3rd ed. Philadelphia, PA: Saunders, 2002.

Kabir, K., J. Sheeder, and L. S. Kelly. "Identifying Postpartum Depression: Are 3 Questions as Good as 10?" *Pediatrics* 122, no. 3 (September 2008): 696–702.

Kachlany, Scott C. *Infectious Diseases of the Mouth.* New York: Chelsea House, 2007.

Kalb, Kate Bracy. *The Everything Health Guide to Menopause: Reassuring Advice and Up-to-date Information to Keep You Healthy and Happy,* 2nd ed. Avon, MA: Adams Media, 2007.

Kalb, Rosalind C., ed. *Multiple Sclerosis: The Questions You Have—The Answers You Need,* 4th ed. New York: Demos Medical, 2008.

Kandeel, Fouad R. *Male Sexual Dysfunction: Pathophysiology and Treatment.* New York: Informa Healthcare, 2007.

Kandel, Joseph, and David Sudderth. *The Headache Cure: How to Uncover What's Really Causing Your Pain and Find Lasting Relief.* New York: McGraw-Hill, 2006.

Kant, Jared. *The Thought that Counts: A Firsthand Account of One Teenager's Experience with Obsessive-Compulsive Disorder.* New York: Oxford University Press, 2008.

Kantor, Martin. *The Psychopathy of Everyday Life: How Antisocial Personality Disorder Affects All of Us.* Westport, CT: Praeger, 2006.

Kaplowitz, Paul, and Jeffrey Baron. *The Short Child: A Parents' Guide to the Causes, Consequences and*

Treatment of Growth Problems. New York: Warner Wellness, 2006.

Karp, Gary. *Life on Wheels: The A-to-Z Guide to Living Fully with Mobility Issues,* 2nd ed. New York: Demos Health, 2009.

Karst, Karlene. *The Metabolic Syndrome Program: How to Lose Weight, Beat Heart Disease, Stop Insulin Resistance and More.* Toronto: Wiley Canada, 2006.

Kastor, John A. *You and Your Arrhythmia: A Guide to Heart Rhythm Problems for Patients and Their Families.* Sudbury, MA: Jones and Bartlett, 2006.

Katz, Aaron E. *Dr. Katz's Guide to Prostate Health: From Conventional to Holistic Therapies.* Topanga, CA: Freedom Press, 2006.

Kaufman, Howard L. *The Melanoma Book: A Complete Guide to Prevention and Treatment.* New York: Gotham Books, 2005.

Kaufman, Miriam. *Easy for You to Say: Q and As for Teens Living with Chronic Illness or Disability.* Buffalo, NY: Firefly Books, 2005.

Kaye, Cathryn Berger. *A Kid's Guide to Hunger and Homelessness: How to Take Action.* Minneapolis, MN: Free Spirit, 2007.

Keating-Velasco, Joanna L. *In His Shoes: A Short Journey Through Autism.* Shawnee Mission, KS: Autism Asperger, 2008.

Kehret, Peg. *Small Steps: The Year I Got Polio,* anniversary ed. Morton Grove, IL: Albert Whitman, 2006.

Kelly, Evelyn B. *Alzheimer's Disease.* New York: Chelsea Press, 2007.

This book covers current research on Alzheimer's disease, including the genetics and latest treatments, written at a seventh-grade reading level.

Kelnar, Christopher J. H., Martin O. Savage, P. Saenger, et al. *Growth Disorders,* 2nd ed. London: Hodder Arnold, 2007.

Kerr, Alison, and Ingegerd Witt Engerstrom, eds. *Rett Disorder and the Developing Brain.* New York: Oxford University Press, 2005.

Kerr, Jim. *Diet and Obesity.* Mankato, MN: Sea-to-Sea, 2010.

Keystone, Jay. *Travel Medicine: Expert Consult,* 2nd ed. St. Louis, MO: Mosby, 2008.

Kidd, J. S., and R. A. Kidd. *New Genetics: The Study of Lifelines.* New York: Chelsea House, 2006.

This survey written for young adults discusses the evolution of the study of genetics.

Killilea, Marie. *Karen.* New York: Buccaneer Books, 1993.

For young readers and their parents, this classic book (originally published in 1952) is an intelligent, very human account of what it is like to have cerebral palsy.

Kita, Joe, ed. *Sports Injuries Handbook.* Emmaus, PA: Rodale, 2005.

Kitchen, Clyde K. *Fact and Fiction of Healthy Vision: Eye Care for Adults and Children.* Westport, CT: Praeger, 2007.

Klippel, John. *Primer on the Rheumatic Diseases,* 13th ed. New York: Springer, 2008.

Klitzman, Robert. *The Trembling Mountain: A Personal Account of Kuru, Cannibals, and Mad Cow Disease.* New York: Plenum Trade, 1998.

Klosterman, Lorrie. *Drug Dependence to Treatment.* New York: Marshall Cavendish Benchmark, 2008.

Klosterman, Lorrie. *Drug-Resistant Diseases and Superbugs.* Tarrytown, NY: Marshall Cavendish Benchmark, 2010.

Klosterman, Lorrie. *Meningitis.* New York: Marshall Cavendish Benchmark, 2007.

Klosterman, Lorrie. *Rabies.* New York: Marshall Cavendish Benchmark, 2008.

Klosterman, Lorrie. *The Facts About Caffeine.* New York: Marshall Cavendish Benchmark, 2006.

Klosterman, Lorrie. *The Facts About Drugs and the Body.* New York: Marshall Cavendish Benchmark, 2008.

Koegel, Lynn Kern, and Claire LaZebnik. *Growing Up on the Spectrum: A Guide to Life, Love, and Learning for Teens and Young Adults with Autism and Asperger's.* New York: Viking, 2009.

Kolata, Gina. *Flu: The Story of the Great Influenza Pandemic of 1918 and the Search for the Virus that*

Caused It. New York: Farrar, Straus, and Giroux, 2001.

A highly readable history of influenza and the scientists who have worked to understand it.

Kollar, Linda, and Brian Schmaefsky. *Gonorrhea.* Philadelphia, PA: Chelsea House, 2005.

Konshin, Victor. *Beating Gout: A Sufferer's Guide to Living Pain Free.* Williamsville, NY: Ayerware, 2008.

Korf, Bruce R., and Allan E. Rubenstein. *Neurofibromatosis: A Handbook for Patients, Families, and Health Care Professionals,* 2nd ed. New York: Thieme Medical, 2005.

Krakow, Barry. *Sound Sleep, Sound Mind: 7 Keys to Sleeping Through the Night.* Hoboken, NJ: Wiley, 2007.

Kramer, Gerri Freid, and Shari Maurer. *The Parent's Guide to Children's Congenital Heart Defects: What They Are, How to Treat Them, How to Cope with Them.* Three Rivers, MI: Three Rivers Press, 2001.

Krane, Elliot J., with Deborah Mitchell. *Relieve Your Child's Chronic Pain: A Doctor's Program to Easing Headaches, Abdominal Pain, Fibromyalgia, Juvenile Rheumatoid Arthritis, and More.* New York: Simon & Schuster, 2005.

Krotec, Joesph W., and Sharon Perkins. *Endometriosis for Dummies.* Hoboken, NJ: Wiley, 2007.

Kruel, Donald. *Trypanosomiasis.* New York: Chelsea House, 2007.

Kübler-Ross, Elisabeth. *On Death and Dying.* New York: Macmillan, 1969.

Kucik, Corry Jeb, Gary L. Martin, and Brett V. Sortor. "Common Intestinal Parasites." *American Family Physician* 69, no. 5 (March 1, 2004): 1161–68. Also available at http://www.aafp.org/afp/20040301/1161.html.

Kumar, P. Dileep. *Rabies.* Westport, CT: Greenwood Press, 2008.

Kunin, Audrey, with Bill Gottlieb. *The Dermadoctor Skinstruction Manual: The Smart Guide to Healthy Beautiful Skin and Looking Good at Any Age.* New York: Simon & Schuster, 2005.

Kunkel, Robert S. *Headaches: A Cleveland Clinic Handbook.* Cleveland, OH: Cleveland Clinic Press, 2007.

Kutscher, Martin L. *Children with Seizures: A Guide for Parents, Teachers, and Other Professionals.* Philadelphia, PA: Jessica Kingsley, 2006.

Lacey, J. Hubert, Christine Craggs-Hinton, and Kate Robinson. *Overcoming Anorexia.* London: Sheldon Press, 2007.

Landau, Elaine. *Bites and Stings.* New York: Marshall Cavendish Benchmark, 2009.

Landau, Elaine. *Nosebleeds.* New York: Marshall Cavendish Benchmark, 2010.

Landau, Elaine. *Pink Eye.* New York: Marshall Cavendish Benchmark, 2010.

Lang, Denise, with Kenneth B. Liegner. *Coping with Lyme Disease: A Practical Guide to Dealing with Diagnosis and Treatment,* 3rd ed. New York: Holt, 2004.

Langer, Paul. *Great Feet for Life: Footcare and Footwear for Healthy Aging.* Minneapolis, MN: Fairview Press, 2007.

This easy-to-follow book discusses how proper foot care and footwear can help adults maintain an active lifestyle.

Langley, Richard. *Psoriasis: Everything You Need to Know.* Buffalo, NY: Firefly Books, 2005.

Laskey, Elizabeth. *Fifth Disease.* Chicago: Heinemann Library, 2003.

Laskey, Elizabeth. *Mumps.* Chicago: Heinemann Library, 2003.

Laskey, Elizabeth. *Whooping Cough.* Chicago: Heinemann Library, 2003.

Lawton, Sandra Augustyn, ed. *Learning Disabilities Information For Teens: Health Tips About Academic Skills Disorders and Other Disabilities that Affect Learning, including Information About Common Signs of Learning Disabilities, School Issues, Learning to Live with a Learning Disability, and Other Related Issues.* Detroit, MI: Omnigraphics, 2006.

Lead Poisoning: What It Is and What You Can Do About It. New Brunswick, NJ: Legal Services of New Jersey, 2006.

Leary, Warren E. "New Therapy Offers Promise in Treatment of Pedophiles." *New York Times* February 12, 1998. http://query.nytimes.com/gst/fullpage.html?res=9C04E6DB153CF931A25751C0A96E958260&sec=health&spon=&pagewanted=1.

Lennard-Brown, Sarah. *Sports Injuries.* Chicago: Raintree, 2005.

Leuenroth, Stephanie J. *Hantavirus Pulmonary Syndrome.* New York: Chelsea House, 2006.

Levete, Sarah. *Learning Difficulties.* North Mankato, MN: Stargazer Books, 2007.

Levin, Judith. *Anxiety and Panic Attacks.* New York: Rosen, 2009.

Levinson, David, and Marcy Ross, eds. *Homelessness Handbook.* Great Barrington, MA: Berkshire Publishing Group, 2007.

Levinthal, Charles F. *Drugs, Behavior, and Modern Society,* 5th ed. Boston: Pearson/Allyn and Bacon, 2008.

Lew, Kristi. *Mosquito-borne Illnesses.* New York: Marshall Cavendish Benchmark, 2010.

Libal, Autumn. *Chained: Youth with Chronic Illness.* Broomall, PA: Mason Crest, 2004.

Libal, Joyce. *Finding My Voice: Youth with Speech Impairment.* Broomall, PA: Mason Crest Publishers, 2004.

Libby, P., et al. *Braunwald's Heart Disease,* 8th ed. Philadelphia, PA: Saunders, 2007.

Lillrank, Sonja M. *Psychological Disorders: Alzheimer's Disease and Other Dementias.* New York: Chelsea House, 2007.

Lindberg, Barbro. *Understanding Rett Syndrome: A Practical Guide For Parents, Teachers, and Therapists,* 2nd rev. ed. Cambridge, MA: Hogrefe & Huber, 2006.

Lindesay, James, Kenneth Rockwood, and Alastair Macdonald, eds. *Delirium in Old Age.* New York: Oxford University Press, 2002.

Lindley, Richard I. *Stroke.* Oxford, UK: Oxford University Press, 2008.

Link, John. *Breast Cancer Survival Manual: A Step-by-Step Guide for the Woman With Newly Diagnosed Breast Cancer,* 4th ed. New York: Holt Paperbacks, 2007.

Liu, Aimee. *Gaining: The Truth About Life after Eating Disorders.* New York: Grand Central, 2007.
This book explores many of the myths surrounding eating disorders.

Livoti, Carol, and Elizabeth Topp. *The Stress-Free Pregnancy Guide: A Doctor Tells You What to Really Expect.* New York: AMACOM, 2009.

Lock, James, and Daniel le Grange. *Help Your Teenager Beat an Eating Disorder.* New York: Guilford Press, 2005.
This book discusses the management of eating disorders, their complexity, the thinking behind teenage sufferers' behavior, and what research shows about the efficacy of treatment methods.

Long, Jody E., Nicholas J. Long, and Signe Whitson. *The Angry Smile: The Psychology of Passive-Aggressive Behavior in Families, Schools, and Workplaces,* 2nd ed. Austin, TX: Pro-Ed, 2009.

Lorig, Kate, et al. *Living a Healthy Life with Chronic Conditions: Self-management of Heart Disease, Arthritis, Diabetes, Asthma, Bronchitis, Emphysema & Others,* 3rd ed. Boulder, CO: Bull Publishing Company, 2006.

Lorig, Kate, James Fries, and Maureen R. Gecht. *The Arthritis Helpbook: A Tested Self-Management Program for Coping with Arthritis and Fibromyalgia,* 6th ed. Cambridge, MA: Da Capo Lifelong, 2006.

Love, Susan M. *Dr. Susan Love's Breast Book,* 4th ed. Cambridge, MA: Da Capo Lifelong Books, 2005.

Lucas, Alexander R. *Demystifying Anorexia Nervosa: An Optimistic Guide to Understanding and Healing.* New York: Oxford University Press, 2008.

Luesley, David M., Frank Lawton, and Andrew Berchuck, eds. *Uterine Cancer.* New York: Taylor and Francis Group, 2006.

Luterman, David. *Children with Hearing Loss: A Family Guide.* Sedona, AZ: Auricle Ink, 2006.

Lutkenhoff, Marlene. *Children with Spina Bifida: A Parents' Guide,* 2nd ed. Bethesda, MD: Woodbine House, 2007.

Lynette, Rachel. *Leprosy.* Farmington Hills, MI: KidHaven Press, 2006.

MacKay, Jenny. *Amnesia.* Detroit, MI: Lucent Books, 2009.

MacKay, Jenny. *Phobias.* Detroit, MI: Lucent Books, 2009.

Maccaro, Janet. *Brain-Boosting Foods.* Lake Mary, FL: Siloam, 2008.

Madaras, Lynda, and Area Madaras. *My Body, My Self for Boys,* 2nd rev. ed. New York: Newmarket Press, 2007.

Madaras, Lynda, and Area Madaras. *My Body, My Self for Girls,* 2nd rev. ed. New York: Newmarket Press, 2007.

Mandell, Gerald, John Bennett, and Raphael Dolin. *Principles and Practice of Infectious Diseases,* 6th ed. London: Churchill Livingstone, 2005.

Marcovitz, Hal. *Caffeine.* San Diego, CA: Lucent Books, 2006.

Marcovitz, Hal. *Infectious Mononucleosis.* Detroit, MI: Lucent Books, 2008.

Marcovitz, Hal. *Meningitis.* San Diego, CA: ReferencePoint Press, 2009.

Marcovitz, Hal. *Sleep Disorders.* San Diego, CA: ReferencePoint Press, 2008.

Marcovitz, Hal. *Teens and Suicide.* Philadelphia, PA: Mason Crest, 2004.

Marcus, Bernard A. *Malaria,* 2nd ed. New York: Chelsea House, 2009.

Marcus, Dawn A. *10 Simple Solutions to Migraines: Recognize Triggers, Control Symptoms, and Reclaim Your Life.* Oakland, CA: New Harbinger, 2006.

Margulies, Phillip. *Everything You Need to Know About Rheumatic Fever.* New York: Rosen, 2004.

Markovic, Nenad, and Olivera Markovic. *What Every Woman Should Know About Cervical Cancer.* New York: Springer, 2008.

Marotz, Lynn R. *Health, Safety, and Nutrition for the Young Child.* Clifton Park, NY: Thomson Delmar Learning, 2005.

Marr, Lisa. *Sexually Transmitted Diseases: A Physician Tells You What You Need to Know,* 2nd ed. Baltimore, MD: Johns Hopkins University Press, 2007.

Marsh, Tracy. *Children with Tourette Syndrome: A Parents' Guide,* 2nd ed. Bethesda, MD: Woodbine House, 2007.

Martin, Sieglinde. *Teaching Motor Skills to Children with Cerebral Palsy and Similar Movement Disorders: A Guide for Parents and Professionals.* Bethesda, MD: Woodbine House, 2006.

Marx, John A., et al. *Rosen's Emergency Medicine,* 6th ed. St. Louis, MO: Mosby, 2006.

Mason, Robert J., V. Courtney Broaddus, John F. Murray, et al. *Murray & Nadel's Textbook of Respiratory Medicine,* 4th ed. Philadelphia, PA: Saunders, 2005.

Maurer, Konrad, and Ulrike Mauer. *Alzheimer: The Life of a Physician & the Career of a Disease.* New York: Columbia University Press, 2003.

This biography of Alois Alzheimer includes his discovery of the disease that bears his name.

Max, D. T. *The Family that Couldn't Sleep: A Medical Mystery.* New York: Random House, 2006.

Mayell, Mark. *Nuclear Accidents.* San Diego, CA: Lucent Books, 2004.

Mayes, Maureen D. *The Scleroderma Book: A Guide for Patients and Families.* New York: Oxford University Press, 2005.

Mayo Clinic Guide to Preventing and Treating Osteoporosis. Rochester, MN: Mayo Clinic, 2008.

Mayo Clinic on Managing Incontinence. Rochester, MN: Mayo Clinic, 2005.

McCallum, Jack. "Steroids in America." *Sports Illustrated* March 11, 2008.

McCann-Beranger, Judith. *A Caregiver's Guide to Alzheimer's and Related Diseases.* New York: B&B Personal Wellness, 2008.

McCarthy, Jenny. *Louder than Words: A Mother's Journey in Healing Autism.* New York: Dutton, 2007.

Actress Jenny McCarthy describes the frustrations and joys of raising her autistic son.

McClay, Edward F., Mary-Eileen T. McClay, and Jodie Smith. *100 Questions & Answers About Melanoma and Other Skin Cancers*. Boston, MA: Jones and Bartlett, 2004.

McHolm, Angela E., Charles E. Cunningham, and Melanie K. Vanier. *Helping Your Child with Selective Mutism: Practical Steps to Overcome a Fear of Speaking*. Oakland, CA: New Harbinger Publications, 2005.

McIntosh, Kenneth, and Phyllis Livingston. *Youth with Conduct Disorder: In Trouble with the World*. Philadelphia, PA: Mason Crest, 2008.

McIntosh, Kenneth, and Phyllis Livingston. *Youth with Juvenile Schizophrenia: The Search for Reality*. Philadelphia, PA: Mason Crest, 2008.

McLay, Evelyn, and Ellen P. Young. *Mom's OK, She Just Forgets: The Alzheimer's Journey from Denial to Acceptance*. Amherst, NY: Prometheus Books, 2007.

Medifocus Guidebook: Hereditary Hemochromatosis. Silver Spring, MD: Medifocus.com, 2008.

Mercer, Renee. *Seven Steps to Nighttime Dryness: A Practical Guide for Parents of Children with Bedwetting*. Ashton, MD: Brookeville Media, 2004.

Metz, Michael E., and Barry W. McCarthy. *Coping with Erectile Dysfunction: How to Regain Confidence and Enjoy Great Sex*. Oakland, CA: New Harbinger, 2004.

Two of the nation's most respected sex therapists wrote this self-help resource on erectile dysfunction.

Metzger, Boyd. *American Medical Association Guide to Living with Diabetes: Preventing and Treating Type 2 Diabetes*. New York: Wiley, 2007.

Meyer, Donald J. *Views From Our Shoes: Growing Up with a Brother or Sister with Special Needs*. Bethesda, MD: Woodbine House, 1997.

In these unpretentious, honest short pieces, 45 children ranging in age from 4 to 18 describe their siblings and their feelings.

Michaud, Christopher. *Gonorrhea*. New York: Rosen, 2007.

Middleman, Amy B., ed. *American Medical Association Boy's Guide to Becoming a Teen*. San Francisco: Jossey-Bass, 2006.

Middleman, Amy B., ed. *American Medical Association Girl's Guide to Becoming a Teen*. San Francisco: Jossey-Bass, 2006.

Middlemiss, Prisca. *What's That Rash? How to Identify and Treat Childhood Rashes*. London: Hamlyn, 2002.

Miller, Debbie S. *The Great Serum Race: Blazing the Iditarod Trail*. New York: Walker, 2002.

Written for children, this beautifully illustrated book tells the story of Alaska's 1925 diphtheria outbreak and the commemorative Iditarod Trail Sled Dog Race.

Miller, Edward. *The Tooth Book: A Guide to Healthy Teeth and Gums*. New York: Holiday House, 2008.

Miller, Freeman, and Steven Bachrach. *Cerebral Palsy: A Complete Guide for Caregiving*, 2nd ed. Baltimore, MD: Johns Hopkins University Press, 2006.

Miller, Orson K., Jr., and Hope Miller. *North American Mushrooms: A Field Guide to Edible and Inedible Fungi*. Guilford, CT: Falcon Guide, 2006.

Mindell, Earl, and Hester Mundis. *Earl Mindell's New Vitamin Bible: 25th Anniversary Edition*. New York: Grand Central, 2004.

Miskovitz, Paul, and Marian Betancourt. *The Doctor's Guide to Gastrointestinal Health: Preventing and Treating Acid Reflux, Ulcers, Irritable Bowel Syndrome, Diverticulitis, Celiac Disease, Colon Cancer, Pancreatitis, Cirrhosis, Hernias and More*. Hoboken, NJ: Wiley, 2005.

Mitman, Gregg. *Breathing Space: How Allergies Shape Our Lives and Landscapes*. New Haven, CT: Yale University Press, 2007.

Moalem, Sharon. "Survival of the Sickest." *New Scientist* 193 (February 17–23, 2007): 42–45.

Moats, Louisa Cook, and Karen E. Dakin. *Basic Facts About Dyslexia and Other Reading Problems*. Baltimore, MD: International Dyslexia Association, 2008.

Moe, Barbara. *Coping with Tourette Syndrome and Tic Disorders*, rev. ed. New York: Rosen, 2004.

Moffett, Shannon. *The Three-Pound Enigma: The Human Brain and the Quest to Unlock Its Mysteries*. Chapel Hill, NC: Algonquin Books of Chapel Hill, 2006.

Monteverde, Matthew. *Making Smart Choices About Violence, Gangs, and Bullying.* New York: Rosen Publishings Rosen Central, 2008.

Moore, Michele C. *The Only Menopause Guide You'll Need.* Baltimore, MD: Johns Hopkins University Press, 2004.

Moore-Mallinos, Jennifer. *It's Called Dyslexia.* Hauppauge, NY: Barron's, 2007.

Morrell, Maureen F., and Ann Palmer. *Parenting Across the Autism Spectrum: Unexpected Lessons We Have Learned.* Philadelphia, PA: Jessica Kingsley, 2006.

Mughal, Tariq I., John M. Goldman, and Sabena T. Mughal. *Understanding Leukemias, Lymphomas, and Myelomas.* London: Taylor and Francis, 2006.

A reference book that explains blood cancers in layman's terms, especially with regards to diagnostic procedures, prognoses, and treatments.

Munro, Alistair. *Delusional Disorder: Paranoia and Related Illnesses.* Cambridge, UK: Cambridge University Press, 2006.

Murkoff, Heidi, and Sharon Mazel. *What to Expect When You're Expecting,* 4th ed. New York: Workman, 2008.

Murphy, Joseph. *Mayo Clinic Cardiology: Concise Textbook,* 3rd ed. New York: Informa HealthCare, 2006.

Murray, Frank. *How to Prevent Prostate Problems: A Complete Guide to the Essentials of Prostate Health.* Laguna Beach, CA: Basic Health, 2009.

Myers, David. *A Quiet World: Living with Hearing Loss.* New Haven, CT: Yale University Press, 2000.

Nadeau, Kathleen G. *Survival Guide for College Students with ADHD or LD,* 2nd ed. Washington, DC: Magination Press, 2006.

Nadeau, Kathleen G., and Ellen B. Dixon. *Learning to Slow Down and Pay Attention: A Book for Kids About ADD,* 3rd ed. Washington, DC: Magination Press, 2004.

Nardo, Don. *Human Papillomavirus (HPV).* Detroit, MI: Lucent Books, 2007.

Nase, Geoffrey. *Beating Rosacea: Vascular, Ocular, and Acne Forms.* Indianapolis, IN: Nase Publications, 2001.

Navarra, Tova. *Encyclopedia of Vitamins, Minerals, and Supplements,* 2nd ed. New York: Facts On File, 2004.

Newby, Robert F., with Carol A. Turkington. *Your Struggling Child: A Guide to Diagnosing, Understanding, and Advocating for Your Child with Learning, Behavior or Emotional Problems.* New York: Collins, 2006.

Newman, Diane K., and Alan J. Wein. *Overcoming Overactive Bladder: Your Complete Self-Care Guide.* Oakland, CA: New Harbinger, 2004.

Northrup, Christiane. *The Wisdom of Menopause: Creating Physical and Emotional Health and Healing During the Change,* 2nd ed. New York: Bantam, 2006.

O'Connor, Frances. *Frequently Asked Questions About Stuttering.* New York: Rosen, 2008.

O'Donnell, Judith A. *Pelvic Inflammatory Disease.* Philadelphia, PA: Chelsea House, 2005.

Ollhof, Jim. *Malaria.* Edina, MN: ABDO, 2010.

O'Neal, Claire. *The Influenza Pandemic of 1918.* Hockessin, DE: Mitchell Lane, 2008.

O'Reilly, Eileen, and Joanne Frankel Kelvin. *100 Questions & Answers About Pancreatic Cancer.* Sudbury, MA: Jones and Bartlett, 2003.

Orenstein, David M. *Cystic Fibrosis: A Guide for Patient and Family,* 3rd ed. Philadelphia, PA: Lippincott Williams & Wilkins, 2004.

Orr, Tamra. *Ovarian Tumors and Cysts.* New York: Rosen, 2009.

Pagel, James F., and S. R. Pandi-Perumal. *Primary Care Sleep Medicine: A Practical Guide.* Totowa, NJ: Humana Press, 2007.

Pan, Philip P. "The Last Hero of Tiananmen." *The New Republic* 238, no. 12 (July 9, 2008): 16.

Parascandola, John. *Sex, Sin, and Science: A History of Syphilis in America.* Westport, CT: Praeger, 2008.

Parham, Peter. *The Immune System,* 3rd ed. New York: Garland Science, 2009.

Parker, James N., and Philip M. Parker. *The Official Patient's Sourcebook on Bell's Palsy.* San Diego, CA: Icon Health, 2003.

Parker, James N., and Philip M. Parker. *The Official Patient's Sourcebook on Narcolepsy.* New York: Icon Health, 2002.

Parker, Katrina. *Living with Diabetes.* New York: Facts On File, 2008.

Parker, Steve. *Allergies.* Chicago: Heinemann Library, 2004.

Parks, Peggy J. *SIDS.* Detroit, MI: Lucent Books, 2009.

Pascarelli, Emil. *Dr. Pascarelli's Complete Guide to Repetitive Strain Injury: What you Need to Know About RSI and Carpal Tunnel Syndrome.* Hoboken, NJ: Wiley, 2004.

Pascoe, Elaine. *Spreading Menace: Salmonella Attack and the Hunger Craving (Body Story).* San Diego, CA: Blackbirch Press, 2004.

Pascualy, Ralph A. *Snoring and Sleep Apnea: Sleep Well, Feel Better,* 4th ed. New York: Demos Health, 2008.

Pass, Harvey I., Laura Roy, and Susan Vento. *100 Questions & Answers About Mesothelioma.* Sudbury, MA: Jones and Bartlett, 2005.

Peak, Lizabeth. *Growth Disorders.* Detroit, MI: Lucent Books, 2007.

Peak, Lizabeth. *Sickle Cell Disease.* Detroit, MI: Lucent Books, 2008.

Peikin, Steven R. *Gastrointestinal Health: The Proven Nutritional Program to Prevent, Cure, or Alleviate Irritable Bowel Syndrome (IBS), Ulcers, Gas, Constipation, Heartburn, and Many Other Digestive Disorders,* 3rd ed. New York: HarperCollins, 2004.

Peña, Kristin S., and Jo Ann Rosenfeld. "Evaluation and Treatment of Galactorrhea." *American Family Physician* 63, no. 9 (May 1, 2001): 1763–70. Also available at http://www.aafp.org/afp/20010501/1763.html.

Penney, David G., ed. *Carbon Monoxide Poisoning.* Boca Raton, FL: CRC Press, 2008.

Penzel, Fred. *The Hair-Pulling Problem: A Complete Guide to Trichotillomania.* New York: Oxford University Press, 2003.

Perkins, Sharon, and Jackie Meyers-Thompson. *Infertility for Dummies.* Hoboken, NJ: Wiley, 2007.

Peters, Stephanie True. *Epidemic! Smallpox in the New World.* New York: Benchmark Books, 2005.

Peters, Stephanie True. *The Black Death.* New York: Benchmark Books, 2005.

Peterson, Judy Monroe. *Sickle Cell Anemia.* New York: Rosen, 2009.

Peurifoy, Reneau Z. *Anxiety, Phobias, and Panic,* rev. and updated. New York: Warner Books, 2005.

Pfeiffer, Ronald P., Alton Thygerson, Nicholas F. Palmieri, and American Academy of Orthopaedic Surgeons. *Sports First Aid and Injury Prevention.* Sudbury, MA: Jones and Bartlett, 2008.

Phillips, Katharine A. *The Broken Mirror: Understanding and Treating Body Dysmorphic Disorder.* New York: Oxford University Press, 2005.

Phillips, Katharine A., ed. *Somatoform and Factitious Disorders (Review of Psychiatry).* Arlington, VA: American Psychiatric, 2001.

Pierce, John R., and Jim Writer. *Yellow Jack: How Yellow Fever Ravaged America and Walter Reed Discovered Its Deadly Secrets.* Hoboken, NJ: Wiley, 2005.

Pinker, Steven. "The Mystery of Consciousness." *Time* 169.5 (January 29, 2007): 58.

Piper, Ross. *Death Zone: Can Humans Survive at 26,000 Feet?* Mankato, MN: Capstone Press, 2009.

Pletcher, Claudine, and Sally Bartolameolli. *Relationships from Addiction to Authenticity.* Deerfield Beach, FL: Health Communications, 2008.

Poe, Dennis, ed. *The Consumer Handbook on Dizziness and Vertigo.* Sedona, AZ: Auricle Ink, 2005.

Poole, Catherine M. *Melanoma: Prevention, Detection, and Treatment,* 2nd ed. New Haven, CT: Yale University Press, 2005.

This is a book written for patients by a melanoma survivor.

Powell, Jillian. *Alcohol and Drug Abuse.* Pleasantville, NY: Gareth Stevens, 2009.

Powell, Jillian. *Self-Harm and Suicide.* Pleasantville, NY: Gareth Stevens, 2009.

Powell, Jillian. *Sore Throat.* North Mankato, MN: Cherrytree Books, 2007.

Powell, Michael, and Oliver Fischer. *101 Diseases You Don't Want to Get.* New York: Thunder's Mouth Press, 2005.

Preston, Richard. *The Hot Zone.* New York: Random House, 1994.

A dramatic account of the destructive effects of Ebola virus, including the story of Ebola-Reston, the virus that infected monkeys in a suburban Washington, DC, laboratory.

Quarrell, Oliver. *Huntington's Disease,* 2nd ed. New York: Oxford University Press, 2008.

Quick Facts Colorectal Cancer: What You Need to Know—Now. From the Experts at the American Cancer Society, 2nd ed. Atlanta, GA: American Cancer Society, 2008.

Quick Facts Lung Cancer: What You Need to Know—Now, from the Experts at the American Cancer Society. Atlanta, GA: American Cancer Society, 2007.

Quickfacts Thyroid Cancer: What You Need to Know Now. Atlanta, GA: American Cancer Society, 2009.

Quigley, Christine. *Conjoined Twins: An Historical, Biological, and Ethical Issues Encyclopedia.* Jefferson, NC: McFarland, 2003.

Quinn, Campion E. *100 Questions & Answers About Chronic Obstructive Pulmonary Disease (COPD).* Sudbury, MA: Jones and Bartlett, 2006.

Quinn, Patricia O., and Judith M. Stern. *Putting on the Brakes: Understanding and Taking Control of Your ADD or ADHD,* 2nd ed. Washington, DC: Magination Press, 20091.

Raabe, Michelle. *Hemophilia.* New York: Chelsea House, 2008.

Radziszewicz, Tina. *Ready or Not? A Girl's Guide to Making Her Own Decisions About Dating, Love, and Sex.* New York: Walker, 2006.

Raez, Luis E., and Orlando E. Silva. *Lung Cancer: A Practical Guide.* Edinburgh, NY: Saunders, 2008.

Raghavan, Derek. *Bladder Cancer: A Cleveland Clinic Guide: Information for Patients and Caregivers.* Cleveland, OH: Cleveland Clinic Press, 2008.

Rangamani, G. N. *Managing Speech and Swallowing Problems: A Guidebook for People with Ataxia,* 2nd ed. Minneapolis, MN: National Ataxia Foundation, 2006.

Raoult, Didier, and Philippe Parola, eds. *Rickettsial Diseases.* New York: Informa Healthcare, 2007.

Rebman, Renee C. *Addictions and Risky Behaviors: Cutting, Bingeing, Snorting, and Other Dangers.* Berkeley Heights, NJ: Enslow, 2006.

Redd, Nancy. *Body Drama: Real Girls, Real Bodies, Real Issues, Real Answers.* New York: Gotham, 2007.

Redwine, David B. *100 Questions & Answers About Endometriosis.* Sudbury, MA: Jones and Bartlett, 2009.

Reeve, Christopher. *Nothing Is Impossible: Reflections on a New Life.* New York: Random House, 2002.

Reid, David M., Alison J. Black, and Rena Sandison. *Osteoporosis.* New York: Oxford University Press, 2009.

Richardson, Malcolm D., and Elizabeth Johnson. *Pocket Guide to Fungal Infection.* Malden, MA: Blackwell, 2005.

Ricks, Delthia. *100 Questions and Answers About Influenza.* Sudbury, MA: Jones and Bartlett, 2009.

Ricotta, Mary C. *A Consumer's Guide to Laboratory Tests.* Amherst, NY: Prometheus Books, 2005.

Rigo, Jacques, and Ekhard E. Ziegler, eds. *Protein and Energy Requirements in Infancy and Childhood.* Basel, Switzerland: Karger, 2006.

Rinzler, Carol Ann, with Ken DeVault. *Heartburn & Reflux for Dummies.* Hoboken, NJ: Wiley, 2004.

Ritter, Rick. *Coping with Physical Loss and Disability: A Workbook.* Ann Arbor, MI: Loving Healing Press, 2006.

This question-and-answer workbook provides individuals with exercises designed to help them explore and understand how disability arising from accidents, injury, and disease may challenge and affect their lives both mentally and physically.

Rodman, John S., et al. *No More Kidney Stones: The Experts Tell You All You Need to Know About Prevention and Treatment,* Rev. ed. Hoboken, NJ: Wiley, 2007.

Rodríguez, Ana María. *Autism and Asperger Syndrome.* Minneapolis, MN: Twenty-First Century Books, 2009.

Bibliography

Roloff, Matt, and Tracy Sumner. *Against Tall Odds: Being a David in a Goliath World.* Sisters, OR: Multnomah, 1999.

Romanelli, Marco, Michael Clark, George W. Cherry, et al., eds. *Science and Practice of Pressure Ulcer Management.* London: Springer-Verlag, 2006.

Romano, Amy. *Germ Warfare.* New York: The Rosen Publishing Group, 2004.

Rosaler, Maxine. *Measles.* New York: Rosen, 2005.

Rosenthal, M. Sara. *The Thyroid Cancer Book* 2nd ed. Canada: Your Health Press, 2006.

This consumer book on thyroid cancer is written in plain language, and it contains a low iodine cookbook.

Rosenthal, Norman E. *Winter Blues: Everything you Need to Know to Beat Seasonal Affective Disorder,* rev. ed. New York: Guilford Press, 2006.

Rosner, Louis J., and Shelley Ross. *Multiple Sclerosis: New Hope and Practical Advice for People with MS and Their Families,* updated ed. New York: Fireside Book, 2008.

Ross, Jonathan H., and Robert Kay. "Pediatric Urinary Tract Infection and Reflux" in *American Family Physician*, Volume 59 Number 6, March 15, 1999, 1472–1488. Also available at http://www.aafp.org/afp/990315ap/1472.html.

Rotbart, Harley A. *Germ Proof Your Kids: The Complete Guide to Protecting (Without Overprotecting) Your Family from Infections.* Washington, DC: ASM Press, 2008.

Royston, Angela. *Broken Bones.* Chicago: Heinemann Library, 2004.

Royston, Angela. *Burns and Blisters.* Chicago: Heinemann Library, 2004.

Royston, Angela. *Stings and Bites.* Chicago: Heinemann Library, 2004.

Royston, Angela. *Tooth Decay.* Mankato, MN: Black Rabbit Books, 2009.

Royston, Angela. *Warts.* Chicago: Heinemann Library, 2002.

Rubin, Jordan, with Joseph Brasco. *The Great Physician's Rx for Heartburn and Acid Reflux.* Nashville, TN: Thomas Nelson, 2007.

Rudy, Lisa Jo. *Bioterror: Deadly Invisible Weapons.* New York: Franklin Watts, 2008.

Ruggiero, Roberta. *Do's and Don'ts of Hypoglycemia: An Everyday Guide to Low Blood Sugar.* Hollywood, FL: Frederick Fell, 2003.

Rushing, Lynda, and Nancy Joste. *Abnormal Pap Smears: What Every Woman Needs to Know.* Amherst, NY: Prometheus Books, 2008.

Sachs, Jessica Snyder. *Good Germs, Bad Germs: Health and Survival in a Bacterial World.* New York: Hill and Wang, 2008.

The author discusses microorganisms and infections, antibiotic use, and approaches to antibiotic therapies.

Saffer, Barbara. *Measles and Rubella.* Detroit, MI: Lucent Books, 2006.

Saks, Elyn R. *The Centre Cannot Hold: A Memoir of My Schizophrenia.* London: Virago, 2007.

Saltz, Gail. *Changing You: A Guide to Body Changes and Sexuality.* New York: Dutton Children's Books, 2007.

Sandler, Adrian. *Living with Spina Bifida: A Guide for Families and Professionals.* Chapel Hill: University of North Carolina Press, 2003.

Saunders, Geraldine. *Hypoglycemia.* New York: Kensington, 2002.

The author provides 120 recipes for hypoglycemia sufferers, as well as personal stories from people who have transformed their lives while coping with the condition.

Sauvain-Dugerdil, Claudine, Henri Léridon, and Nicholas Mascie-Taylor, eds. *Human Clocks: The Bio-Cultural Meanings of Age.* Bern: Peter Lang, 2006.

Schachter, Neil. *The Good Doctor's Guide to Colds and Flu.* New York: Collins, 2005.

Schaefer, Lola M. *Hair.* Chicago: Heinemann, 2003.

Schimpff, Stephen C. *The Future of Medicine: Megatrends in Health Care that Will Improve Your Quality of Life.* Nashville, TN: Thomas Nelson, 2007.

Schiraldi, Glenn R. *The Post-Traumatic Stress Disorder Sourcebook,* 2nd ed. New York: McGraw-Hill, 2009.

Schnurbush, Barbara. *Striped Shirts and Flowered Pants: A Story About Alzheimer's Disease for Young Children.* Washington, DC: Magination Press, 2007.

Schreiber, Flora Rheta. *Sybil.* New York: Warner Books, 1995.

Schrier, Robert W., ed. *Diseases of the Kidney and Urinary Tract.* Philadelphia, PA: Wolters Kluwer Health/Lippincott Williams and Wilkins, 2007.

Schwartzenberger, Tina, ed. *Substance Use and Abuse.* New York: Weigl, 2007.

Schwarz, Alan. "Lineman, Dead at 36, Exposes Brain Injuries." *New York Times,* June 15, 2007. http://www.nytimes.com/2007/06/15/sports/football/15brain.html?_r=1.

Schwarz, Shelley Peterman. *Arthritis: 330 Tips for Making Life Easier.* New York: Demos Medical, 2009.

This book focuses on living with arthritis and describes ways to make homes more accessible to people with arthritis.

Scott, Elizabeth, and Paul Sockett. *How to Prevent Food Poisoning: A Practical Guide to Safe Cooking, Eating, and Food Handling.* New York: Wiley, 2001.

Sehgal, Alfica. *Leprosy.* Philadelphia, PA: Chelsea House, 2006.

Seligman, Linda, and Lourie W. Reichenberg. *Selecting Effective Treatments: A Comprehensive, Systematic Guide to Treating Mental Disorders.* San Francisco: Jossey-Bass, 2007.

This book is a reference guide on treating various mental disorders, including assessment, prognosis, and intervention strategies.

Selikowitz, Mark. *Down Syndrome: The Facts,* 3rd ed. New York: Oxford University Press, 2008.

Senelick, Richard C., and Karla Dougherty. *Living with Stroke: A Guide for Families,* 3rd ed. Clifton Park, NY: Delmar Cengage Learning, 2001.

Sertori, Trisha. *Vitamins and Minerals.* New York: Marshall Cavendish Benchmark, 2009.

Sfakianos, Jeffrey N. *West Nile Virus.* Philadelphia, PA: Chelsea House, 2005.

Shah, Manish A., Natasha Pinheiro, and Brinda M. Shah. *100 Questions & Answers About Gastric Cancer.* Sudbury, MA: Jones and Bartlett, 2008.

Shannon, Joyce Brennfleck, ed. *Endocrine and Metabolic Disorders Sourcebook: Basic Consumer Health Information About Hormonal and Metabolic Disorders that Affect the Body's Growth, Development, and Functioning, Including Disorders of the Pancreas, Ovaries and Testes...,* 2nd ed. Detroit, MI: Omnigraphics, 2007.

Shannon, Joyce Brennfleck, ed. *Suicide Information for Teens: Health Tips About Suicide Causes and Prevention: Including Facts About Depression, Risk Factors, Getting Help, Survivor Support, and More.* Detroit, MI: Omnigraphics, 2005.

Sharp, Katie John. *Smokeless Tobacco: Not a Safe Alternative.* Broomall, PA: Mason Crest, 2009.

Sheen, Barbara. *Birth Defects.* San Diego, CA: Lucent Books, 2005.

Sheen, Barbara. *Toxic Shock Syndrome.* San Diego, CA: Lucent Books, 2006.

Shimberg, Elaine Fantle. *Coping with Chronic Obstructive Pulmonary Disease.* New York: St. Martin's Griffin, 2003.

Shmaefsky, Brian R. *Rubella and Rubeola.* New York: Chelsea House, 2009.

Shors, Teri. *Understanding Viruses.* Sudbury, MA: Jones and Bartlett, 2009.

Shotel, Jay, and Sue Shotel. *It's Good to Know a Miracle: Dani's Story: One Family's Struggle with Leukemia.* New York: Gordian Knot Books, 2008.

Shrier, Lydia. "Breakthrough HPV Vaccine." *Pediatric Views* (December 2006).

Sicile-Kira, Chantal. *Adolescents on the Autism Spectrum: A Parent's Guide to the Cognitive, Social, Physical and Transition Needs of Teenagers with Autism Spectrum Disorders.* New York: Perigee, 2006.

Siderovski, Susan Hutton. *Tularemia.* Philadelphia, PA: Chelsea House, 2006.

Siegel, Bryna. *Getting the Best for Your Child with Autism: An Expert's Guide to Treatment.* New York: Guilford Press, 2008.

Bibliography

Siegel, Mary-Ellen, and Gray Williams. *Shingles: New Hope for an Old Disease,* updated ed. Lanham, MD: M. Evans, 2008.

Silberstein, Stephen. *Wolff's Headache and Other Pain,* 8th ed. New York: Oxford University Press, 2008.

Silver, Julie K. *After Cancer Treatment: Heal Faster, Better, Stronger.* Baltimore, MD: Johns Hopkins University Press, 2006.

A hands-on guide to survival issues: exercise, diet, fatigue, mental health, spirituality, and how to seek assistance from both Western and alternative medicine.

Silverstein, Alvin, Virginia Silverstein, and Laura Silverstein Nunn. *Cancer.* Minneapolis, MN: Twenty-First Century Books, 2006.

Silverstein, Alvin, Virginia Silverstein, and Laura Silverstein Nunn. *Pains and Strains.* New York: Franklin Watts, 2003.

Silverstein, Alvin, Virginia Silverstein, and Laura Silverstein Nunn. *Scoliosis.* New York: Franklin Watts, 2002.

Silverstein, Alvin, Virginia Silverstein, and Laura Silverstein Nunn. *The AIDS Update.* Berkeley Heights, NJ: Enslow, 2008.

Silverstein, Alvin, Virginia Silverstein, and Laura Silverstein Nunn. *The Eating Disorders Update: Understanding Anorexia, Bulimia, and Binge Eating.* Berkeley Heights, NJ: Enslow, 2009.

Silverstein, Alvin, Virginia Silverstein, and Laura Silverstein Nunn. *The Food Poisoning Update.* Berkeley Heights, NJ: Enslow, 2008.

Silverstein, Alvin, Virginia Silverstein, and Laura Silverstein Nunn. *The STDs Update.* Berkeley Heights, NJ: Enslow Elementary, 2006.

Silverstein, Alvin, Virginia Silverstein, and Laura Silverstein Nunn. *The Sickle Cell Anemia Update.* Berkeley Heights, NJ: Enslow, 2006.

Skallerup, Susan J., ed. *Babies with Down Syndrome: A New Parents' Guide,* 3rd ed. Bethesda, MD: Woodbine House, 2008.

Skinner, Harry. *Current Diagnosis and Treatment in Orthopedics.* New York: McGraw-Hill, 2006.

Sklar, Jill. *Crohn's Disease and Ulcerative Colitis: An Essential Guide for the Newly Diagnosed.* New York: Marlowe, 2007.

Sklar, Jill. *The First Year: Crohn's Disease and Ulcerative Colitis: An Essential Guide for the Newly Diagnosed.* New York: Marlowe, 2007.

This book includes current research and insights to help individuals who are newly diagnosed with IBD come to terms with their condition and the accompanying lifestyle changes.

Slaughter, Lynn. *Teen Rape.* San Diego, CA: Lucent Books, 2004.

Slone, Laurie B., and Matthew J. Friedman. *After the War Zone: A Practical Guide for Returning Troops and Their Families.* Cambridge, MA: Da Capo Lifelong, 2008.

Smith, Patricia B., Mary Kenan, and Mark Edwin Kunik. *Alzheimer's for Dummies.* Hoboken, NJ: Wiley, 2004.

Smith, Tara C. *Streptococcus (Group B).* New York: Chelsea House, 2007.

Snedden, Robert. *Explaining Autism.* Mankato, MN: Smart Apple Media, 2010.

Sniderman, A., and Paul N. Durrington. *Fast Facts: Hyperlipidemia,* 4th ed. Abingdon, Oxford, UK: Health Press, 2008.

So Po-Lin. *Skin Cancer.* New York: Chelsea House, 2008.

Solomon, Gary S., Karen M. Johnston, and Mark R. Lovell. *The Heads-up on Sport Concussion.* Champaign, IL: Human Kinetics, 2006.

Sommers, Michael. *Yeast Infections, Trichomoniasis, and Toxic Shock Syndrome.* New York: Rosen Central, 2008.

Sonenklar, Carol. *Virus Hunters.* Brookfield, CT: Twenty-First Century Books, 2003.

Soper, Kathryn, ed. *Gifts: Mothers Reflect on How Children with Down Syndrome Enrich Their Lives.* Bethesda, MD: Woodbine House, 2007.

Souza, D. M. *Packed with Poison! Deadly Animal Defenses.* Minneapolis, MN: Millbrook Press, 2006.

Sparks, Beatrice, ed. *It Happened to Nancy by an Anonymous Teenager, A True Story from Her Diary,* rev. ed. New York: Avon Books, 2005.

"Special Issue: HIV/AIDS." *Science* 321, no. 5888 (July 25, 2008).

Spevak, Peter A., and Maryann Karinch. *Empowering Underachievers: New Strategies to Guide Kids (8–18) to Personal Excellence,* rev. and expanded ed. Far Hills, NJ: New Horizon Press, 2006.

Spilsbury, Louise. *Why Should I Wash My Hair? and Other Questions About Healthy Skin and Hair.* Chicago: Heinemann Library, 2003.

Squire, Larry, and Eric Kandel. *Memory: From Mind to Molecules,* 2nd ed. Greenwood Village, CO: Roberts, 2008.

This book explains some of the most important concepts of how memory works and what can go wrong. It was written by scientists engaged in memory research.

Stanberry, Lawrence R. *Understanding Herpes,* revised 2nd ed. Jackson: University Press of Mississippi, 2006.

Standiford, Natalie. *The Bravest Dog Ever: The True Story of Balto.* New York: Random House, 2003.

This children's book tells the story of Balto, one of the sled dogs used during the 1925 Alaska diphtheria outbreak.

State of Connecticut. *Connecticut's Lawsuit against the Tobacco Companies.* Text available at http://www.ct.gov/ag/cwp/view.asp?A=1771&Q=291124.

Stavrou, Maria, ed. *Bulimics on Bulimia.* London: Jessica Kingsley, 2009.

Steffen, Robert. *Manual of Travel Health and Medicine,* 3rd ed. Hamilton, Ontario: BC Decker, 2007.

Stein, Joel. *Stroke and the Family: A New Guide.* Cambridge, MA: Harvard University Press, 2004.

Stein, Paul. *Pulmonary Embolism,* 2nd ed. Malden, MA: Blackwell, 2007.

This book covers research data, methods of diagnosis, and medical treatment for pulmonary embolism, written from a clinical perspective.

Steinhart, Allan Hillary. *Crohn's and Colitis: Understanding and Managing IBD.* Toronto, Canada: R. Rose, 2006.

Stewart, Gail B. *Fetal Alcohol Syndrome.* Detroit, MI: Lucent Books, 2005.

Stewart, Melissa. *Germ Wars! The Secrets of the Immune System.* New York: Marshall Cavendish Benchmark, 2009.

Stewart, Melissa. *Why Do We See Rainbows?* New York: Marshall Cavendish Benchmark, 2009.

Stratton, Rebecca J. *Disease-related Malnutrition.* Cambridge, MA: CABI, 2003.

Straus, Eugene, and Alex W. Straus. *Medical Marvels: The 100 Greatest Advances in Medicine.* Amherst, NY: Prometheus Books, 2006.

Strickman, Daniel, Stephen P. Frances, and Mustapha Debboun. *Prevention of Bug Bites, Stings, and Disease.* New York: Oxford University Press, 2009.

Stuttering and Your Child: Questions and Answers, 3rd ed. Memphis, TN: Stuttering Foundation of America, 2007.

Styron, William. *Darkness Visible: A Memoir of Madness.* New York: Random House, 1990.

Well-known author Styron tells about his battle with depression.

Subauste, Carlos S. *Toxoplasmosis and HIV.* HIV InSite Knowledge Base Chapter available at http://hivinsite.ucsf.edu/InSite?page=kb-05-04-03.

Sutton, Amy L., ed. *Allergies Sourcebook,* 3rd ed. Detroit, MI: Omnigraphics, 2007.

Sutton, Amy L., ed. *Blood and Circulatory Disorders Sourcebook,* 2nd ed. Detroit, MI: Omnigraphics, 2005.

Sutton, Amy L., ed. *Eye Care Sourcebook,* 3rd ed. Detroit, MI: Omnigraphics, 2008.

The book provides basic consumer health information about the prevention, diagnosis, and treatment of eye diseases, disorders, and injuries.

Swarts, Katherine, ed. *The Aging Population.* Detroit, MI: Greenhaven Press, 2009.

Talbot, Kevin, and Rachael Marsden. *Motor Neuron Disease (The Facts).* New York: Oxford University Press, 2008.

An adult but mostly non-technical book about ALS.

Tames, Richard. *Hiroshima: The Shadow of the Bomb,* rev. and updated. Chicago, IL: Heinemann Library, 2006.

Bibliography

Targan, Stephen R., Fergus Shanahan, Loren C. Karp, eds. *Inflammatory Bowel Disease: From Bench to Bedside.* New York: Springer Science and Business Media, 2003.

This book presents comprehensive reviews by individual authors on the varied aspects of inflammatory bowel diseases.

Temes, Roberta. *Living with an Empty Chair: A Guide Through Grief.* Amherst, MA: Mandala, 1977.

Tewari, Krishnansu Sujata Tewari, and Bradley J. Monk. *Myths & Facts About Cervical Cancer: What You Need to Know.* Manhasset, NY: Oncology Group, CMPMedica, 2007.

Thacker, Holly L. *The Cleveland Clinic Guide to Menopause.* New York: Kaplan, 2009.

Thames, Susan. *Our Immune System.* Vero Beach, FL: Rourke, 2008.

Thomas, Lee. *Turning White: A Memoir of Change.* Troy, MI: Momentum Books, 2007.

African American television journalist Lee Thomas tells of his life with vitiligo.

Thomas, Pat. *Why Am I So Tired? A First Look at Childhood Diabetes.* Hauppauge, NY: Barron's, 2008.

Thomas, Pat. *Why Is It So Hard to Breathe? A First Look at Asthma.* Hauppauge, NY: Barrons, 2008.

Thomas, Peggy. *Post Traumatic Stress Disorder.* Farmington Hills, MI: Lucent Books, 2008.

Thompson, A.E., and J.E. Pope. "Calcium Channel Blockers for Primary Raynaud's Phenomenon: A Meta-analysis." *Rheumatology* (Oxford, England) 44, no. 2 (2005): 145–50.

Thompson, Richard F., and Stephen A. Madigan. *Memory: The Key to Consciousness.* Washington, DC: Joseph Henry Press, 2005.

Thompson, Tricia. *Celiac Disease Nutrition Guide.* Chicago: American Dietetic Association, 2003.

Thomson, Anne, and Ann Harris. *Cystic Fibrosis: The Facts,* 2nd ed. New York: Oxford University Press, 2008.

Tilden, Thomasine E. Lewis. *Belly-Busting Worm Invasions! Parasites That Love Your Insides!* New York: Franklin Watts, 2008.

Tilden, Thomasine E. Lewis. *Help! What's Eating My Flesh? Runaway Staph and Strep Infections!* New York: Franklin Watts, 2008.

Tocci, Salvatore. *Jonas Salk: Creator of the Polio Vaccine.* Enslow, 2003.

Toporek, Chuck, and Kellie Robinson. *Hydrocephalus: A Guide for Patients, Families, and Friends.* O'Reilly and Associates, 1999.

Toriello, James. *The Human Genome Project.* New York: Rosen Group, 2003.

This book describes this international project and the scientists who engaged in the research.

Torrey, E. Fuller, and Robert H. Yolken. *Beasts of the Earth: Animals, Humans, and Disease.* New Brunswick, NJ: Rutgers University Press, 2005.

Torrey, E. Fuller. *Surviving Schizophrenia: A Manual for Families, Patients, and Providers,* 5th ed. New York: Collins, 2006.

Tracy, Kathleen. *Robert Koch and the Study of Anthrax.* Hockessin, DE: Mitchell Lane Publishers, 2005.

Traig, Jennifer. *Devil in the Details: Scenes from an Obsessive Girlhood.* New York: Little, Brown, 2004.

Traig, Jennifer. *Well Enough Alone.* New York: Riverhead, 2008.

This book gives a first-person account of what it is like to have hypochondria.

Tretbar, Lawrence L. *Lymphedema: Diagnosis and Treatment.* London: Springer, 2008.

Tridas, Eric Q., ed. *From ABC to ADHD: What Parents Should Know About Dyslexia and Attention Problems.* Baltimore, MD: International Dyslexia Association, 2007.

"Triglycerides and Heart Disease." *Mayo Clinic Health Letter* 26, no. 8 (August 2008): 6.

Trock, David H., and Frances Chamberlain. *Living with Fibromyalgia.* Hoboken, NJ: Wiley, 2006.

Trope, Graham E. *Glaucoma: A Patient's Guide to the Disease,* 3rd ed. Toronto: University of Toronto Press, 2004.

Turkington, Carol, and Joseph R. Harris. *Understanding Learning Disabilities: The Sourcebook for*

Causes, Disorders, and Treatments. New York: Checkmark Books, 2003.

Tyler, Richard S., ed. *The Consumer Handbook on Tinnitus.* Sedona, AZ: Auricle Ink, 2008.

Underwood, Deborah. *Has a Cow Saved Your Life?* Chicago: Raintree, 2007.

Updike, John. *Self-consciousness: Memoirs.* New York: Knopf, 1989.

Urbano, Mary Theresa. *The Complete Bioterrorism Survival Guide: Everything You Need to Know Before, During and After an Attack.* Boulder, CO: Sentient Publications, 2006.

Van der Keur, Henk. "PSR Minimizes Depleted Uranium Health Hazards," *Nuclear Monitor,* December 23, 2005.

Van der Wijngaard, Marianne. *Reinventing the Sexes: Biomedical Construction of Femininity and Masculinity.* Indianapolis: Indiana University Press, 1997.

Van Nostrand, Douglas, Gary Bloom, and Leonard Wartofsky, eds. *Thyroid Cancer: A Guide for Patients.* Pasadena, MD: Keystone Press, 2004.

Vanderhoof-Forschner, Karen. *Everything You Need to Know About Lyme Disease and Other Tick-Borne Disorders,* 2nd ed. Hoboken, NJ: Wiley, 2003.

Vanderpump, Mark P. J, and W. Michael G. Tunbridge. *Thyroid Disease: The Facts,* 4th ed. New York: Oxford University Press, 2008.

Veague, Heather Barnett. *Schizophrenia.* New York: Chelsea House, 2007.

Venis, Joyce A., and Suzanne McCloskey. *Postpartum Depression Demystified: An Essential Guide to Understanding and Overcoming the Most Common Complication after Childbirth.* New York: Marlowe, 2007.

Verville, Kathleen. *Testicular Cancer.* New York: Chelsea House, 2009.

Viegas, Jennifer. *Fungi and Molds.* New York: Rosen, 2004.

Viegas, Jennifer. *Parasites.* New York: Rosen, 2004.

Voight, Joseph. *My Grandma Has Alzheimer's, Too.* Eagleville, PA: DNA Press, 2007.

In his own words and illustrations, 11-year-old Joseph expresses the fears and frustrations of living with an elderly relative afflicted by Alzheimer's disease.

Walker, David H. *Rocky Mountain Spotted Fever.* New York: Chelsea House, 2008.

Walker, Herschel. *Breaking Free: My Life with Dissociative Identity Disorder.* New York: Simon and Schuster, 2008.

A former professional football player, Walker writes an account of his struggle with DID.

Walker, Julie. *Tay-Sachs Disease.* New York: Rosen, 2007.

Walker, W. Allan. *Eat, Play, and Be Healthy: The Harvard Medical School Guide to Healthy Eating for Kids.* New York: McGraw-Hill, 2005.

Wall, Mary. *Lyme Disease Is No Fun: Let's Get Well!* Jackson, NJ: Lyme Disease Association, 2004.

Watson, Stephanie. *Anorexia.* New York: Rosen, 2007.

Watson, Stephanie. *Bulimia.* New York: Rosen, 2007.

Weiner, William J., Lisa M. Shulman, and Anthony E. Lang. *Parkinson's Disease: A Complete Guide For Patients and Families,* 2nd ed. Baltimore, MD: Johns Hopkins University Press, 2007.

Weinstein, Howard J., Melissa M. Hudson, and Michael P. Link, eds. *Pediatric Lymphomas.* Berlin: Springer, 2006.

A clinical book that explains various aspects of blood cancers that occur among children.

Weisman, Roanne, with John D. Mark. *Your Sick Child: Fever, Allergies, Ear Infections, Colds, and More.* Deerfield Beach, FL: Health Communications, 2006.

Weschler, Toni. *Cycle Savvy: The Smart Teen's Guide to the Mysteries of Her Body.* New York: Collins Living, 2006.

West, Krista. *Urinary Tract Infections.* New York: Rosen, 2007.

White, Katherine. *Dengue Fever.* New York: Rosen, 2004.

Whiteside, Alan. *HIV/AIDS: A Very Short Introduction.* New York: Oxford University Press, 2008.

Bibliography

Whiting, Jim. *Bubonic Plague.* Hockessin, DE: Mitchell Lane, 2007.

Wilkerson, James A. *Hypothermia, Frostbite, and Other Cold Injuries: Prevention, Recognition, Rescue, and Treatment,* 2nd ed. Seattle: Mountaineers Books, 2006.

Williams, Dale F. *Stuttering Recovery: Personal and Empirical Perspectives.* Mahwah, NJ: Erlbaum, 2006.

Wilner, Andrew N. *Epilepsy: 199 Answers. A Doctor Responds to His Patients' Questions,* 3rd ed. New York: Demos Medical, 2007.

Wilson, Michael R. *Pelvic Inflammatory Disease.* New York: Rosen, 2009.

Wilson, Sue, and David Nutt. *Sleep Disorders.* New York: Oxford University Press, 2008.

This book is a resource to individuals seeking basic to advanced research information about sleep disorders. In particular, it addresses sleep disorders in relation to mood disturbance, sleep dysfunction, and sleep physiology, as well as diagnosis and treatment of sleep disorders.

Winters, Adam. *Syphilis.* New York: Rosen, 2007.

Wiseman, Nancy D., with Robert L. Rich. *The First Year: Autism Spectrum Disorders: An Essential Guide for the Newly Diagnosed Child: A Parent-Expert Walks You Through Everything You Need to Learn and Do.* Cambridge, MA: Da Capo Press, 2009.

Wong, Agnes. *Eye Movement Disorders.* New York: Oxford University Press, 2008.

Wood, Lawrence C., David S. Cooper, and E. Chester Ridgway. *Your Thyroid: A Home Reference,* 4th ed. New York: Ballantine Books, 2006.

Woods, Douglas. *Managing Tourette Syndrome: A Behavioral Intervention for Children and Adults.* New York: Oxford University Press, 2008.

Wright, Judith. *The Soft Addiction Solution.* New York: Jeremy Tarcher/Penguin, 2006.

Wyborny, Sheila. *Anxiety Disorders.* Detroit, MI: Lucent Books, 2009.

Wyllie, Elaine. *Epilepsy: Information for You and Those who Care About You.* Cleveland, OH: Cleveland Clinic Press, 2008.

Wynn, Rhoda, and Winston C. Vaughan. *100 Questions & Answers About Sinusitis and Other Sinus Diseases.* Sudbury, MA: Jones and Bartlett, 2008.

Yam, Philip. *The Pathological Protein: Mad Cow, Chronic Wasting, and Other Deadly Prion Diseases.* New York: Copernicus, 2003.

Yamazaki, James N. *Children of the Atomic Bomb: An American Physician's Memoir of Nagasaki, Hiroshima, and the Marshall Islands.* Durham, NC: Duke University Press, 1995.

Yancey, Diane. *Tuberculosis.* Minneapolis, MN: Twenty-First Century Books, 2008.

Yanoff, Myron, and Jay S. Duker. *Ophthalmology: Expert Consult,* 3nd ed. St. Louis, MO: Mosby, 2008.

Yoste, Merle James. *Demystifying Gynecomastia: Men with Breasts.* Woodland Hills, CA: Advanstar Communications, 2006.

Young, Kimberly S. *Caught in the Net: How to Recognize the Signs of Internet Addiction—and a Winning Strategy for Recovery.* New York: Wiley, 1998.

Zallen, Doris. *To Test or Not to Test: A Guide to Genetic Screening and Risk.* Piscataway, NJ: Rutgers University Press, 2008.

This book examines the uses for, the limitations of, and the ethical issues surrounding genetic testing.

Zelinger, Laurie. *The "O, My" in Tonsillectomy & Adenoidectomy: How to Prepare Your Child for Surgery, a Parent's Manual.* Ann Arbor, MI: Loving Healing Press, 2009.

Zimmerman Rutledge, Jill S. *Picture Perfect: What You Need to Feel Better About Your Body.* Deerfield Beach, FL: Health Communications, 2007.

Zinsser, Hans. *Rats, Lice and History: A Study in Biography.* New Brunswick, NJ: Aldine Transaction, 2007.

Zonderman, Jon, and Ronald S. Vender. *Understanding Crohn Disease and Ulcerative Colitis.* Jackson: University Press of Mississippi, 2006.

This book presents an overview of the nature and treatments of IBD and describes various medical, surgical, nutritional, and spiritual treatments.

Zonderman, Jon, and Laurel Shader. *Legionnaires' Disease.* New York: Chelsea House, 2006.

Glossary

The following is an alphabetical compilation of the terms and definitions that appear in the main body entries. Although the list is comprehensive, it is by no means exhaustive and is intended to serve as a starting point for further research.

abdomen (AB-do-men) the portion of the body between the thorax (THOR-aks) and the pelvis. Also called the belly.

abdominal (ab-DAH-mih-nul) the area of the body below the ribs and above the hips that contains the stomach, intestines, and other organs.

abscess (AB-ses) a localized or walled off accumulation of pus caused by infection that can occur anywhere in the body.

acetaminophen (uh-see-teh-MIH-noh-fen) a medication commonly used to reduce fever and relieve pain.

acid reflux a condition in which stomach acid flows upward into the esophagus, often causing a burning sensation (so-called heartburn) in the upper abdomen or chest.

acne (AK-nee) a condition in which pimples, blackheads, whiteheads, and sometimes deeper lumps occur on the skin.

Acquired Immunodeficiency Syndrome (or AIDS) an infection that severely weakens the immune system; it is caused by the human immunodeficiency virus (HIV).

acromegaly (akro-MEG-al-ee) a disease in which the pituitary gland secretes too much growth hormone with the effect of gradual and permanent enlargement of flat bones, the hands and feet, abdominal organs, and some facial features.

acute an infection or other illness that comes on suddenly and usually does not last very long.

addiction (a-DIK-shun) a strong physical or psychological dependence on a physical substance.

adenoids (AH-din-oyds) the fleshy lumps of tissue behind the nose that contain collections of infection-fighting cells of the immune system.

adenovirus (ah-deh-no-VY-rus) a type of virus that can produce a variety of symptoms, including upper respiratory disease, when it infects humans.

ADHD (or Attention Deficit Hyperactivity Disorder) a condition that makes it hard for a person to pay attention, sit still, or think before acting.

adrenal glands (a-DREEN-al glands) the pair of endocrine organs located near the kidneys.

adrenaline (a-DREN-a-lin) a hormone, or chemical messenger, that is released in response to fear, anger, panic, and other emotions. It readies the body to respond to threat by increasing heart rate, breathing rate, and blood flow to the arms and legs. These and other effects prepare the body to run away or fight. Also called epinephrine (ep-e-NEF-rin).

aerobic exercise (air-O-bik) exercise designed to increase oxygen consumption by the body; it helps keep the heart and lungs in shape.

aerosolize (AIR-o-suh-lize) to put something, such as a medication, in the form of small particles or droplets that can be sprayed or released into the air.

AIDS (or Acquired Immunodeficiency (ih-myoo-no-dih-FIH-shen-see) Syndrome) an infection that severely weakens the immune system; it is caused by the human immunodeficiency virus (HIV).

allergens substances that provoke a response by the body's immune system or cause a hypersensitive reaction.

allergy (AL-uhr-jee) an immune system-related sensitivity to certain substances, for example, cat dander or the pollen of certain plants, that cause various reactions, such as sneezing, runny nose, wheezing, or swollen, itchy patches on the skin, called hives.

alopecia areata (al-o-PEA-shah a-ree-AH-ta) a condition that leads to sudden hair loss, often in small, round patches on the scalp. The cause is not known.

alpha-fetoprotein (AL-fah-FEE-toe-PRO-teen) a substance produced by a fetus and present in maternal blood and amniotic fluid, measured to determine likelihood of neural tube defects.

Alzheimer's disease (ALTS-hy-merz) a condition that leads to gradually worsening loss of mental abilities, including memory, judgment, and abstract thinking, as well as changes in personality.

amebas (a-MEE-buz) small, one-celled animals that live in fresh and salt water. Amebas can be seen only with a microscope. Also spelled amoebas.

amino acids (a-MEE-no acids) the chief building blocks of proteins. In humans, certain amino acids are required to sustain life.

amnesia (am-NEE-zha) the loss of memory about one or more past experiences that is more than normal forgetfulness.

amniocentesis (am-nee-o-sen-TEE-sis) a test in which a long, thin needle is inserted in the mother's uterus to obtain a sample of the amniotic fluid from the sac that surrounds the fetus. The fetal cells in the fluid are then examined for genetic defects.

amniotic sac (am-nee-AH-tik SAK) the sac formed by the amnion, the thin but tough membrane that lines the outside of the embryo in the uterus and is filled with fluid to cushion and protect the embryo as it grows.

amoebas (a-MEE-buz) small, one-celled animals that live in fresh and salt water. Amoebas can be seen only with a microscope. Also spelled amebas.

amphetamines (am-FET-a-meenz) drugs that produce a temporary feeling of alertness, energy, and euphoria.

amputation (am-pyoo-TAY-shun) the removal of a limb or other appendage or outgrowth of the body.

amygdala (a-MIG-da-la) a small almond-shaped structure in the brain that plays a part in processing emotions.

amyloidosis a condition in which excessive amounts of a protein known as amyloid are created by the body and deposited in tissues causing damage.

anal of or referring to the anus, the opening at the end of the digestive system through which waste leaves the body.

androgen deficiency (AN-dro-gen de-FISH-ens-see) reduced male hormones in men. Also called male menopause.

androgynous (an-DRAW-gin-us) having characteristics of both sexes.

anemia (uh-NEE-me-uh) a blood condition in which there is a decreased hemoglobin in the blood and, usually, fewer than normal numbers of red blood cells.

anencephaly (an-en-SEF-uh-lee) a condition present at birth in which most of the brain is missing.

anesthesia (an-es-THEE-zha) a state in which a person is temporarily unable to feel pain while under the influence of a medication.

anesthetic (an-es-THET-ik) a medicine that decreases the sensation of pain.

angiogram (AN-jee-o-gram) a test in which x-rays are taken as dye is injected into the body, showing the flow of blood through the heart and blood vessels.

anorexia nervosa (an-o-REK-se-a ner-VO-sa) an emotional disorder characterized by dread of gaining weight, leading to self-starvation and dangerous loss of weight and malnutrition.

antagonist (an-TAG-oh-nist) a chemical that acts within the body to reduce or oppose the effects of another chemical.

anthrax (AN-thraks) a rare infectious disease caused by the bacterium *Bacillus anthracis*.

antibiotic (an-tie-by-AH-tik) a drug that kills or slows the growth of bacteria.

antibiotic resistance occurs when bacteria evolve to withstand attack by antibiotics.

antibody (AN-tih-bah-dee) a protein molecule produced by the body's immune system to help fight a specific infection caused by a microorganism, such as a bacterium or virus.

anticholinergics (AN-ti-koll-in-ER-giks) medications given to counteract a chemical in the central nervous system that controls muscles, sweat glands, and some glands that secrete mucus.

anticonvulsants (an-tie-kon-VUL-sents) medications that affect the electrical activity in the brain and are given to prevent or stop seizures.

antidepressant medications medications used for the treatment and prevention of depression.

antifungal drugs (an-ty-FUN-gal) medications that kill fungi.

antigen (AN-tih-jen) a substance that is recognized as a threat by the body's immune system, which triggers the formation of specific antibodies against the substance.

antihistamines (an-tie-HIS-tuh-meens) drugs used to combat allergic reactions and relieve itching.

antimony (AN-tih-mo-nee) an element that has properties of both metals and nonmetals and can kill or inhibit the growth of certain bacteria.

antipsychotic drugs medications that counteract or reduce the symptoms of a severe mental disorder such as schizophrenia.

antisocial behaving in ways that purposefully disregard the rights of others and break society's rules or laws.

antisocial behavior behavior that differs significantly from the norms of society and is considered harmful to society.

antitoxin (an-tih-TOK-sin) counteracts the effects of toxins, or poisons, on the body. It is produced to act against specific toxins, such as those made by the bacteria that cause botulism or diphtheria.

antivenin an antibody (protein) capable of neutralizing a specific venom.

anus (A-nus) the opening at the end of the digestive system, through which waste leaves the body.

anxiety (ang-ZY-e-tee) can be experienced as a troubled feeling, a sense of dread, fear of the future, or distress over a possible threat to a person's physical or mental well-being.

anxiety disorders (ang-ZY-e-tee dis-OR-derz) a group of conditions that cause people to feel extreme fear or worry that sometimes is accompanied by symptoms such as dizziness, chest pain, or difficulty sleeping or concentrating,

aorta (ay-OR-ta) the major large artery that carries blood from the heart to the rest of the body.

aortic aneurysm (ay-OR-tik AN-yoo-rizm) a weak spot in the aorta, the body's largest blood vessel. The weak spot can rupture or break, causing massive internal bleeding.

apnea (AP-nee-uh) the temporary stopping of breathing.

appendectomy (ah-pen-DEK-toe-me) a surgical procedure in which the appendix is removed.

appendicitis (ah-pen-dih-SY-tis) an inflammation of the appendix.

appendix (ah-PEN-diks) the narrow, finger-shaped organ that branches off the part of the large intestine in the lower right side of the abdomen. Although the organ is not known to have any vital function, the tissue of the appendix is populated by cells of the immune system.

arbovirus (ar-buh-VY-rus) a member of a family of viruses that multiply in blood-sucking organisms, such as mosquitoes and ticks, and spread through their bites.

arteriosclerosis (ar-teer-e-o-sklah-RO-sis) a condition in which arteries of the body become narrowed and hardened from the buildup of calcium, cholesterol, and other substances, causing decreased blood flow through these vessels.

artery a vessel that carries blood from the heart to tissues in the body.

arthritis (ar-THRY-tis) any of several disorders characterized by inflammation of the joints.

arthropod a member of a group of organisms that lack a spinal column and have a segmented body and jointed limbs. This group includes various insects, ticks, spiders, lice, and fleas.

aseptic meningitis (a-SEP-tik meh-nin-JY-tis) a milder, non-bacterial form of meningitis that is usually caused by a virus.

Asperger's syndrome a pervasive developmental disorder in which a child does not learn to communicate and interact socially with others in a typical way. Children with Asperger's syndrome have normal intelligence and generally good language development.

aspiration (as-puh-RAY-shun) the sucking of fluid or other material out of the body, such as the removal of a sample of joint fluid through a needle inserted into the joint.

asthma (AZ-mah) a condition in which the airways of the lungs repeatedly become narrowed and inflamed, causing breathing difficulty.

ataxia a disorder involving an unsteady gait.

atopy (AT-uh-pee) an allergic hypersensitivity that affects parts of the body not in direct contact with the allergen, such as hay fever, asthma, or eczema.

atrial fibrillation (AY-tree-al fib-ri-LAY-shun) the arrhythmic or irregular beating of the left upper chamber of the heart. This leads to an irregular flow of blood and to the formation of blood clots that can leave the heart and travel to the brain, causing a stroke.

Attention Deficit Hyperactivity Disorder (or ADHD) a condition that makes it hard for a person to pay attention, sit still, or think before acting.

aura a warning sensation that precedes a seizure or other neurological event.

autism (AW-tih-zum) a developmental disorder in which a person has difficulty interacting and communicating with others and usually has severely limited interest in social activities.

autoimmune disease (aw-toh-ih-MYOON) a disease in which the body's immune system attacks some of the body's own normal tissues and cells.

autonomic nervous system a branch of the peripheral nervous system that controls various involuntary body activities such as body temperature, metabolism, heart rate, blood pressure, breathing, and digestion. The autonomic nervous system has two parts—the sympathetic and parasympathetic branches.

autopsy (AW-top-see) an examination of a body after death to look for the cause of death or the effects of a disease.

autosomal dominant a mode of inheritance in which only one copy of an abnormal gene is necessary to cause disease.

bacteremia (bak-tuh-REE-me-uh) the presence of bacteria in the blood.

bacteria (bak-TEER-ee-a) single-celled micro-organisms which typically reproduce by cell division. Some, but not all, types of bacteria can cause disease in humans. Many types can live in the body without causing harm.

bacterial vaginosis (back-TER-i-all vag-in-OH-sis) a condition of the vagina caused by an overgrowth of normal bacteria. Symptoms include an abnormal discharge and fishy odor. This condition is treated with oral antibiotics and vaginal gels.

Bartholin glands (BAR-tha-lin) two very small glands, inside the vagina, that are important for vaginal lubrication during sexual intercourse.

battery a group of related tests that are given together.

bedsores skin sores caused by prolonged pressure on the skin and typically are seen in people who are confined by illness or paralysis to beds or wheelchairs. Also called pressure sores.

behavior therapy a type of counseling that works to help people change their actions.

behavioral related to the way a person acts.

Bell's palsy (PAWL-zee) a condition in which there is weakness or loss of function of muscles on one side of the face.

benign (be-NINE) a condition that is not cancerous or serious and will probably improve, go away, or not get worse.

bifocals prescription eyeglasses that have lenses divided into two or more sections. The bottom section allows a person to see things clearly that are close, and the top section allows a person to see things clearly that are far away. Also called multifocal (progressive) lenses.

bile a greenish-brown fluid manufactured in the liver that is essential for digesting food. Bile is stored in the gallbladder, which contracts and discharges bile into the intestine to aid digestion of fats after a person eats.

bile duct a passageway that carries bile, a substance that aids the digestion of fat, from the liver to the gallbladder (a small pouch-like organ where the bile is temporarily stored) and from the gallbladder to the small intestine.

biliary tract (BIH-lee-ah-ree) the organs and ducts, including the liver and gallbladder, that produce, store, and transport bile, a substance which aids in digestion.

bilirubin (bih-lih-ROO-bin) a substance that the body produces when hemoglobin, an iron-containing component of the blood, is broken down.

binge drinking having five or more drinks in a row within a few hours.

biochemical relating to the chemistry of living organisms.

biofeedback a technique that helps people gain some voluntary control over normally involuntary body functions.

biohazard a biological agent or condition that causes a threat to humans.

biological warfare a method of waging war by using harmful microorganisms to purposely spread disease to many people.

biopsy (BI-op-see) a test in which a small sample of skin or other body tissue is removed and examined for signs of disease.

bipolar disorder a group of mood disorders that are characterized by alternating episodes of depression and mania.

bisexual (bi-SEK-shoo-al) sexually attracted to both sexes.

bladder (BLAD-er) the sac that stores urine produced by the kidneys prior to discharge from the body.

blood clot a thickening of the blood into a jelly-like substance that helps stop bleeding. Clotting of the blood within a blood vessel can lead to blockage of blood flow.

blood transfusion the process of giving blood (or certain cells or chemicals found in the blood) to a person who needs it due to illness or blood loss.

blood-brain barrier a biological shield in the body that helps prevent germs or other potentially harmful materials in the blood from entering the brain and spinal cord.

body dysmorphic disorder (dis-MORE-fik) (or BDD) an extremely distressing, obsessive preoccupation with perceived flaws in one's appearance.

body image a person's impressions, thoughts, feelings, and opinions about his or her body.

boils skin abscesses or collections of pus in the skin.

bone marrow the soft tissue inside bones where blood cells are made.

brain stem the part of the brain that connects to the spinal cord. The brain stem controls the basic functions of life, such as breathing and blood pressure.

bronchi (BRONG-kye) the larger tube-like airways that carry air in and out of the lungs.

bronchitis (brong-KYE-tis) a disease that involves inflammation of the larger airways in the respiratory tract, which can result from infection or other causes.

bronchodilator (brong-ko-DYE-lay-tor) a medication that helps improve air flow through the lungs by widening narrowed airways.

bronchoscopy (brong-KOS-ko-pee) a procedure used to examine the bronchi with an instrument called a bronchoscope, which is a tool for looking inside the lungs that is made up of a lighted tube with viewing lenses. A bronchoscope has channels through which samples of material can be taken from the lungs for study in the laboratory.

bulimia (bu-LEE-me-a) an eating disorder in which a person has episodes of out-of-control overeating, or binges, and then tries to make up for them by making themselves vomit, by taking laxatives, or by exercising to excess to avoid gaining weight.

bullying when a person repeatedly intimidates or acts aggressively toward those with less power or ability to defend themselves.

caisson (KAY-son) a watertight container that divers or construction workers use under water.

calorie (KAL-or-ee) a unit of energy used to describe both the amount of energy in food and the amount of energy the body uses.

cancer a condition characterized by abnormal overgrowth of certain cells, which may be fatal.

candidiasis (kan-dih-DYE-uh-sis) an overgrowth of *Candida,* a type of yeast, in or on the body.

carbohydrates the nutrients in food that help provide energy to the body.

carbon dioxide (CAR-bon dy-OK-side) an odorless, colorless gas that is formed in the tissues and breathed out through the lungs.

carcinogens (kar-SIH-no-jenz) substances or agents that can cause cancer.

carcinoma (kar-sih-NO-muh) a cancerous tumor that arises in the epithelium (eh-puh-THEE-lee-um), the sheets of cells that line body surfaces, such as the insides of hollow organs and cavities.

cardiovascular system (kar-dee-o-VAS-ku-lur) the heart and blood vessels.

carrier a person who has in his body a bacterium or virus or gene for a disease that he can transmit to other people without getting sick himself.

cataracts (KAH-tuh-rakts) areas of cloudiness of the lens of the eye that can interfere with vision.

catatonic (kat-a-TON-ik) an extreme disturbance in movement that has a psychological cause. Catatonic people can develop a wide range of symptoms, including: becoming very inactive and withdrawn, displaying excessive activity with no purpose, refusing to talk or follow instructions, becoming rigid if others try to move them, adopting strange gestures and facial expressions, and repeating the words or copying the movements of others.

catecholamines (kat-e-KO-la-meens) hormones and neurotransmitters such as epinephrine, norepinephrine, and dopamine.

catheter (KAH-thuh-ter) a small plastic tube placed through a body opening into an organ (such as the bladder) or through the skin directly into a blood vessel. It is used to give fluids to or drain fluids from a person.

cecum (SEE-kum) the pouch-like start of the large intestine that connects it to the small intestine.

cell division the process by which a cell divides to form new cells, each of which contains the same genetic material as the original cell.

cellular (cell-U-lar) relating to or consisting of cells, cell-mandated, as in cellular immunity.

cellulitis (sel-yoo-LYE-tis) an infection of the skin and the tissues beneath it.

centenarians people who are at least 100 years old.

central nervous system (SEN-trul NER-vus SIS-tem) the part of the nervous system that includes the brain and spinal cord.

cerebellum (se-re-BEL-um) the portion of the brain that is responsible for muscle coordination and balance.

cerebral cortex (suh-REE-brul KOR-teks) the part of the brain that controls functions such as conscious thought, listening, and speaking.

cerebral palsy (se-RE-bral PAL-zee) a group of conditions, all of which affect a person's ability to move. They are caused by injury to the brain before or during the birth process.

cerebrum (se-RE-brum) the largest, front and upper part of the brain that is responsible for mental processes.

cerebrospinal fluid (seh-ree-bro-SPY-nuhl) the fluid that surrounds the brain and spinal cord.

cervical referring to the cervix

cervix (SIR-viks) the lower, narrow end of the uterus that opens into the vagina.

cesarean section (si-ZAR-ee-an SEK-shun) the surgical incision of the walls of the abdomen and uterus to deliver offspring in cases where the mother cannot deliver through the vagina.

chancre (SHANG-ker) a usually painless sore or ulcer that forms where a disease-causing germ enters the body, such as with syphilis.

chancroid (SHANG-kroid) a bacterial infection that causes painful sores in the genital region. Relatively rare in the United States, it mostly occurs in tropical and subtropical areas.

chelation therapy (kee-LAY-shun) a technique used to treat patients with lead or mercury poisoning by administering medications that combine with the metal to keep the body from absorbing it.

chemotherapy (KEE-mo-THER-a-pee) the treatment of cancer with powerful drugs that kill cancer cells.

chlamydia (kla-MIH-dee-uh) microorganisms that can infect the urinary tract, genitals, eye, and respiratory tract, including the lungs.

chlamydial infection (kla-MIH-dee-ul) occurs in various forms in which the bacteria can invade the urinary and genital systems of the body, as well as the eyes and lungs. One of its most common forms is a sexually transmitted disease (STD), usually passed from one person to another through unprotected sexual intercourse.

cholera (KAH-luh-ruh) an infection of the small intestine that can cause severe diarrhea.

cholesterol (ko-LES-ter-ol) a fatlike substance found in the blood and body tissues.

chorionic villus sampling (KOR-ee-on-ik VIL-lus) a test in which a small tube is inserted through the cervix and a small piece of the placenta supporting the fetus is removed for genetic testing.

chromosome (KRO-mo-zom) a unit or strand of DNA, the chemical substance that contains the genetic code to build and maintain a living being. Humans have 23 pairs of chromosomes, for a total of 46.

chromosomes (KRO-mo-somz) threadlike chemical structures inside cells on which the genes are located. There are 46 (23 pairs) of chromosomes in normal human cells. Genes on the X and Y chromosomes (known as the sex chromosomes) help determine whether a person is male or female, Females have two X chromosomes; males have one X and one Y chromosome.

chrondrodystrophy (kon-dro-DIS-trof-ee) abnormal growth at the ends of the bones.

chronic (KRAH-nik) lasting a long time or recurring frequently.

chronic fatigue syndrome (KRON-ik fat-TEEG) a debilitating and complicated disorder in which individuals feel intense fatigue that lasts six months or longer. Symptoms may include insomnia, muscle pain, and impaired concentration. Because other illnesses have these symptoms, doctors must rule out a number of conditions in order to make a diagnosis.

chronic illness (KRAH-nik) an illness with symptoms that last a long time or that recur frequently.

circulatory system (SIR-kyoo-luh-tor-e) the system composed of the heart and blood vessels that moves blood throughout the body.

circumcision a surgical procedure in which the fold of skin covering the end of the penis is removed.

cirrhosis (sir-O-sis) a condition that affects the liver, involving long-term inflammation and scarring, which can lead to problems with liver function.

cleft palate a gap or split in the roof of the mouth (the palate). It occurs when the palate of a fetus does not develop properly during the first months of pregnancy.

clinical psychologist a mental health professional who has earned a non-medical doctoral degree. Clinical psychologists can do psychological evaluation and provide mental health counseling and therapy.

cloning (KLOH-ning) a process in which a group of cells or even an entire organism is grown from a single stem cell and is genetically identical to it.

clot as a verb: the process by which the body forms a thickened mass of blood cells and protein to stop bleeding; as a noun: the result of that process.

cocaine (ko-KAYN) a drug that produces a temporary feeling of alertness, energy, and euphoria.

cognitive associated with thinking, learning, perception, awareness, and judgment.

cognitive behavioral therapy (KOG-nih-tiv be-HAY-vyuh-rul THAIR-uh-pee) treatment that helps people identify negative ways of thinking and behaving and change them to more positive approaches.

cognitive therapy a form of counseling that helps people work to change distorted attitudes and ways of thinking.

colitis, ulcerative (ko-LIE-tis, UL-sir-ah-tiv) a common form of inflammatory bowel disease that causes inflammation with sore spots or breaks in the inner lining of the large intestine (colon). Symptoms include cramping, bleeding from the rectum, and diarrhea.

colon (KO-lin) the muscular tube through which food passes as it is digested, just before it moves into the rectum and out of the body through the anus. Also called the large intestine.

colonized means that a group of organisms, particularly bacteria, are living on or inside the body without causing symptoms of infection.

colostomy (ko-LOS-to-mee) a surgical procedure in which a part of the large intestine is removed, and the end of the intestine is attached to an opening made in the abdomen. The stool is passed through this opening into a special bag.

coma (KO-ma) an unconscious state, like a very deep sleep. A person in a coma cannot be awakened, and cannot move, see, speak, or hear.

comedo (KOM-e-do) an acne pimple. A blackhead is an open comedo. A whitehead is a closed comedo. Cosmetics that are labeled non-comedogenic (non-kom-e-do-JEN-ik) are less likely to cause pimples.

communication disorder a condition affecting a person's ability to use or understand speech and language.

complement proteins proteins that circulate in the blood and play a role in the immune system's response to infections. More than 20 complement proteins have been identified.

computerized tomography (kom-PYOO-ter-ized toe-MAH-gruh-fee), or CT, a technique in which a machine takes many x-rays of the body to create a three-dimensional picture. Also called computerized axial tomography (CAT).

concussion (kon-KUH-shun) an injury to the brain, produced by a blow to the head or violent shaking.

conduct disorder is diagnosed in children and adolescents who have had serious problems with lying, stealing, and aggressive behavior for at least six months.

confabulation filling in gaps in memory by making up or fabricating facts. The gaps occur because the memory function is impaired.

congenital (kon-JEH-nih-tul) present at birth

congestive (kon-JES-tiv) characterized by accumulation of too much fluid.

congestive heart failure (kon-JES-tiv) a condition in which a damaged or overworked heart cannot pump enough blood to meet the oxygen and nutrient needs of the body. People with heart failure may find it hard to exercise due to the insufficient blood flow, but many people live a long time with this condition. Also called heart failure.

conjunctivitis (kon-jung-tih-VY-tis) an inflammation of the thin membrane that lines the inside of the eyelids and covers the surface of the eyeball. Conjunctivitis can be caused by viruses, bacteria, allergies, chemical irritation, and other conditions or diseases that cause inflammation. Also called pinkeye

connective tissue helps hold the body together, is found in skin, joints and bones.

consensual sex sexual activity in which both people freely agree to participate.

constipation the sluggish movement of the bowels, usually resulting in infrequent, hard stools.

contagious (kon-TAY-jus) transmittable from one person to another, usually referring to an infection.

contraception (kon-tra-SEP-shun) the deliberate prevention of conception or impregnation.

controversy discussions with many different and opposing points of view.

conversion disorder a mental disorder in which psychological symptoms are converted to physical symptoms, such as blindness, paralysis, or seizures. A person with conversion disorder does not intentionally produce symptoms.

convulsions (kon-VUL-shuns) sudden bursts of disorganized electrical activity that interrupt the normal functioning of the brain, often leading to uncontrolled movements in the body and sometimes a temporary change in consciousness. Also called seizures.

cornea (KOR-nee-uh) the transparent circular layer of cells over the central colored part of the eyeball (the iris) through which light enters the eye.

coronary aneurysm (KOR-uh-nair-e AN-yuh-rih-zum) an abnormal stretching and weakening of a blood vessel that supplies blood to the heart. If it breaks open, it may cause serious damage to the heart, sometimes leading to death.

coronary arteries (KOR-uh-nair-e AR-tuh-reez) the blood vessels that directly supply blood to the heart.

correlated linked in a way that can be measured and predicted.

cortex (KOR-teks) the top outer layer of the brain. It controls the brain's higher functions, such as thinking, learning, and personality.

corticosteroids (kor-tih-ko-STIR-oyds) chemical substances made by the adrenal glands that have several functions in the body, including maintaining blood pressure during stress and controlling inflammation. They can also be given to people as medication to treat certain illnesses.

cortisol (KOR-ti-sol) a hormone that helps control blood pressure and metabolism, the process of converting food into energy and waste products. It plays a part in the stress response.

cortisone (KOR-ti-zone) a medication used to relieve inflammation.

Crohn's disease (KRONZ) an often inherited, chronic inflammatory disease that typically affects the small and/or large intestine but which can affect any part of the digestive system. The disease causes crater-like ulcers or sores in the inner surface of the bowel. Mild cases may be treated with medication; serious cases may be treated with surgery.

cri du chat (kree-doo-SHA), French for *cat's cry,* a genetic disorder that can cause mental retardation, a small head, and a cat-like whine.

croup (KROOP) an infection involving the trachea (windpipe) and larynx (voice box) that typically occurs in childhood. It causes inflammation and narrowing of the upper airway, sometimes making it difficult to breathe. The characteristic symptom is a barking cough.

CT scan the shortened name for computerized axial tomography (to-MOG-ra-fee), which uses computers to view structures inside the body. Also called CAT scan.

culture (KUL-chur) a test in which a sample of fluid or tissue from the body is placed in a dish containing material that supports the growth of certain organisms. Typically, within days the organisms will grow and can be identified.

cutaneous (kyoo-TAY-nee-us) related to or affecting the skin.

cyanosis (sye-uh-NO-sis) a bluish or purplish discoloration of the skin and mucous membranes due to a lack of oxygen in the blood.

cystic fibrosis (SIS-tik fy-BRO-sis) a disease that causes the body to produce thick mucus that clogs passages in many of the body's organs, including the lungs.

cysts (SISTS) shell-like enclosures that contain small organisms in a resting stage.

cytomegalovirus infection (sy-tuh-MEH-guh-lo-vy-rus) (CMV) a common infection usually causing no symptoms. It poses little risk for healthy people, but it can lead to serious illness in people with weak immune systems.

debilitating (de-BI-li-tay-ting) making weak or sapping strength.

DEET (abbreviation for N,N-Diethyl-meta-toluamide) the active ingredient in many insect repellants.

defiant (dee-FY-ent) an attitude of challenging the rules in a hostile way or of being disobedient on purpose.

degenerative (dee-JEN-er-uh-tiv) progressively worsening or becoming more impaired.

dehydration (dee-hi-DRAY-shun) a condition in which the body is depleted of water, usually caused by excessive and unreplaced loss of body fluids, such as through sweating, vomiting, or diarrhea.

delinquent a legal term that refers to a juvenile (someone under the age of 18) who has committed an illegal act. Delinquent behavior includes any behavior that would be considered a crime if committed by an adult as well as specific behaviors that are illegal for youth, such as school truancy, violating curfew, or running away.

delirious (dee-LEER-ee-us) an acute mental syndrome characterized by confusion, disordered thinking, and hallucinations (ha-loo-si-NAY-shunz).

delirium (dih-LEER-e-um) a condition in which a person is confused, is unable to think clearly, and has a reduced level of consciousness.

delirium tremens also called the DTs or Alcohol Withdrawal Delirium. The DTs may occur two to three days after a person with long-term alcoholism stops drinking. Symptoms include rapid heartbeat, sweating, abnormally high blood pressure, an irregular tremor, delusions, hallucinations, and agitated or wild behavior. The delirium and other withdrawal symptoms usually subside in three or four days.

delusion (de-LOO-zhun) a false belief or judgment that remains even in the face of proof that it is not true.

dementia (dih-MEN-sha) a loss of mental abilities, including memory, understanding, and judgment.

depersonalization (de-per-son-al-i-ZAY-shun) a mental condition in which people feel that they are living in a dream or are removed from their body and are watching themselves live.

depression (de-PRESH-un) a mental state characterized by feelings of sadness, despair, and discouragement.

depressive disorders a collection of mental disorders that involve long periods of excessive sadness and affect a person's feelings, thoughts, and behavior.

derealization (de-reel-i-ZAY-shun) a mental condition in which people feel that the external world is strange or unreal.

dermatitis a skin condition characterized by a red, itchy rash. It may occur when the skin comes in contact with something to which it is sensitive.

desensitization (de-sens-ih-tih-ZAY-shun) a method for reducing a person's reaction to an allergen.

detoxification (de-tox-i-fi-KAY-shun) the process of breaking dependence on an addictive substance.

deviated septum a condition in which the wall of tissue between the passages, the septum, divides the passage-ways unevenly, sometimes causing breathing difficulties and blockage of sinus drainage.

dextrocardia mirror image rotation that is confined to the heart.

diabetes (dye-uh-BEE-teez) a condition in which the body's pancreas does not produce enough insulin or the body cannot use the insulin it makes effectively, resulting in increased levels of sugar in the blood. This can lead to increased urination, dehydration, weight loss, weakness, and a number of other symptoms and complications related to chemical imbalances within the body.

dialysis (dye-AL-uh-sis) a process that removes waste, toxins (poisons), and extra fluid from the blood. Usually dialysis is done when a person's kidneys are unable to perform these functions normally.

diaphragm (DY-a-fram) the muscle that separates the chest and abdominal cavities. It is the chief muscle used in breathing.

diarrhea (di-ah-RE-a) frequent, watery stools (bowel movements).

differentiation (dif-feh-rent-see-AY-shun) the process in which embryonic or adult stem cells give rise to more specialized cells.

digestive system the system that processes food. It includes the mouth, esophagus, stomach, intestines, colon, rectum, and other organs involved in digestion, including the liver and pancreas.

dilate (DY-late) to become enlarged or stretched beyond the usual boundaries.

diphtheria (dif-THEER-e-uh) an infection of the lining of the upper respiratory tract (the nose and throat). It can cause breathing difficulty and other complications, including death.

disseminated a disease that has spread widely in the body.

dissociative identity disorder (DID) a severe psychiatric condition in which a person has two or more distinct sub-personalities that periodically take control of his or her behavior. The sub-personalities are thought to be caused by repeated episodes of an extreme form of dissociation. Formerly known as multiple personality disorder (MPD).

diuretics (dye-yoor-EH-tiks) medications that increase the body's output of urine.

dizygotic (dye-zye-GOT-ik) derived from two different fertilized eggs.

DNA or deoxyribonucleic acid (dee-OX-see-ry-bo-nyoo-KLAY-ik AH-sid), the specialized chemical substance that contains the genetic code necessary to build and maintain the structures and functions of living organisms.

dopamine (DOE-puh-meen) a neurotransmitter in the brain that is involved in the brain structures that control motor activity (movement).

double vision a vision problem in which a person sees two images of a single object.

Down syndrome a genetic disorder that can cause mental retardation, shortness, and distinctive facial characteristics, as well as many other features.

DSM-IV The *Diagnostic and Statistical Manual of Mental Disorders,* 4th revision, published by the American Psychiatric Association. This is the system of classification and diagnosis of mental conditions used in the United States.

duodenal (do-uh-DEE-nul) the upper part of the small intestine.

duodenum (dew-eh-DEE-num) the first part of the small intestine that connects to the stomach.

dura mater (DUR-uh MAY-ter) the outermost of three membranes covering the brain and spinal cord.

dust mites tiny insects that live in dust and in materials such as carpets, pillows, mattresses and furniture.

dysplasia (dis-PLAY-zha) abnormal growth or development.

ear wax the wax-like substance in the ear that traps dust and other particles to prevent them from damaging the inner ear. Also known as cerumen (se-ROO-men).

eating disorder a condition in which a person's eating behaviors and food habits are so unbalanced that they cause physical and emotional problems.

echocardiogram (eh-ko-KAR-dee-uh-gram) a diagnostic test that uses sound waves to produce images of the heart's chambers and valves and blood flow through the heart.

echoviruses a group of viruses found in the intestinal tract. The word echo in the name is acronym for enteric cytopathic human orphan viruses. When these viruses were named, they were not associated with any disease, hence the use of the word orphan. However, later these viruses were associated with various diseases, including meningitis and encephalitis.

ectopic pregnancy (ek-TAH-pik) an abnormal pregnancy in which the fertilized egg develops outside the uterus, usually within one of the fallopian tubes.

eczema (EG-ze-mah) an inflammatory skin condition characterized by redness, itchiness, and oozing blisters that become crusty and hard.

edema (e-DEE-ma) swelling in the body's tissues caused by excess fluids.

effusion (ih-FYOO-zhun) an excessive accumulation of body fluid in a body space or cavity, such as the middle ear.

ejaculate (e-JAH-kyoo-late) to discharge semen from the penis.

elasticity the ability to be stretched and to return to original shape.

electrocardiogram (e-lek-tro-KAR-dee-o-gram) a test that records and displays the electrical activity of the heart. Also known as an EKG.

electroconvulsive therapy involves sending small, carefully controlled pulses of electric current to the brain, which leads to brief seizures. It is a fast treatment for severe depression. Popularly known as shock therapy

electroencephalogram an instrument that records the electrical activity of the brain.

electrolysis (ee-lek-TRAW-li-sis) a method of destroying hair roots by passing an electric current through them.

electromyogram (ee-lek-tro-MY-eh-gram) (EMG) a visual record made by an electromyograph, which measures the electrical activity associated with functioning muscle.

elephantiasis (eh-luh-fan-TIE-uh-sis) the significant enlargement and thickening of body tissues caused by an infestation of parasites known as filaria.

embolism a blockage in a blood vessel caused by a blood clot, air bubble, fatty tissue, or other substance that traveled through the bloodstream from another part of the body.

embryo (EM-bree-o), in humans, the developing organism from the end of the second week after fertilization to the end of the eighth week.

empathy the action of being aware or understanding the feelings of others without having those feelings explained.

emphysema (em-fuh-ZEE-mah) a lung disease in which the tiny air sacs in the lungs become permanently damaged and are unable to maintain the normal exchange of oxygen and other respiratory gases with the blood, often causing breathing difficulty.

encephalitis (en-seh-fuh-LYE-tis) an inflammation of the brain, usually caused by a viral infection.

endemic (en-DEH-mik) a disease or condition that is present in a population or geographic area at all times.

endocarditis (en-do-kar-DYE-tis) an inflammation of the valves and internal lining of the heart, known as the endocardium (en-doh-KAR-dee-um), usually caused by an infection.

endocrine (EN-do-krin) a group of glands, such as the thyroid, adrenal, and pituitary glands, and the hormones they produce. The endocrine glands secrete their hormones into the bloodstream, and the hormones travel to the cells that have receptors for them. Certain hormones have effects on mood and sometimes cause emotional swings.

endocrine system a system of ductless glands, including the thyroid and pituitary among others, that secrete hormones and control many bodily functions.

endocrinologist (en-do-krin-OL-o-jist) a doctor who specializes in treating patients with hormone-related disorders.

endoscope (EN-doh-skope) a tool for looking inside parts of the body. It consists of a lighted tube and optical fibers and/or lenses.

endoscopy (en-DOS-ko-pee) a type of diagnostic test in which a lighted tube-like instrument is inserted into a part of the body.

enema (EH-nuh-muh) a procedure in which liquid is injected through the anus into the intestine, usually to flush out the intestines.

enterovirus (en-tuh-ro-VY-rus) a group of viruses that can infect the human gastrointestinal tract and spread through the body causing a number of symptoms.

enzyme (EN-zime) a protein that helps speed up a chemical reaction in cells or organisms.

epidemic (eh-pih-DEH-mik) an outbreak of disease, especially infectious disease, in which the number of cases suddenly becomes far greater than usual. Usually epidemics are outbreaks of diseases in specific regions, whereas widespread epidemics are called pandemics.

epididymitis (eh-pih-dih-duh-MY-tis) a painful inflammation of the epididymitis, a structure attached to the testicles.

epidural (ep-I-DOO-ral) above or outside the dura, the covering of the brain.

epiglottis (eh-pih-GLAH-tis) the soft flap of tissue that covers the opening of the trachea (windpipe) when a person swallows to prevent food or fluid from entering the airway and lungs.

epiglottitis (eh-pih-glah-TIE-tis) a condition involving life-threatening swelling of the epiglottis, which is usually caused by a bacterial infection of the epiglottis. The condition can result in a blockage of the trachea and severe breathing difficulty.

epilepsy (EP-i-lep-see) a condition of the nervous system characterized by recurrent seizures that temporarily affect a person's awareness, movements, or sensations. Seizures occur when powerful, rapid bursts of electrical energy interrupt the normal electrical patterns of the brain.

epinephrine (eh-pih-NEH-frin) a chemical substance produced by the body that can also be given as a medication to constrict, or narrow, small blood vessels, stimulate the heart, and cause other effects, such as helping to open narrowed airways in conditions such as asthma and croup.

Epstein-Barr virus (EP-stine-BAHR VI-rus) a common virus that causes infectious mononucleosis.

ergonomics (er-go-NOM-iks) a science that helps people to know the best postures and movements to use while working, in order to avoid injury and discomfort.

esophagus (eh-SAH-fuh-gus) the soft tube that, with swallowing, carries food from the throat to the stomach.

esteomyelitis (ah-stee-o-my-uh-LYE-tis) a bone infection that is usually caused by bacteria. It can involve any bone in the body, but it most commonly affects the long bones in the arms and legs.

estrogen (ES-tro-jen) a steroid hormone that stimulates the development of female sexual characteristics and maintenance of the female reproductive system.

ethical having to do with questions of what is right and wrong, or with moral values.

ethics a guiding set of principles for conduct, a system of moral values.

euphoria (yoo-FOR-ee-uh) an abnormally high mood with the tendency to be overactive and overly talkative, and to have racing thoughts and overinflated self-confidence.

eustachian tube (yoo-STAY-she-un) the tiny channel that connects and allows air to flow between the middle ear and the throat.

exotoxin (ek-so-TOK-sin) a substance produced by bacteria that has harmful effects on the infected person.

factitious false.

failure to thrive a condition in which an infant fails to gain weight and grow at the expected rate.

fallopian tubes (fa-LO-pee-an tubes) the two slender tubes that connect the ovaries and the uterus in females. They carry the ova, or eggs, from the ovaries to the uterus.

feces (FEE-seez) the excreted waste from the gastrointestinal tract.

fetal alcohol syndrome occurs if the fetus is exposed to alcohol and is a condition that can be associated with mental, physical, and behavioral differences. Oppositional behavioral problems, learning difficulties, intellectual disability, and retarded growth can occur in the children of women who drink alcohol while they are pregnant.

fetus (FEE-tus) an unborn human after it is an embryo, from 9 weeks after fertilization until childbirth.

fibromyalgia (fi-bro-my-AL-ja) a group of disorders that are characterized by achy, tender, and stiff muscles.

fistulas (FIS-tu-las) abnormal connections between two organs or leading from an internal organ to the surface of the body.

flashbacks intensely vivid, recurring mental images of a past traumatic event. People may feel or act as if they were reliving the experience.

flavivirus family (FLAY-vih-vy-rus) a group of viruses that includes those that cause dengue fever and yellow fever.

fluoridation the process of adding fluoride to drinking water to help prevent tooth decay.

follicles tiny pits in the skin from which hair grows.

food chain the eating relationships between different organisms in a specific environment.

foreign coming from outside a person's body.

formula a prepared, nutritious drink or a dry drink mix designed specifically for infants.

fragile X syndrome a disorder associated with a faulty X chromosome (a chromosome is a structure inside the body's cells that contains DNA, which is the genetic material that helps determine characteristics such as hair and eye color; females have two X chromosomes whereas males have only one). Fragile X syndrome is associated with mental retardation, especially in males.

fraternal twins twins who are born at the same time but develop from two separate fertilized eggs. Unlike identical twins, who develop from only one fertilized egg that splits into two and who look exactly alike, fraternal twins may not look the same at all or be the same

gender. Identical twins have the same genes, but fraternal twins are no more likely to share genes than non-twin siblings.

frostbite damage to tissues resulting from exposure to low environmental temperatures. It is also called congelation (kon-jeh-LAY-shun).

fugue (FYOOG) a psychiatric condition in which people wander or travel and may appear to be functioning normally, but they are unable to remember their identity or details about their past.

fulminant (FUL-mi-nant) occurring suddenly and with great severity.

fungus (FUN-gus) a microorganism that can grow in or on the body, causing infections of internal organs or of the skin, hair, and nails. The plural form is fungi (FUNG-eye).

gall bladder a small pear-shaped organ on the right side of the abdomen that stores bile, a liquid that helps the body digest fat.

gallstones (GAWL-stonz) hard masses that form in the gallbladder or bile duct.

gamma globulin (GAH-muh GLAH-byoolin) a type of protein in the blood that contains the antibodies produced by the cells of the body's immune system that help defend the body against infection-causing germs, such as bacteria and viruses.

gangrene (GANG-green) the decay or death of living tissue caused by a lack of oxygen supply to the tissue and/or bacterial infection of the tissue.

gastrointestinal (gas-tro-in-TES-tih-nuhl) pertaining to the organs of the digestive system, the system that processes food. It includes the mouth, esophagus, stomach, intestines, colon, and rectum and other organs involved in digestion, including the liver and pancreas.

gene therapy a treatment that works by altering genes.

general anesthesia (an-es-THE-zha) using drugs or inhaled gases to create a state of unconsciousness and muscle relaxation throughout the body to block pain during surgery. Local anesthesia blocks or numbs pain in one part of the body while patients remain awake.

genes (JEENS) chemical structures composed of deoxyribonucleic acid (DNA) that help determine a person's body structure and physical characteristics such as hair or eye color. Inherited from a person's parents, genes are contained in the chromosomes found in the body's cells.

genetic (juh-NEH-tik) refers to heredity and the ways in which genes control the development and maintenance of organisms.

genetic predisposition the tendency to get a certain disease that is inherited from a person's parents.

genetics (juh-NEH-tiks) the branch of science that deals with heredity and the ways in which genes control the development and maintenance of organisms.

genital (JEH-nih-tul) the external sexual organs.

genital herpes (GEN-eh-tal her-PEES) a viral infections transmitted by intimate contact with an infected person. The herpes simplex type 2 virus enters the mucous membrane and settles in nerves near the spinal column. When an infected person has an outbreak, the virus causes blisters at the infection site.

gestational (jes-TAY-shun-al) relating to pregnancy.

gestational age the length of time a fetus has remained developing within the womb.

gland an organ that produces substances such as hormones and chemicals that regulate body functions.

glaucoma a group of disorders that cause pressure to build in the eye, which may result in vision loss.

glomerulus (glom-ER-you-lus) a knot of blood vessels that have the job of filtering the blood. From a Greek word meaning filter.

gonorrhea (gah-nuh-REE-uh) a sexually transmitted disease (STD) spread through all forms of sexual intercourse. The bacteria can also be passed from an infected mother to her baby during childbirth. Gonorrhea can affect the genitals, urethra, rectum, eyes, throat, joints, and other tissues of the body.

Goodpasture's syndrome an autoimmune disorder of unknown cause, characterized by circulating antibodies in the blood that attack the membrane of the kidney's glomeruli and the lung's alveoli.

gout occurs when deposits of uric acid in the joints cause inflammation and pain.

grafts tissue or organ transplants.

granuloma (gran-yoo-LO-muh) chronically inflamed and swollen tissue that often develops as the result of an infection.

growth hormone a chemical substance produced by the pituitary gland that regulates growth and other body functions.

gum disease an infection caused by bacteria that affect the tissues surrounding and supporting the teeth.

gynecologist (gy-ne-KOL-o-jist) a doctor who specializes in the reproductive system of women.

Haemophilus influenzae type B bacteria that can cause serious illnesses, including meningitis, pneumonia, and other infections.

hantavirus a group of viruses transmitted to humans through the saliva or excrement of rodents, such as field mice, and which causes hemorrhagic fever and pneumonia.

hair follicle (FAH-lih-kul) the skin structure from which hair develops and grows.

hallucinate (ha-LOO-sin-ate) to hear, see, or otherwise sense things that are not real.

hallucinations (ha-LOO-sin-AY-shuns) occur when a person sees or hears things that are not really there. Hallucinations can result from nervous system abnormalities, mental disorders, or the use of certain drugs.

hallucinogenic drugs substances that cause a person to have hallucinations.

heart attack a general term that usually refers to a sudden, intense episode of heart injury. It is usually caused by a blockage of a coronary artery, which stops blood from supplying the heart muscle with oxygen.

heart disease a broad term that covers many conditions that prevent the heart from working properly to pump blood throughout the body.

heart failure a condition in which a damaged heart cannot pump enough blood to meet the oxygen and nutrient demands of the body. People with heart failure may find if hard to exercise due to the insufficient blood flow, but many people live a long time with heart failure. Also called congestive heart failure.

heart murmur an abnormal sound from the heart, heard with a stethoscope, that is usually related to the flow of blood through the heart. Some murmurs indicate a problem with a heart valve or other part of the heart's structures, but many murmurs do not indicate any problem.

heel spur a bony growth under the heel that causes pain when a person walks.

Helicobacter pylori (HEEL-ih-ko-bak-ter pie-LOR-eye) a bacterium that causes inflammation and ulcers, or sores, in the lining of the stomach and the upper part of the small intestine.

hemodialysis (HEE-mo-dye-AL-is-is) a method for removing waste products from the blood in patients with kidney failure.

hemoglobin (HE-muh-glo-bin) the oxygen-carrying pigment of the red blood cells.

hemolytic (he-mo-LIT-ik) destruction of red blood cells with the release of hemoglobin into the bloodstream.

hemophilia (hee-mo-FIL-e-a) a hereditary disease that results in abnormal bleeding because the blood fails to clot. It occurs almost exclusively in males.

hemorrhage (HEH-muh-rij) uncontrolled or abnormal bleeding.

hemorrhoids (HEM-o-roidz) a mass of dilated veins in swollen tissue at the margin of the anus or nearby within the rectum.

hepatitis (heh-puh-TIE-tis) an inflammation of the liver. Hepatitis can be caused by viruses, bacteria, and a number of other noninfectious medical conditions.

hepatitis A (heh-puh-TIE-tis A) an inflammation of the liver that is caused by an infection with the hepatitis A virus.

hepatocellular (hep-a-to-SEL-ular) the cells of the liver.

hernia (HER-nee-ah) a protrusion of an organ through connective tissue or a cavity wall.

heroin a narcotic, an addictive painkiller that produces a high, or a euphoric effect. Euphoria (yoo-FOR-ee-a) is an abnormal, exaggerated feeling of well-being.

herpes (HER-peez) a viral infection that can produce painful, recurring skin blisters around the mouth or the genitals, and sometimes symptoms of infection elsewhere in the body.

herpes simplex (HER-peez SIM-plex) a virus that can cause infections of the skin, mouth, genitals, and other parts of the body.

herpesvirus family (her-peez-VY-rus) a group of viruses that can store themselves permanently in the body. The family includes varicella zoster virus, Epstein-Barr virus, and herpes simplex virus.

heterosexual (he-te-ro-SEK-shoo-al) a tendency to be sexually attracted to the opposite sex.

high blood pressure a condition in which the pressure of the blood in the arteries is above normal. Also called hypertension.

hippocampus (hip-o-KAM-pus) the part of the brain that is involved in learning and memory.

histamine (HIS-tuh-meen) a substance released by the body during inflammation. It causes blood vessels to expand and makes it easier for fluid and other substances to pass through vessel walls.

HIV human immunodeficiency virus (HYOO-mun ih-myoo-no-dih-FIH-shen-see) the virus that causes AIDS (acquired immunodeficiency syndrome), an infection that severely weakens the immune system.

hives swollen, itchy patches on the skin.

hormone a chemical substance that is produced by a gland and sent into the bloodstream carrying messages that have certain effects on other parts of the body.

host an organism that provides another organism (such as a parasite or virus) with a place to live and grow.

HTLV-1 (short for human T-cell lymphotropic virus type 1) a virus that is associated with certain kinds of adult leukemia and lymphoma.

human immunodeficiency virus (HYOO-mun ih-myoo-no-dih-FIH-shen-sce), or HIV, the virus that causes AIDS (acquired immunodeficiency syndrome), an infection that severely weakens the immune system.

humoral (HUM-eh-ral) relating to a hormone, relating to or part of an immune response that involves antibodies secreted by B cells and circulating in bodily fluids.

Huntington's disease a genetic condition that leads to involuntary twitching or jerking of the muscles in the face, arms, and legs along with a gradual loss of mental abilities.

hydrocephalus (hy-droe-SEF-uh-lus) a condition, sometimes present at birth, in which there is an abnormal buildup of fluid within the skull, leading to enlargement of the skull and pressure on the brain.

hydrocephaly (hi-dro-SEH-fah-lee) having an abnormally large amount of cerebrospinal fluid in the brain, resulting in an enlarged skull and brain atrophy.

hyperactivity (hy-per-ak-TI-vi-tee) overly active behavior, which makes it hard for a person to sit still.

hyperglycemia (hi-per-gly-SEE-mee-uh) an excess of blood sugar.

hypersensitivity excessively sensitive or abnormally susceptible physically to a specific agent such as a drug.

hypertension (HI-per-ten-chen) abnormally high arterial blood pressure.

hyperthermia (hi-per-THER-me-ah) a state in which the body either produces or absorbs more heat than it can dissipate resulting in a significantly raised body temperature.

hyperthyroidism (hi-per-THY-royd-ih-zum) excessive activity of the thyroid gland, characterized by an enlarged thyroid gland, increased metabolic rate, rapid heartbeat, and high blood pressure.

hypnosis a trance-like state, usually induced by another person. The person under hypnosis may recall forgotten or suppressed memories and be unusually responsive to suggestions,

1861

hypochondria (hy-po-KON-dree-a) a mental disorder in which people believe that they are sick, but their symptoms are not related to any physical illness.

hypoglycemia (hi-po-gly-SEE-mee-uh) a condition that occurs when the amount of glucose, or sugar, in the blood becomes too low. Symptoms can include dizziness, trembling, sweating, and confusion.

hypothalamus (hy-po-THAL-uh-mus) a brain structure located deep within the brain that regulates automatic body functions such as heart rate, blood pressure, temperature, respiration, and the release of hormones.

hypothyroidism (hi-po-THY-royd-ih-zum) an impairment of the functioning of the thyroid gland that causes too little thyroid hormone to be produced by the body. Symptoms of hypothyroidism can include tiredness, paleness, dry skin, and in children, delayed growth and mental and sexual development.

hypoxia (hip-AK-see-ah) occurs when insufficient oxygen reaches the tissues of the body.

ibuprofen (eye-bew-PRO-fin) a nonsteroidal anti-inflammatory drug (NISAD) used to reduce fever and relieve pain or inflammation.

identical twins twins produced when a single egg from the mother is fertilized and divides to form two separate embryos of the same sex with nearly identical DNA.

immune (ih-MYOON) resistant to or not susceptible to a disease.

immune globulin (ih-MYOON GLAH-byoo-lin) the protein material that contains antibodies. Also called gamma globulin.

immune system (im-YOON SIS-tem) the system of the body composed of specialized cells and the substances they produce that helps protect the body against disease-causing germs.

immunity (ih-MYOON-uh-tee) the condition of being protected against an infectious disease. Immunity often develops after a germ has entered the body. One type of immunity occurs when the body makes special protein molecules called antibodies to fight the disease-causing germ. The next time that germ enters the body, the antibodies quickly attack it, usually preventing the germ from causing disease.

immunoglobulins (im-mune-o-GLOB-u-linz) types of antibodies.

immunology (ih-myoo-NOL-uh-jee) the science of the system of the body composed of specialized cells and the substances they produce that help protect the body against disease-causing germs.

immunosuppressants (im-yoo-no-su-PRES-ants) substances that weaken the body's immune system.

impetigo (im-pih-TEE-go) a bacterial skin infection that usually occurs around the nose and mouth and causes itching and fluid-filled blisters that often burst and form yellowish crusts.

impotence (IM-po-tens) the failure of a man to achieve or to maintain an erection.

impulsive acting quickly before thinking about the effect of a certain action or behavior.

in vitro in the laboratory or other artificial environment rather than in the living body.

inborn present from birth, or inherited.

incidence rate of occurrence.

incontinence (in-KON-ti-nens) loss of control of urination or bowel movement.

incontinent unable to control urination or bowel movements.

incubation (ing-kyoo-BAY-shun) the period of time between infection by a germ and when symptoms first appear. Depending on the germ, this period can be from hours to months.

infectious able to spread to others.

infertility (in-fer-TIH-lih-tee) the inability of females to become pregnant or of males to cause pregnancy.

infestations illnesses caused by multi-celled parasitic organisms, such as tapeworms, roundworms, or protozoa living on or in the body tissues of a human or other host.

inflammation (in-fla-MAY-shun) the body's reaction to irritation, infection, or injury that often involves swelling, pain, redness, and warmth.

influenza (in-floo-EN-zuh) a contagious viral infection that attacks the respiratory tract, including the nose, throat, and lungs. Also known as the flu.

influenza A (in-floo-EN-zuh A) one member of a family of viruses that attack the respiratory tract.

inhalants (in-HAY-lunts) substances that a person can sniff, or inhale, to get high.

inhaler (in-HAY-ler) a hand-held device that produces a mist that is breathed in through the mouth.

insecticides chemicals used to kill insects and prevent infestation.

insomnia abnormal inability to get adequate sleep.

insulin a hormone, or chemical produced in the body, that is crucial in controlling the level of glucose (sugar) in the blood and in helping the body use glucose to produce energy. When the body cannot produce or use insulin properly, a person must take insulin or other medications.

intelligence quotient test a test designed to estimate a person's intellectual potential. Also known as an IQ test.

intestines the muscular tubes that food passes through during digestion after it exits the stomach.

intolerance lacking an ability to endure exposure to some environmental feature, such as sunlight, or an exceptional sensitivity, for example to milk, so that the food cannot be properly metabolized, as in glucose intolerance.

intravenous (in-tra-VEE-nus) or IV, means within or through a vein. For example, medications, fluid, or other substances can be given through a needle or soft tube inserted through the skin's surface directly into a vein.

intubation (in-too-BAY-shun) the insertion of a tube into the windpipe to allow air and gases to flow into and out of the lungs in a person who needs help breathing.

ions positively or negatively charged elements or compounds, such as hydrogen, sodium, potassium, and phosphate, which are necessary for cellular metabolism.

ischemic stroke events that occur when a blood vessel bringing oxygen and nutrients to the brain becomes clogged by a blood clot or other particle. As a result, nerve cells in the affected area of the brain cannot function properly.

jaundice (JON-dis) a yellowing of the skin, and sometimes the whites of the eyes, caused by a buildup in the body of bilirubin, a chemical produced in and released by the liver. An increase in bilirubin may indicate disease of the liver or certain blood disorders.

joint the structure where two or more bones come together, allowing flexibility and motion of the skeleton.

juvenile rheumatoid arthritis a joint disease in children with symptoms of high fever, rash, swollen lymph glands, enlarged spleen and liver, and inflammation around the heart and of the lungs. Arthritis in the joints appears later. This disease is also known as systemic-onset chronic arthritis or Still's disease.

ketones (KEE-tones) the chemicals produced when the body breaks down fat for energy.

kidney stone a hard structure that forms in the urinary tract. This structure is composed of crystallized chemicals that have separated from the urine. It can obstruct the flow of urine and cause tissue damage and pain as the body attempts to pass the stone through the urinary tract and out of the body.

kidneys the pair of organs that filter blood and remove waste products and excess water from the body in the form of urine.

kuru (KUR-ew) a progressive, fatal brain disease characterized by tremors and loss of muscle coordination that is caused by eating contaminated brain tissue from other humans who had the disease.

laparoscope (LAP-a-ro-skope) a fiber-optic instrument inserted into an incision in the abdominal wall to perform a visual examination.

laparoscopy (lap-uh-ROS-kuh-pee) a type of surgery in which a small fiberoptic instrument is inserted through a very small incision to examine the inside of the abdomen or remove small amounts of tissue. Also called minimally invasive surgery.

large intestine the part of the intestine that contains the colon and rectum.

larva (LAR-vuh) the immature form of an insect or worm that hatches from an egg. The plural form is larvae (LAR-vee).

laryngitis (lair-in-JY-tis) an inflammation of the vocal cords that causes hoarseness or a temporary loss of voice.

larynx (LAIR-inks) the voice box (which contains the vocal cords) and is located between the base of the tongue and the top of the windpipe.

laser surgery uses a very narrow and intense beam of light that can destroy body tissue.

latent dormant illnesses that may or may not show the signs and symptoms of active diseases.

latex (LAY-tex) a substance made from a rubber tree and is used in such things as medical equipment (especially gloves), toys, and other household products.

learning disability a disorder in the basic mental processes used for language or math. The disorder occurs in people of normal or above-normal intelligence. It is not the result of an emotional disturbance or of an impairment in sight or hearing.

lesion (LEE-zhun) a general term referring to a sore or a damaged or irregular area of tissue.

leukemia (loo-KEE-me-uh) a form of cancer characterized by the body's uncontrolled production of abnormal white blood cells.

leukocytes (LOO-ko-sites) white blood cells sent by the body's immune system to fight infection.

ligaments (LIG-a-ments) bands of fibrous tissue that connect bones or cartilage, supporting and strengthening the joints. Ligaments in the mouth hold the roots of teeth in the tooth sockets.

listeriosis (lis-teer-e-O-sis) a bacterial infection that can cause a form of meningitis in infants and other symptoms in children and adults.

liver a large organ located beneath the ribs on the right side of the body. The liver performs numerous digestive and chemical functions essential for health.

local anesthesia (an-es-THEE-zha) using medicine to block or numb pain in one part of the body while the patient remains awake. General anesthesia blocks pain over the entire body while the patient sleeps.

low birth weight born weighing less than normal. In humans, it refers to a full-term (pregnancy lasting 37 weeks or longer) baby weighing less than 5 pounds.

LSD short for lysergic acid diethylamide (ly-SER-jik A-sid dy-e-thel-AM-eyed), a hallucinogen, a drug that distorts a person's view of reality and causes hallucinations.

lupus (LOO-pus) a chronic, or long-lasting, disease that causes inflammation of connective tissue, the material that holds together the various structures of the body.

Lyme disease (LIME) a bacterial infection that is spread to humans by the bite of an infected tick. It begins with a distinctive rash and/or flulike symptoms and, in some cases, can progress to a more serious disease with complications affecting other body organs.

lymph node (LIMF) a small, bean-shaped mass of tissue containing immune system cells that fight harmful microorganisms. The lymph node may swell during infections.

lymphadenitis (lim-fah-den-EYE-tis) inflammation of the lymph nodes and channels of the lymphatic system.

lymphangitis (lim-fan-JIE-tis) inflammation of the lymphatic system, the system that carries lymph through the body. Lymph is a clear fluid that contains white blood cells.

lymphatic system (lim-FAH-tik) the system that contains lymph nodes and a network of channels that carry fluid and cells of the immune system through the body.

lymphatic tissue the tissue where white blood cells fight invading germs.

lymphocytes (LIM-fo-sites) white blood cells, which play a part in the body's immune system, particularly the production of antibodies and other substances to fight infection.

lymphoma (lim-FO-muh) a cancerous tumor of the lymphocytes, cells that normally help the body fight infection.

macrocephaly (ma-kro-SEH-fah-lee) having an abnormally large head.

magnetic resonance imaging (or MRI) uses magnetic waves, instead of x-rays, to scan the body and produce detailed pictures of the body's structures.

malaria (mah-LAIR-e-uh) a disease spread to humans by the bite of an infected mosquito.

malformation (mal-for-MAY-shun) an abnormal formation of a body part.

malignant (ma-LIG-nant) a condition that is severe and progressively worsening.

malingering (ma-LING-er-ing) intentionally pretending to be sick or injured to avoid work or responsibility.

mammals warm-blooded animals with backbones, who usually have fur or hair. Female mammals secrete milk from mammary glands to feed their young. Humans are mammals.

mammography (mam-MOG-ra-fee) an x-ray examination of the breasts. A mammogram is used in the diagnosis of breast cancer. It may show changes that indicate a possibility of cancer, and medical professionals will then run other tests to check for other signs of the disease.

mapping locates the positions of all the genes on a chromosome.

marijuana (mar-a-WA-na) a mixture of dried, shredded flowers and leaves from the hemp plant that a person can smoke or eat to get high.

marrow (MAR-o) the soft tissue that fills the cavities of the bones.

mastectomy (mas-TEK-to-mee) the surgical removal of the breast.

mastoiditis (mas-toy-DYE-tis) an infection of the mastoid bone, located behind the ear.

measles (ME-zuls) a viral respiratory infection that is best known for the rash of large, flat, red blotches that appear on the arms, face, neck, and body.

meiosis (my-OH-sis) the process of reduction division in which the number of chromosomes per cell is cut in half.

membrane (MEM-brain) a thin layer of tissue that covers a surface, lines a cavity, or divides a space or organ.

meninges (meh-NIN-jeez) the membranes that enclose and protect the brain and the spinal cord.

meningitis (meh-nin-JY-tis) an inflammation of the mcninges, the membranes that surround the brain and the spinal cord. Meningitis is most often caused by infection with a virus or a bacterium.

menopause (MEN-o-pawz) the end of menstruation.

mesothelium (me-zo-THEE-le-um) epithelium derived from embryonic mesoderm that lines the body cavities.

menstrual (MEN-stroo-al) refers to menstruation (men-stroo-AY-shun).

menstrual cycle (MEN-stroo-al SYkul) culminates in menstruation (men-stroo-AY-shun), the discharging through the vagina of blood, secretions, and tissue debris from the uterus that recurs at approximately monthly intervals in females of reproductive age.

menstrual period (MEN-stroo-al PE-re-od) the discharging through the vagina (va-JY-na) of blood, secretions, and tissue debris from the uterus (YOO-ter-us) that recurs at approximately monthly intervals in females of breeding age.

menstruation (men-stroo-AY-shun) is the discharge of the blood-enriched lining of the uterus. Menstruation normally occurs in females who are physically mature enough to bear children. Most girls have their first period between the age of 9 and 16. Menstruation ceases during pregnancy and with the onset of menopause. Because it usually occurs at about four-week intervals, it is often called the monthly period.

mental health counseling involves talking about feelings with a trained professional. The counselor can help the person change thoughts, actions, or relationships that play a part in the illness. Also known as psychotherapy.

mental retardation a condition in which people have below average intelligence that limits their ability to function normally. Also known as intellectual disability.

metabolic (meh-tuh-BALL-ik) the process in the body (metabolism) that converts food into energy and waste products.

metabolism (meh-TAB-o-liz-um) the process in the body that converts foods into the energy necessary for body functions.

metastases (me-TAS-ta-seez) tumors formed when cancer cells from a tumor spread to other parts of the body.

microbes (MY-krobes) microscopic living organisms, such as bacteria, viruses and fungi.

microcephaly (my-kro-SEH-fah-lee) the condition of having an abnormally small head, which typically results from having an underdeveloped or malformed brain.

microorganism a tiny organism that can be seen only by using a microscope. Types of microorganisms include fungi, bacteria, and viruses.

miscarriage (MIS-kare-ij) the end of a pregnancy through the death of the embryo or fetus before birth.

mittelschmerz (MITT-el-shmairts) cramping pain that some women experience at the mid-point in their menstrual cycle when one of their ovaries releases an egg.

mononucleosis (mah-no-nu-klee-O-sis) an infectious illness caused by a virus with symptoms that typically include fever, sore throat, swollen glands, and tiredness.

monozygotic (mah-no-zye-GOT-ik) derived from a single fertilized egg.

mood disorder a mental disorder that involves a disturbance in the person's internal emotional state. Depressive disorders, bipolar disorders, and mood disorders are associated with the use of drugs or medical illnesses.

morbidly obese weighing two or more times a person's ideal body weight.

morphine (MOR-feen) a narcotic, an addictive painkiller that produces a high.

motor skills muscular movements or actions.

MRI (short for magnetic resonance imaging) produces computerized images of internal body tissues based on the magnetic properties of atoms within the body.

mucosa (mu-KOH-sa) the moist tissue that lines some organs and body cavities. It makes mucus, a thick, slippery fluid.

mucous membranes the thin layers of tissue found inside the nose, ears, cervix (SER-viks) and uterus, stomach, colon and rectum, on the vocal cords, and in other parts of the body.

mucus (MYOO-kus) a thick, slippery substance that lines the insides of many body parts.

multiple personality disorder (MUL-ti-pul per-so-NAL-i-tee dis-OR-der) a mental disorder in which a person displays two or more distinct identities that take control of behavior in turn. Also known as dissociative identity disorder.

multiple sclerosis (skluh-RO-sis) (or MS) an inflammatory disease of the nervous system that disrupts communication between the brain and other parts of the body. MS can result in paralysis, loss of vision, and other symptoms.

mumps a contagious viral infection that causes inflammation and swelling in the glands of the mouth that produce saliva.

Munchausen syndrome (MOON-chow-zen SIN-drome) a mental disorder in which a person pretends to have symptoms or causes symptoms of a disease in order to be hospitalized or receive tests, medication, or surgery.

muscular dystrophy (DIS-tro-fee) a group of inherited disorders that causes muscle weakening that worsens over time.

mutation (myoo-TAY-shun) is a change in an organism's gene or genes.

mycobacteria (my-ko-bak-TEER-e-uh) a family of bacteria called fungus bacteria because they are found in wet environments.

myocarditis (my-oh-kar-DYE-tis) an inflammation of the muscular walls of the heart.

myositis (my-oh-SY-tis) an inflammation of the muscles.

nasal (NA-zal) of or relating to the nose.

nasopharyngeal (nay-zo-fair-in-JEE-ul) the nose and pharynx (FAIR-inks), or throat.

nausea (NAW-zha) a feeling of being sick to one's stomach or needing to vomit.

neonatal (ne-o-NAY-tal) pertaining to the first 4 weeks after birth.

nervous system a network of specialized tissue made of nerve cells, or neurons, that processes messages to and from different parts of the human body.

neuritis (nuh-RYE-tis) an inflammation of the nerves that disrupts their function.

neurocutaneous (nur-o-kyoo-TAY-nee-us) affecting the skin and nerves.

neurologic exam a battery of systematic tests to determine how well various parts of the nervous system are functioning.

neurological (nur-a-LAH-je-kal) referring to the nervous system, which includes the brain, spinal cord, and the nerves that control the senses, movement, and organ functions throughout the body.

neurologist (new-RHAL-eh-jist) a physician who specializes in diagnosing and treating diseases of the nervous system.

neurons nerve cells. Most neurons have extensions called axons and dendrites through which they send and receive signals from other neurons.

neuroscientists scientists who study the nerves and nervous system, especially their relationship to learning and behavior.

neurotransmitter (NUR-o-tranz-mit-er) a chemical substance that transmits nerve impulses, or messages, throughout the brain and nervous system and is involved in the control of thought, movement, and other body functions.

night terrors occur during deep (stage 4) sleep, usually within an hour after a person goes to bed. People experiencing night terrors may sit up in bed, scream, cry, sweat, and appear to be extremely frightened, but they are still asleep and are unaware of their environment. Night terrors most commonly affect young children, although anyone can experience them.

nipah virus a virus that infects pigs and humans, and in people it can cause a sometimes fatal form of viral encephalitis. The transmission is not understood, but it may be transmitted from pigs to humans by infected mosquitoes.

nitrates (NYE-trayts) chemical substances that can be produced by the breakdown of proteins by certain bacteria.

norepinephrine (NOR-e-pi-ne-frin) a body chemical that can increase the arousal response, heart rate, and blood pressure.

nucleic acids the cell structures that transfer genetic information DNA (deoxyribonucleic acid) transfers information to RNA (ribonucleic acid), which leads to the production of body proteins.

nucleus the part of the cell that contains its genetic information.

nutrients the components of food (protein, carbohydrate, fat, vitamins, and minerals) needed for growth and maintenance of the body.

obesity (o-BEE-si-tee) an excess of body fat. People are considered obese if they weigh more than 30 percent above what is healthy for their height.

obsessions (ob-SESH-unz) repeated disturbing thoughts or urges that a person cannot ignore and that will not go away.

obsessive-compulsive disorder a condition that causes people to become trapped in a pattern of repeated, unwanted thoughts, called obsessions (ob-SESH-unz), and a pattern of repetitive behaviors, called compulsions (kom-PUL-shunz).

oncotic pressure the pressure difference of blood plasma and tissue fluid.

ophthalmologic (off-thal-MOLL-o-jik) related to the function, structure, and diseases of the eye.

ophthalmologist (off-thal-MOLL-o-jist) a medical doctor who specializes in treating diseases of the eye.

opiates (O-pea-atz) painkilling chemicals that can cause sleepiness and loss of sensation.

opportunistic infections infections caused by infectious agents that usually do not produce disease in people with healthy immune systems but can cause widespread and severe illness in patients with weak or faulty immune systems.

oppositional (op-po-ZI-shun-al) an attitude of going against something or refusing in a combative way.

oppositional defiant disorder (op-uh-ZIH-shun-ul de-FY-unt dis-OR-der) a disruptive behavior disorder that can be diagnosed in children as young as preschoolers who demonstrate hostile or aggressive behavior and who refuse to follow rules.

optic nerve the nerve that sends messages, or conducts impulses, from the eyes to the brain, making it possible to see. The optic nerve is also referred to as the second cranial nerve.

optometrist a licensed specialist who practices optometry, a healthcare profession that specializes in eye examinations and prescribing corrective lenses.

oral by mouth or referring to the mouth.

orthotic a support or brace for weak or ineffective joints or muscles.

osteoarthritis (os-tee-o-ar-THRY-tis) a common disease that involves inflammation and pain in the joints (places where bones meet), especially those in the knees, hips, and lower back of older people.

osteomyelitis (ah-stee-o-my-uh-LYE-tis) a bone infection that is usually caused by bacteria. It can involve any bone in the body, but it most commonly affects the long bones in the arms and legs.

osteoporosis (os-te-o-por-O-sis) the loss of material from the bone. This makes the bones weak and brittle.

outpatient 1) a medical procedure that is conducted in a doctor's office or hospital for treatment but does not require an overnight stay in a hospital bed; 2) the patient who is treated in a doctor's office or hospital but does not stay overnight in a hospital bed.

ovaries (O-vuh-reez) the sexual glands from which ova, or eggs, are released in women.

ovulation (ov-yoo-LAY-shun) the release of a mature egg from the ovary.

oxygen (OK-si-jen) an odorless, colorless gas essential for the human body. It is taken in through the lungs and delivered to the body by the bloodstream.

pacemaker a device whose function is to send electrical signals that control the heartbeat. The heart's natural pacemaker is the sinoatrial node, a special group of cells. Sometimes it is necessary to implant a battery-powered pacemaker that sends small electrical charges through an electrode placed next to the wall of the heart.

palate (PAL-it) the structure at the roof of the mouth. Damage or poor functioning of the palate can affect swallowing, the voice, and breathing.

palliative (PAL-ee-at-iv) to ease or relieve without curing.

palpitation the sensation of a rapid or irregular heartbeat.

pancreas (PAN-kree-us) the gland located behind the stomach that produces enzymes and hormones necessary for digestion and metabolism.

pandemic (pan-DEHM-ik) a worldwide outbreak of disease, especially infectious disease, in which the number of cases suddenly becomes far greater than usual.

panic attack a period of intense fear or discomfort with a feeling of doom and a desire to escape. The person may shake, sweat, be short of breath, and experience chest pain

Pap smear a common diagnostic test used to look for cancerous cells in the tissue of the cervix.

parainfluenza (pair-uh-in-floo-EN-zuh) a family of viruses that cause respiratory infections.

paralysis (pah-RAHL-uh-sis) the loss or impairment of the ability to move some part of the body.

paranoia (pair-a-NOY-a) either an unreasonable fear of harm by others (delusions of persecution) or an unrealistic sense of self-importance (delusions of grandeur).

paranoid (PARE-a-noyd) behavior that is based on delusions of persecution or grandeur. People with persecution delusions falsely believe that other people are out to get them. People with delusions of grandeur falsely believe that they have great importance, power, wealth, intelligence, or ability.

parasite (PAIR-uh-site) an organism such as protozoa (one-celled animals), worms, or insects that must live on or inside a human or other organism to survive. An animal or plant harboring a parasite is called its host. Parasites live at the expense of the host and may cause illness. The adjectival form is parasitic.

Parkinson's disease a disorder of the nervous system that causes shaking, rigid muscles, slow movements, and poor balance.

parkinsonism a neurological condition with various causes with symptoms similar to those seen in Parkinson's disease.

parotid gland (puh-RAH-tid) the salivary gland located in the jaw just beneath and in front of each ear.

pasteurize (PAS-cha-rise) to sterilize a substance, generally a liquid such as milk, by bringing it to high temperature and keeping it at that temperature long enough to destroy unhealthy organisms in it without changing its other characteristics.

pathogens (PAH-tho-jens) microorganisms that can cause disease in another living organism.

PCP short for phencyclidine (fen-SY-kle-deen), a hallucinogen, a drug that distorts a person's view of reality.

pelvic exam an internal examination of a woman's reproductive organs.

pelvic inflammatory disease an infection of a woman's internal reproductive organs, including the fallopian tubes, uterus, cervix, and ovaries.

penile (PEE-nile) refers to the penis, the external male sexual organ.

perianal (pair-e-A-nul) the area of skin surrounding the anus.

pericarditis (per-ih-kar-DYE-tis) an inflammation of the sac surrounding the heart.

perinatal (per-ee-NAY-tal) existing or occurring around the time of birth, with reference to the fetus.

period the monthly flow, or discharge, of the blood-enriched lining of the uterus that normally occurs in women who are physically mature enough to bear children. Most girls have their first period between the ages of 9 and 16. Because it usually occurs at four-week intervals, it is often called the monthly period. Also called menstruation (men-stroo-AY-shun).

periodontal (pare-e-o-DON-tul) located around a tooth.

peripheral nerves (puh-RIH-fer-ul) a network of nerve fibers throughout the body that send and receive messages to and from the central nervous system (the brain and spinal cord).

perishable able to spoil or decay, as in perishable foods.

peritoneum the membrane that lines the abdominal cavity.

peritonitis (per-i-to-NI-tis) an inflammation of the peritoneum.

personality disorders a group of mental disorders characterized by long-term patterns of behavior that differ from those expected by society. People with personality disorders have patterns of emotional response, impulse control, and perception that differ from those of most people.

pertussis (per-TUH-sis) a bacterial infection of the respiratory tract that causes severe coughing. Also called whooping cough.

pet dander microscopic parts of the pet's skin that flake off and get into the air people breathe.

pharyngitis (far-in-JI-tis) inflammation of the pharynx, part of the throat.

phenylketonuria (fen-ul-ke-ton-U-ree-a) (or PKU) a genetic disorder of body chemistry that, if left untreated, causes mental retardation.

phlebitis (fle-BY-tis) inflammation of a vein.

phobia an intense, persistent, unreasonable fear of (and avoidance of) a particular thing or situation.

phonemes (FO-neemz) the smallest units of spoken language, such as the puh' sound at the start of the word pat.

photosensitive responsive to light.

physical and occupational therapists professionals who are trained to treat injured people by means of activities designed to help them recover or relearn specific functions or movements and restore their abilities to perform the tasks of daily living.

physiologic (fiz-ee-o-LOJ-ik) an organism's healthy and normal functioning.

pigment (PIG-ment) a substance that imparts color to another substance.

pituitary (pih-TOO-ih-tare-e) a small oval-shaped gland at the base of the skull that produces several hormones—substances that affect various body functions, including growth.

placenta (pluh-SEN-ta) an organ that provides nutrients and oxygen to a developing baby; it is located within the womb during pregnancy.

plague (PLAYG) a serious bacterial infection that is spread to humans by infected rodents and their fleas.

plaque (PLAK) a raised patch or swelling on a body surface. Arterial plaque occurs on the inner surface of an artery and is produced by fatty deposits.

plastic surgery the surgical repair, restoration, or improvement in the shape and appearance of body parts.

platelets (PLATE-lets) tiny disk-shaped particles within the blood that play an important role in clotting.

pneumonia (nu-MO-nyah) inflammation of the lungs.

podiatrist (po-DIE-uh-trist) a specialist in the medical care of the foot, ankle, and lower leg.

poliomyelitis (po-lee-o-my-uh-LYE-tis) a condition caused by the polio virus that involves damage of nerve cells. It may lead to weakness and deterioration of the muscles and sometimes paralysis.

polyps (PAH-lips) bumps or growths usually on the lining or surface of a body part (such as the nose or intestine). Their size can range from tiny to large enough to cause pain or obstruction. They may be harmless, but they also may be cancerous.

pornography (por-NAH-gra-fee) any material, such as magazines or videos, that shows sexual behavior and is meant to cause sexual excitement.

1871

positron emission tomography (POZ-i-tron i-MISH-en toe-MAH-gruh-fee) uses a radiotracer that accumulates in an area of the body and emits gamma rays that are detected as diagnostic images. Also called PET imaging or PET scanning.

post-traumatic stress disorder (post-traw-MAT-ik STRES dis-OR-der) a mental disorder that interferes with everyday living and occurs in people who survive a terrifying event, such as school violence, military combat, or a natural disaster.

premalignant a disease or condition considered highly associated with future cancer.

premature birth (pre-ma-CHUR) born too early. In humans, it means being born after a pregnancy term lasting less than 37 weeks.

premature labor labor (the birth process) that begins too early, before the fetus has developed fully in the womb.

prenatal (pre-NAY-tal) existing or occurring before birth, with reference to the fetus.

prevalence (of a disease or condition) how common it is in a population of people.

progesterone (pro-JES-teh-ron) a female steroid sex hormone that prepares for and supports pregnancy.

pronation the rotation of the foot inward and downward so that, in walking, the foot comes down on its inner edge.

prophylactic (pro-fih-LAK-tik) something that is used to prevent an illness or other condition, such as an infection or pregnancy.

prophylaxis (pro-fih-LAK-sis) taking specific measures, such as using medication or a device (such as a condom), to help prevent infection, illness, or pregnancy.

prostate (PRAH-state) a male reproductive gland located near where the bladder joins the urethra. The prostate produces the fluid part of semen.

prosthesis (pros-THEE-sis) an artificial substitute for a missing body part. It can be used for appearance only or to replace the function of the missing part (as with a prosthetic leg).

protooncogene (pro-toe-AN-keh-gene) a gene that is used to divide normal cells for specialized uses.

protozoa (pro-tuh-ZOH-uh) single-celled microorganisms (tiny organisms), some of which are capable of causing disease in humans.

psychiatrist (sy-KY-uh-trist) a medical doctor who has completed specialized training in the diagnosis and treatment of mental illness. Psychiatrists can diagnose mental illnesses, provide mental health counseling, and prescribe medications.

psychoactive (sy-ko-AK-tiv) affecting a person's mood, behavior, perceptions, or consciousness.

psychoanalysis (sy-ko-a-NAL-i-sis) a method of treating a person with psychological problems, based on the theories of Sigmund Freud. It involves sessions in which a therapist encourages a person to talk freely about personal experiences, and the psychoanalyst interprets the patient's ideas and dreams.

psychogenic (SIGH-ko-JEN-ik) originating in the mind as a result of emotional conflict.

psychological (SI-ko-LOJ-i-kal) mental processes, including thoughts, feelings, and emotions.

psychologist (sy-KOL-o-jist) a mental health professional who treats mental and behavioral disorders by support and insight to encourage healthy behavior patterns and personality growth. Psychologists also study the brain, behavior, emotions, and learning.

psychosis (sy-KO-sis) a mental disorder in which the sense of reality is so impaired that a patient can not function normally. People with psychotic disorders may experience delusions (exaggerated beliefs that are contrary to fact), hallucinations (something that a person perceives as real but that is not actually caused by an outside event), incoherent speech, and agitated behavior, but they usually are not aware of their altered mental state.

psychotherapist (sy-ko-THER-a-pist) any mental health professional who works with people to help them change thoughts, actions, or relationships that play a part in their emotional or behavioral problems.

psychotherapy (sy-ko-THER-a-pea) the treatment of mental and behavioral disorders by support and insight to encourage healthy behavior patterns and personality growth.

psychotic disorders (sy-KOT-ik) mental disorders, such as schizophrenia, in which the sense of reality is so impaired that a person can not function normally. People with psychotic disorders may experience delusions, hallucinations, incoherent speech, and agitated behavior, but they usually are not aware of their altered mental state.

puberty (PU-ber-tee) the period during which sexual maturity is attained.

pulmonary refers to the lungs.

pulmonary embolism a blockage of the pulmonary artery or one of its branches that is frequently caused by thrombosis, or formation of a blood clot, in the lower extremities.

pulp the sensitive area deep inside the central part of the tooth, where the nerves and blood vessels are located.

pus a thick, creamy fluid, usually yellow or ivory in color, that forms at the site of an infection. Pus contains infection-fighting white cells and other substances.

quarantine the enforced isolation (for a fixed period) of apparently well persons or animals who may have been exposed to infectious disease.

rabies (RAY-beez) a viral infection of the central nervous system that usually is transmitted to humans by the bite of an infected animal.

radiation energy that is transmitted in the form of rays, waves, or particles. Only high-energy radiation, such as that found in x-rays and the sun's ultraviolet rays, has been proven to cause human cancer.

radiation therapy a treatment that uses high-energy radiation from x-rays and other sources to kill cancer cells and shrink cancerous growths.

radiculitis (ruh-dih-kyoo-LYE-tis) numbness, tingling, or burning sensation along the course of a nerve due to irritation or inflammation of the nerve.

radionuclide scans (ray-dee-o-NU-klide) tests that begin by giving a patient a small amount of a radioactive substance. The radioactive substance shows up on a scan, producing a view of the structure or function of the part of the body being studied.

radiotracer a substance that contains radioactive material.

rape when a person forces another person to have sexual intercourse, or engage in other unwanted sexual activities.

Raynaud's disease (ray-NOZE) a condition in which discoloration of the skin typically on the fingers and/or toes occurs when individuals experience changes in temperature or emotional events. An abnormal spasm of blood vessels causes the reduced supply of blood to the affected areas of the body.

reaction speed the time it takes to respond to a stimulus.

reaction time the time it takes a muscle or some other living tissue to respond to a stimulus

receptors   cell structures that form a chemical bond with specific substances, such as neurotransmitters. This leads to a specific effect.

recessive   a gene that is not dominant, one that requires a second identical recessive gene in order for the trait to show in the individual. When a recessive gene is paired with a dominant one, the individual is said to be a carrier of the trait.

rectum   the final portion of the large intestine, connecting the colon to the outside opening of the anus.

rehabilitative therapy   helps people return to more normal physical, mental, or emotional function following an illness or injury. Rehabilitative therapy also helps people find ways to better cope with conditions that interfere with their lives.

relaxation techniques   exercises such as meditation that help people reduce the physical symptoms of stress.

remission   an easing of a disease or its symptoms for a prolonged period.

replicate   (REP-li-kate) to create an identical copy.

respirator   a machine that helps people breathe when they are unable to breathe adequately on their own.

respiratory   (RES-pi-ra-tor-ee) the breathing passages and lungs.

respiratory failure   a condition in which breathing and oxygen delivery to the body are dangerously altered. This may result from infection, nerve or muscle damage, poisoning, or other causes.

respiratory syncytial virus   (RES-puh-ruh-tor-e sin-SIH-she-ul) (or RSV) a virus that infects the respiratory tract and typically causes minor symptoms in adults but can lead to more serious respiratory illnesses in children.

respiratory system   includes the nose, mouth, throat, and lungs. It is the pathway through which air and gases are transported down into the lungs and back out of the body. Also called the respiratory tract.

retina   (RET-i-na) the tissue that forms the inner surface of the back of the eyeballs; it receives the light that enters the eye and transmits it through the optic nerves to the brain to produce visual images.

retinitis   (reh-tin-EYE-tis) an inflammation of the retina, the nerve-rich membrane at the back of the eye on which visual images form.

retrovirus   viruses whose genetic information is found in ribonucleic acid (RNA), a nucleic acid that is found in all living cells.

Reye's syndrome   (RYES SIN-drome) a rare condition that involves inflammation of the liver and brain, and sometimes appears after illnesses such as chicken pox or influenza. It has also been associated with taking aspirin during certain viral infections.

rheumatic fever   (roo-MAH-tik) a condition associated with fever, joint pain, and inflammation affecting many parts of the body, including the heart. It occurs following infection with certain types of strep bacteria.

rheumatoid arthritis   (ROO-mah-toyd ar-THRY-tis) a chronic disease characterized by painful swelling, stiffness, and deformity of the joints.

rheumatologist   (roo-ma-TOL-o-jist) a doctor who specializes in disorders involving the connective tissue structures of the body.

rickets   (RICK-kets) a condition of bones that causes them to soften and bend creating deformity. In the early twentieth century, rickets was caused by lack of sunlight, and the lack of vitamin D, calcium, and phosphorus. As enriched foods and improved diets became more widespread, rickets practically disappeared in industrialized countries.

ringworm   a fungal infection of the skin or scalp that appears as a round, red rash.

risk factor   any factor that increases the chance of developing a disease.

RNA   or ribonucleic acid (ry-bo-nyoo-KLAY-ik AH-sid), the chemical substance through which DNA sends genetic information to build new cells.

root canal   a procedure in which a dentist cleans out the pulp of an infected tooth, removes the nerve, and then fills the cavity with a protective substance.

roundworm   one of several types of cylinder-shaped worms that live in people. Roundworms are also known as nematodes (NEE-muh-todes).

rubella   (roo-BEH-luh) a viral infection that usually causes a rash and mild fever.

salivary glands   (SAL-i-var-ee) the three pairs of glands that produce the liquid called saliva, which aids in the digestion of food.

sarcoma   (sar-COHM-ah) one of a group of tumors that occur in connective tissue and are mostly malignant.

scarlet fever   an infection that causes a sore throat and a rash.

schizophrenia   (skit-so-FREE-nee-ah) a serious mental disorder that causes people to experience hallucinations, delusions, and other confusing thoughts and behaviors, which distort their view of reality.

sciatica   (sy-AT-i-ka) pain along the course of either of the sciatic (sy-AT-ik) nerves, which run through the pelvis and down the backs of the thighs.

scrapie   (SKRAY-pee) a fatal brain disorder of sheep that is characterized by itching of the skin and difficulty walking.

scrotum   (SKRO-tum) the pouch on a male body that contains the testicles.

secondhand smoke   smoke that is inhaled passively or involuntarily by someone who is not smoking. It is a mixture of gases and particles from a burning cigarette, cigar, or pipe and the smoke exhaled by smokers. Also called environmental tobacco smoke or passive smoke.

sedatives   (SAID-uh-tivs) drugs that produce a calming effect or sleepiness.

seizures   (SEE-zhurs) sudden bursts of disorganized electrical activity that interrupt the normal functioning of the brain, often leading to uncontrolled movements in the body and sometimes a temporary change in consciousness. Also called convulsions.

self-esteem   the value that people put on the mental image that they have of themselves.

semen   (SEE-men) the sperm-containing whitish fluid produced by the male reproductive tract.

separation anxiety   the normal fear that babies and young children feel when they are separated from their parents or approached by strangers.

sepsis   a potentially serious spreading of infection, usually bacterial, through the bloodstream and body.

septic shock   shock due to overwhelming infection and is characterized by decreased blood pressure, internal bleeding, heart failure, and, in some cases, death.

septicemia   (sep-ti-SE-me-a) a bacterial infection in the blood that spreads throughout the body, with potentially fatal results.

serotonin   (ser-o-TO-nin) a neurotransmitter, a substance that helps transmit information from one nerve cell to another in the brain. It is associated with feelings of well-being.

between two bones. This fluid lubricates and nourishes the joint.

synovitis (sin-o-VY-tis) inflammation of the membrane surrounding a joint.

synthetic produced artificially or chemically rather than grown naturally.

syphilis (SIH-fih-lis) a sexually transmitted disease that, if untreated, can lead to serious life-long problems throughout the body, including blindness and paralysis.

systemic (sis-TEM-ik) a problem affecting the whole system or whole body, as opposed to a localized problem that affects only one place on the body.

systemic lupus erythematosus (sis-TEM-ik LOO-pus er-i-them-a-TO-sus) (sometimes just called lupus) a chronic inflammatory disease that can affect the skin, joints, kidneys, nervous system, membranes lining body cavities, and other organs.

temperament (TEM-per-uh-ment) the genetically or biologically based part of an individual's personality.

temporal lobe epilepsy a form of epilepsy that affects the part of the brain that is located underneath the sides of the head, near the ears. Epilepsy is a condition of the nervous system characterized by recurrent seizures that temporarily affect a person's awareness, movements, or sensations. Also called complex partial epilepsy.

temporal lobes (TEM-por-al) the side portions of the cortex. They contain the sensory center for hearing and are centers for language function.

tendon (TEN-don) a fibrous cord of connective tissue that attaches a muscle to a bone or other structure.

tertiary (TER-she-air-ee) third stage.

testicles (TES-tih-kulz) the paired male reproductive glands that produce sperm.

tetanus (TET-nus) a serious bacterial infection that affects the body's central nervous system.

thalamus (THAL-uh-mus) a pair of large egg-shaped areas located in the middle of the brain just under the cerebral cortex. The plural form is thalami.

thrombosis the formation or development of a blood clot or thrombus.

thyroid gland (THY-roid GLAND) is located in the lower part of the front of the neck. The thyroid produces hormones that regulate the body's metabolism (me-TAB-o-LIZ-um), the processes the body uses to produce energy, to grow, and to maintain body tissues.

tic a sudden, brain-activated involuntary movement (such as eye blinking or shoulder shrugging) or sound, (words or other sounds, such as sniffing, grunting, throat clearing, or even barking) that is repeated over and over in the same way.

tick a small blood-sucking creature that may transmit disease-causing germs from animals to humans through its bite.

tolerance (TALL-uh-runce) a condition in which a person needs more of a drug to feel the original effects of the drug.

tonsils paired clusters of lymphatic tissue in the throat that help protect the body from bacteria and viruses that enter through a person's nose or mouth.

tourniquet a device, often a bandage twisted tight around an arm or a leg, used to stop blood flow or hemorrhage.

toxin a substance that causes harm to the body.

toxoplasmosis (tox-o-plaz-MO-sis) a parasitic infection that usually causes no symptoms in healthy people, but it can cause serious problems in unborn babies and people with weak immune systems.

trachea (TRAY-kee-uh) the firm, tubular structure that carries air from the throat to the lungs. Also called the windpipe.

tracheostomy (tray-kee-AHS-tuh-me) a small opening through the neck into the trachea, or windpipe, which has been made to allow air to enter the lungs more directly. The surgical procedure to create a tracheostomy is usually performed when a person's upper airway is narrowed or blocked or when there are other problems causing breathing difficulty.

transfusion (trans-FYOO-zhun) a procedure in which blood or certain parts of blood, such as specific cells, is given to a person who needs it due to illness or blood loss.

transgendered a person who identifies with and expresses a gender identity that differs from the one which corresponds to the person's sex at birth.

transient (TRAN-shent) brief or producing effects for a short period of time.

transient ischemic attack (TRAN-shent iss-KEE-mik) a temporary loss of blood supply to a particular area of the brain. Also called a TIA.

transmissible (trans-MIH-sih-bul) able to be transferred or spread.

transplants (TRANS-plantz) organs or tissues from another body used to replace a poorly functioning organ or tissue.

trauma a wound or injury, whether psychological or physical. Psychological trauma refers to an emotional shock that leads to lasting psychological damage.

traumatic causing mental or emotional stress or physical injury.

trichomoniasis (trih-ko-mo-NYE-uh-sis) a common sexually transmitted disease caused by the parasite Trichomonas vaginalis.

triglycerides (try-GLISS-eh-rides) a type of fatty substances found in the blood.

trimester (tri-MES-ter) any of three periods of approximately 3 months each into which a human pregnancy is divided.

truancy staying out of school without permission.

tubal pregnancy (TOO-bal) a condition in which a fertilized egg implants in the fallopian tube instead of the wall of the uterus.

tuberculosis (too-ber-kyoo-LO-sis) a bacterial infection that primarily attacks the lungs but can spread to other parts of the body.

tularemia (too-lah-REE-me-uh) an infection caused by bacteria that can be spread to humans by wild animals. Also called rabbit fever.

tumor (TOO-mor) an abnormal growth of body tissue that has no known cause or physiologic purpose. A tumor may or may not be cancerous.

tumor marker (TOO-mer MARK-er) a substance found in blood, urine, or body tissues whose level rises when a person has cancer. Tumor markers can be used to detect possible cancer.

Turner syndrome a genetic disorder that can cause several physical abnormalities, including short stature and lack of sexual development.

typhoid fever (TIE-foyd FEE-ver) an infection with the bacterium *Salmonella typhi* that causes fever, headache, confusion, and muscle aches.

ulcer an open sore on the skin or the lining of a hollow body organ, such as the stomach or intestine. It may or may not be painful.

ulcerate to become eroded by infection, inflammation, or irritation.

ulcerative colitis (UL-sir-ah-tiv ko-LIE-tis) a common form of inflammatory bowel disease that causes inflammation with sore spots or

Organizations

The following is an alphabetical compilation of organizations listed in the *Resources* section of the main body entries. Although the list is comprehensive, it is by no means exhaustive and is intended to serve as a starting point for further research. Cengage Learning is not responsible for the accuracy of the addresses or the contents of the web sites.

A

Abramson Cancer Center of the University of Pennsylvania
3400 Spruce Street
Philadelphia, PA, 19104
Web site: http://www.oncolink.upenn.edu

ADD Warehouse
200 NW 17th Avenue, Suite 102
Plantation, FL, 33317
Toll free: 800-233-9273
Web site: http://www.addwarehouse.com
The ADD Warehouse offers a wide selection of books and other products that deal with ADHD.

ADDvance
100l Spring Street, Suite 118
Silver Spring, MD, 20910
Toll free: 888-238-8588
Web site: http://www.addvance.com

Agency for Toxic Substances and Disease Registry
1600 Clifton Road
Atlanta, GA, 30333
Toll free: 800-232-4636
Web site: http://www.atsdr.cdc.gov
A part of the Centers for Disease Control and Prevention. Its web site aims to provide trusted health information to prevent harmful exposures and diseases related to toxic substances.

Agenesis of the Corpus Callosum/ ACC Network
University of Maine,
5749 Merrill Hall, Room 118
Orono, ME, 04469-5749
Telephone: 207-581-3119
Web site: http://www.umaine.edu/edhd/research/accnetwork.htm

AIDS Education Global Information Service
32234 Paseo Adelanto, Suite B
San Juan Capistrano, CA, 92675
Telephone: 949-248-5843
Web site: http://www.aegis.com
An online AIDS bulletin board is run by a nonprofit foundation.

aids.gov
Web site: http://www.aids.gov
Managed by the Department of Health & Human Services, aids.gov provides access to federal HIV/AIDS information through a variety of media channels.

Al-Anon/Alateen
1600 Corporate Landing Parkway
Virginia Beach, VA, 23454-5617
Toll free: 888-4AL-ANON
Web site: http://www.al-anon.alateen.org
An international self-help group for family members and friends of people with alcoholism. Alateen is a group especially for teenagers affected by someone else's drinking.

Alcoholics Anonymous
Grand Central Station,
P.O. Box 459
New York, NY, 10163
Telephone: 212-870-3400
Web site: http://www.aa.org
A worldwide self-help organization for alcoholics.

Allergy and Asthma Network/ Mothers of Asthmatics
2751 Prosperity Avenue, Suite 150
Fairfax, VA, 22031
Toll free: 800-878-4403
Web site: http://www.aanma.org

A national nonprofit network of families whose desire is to overcome, not cope with, allergies and asthma.

Alliance for the Prudent Use of Antibiotics
75 Kneeland Street
Boston, MA, 02111-1901
Telephone: 617-636-0966
Web site: http://www.tufts.edu/med/apua
The Alliance for the Prudent Use of Antibiotics promotes the appropriate use of and access to antimicrobials and the control of antimicrobial resistance on a worldwide basis.

ALS Society of Canada
265 Yorkland Boulevard, Suite 300
Toronto, ON, M2J 1S5, Canada
Toll free: 800-267-4ALS
Web site: http://www.als.ca

Alzheimer's Association
225 N. Michigan Avenue,
17th Floor
Chicago, IL, 60601
Toll free: 800-272-3900
Web site: http://www.alz.org

Alzheimer's Disease Education and Referral Center, National Institute on Aging, National Institutes of Health
P.O. Box 8250
Silver Spring, MD, 20907-8250
Toll free: 800-438-4380
Web site: http://www.alzheimers.org
A service of the federal government providing research updates and referrals.

American Academy of Allergy, Asthma, and Immunology
555 East Wells Street, Suite 1100
Milwaukee, WI, 53202-3823

Organizations

Telephone: 414-272-6071
Web site: http://www.aaaai.org

American Academy of Child and Adolescent Psychiatry
3615 Wisconsin Avenue NW
Washington, DC, 20016-3007
Telephone: 202-966-7300
Web site: http://www.aacap.org

American Academy of Dermatology
PO Box 4014
Schaumburg, IL, 60168-4014
Toll free: 866-503-SKIN
Web site: http://www.aad.org

American Academy of Family Physicians
P.O. Box 11210
Shawnee Mission, KS, 66207-1210
Toll free: 800-274-2237
Web site: http://www.aafp.org
Web site: http://www.familydoctor.org
The national association of family doctors that supports a web site for patients (familydoctor.org) providing health information for the entire family.

American Academy of Neurology
1080 Montreal Avenue
St. Paul, MN, 55116
Telephone: 612-695-1940
Web site: http://www.aan.com

American Academy of Ophthalmology
P.O. Box 7424
San Francisco, CA, 94120
Telephone: 415-561-8500
Web site: http://aao.org

American Academy of Orthopedic Surgeons
6300 North River Road
Rosemont, IL, 60018-4262
Toll free: 800-346-2267
Web site: http://www.aaos.org

American Academy of Otolaryngology, Head and Neck Surgery
1650 Diagonal Road
Alexandria, VA, 22314-2857

Telephone: 703-836-4444
Web site: http://www.entnet.org

American Academy of Pediatrics
141 Northwest Point Boulevard
Elk Grove Village, IL, 60007-1098
Telephone: 847-434-4000
Web site: http://www.aap.org

American Academy of Periodontology
737 N. Michigan Avenue, Suite 800
Chicago, IL, 60611-6660
Telephone: 312-787-5518
Web site: http://www.perio.org

American Academy of Psychiatry and the Law
P.O. Box 30, One Regency Drive
Bloomfield, CT, 06002-0030
Toll free: 800-331-1389
Web site: http://www.aapl.org
The American Academy of Psychiatry and the Law promotes scientific and educational research in how psychiatry is applied to legal issues (forensic psychiatry).

American Association for Clinical Chemistry
1850 K Street NW, Suite 625
Washington, DC, 20006
Toll free: 800-892-1400
Web site: http://www.labtestsonline.org
The American Association for Clinical Chemistry's labtestsonline.org web site explains how specific lab tests are done and what the results mean.

American Association for Pediatric Ophthalmology and Strabismus
P.O. Box 193832
San Francisco, CA, 94119-3832
Telephone: 415-561-8505
Web site: http://www.aapos.org
The American Association for Pediatric Ophthalmology and Strabismus provides information on both pediatric and adult strabismus.

American Association of Clinical Endocrinologists
245 Riverside Avenue, Suite 200
Jacksonville, FL, 32202

Telephone: 904-353-7878
Web site: http://www.aace.com

American Association of Neurological Surgeons
5550 Meadowbrook Drive
Rolling Meadows, IL, 60008
Web site: http://www.neurosurgerytoday.org

American Association of Oral and Maxillofacial Surgeons
9700 W. Bryn Mawr Avenue
Rosemont, IL, 60018-570
Telephone: 847-678-6200
Web site: http://www.aaoms.org
Members of the American Association of Oral and Maxillofacial Surgeons care for patients with problem wisdom teeth, facial pain, and misaligned jaws. They treat accident victims suffering facial injuries, place dental implants, care for patients with oral cancer, tumors and cysts of the jaws, and perform facial cosmetic surgery.

American Association of Poison Control Centers
515 King Street, Suite 510
Alexandria, VA, 22314
Telephone: 703-894-1858
Web site: http://www.aapcc.org
The American Association of Poison Control Centers consists of poison control centers across the United States. Poison centers are open 24 hours a day, seven days a week to help both ordinary citizens and medical professional to care for people who have been poisoned. All of the centers use the same Poison Help Hotline number: 1-800-222-1222.

American Association of Retired Persons
601 E Street NW
Washington, DC, 20049
Toll free: 888-687-2277
Web site: http://www.aarp.org

American Association on Intellectual and Developmental Disabilities
444 North Capitol Street
Northwest, Suite 846

Washington, DC, 20001-1512
Toll free: 800-424-3688
Web site: http://www.aaidd.org

American Autoimmune Related Diseases Association
22100 Gratiot Avenue
Eastpointe, MI, 48021
Telephone: 586-776-3900
Web site: http://www.aarda.org

American Brain Tumor Association
2720 River Road
Des Plaines, IL, 60018
Toll free: 800-886-2282
Web site: http://www.abta.org

American Burn Association
625 N. Michigan Avenue,
Suite 2550
Chicago, IL, 60611
Telephone: 312-642-9260
Web site: http://www.ameriburn.org

American Cancer Society
1599 Clifton Road NE
Atlanta, GA, 30329-4251
Toll free: 800-ACS-2345
Web site: http://www.cancer.org

American Celiac Disease Alliance
2504 Duxbury Place
Alexandria, VA, 22308
Telephone: 703-622-3331
Web site: http://americanceliac.org

A non-profit advocacy organization that strives to represent all celiac patients, along with involved physicians, healthcare providers, researchers, food manufacturers, and service providers.

American Chronic Pain Association
P.O. Box 850
Rocklin, CA, 95677
Toll free: 800-533-3231
Web site: http://www.theacpa.org

American College of Allergy, Asthma, and Immunology
85 West Algonquin Road, Suite 550
Arlington Heights, IL, 60005
Telephone: 847-427-1200
Web site: http://www.acaai.org

American College of Cardiology
2400 N Street NW
Washington, DC, 20037
Toll free: 800-253-4636
Web site: http://www.acc.org

American College of Foot and Ankle Surgeons
8725 West Higgins Road, Suite 555
Chicago, IL, 60631-2724
Toll free: 800-421-2237
Web site: http://www.acfas.org

American College of Gastroenterology
P.O. Box 342260
Bethesda, MD, 20827-2260
Telephone: 301-263-9000
Web site: http://www.acg.gi.org

American College of Obstetricians and Gynecologists
409 12th Street SW
P.O. Box 96920
Washington, DC, 20090-6920
Telephone: 202-638-5577
Web site: http://www.acog.org

American College of Occupational and Environmental Medicine
55 West Seegers Road
Arlington Heights, IL, 60005
Telephone: 708-228-6850
Web site: http://www.acoem.org

American College of Physicians
190 N. Independence Mall West
Philadelphia, PA, 19106
Toll free: 800-523-1546
Web site: http://www.acponline.org

American College of Rheumatology
1800 Century Place, Suite 250
Atlanta, GA, 30345-4300
Telephone: 404-633-3777
Web site: http://www.rheumatology.org

American College of Sports Medicine
P.O. Box 1440
Indianapolis, IN, 46206-1440
Telephone: 317-637-9200
Web site: http://www.acsm.org

American Council for Headache Education
19 Mantua Road
Mt. Royal, NJ, 08061
Telephone: 856-423-0258
Web site: http://www.achenet.org

American Council of the Blind
1155 15th Street NW, Suite 1004
Washington, DC, 20005
Toll free: 800-424-8666
Web site: http://www.acb.org

American Dental Association
211 East Chicago Avenue
Chicago, IL, 60611-2678
Telephone: 312-440-2500
Web site: http://www.ada.org

American Diabetes Association
1701 North Beauregard Street
Alexandria, VA, 22311
Toll free: 800-342-2383
Web site: http://www.diabetes.org

American Dietetic Association
216 West Jackson Boulevard,
Suite 800
Chicago, IL, 60606-6995
Toll free: 800-366-1655
Web site: http://www.eatright.org

American Foundation for the Blind
11 Penn Plaza, Suite 300
New York, NY, 10001
Telephone: 212-502-7600
Web site: http://www.afb.org

American Gastroenterological Association
4930 Del Ray Avenue
Bethesda, MD, 20814
Telephone: 301-654-2055
Web site: http://www.gastro.org

American Geriatrics Society
Empire State Building
350 5th Avenue, Suite 801
New York, NY, 10118
Telephone: 212-308-1414
Web site: http://www.americangeriatrics.org
Web site: http://www.healthinaging.org

Organizations

The American Geriatrics Society web site features information on aging. The Society also has a Foundation for Health in Aging which has its own web site.

American Hair Loss Council
30 South Main Street
Shenandoah, PA, 17076
Web site: http://www.ahlc.org

American Headache Society
19 Mantua Road
Mount Royal, NJ, 08061
Telephone: 856-423-0043
Web site: http://www.
americanheadachesociety.org

American Heart Association
7272 Greenville Avenue
Dallas, TX, 75231-4596
Toll free: 800-AHA-USA1
Web site: http://www.americanheart.
org

American Hemochromatosis Society
4044 W. Lake Mary Boulevard,
Unit #104, PMB 416
Lake Mary, FL, 32746-2012
Toll free: 888-655-IRON
Web site: http://www.americanhs.org

American Insomnia Association
One Westbrook Corporate Center,
Suite 920
Westchester, IL, 60154
Telephone: 708-492-0930
Web site: http://www.
americaninsomniaassociation.org

American Institute of Stress
124 Park Avenue
Yonkers, NY, 10703
Telephone: 914-963-1200
Web site: http://www.stress.org

American Liver Foundation
75 Maiden Lane, Suite 603
New York, NY, 10038
Telephone: 212-668-1000
Web site: http://www.liverfoundation.
org

American Lung Association
1301 Pennsylvania Ave. NW,
Suite 800
Washington, DC, 20004
Toll free: 800-LUNG-USA
Web site: http://www.lungusa.org

American Lyme Disease Foundation
P.O. Box 466
Lyme, CT, 06371
Web site: http://www.aldf.com

American Optometric Association
243 N. Lindbergh Boulevard
St. Louis, MO, 63141
Web site: http://www.aoa.org

American Osteopathic College of Dermatology
1501 East Illinois Street,
P.O. Box 7525
Kirksville, MO, 63501
Toll free: 800-449-2623
Web site: http://www.aocd.org
The American Osteopathic College of Dermatology posts information at its web site on many dermatological conditions.

American Parkinson's Disease Association
135 Parkinson Avenue
Staten Island, NY, 10305
Toll free: 800-223-2732
Web site: http://www.apdaparkinson.
org

American Pediatric Surgical Association
111 Deer Lake Road, Suite 100
Deerfield, IL, 60015
Telephone: 847-480-9576
Web site: http://www.eapsa.org
An organization of surgeons who specialize in treating children with complex conditions.

American Physical Therapy Association
1111 North Fairfax Street
Alexandria, VA, 22314-1488
Telephone: 703-684-2782
Web site: http://www.apta.org

American Podiatric Medical Association
9312 Old Georgetown Road
Bethesda, MD, 20814-1621
Toll free: 800-366-8227
Web site: http://www.apma.org

American Porphyria Foundation
4900 Woodway, Suite 780
Houston, TX, 77056-1837
Toll free: 866-273-3635
Web site: http://www.
porphyriafoundation.com

American Pregnancy Association
1431 Greenway Drive, Suite 800
Irving, TX, 75038
Telephone: 972-550-0140
Web site: http://www.
americanpregnancy.org

American Psychiatric Association
1000 Wilson Boulevard, Suite 1825
Arlington, VA, 22209
Toll free: 888-35-PSYCH
Web site: http://www.psych.org

American Psychological Association
750 First Street NE
Washington, DC, 20002-4242
Telephone: 202-336-5500
Web site: http://www.apa.org

American Red Cross, National Headquarters
2025 E Street NW
Washington, DC, 20006
Telephone: 703-206-6000
Web site: http://www.redcross.org

American Rhinologic Society
P.O. Box 495
Warwick, NY, 10990-0495
Telephone: 845-988-1631
Web site: http://www.american-
rhinologic.org

American Sleep Apnea Association
6856 Eastern Avenue, NW,
Suite 203
Washington, DC, 20012
Telephone: 202-293-3650
Web site: http://www.sleepapnea.org

American Social Health Association
P.O. Box 13827
Research Triangle Park, NC, 27709
Telephone: 919-361-8400
Web site: http://www.ashastd.org

Dedicated to improving the health of individuals, families, and communities, with a focus on preventing sexually transmitted diseases and infections (STDs/STIs) and their harmful consequences.

American Society for Deaf Children
P.O. Box 1510
Olney, MD, 20830-1510
Toll free: 800-942-ASDC
Web site: http://www.deafchildren.org

The American Society for Deaf Children supports parents and families of deaf children and the professionals who work with them, stressing the use of sign language in the home, school, and community.

American Society for Dermatologic Surgery
930 N. Meacham Road
Schaumburg, IL, 60173
Toll frcc: 800-441-2737
Web site: http://www.asds-net.org

American Society for Microbiology
1752 N Street, NW
Washington, DC, 20036-2904
Telephone: 202-737-3600
Web site: http://www.microbeworld.org

American Society for Neurochemistry
9037 Ron Den Lane
Windermere, FL, 34786
Telephone: 407-909-9064
Web site: http://asneurochem.org

American Society for Reproductive Medicine
1209 Montgomery Highway
Birmingham, AL, 35216-2809

Telephone: 205-978-5000
Web site: http://www.asrm.org

American Society of Hypertension
148 Madison Avenue, 5th Floor
New York, NY, 10016
Telephone: 212-696-9099
Web site: http://www.ash-us.org

American Speech-Language-Hearing Association
2200 Research Boulevard
Rockville, MD, 20850-3289
Toll free: 800-638-8255
Web site: http://www.asha.org

American Stroke Association, National Center
7272 Greenville Avenue
Dallas, TX, 75231
Toll free: 888-478-7653
Web site: http://strokeassociation.org

American Thyroid Association
6066 Leesburg Pike, Suite 550
Falls Church, VA, 22041
Telephone: 703-998-8890
Web site: http://www.thyroid.org

American Tinnitus Association
P.O. Box 5
Portland, OR, 97207-0005
Toll free: 800-634-8978
Web site: http://www.ata.org

American Trauma Society
7611 South Osborne Road, Suite 202
Upper Marlboro, MD, 20772
Toll free: 800-556-7890
Web site: http://www.amtrauma.org

American Urological Association
1000 Corporate Boulevard
Linthicum, MD, 21090
Toll free: 866-RING-AUA
Web site: http://www.urologyhealth.org

American Veterinary Medical Association
1931 North Meacham Road, Suite 100
Schaumburg, IL, 60173

Telephone: 847-925-8070
Web site: ttp://www.avma.org/animal_health/brochures/rabies/rabies_brochure.asp

The American Veterinary Medical Association has a brochure on rabies available for download on its web site.

amfAR
120 Wall Street, 13th Floor
New York, NY, 10005-3908
Toll free: 800-39-amfAR
Web site: http://www.amfar.org

A nonprofit organization dedicated to the support of HIV/AIDS research, HIV prevention, treatment education, and the advocacy of sound AIDS-related public policy.

Amyotrophic Lateral Sclerosis Association
27001 Agoura Road, Suite 150
Calabasas Hills, CA, 91301
Toll free: 800-782-4747
Web site: http://www.alsa.org

Anencephaly Support Foundation
20311 Sienna Pines Court
Spring, TX, 77379
Web site: http://www.asfhelp.com

Anosmia Foundation of Canada
Web site: http://www.anosmiafoundation.org

This Web-based organization provides extensive information about anosmia along with links to other pages related to smell and smell disorders.

Anxiety Disorders Association of America
8730 Georgia Avenue, Suite 600
Silver Spring, MD, 20910
Telephone: 240-485-1001
Web site: http://www.adaa.org

Anxiety Disorders Health Information Program, National Institute of Mental Health
Science Writing, Press, and Dissemination Branch

6001 Executive Boulevard,
Room 8184, MSC 9663
Bethesda, MD, 20892-9663
Toll free: 866-615-6464
Web site: http://www.nimh.nih.gov/
healthinformation/anxietymenu.cfm

Arc of the United States
1010 Wayne Avenue, Suite 650
Silver Spring, MD, 20910
Telephone: 301-565-3842
Web site: http://www.thearc.org

An organization for people with intellectual and developmental disabilities that provides an array of services and support for families and individuals through 850 chapters across the nation.

Arthritis Foundation
P.O. Box 7669
Atlanta, GA, 30357-0669
Toll free: 800-283-7800
Web site: http://www.arthritis.org

Arthritis Society
393 University Avenue, Suite 1700
Toronto, ON, M5G 1E6, Canada
Telephone: 416-979-7228
http://www.arthritis.ca

Association for Glycogen Storage Diseases
P.O. Box 896
Durant, IA, 52747
Telephone: 563-785-6038
Web site: http://www.agsdus.org

Association for Psychological Science
1133 15th Street NW, Suite 1000
Washington, DC, 20005
Telephone: 202-293-9300
Web site: http://www.
psychologicalscience.org

Association for Repetitive Motion Syndromes
P.O. Box 471973
Aurora, CO, 80047-1973
Telephone: 303-369-0803
Web site: http://www.certifiedpst.
com/arms

Asthma and Allergy Foundation of America
1233 20th Street NW, Suite 402
Washington, DC, 20036
Toll free: 800-7-ASTHMA
Web site: http://www.aafa.org

Autism Research Institute
4182 Adams Avenue
San Diego, CA, 92116
Telephone: 619-281-7165
Web site: http://www.autism.com

A non-profit research, resource, and referral organization that conducts and funds research on the causes of autism and on safe, effective treatments for autism.

Autism Society of America
7910 Woodmont Avenue, Suite 300
Bethesda, MD, 20814-3067
Toll free: 800-3AUTISM
Web site: http://www.autism-society.
org

B

BBC Television Centre
Wood Lane
London, W12 7RJ, UK
Web site: http://www.bbc.co.uk/
health

Britain's BBC Television offers information on many health issues at the health section of its web site.

Bell's Palsy Research Foundation
9121 East Tanque Verde,
Suite 105-286
Tucson, AZ, 85749
Telephone: 520-749-4614

Binghamton University, State University of New York
PO Box 6000
Binghamton, NY, 13902-6000
Web site: http://www2.binghamton.
edu/news/the-newsroom/ask-a-
scientist/archive.html

SUNY Binghamton posts information various health issues at the "Ask A Scientist" section of its web site.

Bohart Museum of Entomology, University of California
1124 Academic Surge

Davis, CA, 95616
Web site: http://delusion.ucdavis.edu

The Bohart Museum of Entomology, founded in 1946, is located on the campus of the University of California, Davis. The museum posts facts about human skin parasites and delusional parasitosis at its web site.

Boomer Esiason Foundation
52 Vanderbilt Avenue, 15th Floor
New York, NY, 10017
Telephone: 646-292-7930
Web site: http://www.esiason.org

The Boomer Esiason Foundation provides information on treatment, resources, research, and care centers for Cystic Fibrosis patients and their families.

Brain Injury Association
1608 Spring Hill Road, Suite 110
Vienna, VA, 20036
Toll free: 800-444-6443
Web site: http://www.biausa.org

Brain Injury Resource Center
P.O. Box 84151
Seattle, WA, 98104-5451
Telephone: 206-621-8558
Web site: http://www.headinjury.com

Breast Cancer and the Environment Research Centers
Web site: http://www.bcerc.org/pubs.
htm

The Breast Cancer and the Environment Research Centers web site includes a list of scientific publications as well as a link to fact sheets and other materials that describe known and possible connections between breast cancer incidence and environmental factors. In addition, its web site posts abstracts and summaries of various presentations made at the annual network meetings.

Breast Cancer Network of Strength
212 W. Van Buren, Suite 1000
Chicago, IL, 60607-3903
Telephone: 312-986-8338
Web site: http://www.
networkofstrength.org

British Hernia Centre
87 Watford Way
London, England, NW4 4RS
Web site: http://www.hernia.org

C

Campaign for Tobacco-Free Kids
1400 Eye Street NW, Suite 1200
Washington, DC, 20005
Telephone: 202-296-5469
Web site: http://www.tobaccofreekids.
org

Canadian Cancer Society
Suite 200, 10 Alcorn Avenue
Toronto ON M4V 3B1 Canada
Telephone: 416-961-7223
Web site: http://www.cancer.ca

Canadian Paediatric Society
2305 St. Laurent Boulevard
Ottawa ON K1G 4J8 Canada
Telephone: 613-526-9397
Web site: http://www.cps.ca

CancerHelp, Cancer Research UK
P.O. Box 123 Lincoln's Inn Fields
London UK
Web site: http://www.cancerhelp.
org.uk

CancerHelp UK is the patient information web site of Cancer Research UK.

Cedars-Sinai Medical Center
8700 Beverly Boulevard
Los Angeles, CA, 90048
Telephone: 310-4-CEDARS
Web site: http://www.csmc.edu

The Cedars-Sinai Medical Center posts information on many medical conditions on its web site.

Celiac Disease Foundation
13251 Ventura Boulevard, Suite 1
Studio City, CA, 91604
Telephone: 818-990-2354
Web site: http://www.celiac.org

Celiac Sprue Association/United States of America
P.O. Box 31700
Omaha, NE, 68131-0700

Toll free: 877-272-4272
Web site: http://www.csaceliacs.org

Center for Civilian Biodefense Strategies, Johns Hopkins University
111 Market Place, Suite 830
Baltimore, MD, 21202
Telephone: 410-223-1667
Web site: http://www.
hopkins-biodefense.org

The Center for Civilian Biodefense Strategies carries information about possible bioweapons and posts news updates on the preparedness and response plans of public health agencies and the work of the Department of Homeland Security.

Center For Consciousness Studies
P.O. Box 210068
Tucson, AZ, 85721-0068
Telephone: 520-621-9317
Web site: http://www.consciousness.
arizona.edu

The aim of the Center for Consciousness Studies at the University of Arizona is to bring together the perspectives of philosophy, the cognitive sciences, neuroscience, the social sciences, medicine, and the physical sciences, the arts and humanities, to move toward an integrated understanding of human consciousness.

Center for Disability Information and Referral
Indiana Institute on Disability and Community, 2853 East 10th Street
Bloomington, IN, 47408-2696
Telephone: 812-855-9396
Web site: http://www.iidc.indiana.edu

The Center for Disability Information and Referral, which is associated with Indiana University, provides referrals for all types of disabilities. It also maintains an educational web site for disabled and non-disabled children.

Center for Effective Collaboration and Practice
1000 Thomas Jefferson Street,
Suite 400
Washington, DC, 20007

Toll free: 888-457-1551
Web site: http://cecp.air.org/
resources/schfail/prevsch.asp

A part of the American Institutes for Research, the Center for Effective Collaboration and Practice posts a collection of articles and fact sheets on strategies to prevent school failure at its web site.

Center for Food Safety and Applied Nutrition, Food and Drug Administration
5100 Paint Branch Parkway
College Park, MD, 20740
Toll free: 888-SAFEFOOD
Web site: http://www.cfsan.fda.gov

Center for Human Genetics, Duke University Medical Center
Box 3445
Durham, NC, 27710
Web site: http://www.chg.duke.edu

Center for Molecular & Behavioral Neuroscience–Rutgers University, Newark Campus
197 University Avenue
Newark, NJ, 07102
Web site: http://www.memory.
rutgers.edu

The Memory Disorders Project, housed at Rutgers University, Newark, involves neuroscientists, psychologists, and other researchers who explore how the human brain creates and stores memories. The web site features easy-to-understand information about memory and memory disorders.

Center for Narcolepsy, Sleep, and Health Research. College of Nursing, Suite 208, University of Illinois at Chicago
845 South Damen Avenue (M/C 802)
Chicago, IL, 60612
Telephone: 312-996-5176
Web site: http://www.uic.edu/
nursing/CNSHR

Center for the Prevention of School Violence
313 Chapanoke Road, Suite 140
Raleigh, NC, 27603

Organizations

Toll free: 800-299-6054
Web site: http://www.ncsu.edu/cpsv
Based at North Carolina State University, this center works to inform the public about school violence and ways to prevent it.

Centers for Disease Control and Prevention
1600 Clifton Road
Atlanta, GA, 30333
Toll free: 800-311-3435
Web site: http://www.cdc.gov
The CDC is the federal authority for information about infectious and other diseases.

Charcot-Marie-Tooth Association
2700 Chester Street
Philadelphia, PA, 19013
Toll free: 800-606-2682
Web site: http://www.charcot-marie-tooth.org

Chicago Center for Jewish Genetic Disorders
Ben Gurion Way,
30 South Wells Street
Chicago, IL, 60606
Telephone: 312-357-4718
Web site: http://www.jewishgeneticscenter.org
The Chicago Center for Jewish Genetic Disorders provides education, information, and prevention strategies.

Child and Adolescent Bipolar Foundation (CABF)
1000 Skokie Boulevard, Suite 570
Wilmette, IL, 60091
Telephone: 847-256-8525
Web site: http://www.bpkids.org

Children and Adults with Attention-Deficit/Hyperactivity Disorder
8181 Professional Place, Suite 201
Landover, MD, 20785
Web site: http://www.chadd.org

Children with Diabetes
8216 Princeton-Glendale Road,
PMB 200

West Chester, OH, 45069-1675
Web site: http://childrenwithdiabetes.com
Children with Diabetes provides an online community for children and young adults with Type I diabetes.

Children's Hospital Boston
300 Longwood Avenue
Boston, MA, 02115
Telephone: 617-355-6000
Web site: http://www.childrenshospital.org
Boston's Children's Hospital posts information on many children's health issues at its web site.

Children's Neuroblastoma Cancer Foundation
P.O. Box 6635
Bloomingdale, IL, 60108
Toll free: 866-671-2623
Web site: http://www.nbhope.org
The mission of Children's Neuroblastoma Cancer Foundation is to support families living with this disease by listing the most current, reliable information and resources available.

Children's PKU Network
3790 Via De La Valle, Suite 120
Del Mar, CA, 92014
Toll free: 800-377-6677
Web site: http://www.pkunetwork.org

Children's Tumor Foundation
95 Pine Street, 16th Floor
New York, NY, 10005
Toll free: 800-323-7938
Web site: http://www.ctf.org

Cleft Palate Foundation
1504 E. Franklin Street, Suite 102
Chapel Hill, NC, 27514-2820
Telephone: 919-933-9044
Web site: http://www.cleftline.org

Cleveland Clinic
9500 Euclid Avenue
Cleveland, OH, 44195
Toll free: 800-223-2273
Web site: http://my.clevelandclinic.org

The Cleveland Clinic's my.clevelandclinic.org web site offers information on many health related topics.

College Drinking: Changing the Culture
Web site: http://www.collegedrinkingprevention.gov
This web site sponsored by the National Institute on Alcohol Abuse and Alcoholism is a comprehensive resource for information on drinking prevention in college-age young people.

Compassionate Friends
P.O. Box 3696
Oak Brook, IL, 60522
Toll free: 877-969-0010
Web site: http://www.compassionatefriends.org
The mission of Compassionate Friends is to assist families toward the positive resolution of grief following the death of a child of any age and to provide information on how others can be supportive.

Congenital Heart Information Network
600 North Third Street
Philadelphia, PA, 19123
Telephone: 215-627-4034
Web site: http://www.tchin.org

Conjoined Twins International
P.O. Box 10895
Prescott, AZ, 86304-0895
Telephone: 928-445-2777
A support group for conjoined twins and their families.

Connecticut Clearinghouse
334 Farmington Avenue
Plainville, CT, 06062
Toll free: 800-232-4424
Web site: http://www.ctclearinghouse.org/Topics/topicView.asp?TopicID=87
Connecticut Clearinghouse provides information as well as referrals to people dealing with fetal alcohol syndrome.

Cooley's Anemia Foundation
330 7th Avenue, No. 900
New York, NY, 10001

Toll free: 800-522-7222
Web site: http://www.thalassemia.org

COPD International
131 DW Highway #627
Nashua, NH, 03060
Web site: http://www.copd-international.com

Creutzfeldt-Jakob Disease Foundation
P.O. Box 5312
Akron, OH, 44334
Toll free: 800-659-1991
Web site: http://cjdfoundation.org

Crohn's and Colitis Foundation of America
386 Park Avenue South, 17th Floor
New York, NY, 10016-8804
Toll free: 800-932-2423
Web site: http://www.ccfa.org

Cushing's Support and Research Foundation
65 East India Row, Suite 22B
Boston, MA, 02110
Telephone: 617-723-3824
Web site: http://www.csrf.net

Cystic Fibrosis Foundation
6931 Arlington Road
Bethesda, MD, 20814
Toll free: 800-FIGHT CF
Web site: http://www.cff.org

D

Department of Health and Human Services
200 Independence Avenue SW
Washington, DC, 20201
Web site: http://www.hhs.gov
Web site: http://www.pandemicflu.gov/index.html
Web site: http://www.4parents.gov/sexdevt/index.html

The Department of Health and Human Services (HHS) is the United States government's principal agency for protecting the health of all Americans and providing essential human services, especially for those who are least able to help themselves. They provide information on

various health issues at their specialized web sites.

Department of Health and Mental Hygiene, Community Health Administration
201 West Preston Street, 3rd Floor
Baltimore, MD, 21201
Telephone: 410-767-5300
Web site: http://www.cha.state.md.us
Web site: http://www.edcp.org

Maryland's Department of Health and Mental Hygiene posts information about health and diseases at its web site.

Department of Health Services
1 West Wilson Street
Madison, WI, 53703
Telephone: 608-266-1865
Web site: http://dhs.wisconsin.gov

The Wisconsin Department of Health Services posts information on many diseases and health issues at its web site.

Depression and Bipolar Support Alliance
730 N. Franklin Street, Suite 501
Chicago, IL, 60610-7224
Toll free: 800-826-3632
Web site: http://www.dbsalliance.org

A patient-directed national organization focusing on bipolar disorder, with a network of nearly 1,000 patient-run support groups across the United States.

Directors of Health Promotion and Education
1015 18th Street NW, 3rd Floor
Washington, DC, 20036
Telephone: 202-659-2230
Web site: http://www.dhpe.org

The Directors of Health Promotion and Education work to strengthen, promote, and enhance the professional practice of health promotion and public health education nationally and within State health departments.

Discovery Communications
One Discovery Place
Silver Spring, MD, 20910
Telephone: 240-662-2000

Web site: http://www.health.discovery.com

Division of Diabetes Translation, National Center for Chronic Disease Prevention and Health Promotion, Centers for Disease Control and Prevention
Mail Stop K-10,
4770 Buford Highway, NE,
Atlanta, GA, 30341-3717
Toll free: 800-232-4636
Web site: http://www.cdc.gov/diabetes

A division of the Centers for Disease Control and Prevention, the Division of Diabetes Translation has the goal of reducing the burden of diabetes in the United States.

Doctors Without Borders
333 7th Avenue, 2nd Floor
New York, NY, 10001
Telephone: 212-679-6800
Web site: http://www.doctorswithoutborders.org

Doctors Without Borders provides treatment for people throughout the world. It is not affiliated with any government.

Dolan DNA Learning Center
334 Main Street
Cold Spring Harbor, NY, 11724
Web site: http://www.ygyh.org

The Dolan DNA Learning Center, a part of the Cold Spring Harbor Laboratory, provides a multimedia guide to genetic disorders at its web site.

DrGreene.com
9000 Crow Canyon Road, Suite S220
Danville, CA, 94506
Telephone: 925-964-1793
Web site: http://www.drgreene.com

This web site offers information for parents.

E

Emergency Services and Disaster Relief Branch, Center for Mental Health Services, Substance Abuse and Mental Health Services Administration
5600 Fishers Lane, Room 17C-20
Rockville, MD, 20857

Telephone: 301-443-4735
Web site: http://www.mentalhealth.org/cmhs/emergencyservices
This government agency helps oversee national efforts to provide mental health services to victims of major disasters.

Emory Orthopaedics, Spine Center & Sports Medicine Center
59 Executive Park South
Atlanta, GA, 30329
Web site: http://www.emoryhealthcare.org
Part of the Robert W. Woodruff Health Sciences Center of Emory University, Emory Healthcare posts information about various orthopaedic conditions on its web site.

Enabled Online
321 Wilton Circle
Sanford, FL, 32773
Telephone: 407-474-3841
Web site: http://www.enabledonline.com
A web site that provides a list of organizations and information links related to disability. The web site also includes news and event resources for and about people with disabilities.

Endocrine Society
8401 Connecticut Avenue, Suite 900
Chevy Chase, MD, 20815
Toll free: 888-363-6274
Web site: http://www.endo-society.org
The Endocrine Society studies and performs research on hormones within the human body in association with the clinical practice of endocrinology.

Endometriosis Association
8585 North Seventy-sixth Place
Milwaukee, WI, 53223-2600
Telephone: 414-355-2200
Web site: http://www.endometriosisassn.org

Environmental Protection Agency/Office of Radiation and Indoor Air, Indoor Environments Division
1200 Pennsylvania Avenue, NW, Mail Code 6609J
Washington, DC, 20460
Telephone: 202-343-9370

Web site: http://www.epa.gov/iedweb00/pubs/coftsht.html
The U.S. Environmental Protection Agency's Indoor Environments Division posts an informative pamphlet called "Protect Your Family and Yourself from Carbon Monoxide Poisoning" on its web site.

Epilepsy Foundation
8301 Professional Place
Landover, MD, 20785
Toll free: 800-332-1000
Web site: http://www.epilepsyfoundation.org

Eunice Kennedy Shriver National Institute of Child Health and Human Development
31 Center Drive, Building 31, Room 2A32, MSC 2425
Bethesda, MD, 20892-2425
Toll free: 800-370-2943
Web site: http://www.nichd.nih.gov

The National Institute of Child Health and Human Development web site has information of all aspects of children's health and development.

F

Family Caregiver Alliance
180 Montgomery Street, Suite 1100
San Francisco, CA, 94104
Toll free: 800-445-8106
Web site: http://www.caregiver.org
The Family Caregiver Alliance offers information helpful to people who are caring for loved ones with dementia.

Fanconi Anemia Research Fund
1801 Willamette Street, Suite 200
Eugene, OR, 97401
Toll free: 888-326-2664
Web site: http://www.fanconi.org

Federal Emergency Management Agency
500 C Street SW
Washington, DC, 20472
Toll free: 800-621-FEMA
Web site: http://www.fema.gov/hazard/chemical/index.shtm

The web site of the Federal Emergency Management Agency posts a list of common hazardous household items, tips to prevent chemical poisonings, and advice on responding to chemical emergencies.

First Candle
1314 Bedford Avenue, Suite 210
Baltimore, MD, 21208
Toll free: 800-221-7437
Web site: http://www.sidsalliance.org

First Candle is a resource for expecting and new parents, and also those who have experienced the death of a baby.

Food and Drug Administration
5600 Fishers Lane
Rockville, MD, 20857
Toll free: 888-INFO-FDA
Web site: http://www.fda.gov

Food Safety and Inspection Service
1400 Independence Avenue SW, Room 2137 South Building
Washington, DC, 20250
Toll free: 800-336-3747
Web site: http://www.fsis.usda.gov

The Food Safety and Inspection Service is the public health agency of the Department of Agriculture.

G

Genetic Alliance
4301 Connecticut Avenue NW, Suite 404
Washington, DC, 20008-2369
Telephone: 202-966-5557
Web site: http://www.geneticalliance.org

A national organization of support groups for people who have or who are at risk for genetic disorders.

GLAAD (Gay & Lesbian Alliance Against Defamation)
5455 Wilshire Boulevard, #1500
Los Angeles, CA, 90036
Telephone: 323-933-2240
Web site: http://www.glaad.org

GLAAD is dedicated to promoting and ensuring fair, accurate, and inclusive representation of people and events in the media as a means of eliminating homophobia and discrimination based on gender identity and sexual orientation. They also have offices in New York City.

Glaucoma Research Foundation
251 Post Street, Suite 600
San Francisco, CA, 94108
Toll free: 800-826-6693
Web site: http://www.glaucoma.org

Gynecologic Cancer Foundation
230 W. Monroe, Suite 2528
Chicago, IL, 60606
Toll free: 800-444-4441
Web site: http://www.thegcf.org

Gynecomastia
2917 McClure Street
Oakland, CA, 94609
Telephone: 510-627-0090
Web site: http://www.gynecomastia.org

H

H.E.A.R. (Hearing Education and Awareness for Rockers)
P.O. Box 460847
San Francisco, CA, 94146
Telephone: 415-773-9590
Web site: http://www.hearnet.com

H.E.A.R. provides information on safe volume levels for music and on ear plugs for musicians and fans.

Health24
P.O. Box 2434
Cape Town 8000 South Africa
Web site: http://www.health24.com/medical

South Africa's leading health and lifestyle web site.

Healthcommunities.com, Inc.
136 West Street
Northampton, MA, 01060
Toll free: 888-950-0808
Web site: http://www.urologychannel.com

Healthcommunities.com, Inc., (HC) provides reliable, physician-developed patient education to consumers, medical web site design services for doctors, and online directories of doctors. The Urology Channel site has in-depth information about the parts of the urinary tract, urinary tract infections, and other urological conditions.

HealthInsite
Editorial Team Service Access
Programs Branch, Department of
Health and Ageing, MD,P 2,
GPO Box 9848
Canberra, ACT, 2601, Australia
Telephone: 02 6289 8488
Web site: http://www.healthinsite.gov.au

An Australian governmental initiative, funded by the Department of Health and Ageing. It aims to improve the health of Australians by providing easy access to quality information about human health.

Heart and Stroke Foundation of Canada
222 Queen Street, Suite 1402
Ottawa, ON, K1P 5V9, Canada
Telephone: 613-569-4361
Web site: http://www.hsf.ca

Helicobacter Research Laboratory
Room 1.11, L Block
QEII Medical Centre
Nedlands, Western Australia
Australia 6009
Telephone: +61 8 9346 4815
Web site: http://www.hpylori.com.au

Hepatitis Foundation International
504 Blick Drive
Silver Spring, MD, 20904
Toll free: 800-891-0707
Web site: http://www.hepfi.org

Hermansky-Pudlak Syndrome Network
One South Road
Oyster Bay, NY, 11771-1905
Toll free: 800-789-9477
Web site: http://www.hermansky-pudlak.org

Human Growth Foundation
997 Glen Cove Avenue
Glen Head, NY, 11545
Toll free: 800-451-6434
Web site: http://www.hgfound.org

Huntington's Disease Society of America
505 8th Avenue, Suite 902
New York, NY, 10018
Toll free: 800-345-HDSA (4372)
Web site: http://www.hdsa.org

Hydrocephalus Association
870 Market Street, Suite 705
San Francisco, CA, 94102
Toll free: 888-598-3789
Web site: http://www.hydroassoc.org

I

Illinois Department of Public Health
535 West Jefferson Street
Springfield, IL, 62761
Telephone: 217-782-4977
Web site: http://www.idph.state.il.us/public

The Illinois Department of Public Health posts information on various diseases and their prevention at its web site.

Immune Deficiency Foundation
40 West Chesapeake Avenue,
Suite 308
Towson, MD, 21204
Toll free: 800-296-4433
Web site: http://www.primaryimmune.org

The Immune Deficiency Foundation promotes education about primary immunodeficiency diseases, as well as research and patient support.

Immunization Action Coalition
1573 Selby Avenue, Suite 234
St. Paul, MN, 55104
Telephone: 651-647-9009
Web site: http://www.immunize.org

The Immunization Action Coalition provides information about infectious diseases and immunization.

International AIDS Society
Avenue Louis Casaï 71, P.O. Box 20
CH - 1216 Cointrin
Geneva, Switzerland
Telephone: 41-(0)22-7 100 800
Web site: http://www.iasociety.org

International Association for CFS/ME
27 N. Wacker Drive, Suite 416
Chicago, IL, 60606
Telephone: 847-258-7248
Web site: http://www.iacfsme.org

International Council on Infertility Information Dissemination
P.O. Box 6836
Arlington, VA, 22206
Telephone: 703-379-9178
Web site: http://www.inciid.org

International Dyslexia Association
40 York Road, 4th Floor
Baltimore, MD, 21204
Telephone: 410-296-0232
Web site: http://www.interdys.org

International Food Information Council
1100 Connecticut Avenue NW,
Suite 430
Washington, DC, 20036
Telephone: 202-296-6540
Web site: http://www.ific.org
This web site posts information about nutrition for adults and for children.

International Foundation for Functional Gastrointestinal Disorders
P.O. Box 170864
Milwaukee, WI, 53217-8076
Toll free: 888-964-2001
Web site: http://www.iffgd.org

International Hyperhidrosis Society
Kellers Church Road, Suite 6121-A
Pipersville, PA, 18947
Web site: http://www.sweathelp.org

International Rett Syndrome Association
4600 Devitt Drive
Cincinnati, OH, 45246

Telephone: 513-874-3020
Web site: http://www.rettsyndrome.org

International Society of Travel Medicine
2386 Clower Street, Suite A-102
Snellville, GA, 30078
Telephone: 770-736-7060
Web site: http://www.istm.org

Intersex Society of North America
979 Golf Course Drive, No. 282
Rohnert Park, CA, 94928
Web site: http://www.isna.org

Iron Disorders Institute
2722 Wade Hampton Boulevard,
Suite A, Greenville, SC, 29615
Toll free: 888-565-IRON
Web site: http://www.irondisorders.org

J

Jeffrey Modell Foundation
747 Third Avenue
New York, NY, 10017
Telephone: 212-819-0200
Web site: http://www.info4pi.org
A nonprofit research foundation devoted to primary immune deficiencies.

Juvenile Diabetes Research Foundation International
120 Wall Street
New York, NY, 10005-4001
Toll free: 800-533-CURE (2873)
Web site: http://www.jdrf.org

K

Karolinska Institutet
SE-171 77
Stockholm, Sweden
Telephone: +46 8 524 800 00
Web site: http://www.mic.ki.se/
Diseases/C02.html
This research institute posts links pertaining to virus diseases on its web site.

Kidney Cancer Association
1988 Momentum Place
Chicago, IL, 60689-5319

Toll free: 800-850-9132
Web site: http://www.kidneycancer.org

L

Lab Tests Online–American Association for Clinical Chemistry
1850 K Street NW, Suite 625
Washington, DC, 20006
Web site: http://labtestsonline.org
Lab Tests Online is the product of a collaboration among professional societies representing the clinical laboratory community. It was designed to help patients and caregivers better understand the many clinical lab tests that are part of routine care as well as diagnosis and treatment of a broad range of conditions and diseases.

Lance Armstrong Foundation
P.O. Box 161150
Austin, TX, 78716
Telephone: 512-236-8820
Web site: http://www.livestrong.org

LD OnLine
2775 S. Quincy Street
Arlington, VA, 22206
Web site: http://www.ldonline.org
LD OnLine seeks to help children and adults reach their full potential by providing accurate and up-to-date information and advice about learning disabilities and ADHD.

Learning Disabilities Association of America
4156 Library Road
Pittsburgh, PA, 15234-1349
Telephone: 412-341-1515
Web site: http://www.ldanatl.org

Leukemia and Lymphoma Society
1311 Mamaroneck Avenue
White Plains, NY, 10605
Telephone: 914-949-5213
Web site: http://www.leukemia.org
Formerly the Leukemia Society of America.

Lighthouse International
111 East 59th Street
New York, NY, 10022-1202

Telephone: 212-821-9200 or 212-821-9713 (TTY)
Web site: http://www.lighthouse.org

A comprehensive resource for those affected by vision impairment.

Little People of America/National Headquarters
P.O. Box 745
Lubbock, TX, 79408
Toll free: 888-LPA-2001
Web site: http://www.lpaonline.org

Little People of America posts information on growth issues at its web site.

Livestrong.com
15801 NE Twenty-fourth St.
Bellevue, WA, 98008
Web site: http://www.livestrong.com

Associated with Lance Armstrong, Livestrong is an online information source for health-related topics.

Lupus Foundation of America
2000 L Street NW, Suite 710
Washington, DC, 20036
Telephone: 202-349-1155
Web site: http://www.lupus.org

Lyme Disease Foundation
P.O. Box 332
Tolland, CT, 06084-0332
Telephone: 860-870-0070
Web site: http://www.lyme.org

Lymphoma Research Foundation of America (New York office)
111 Broadway, 19th Floor
New York, NY, 10006
Toll free: 800-235-6848
Web site: http://lymphoma.org

M

Maple Syrup Urine Disease Family Support Group
Telephone: 740-548-4475
Web site: http://www.msud-support.org

March of Dimes
1275 Mamaroneck Avenue
White Plains, NY, 10605

Toll free: 888-663-4637
Web site: http://www.marchofdimes.com

The mission of this national organization is to improve the health of babies by preventing birth defects and infant mortality. Its web site offers information on the cause and prevention of birth defects as well as "The March of Dimes Global Report on Birth Defects: The Hidden Toll of Dying and Disabled Children".

Massachusetts General Hospital Department of Orthopedic Surgeons
55 Fruit Street
Boston, MA, 02114
Telephone: 617-726-2000
Web site: http://www.massgeneral.org/ORTHO

The Massachusetts General Hospital Department of Orthopedic Surgeons provides information about various orthopedic conditions at its web site.

Mayo Clinic
200 First Street SW
Rochester, MN, 55905
Web site: http://www.mayoclinic.com

The Mayo Clinic provides information for patients on many diseases and conditions and their treatment at its health information web site.

McGowan Institute for Regenerative Medicine
100 Technology Drive, Suite 200
Pittsburgh, PA, 15219-3110
Telephone: 412-235-5100
Web site: http://www.mirm.pitt.edu

The McGowan Institute is a research center in regenerative medicine founded jointly by the University of Pittsburgh School of Medicine and the University of Pittsburgh Medical Center.

McKinley Health Center
1109 S. Lincoln Avenue
Urbana, IL, 61801
Telephone: 217-333-2701
Web site: http://www.mckinley.uiuc.edu/handouts

The University of Illinois McKinley Health Center web site offers information concerning various diseases and conditions at their web site.

Medical College of Wisconsin
8701 Watertown Plank Road
Milwaukee, WI, 53226
Web site: http://www.healthlink.mcw.edu

The Medical College of Wisconsin posts patient information on various diseases at its HealthLink web site.

Melissa's Living Legacy Foundation
3111 Winton Road S.
Rochester, NY, 14623
Web site: http://www.teenslivingwithcancer.org

Written for teens, this foundation's web site describes many cancers and what a patient can expect during diagnosis and treatment. It also has a page where teens can write in their own stories about living with cancer.

Memorial Sloan-Kettering Cancer Center
1275 York Avenue
New York, NY, 10065
Telephone: 212-639-2000
Web site: http://www.mskcc.org

The Memorial Sloan-Kettering Cancer Center posts information many cancers on its web site.

Meningitis Foundation of America
212 W 10th Street, Suite B-330
Indianapolis, IN, 46202
Toll free: 800-668-1129
Web site: http://www.meningitisfoundationofamerica.org

Mental Health America
2000 N. Beauregard St., 6th Floor
Alexandria, VA, 22311
Toll free: 800-969-6642
Web site: http://www.mentalhealthamerica.net

A nonprofit orginazation dedicated to helping all people live mentally healthier lives

Mesothelioma Applied Research Foundation
P.O. Box 91840
Santa Barbara, CA, 93190-1840
Telephone: 805-563-8400
Web site: http://www.curemeso.org

Mothers Against Drunk Driving
P.O. Box 541688
Dallas, TX, 75354-1688
Toll free: 800-GET-MADD
Web site: http://www.madd.org

Mothers Against Drunk Driving is a nonprofit organization that seeks to stop drunk driving, support victims of this crime, and prevent underage drinking.

Mulhauser Consulting
55, De Tracey Park
Newton Abbot, TQ13 9QT, UK
Web site: http://www.
counsellingresource.com/distress/
personality-disorders/foundation/
index.html

This group publishes materials from the former Personality Disorders Foundation at its web site.

Multiple Sclerosis Foundation
6350 North Andrews Avenue
Fort Lauderdale, FL, 33309-2130
Toll free: 888-MSFOCUS
Web site: http://www.msfacts.org

Muscular Dystrophy Association—USA, National Headquarters
3300 E. Sunrise Drive
Tucson, AZ, 85718
Toll free: 800-572-1717
Web site: http://www.mda.org

Muscular Dystrophy Campaign
61 Southwark Street
London, SE1 0HL, UK
Toll free: 0800 652 6352
Web site: http://www.
muscular-dystrophy.org

Muscular Dystrophy Canada
2345 Yonge Street, Suite 900
Toronto ON M4P 2E5 Canada
Toll free: 866-MUSCLE-8
Web site: http://www.muscle.ca

N

Narcolepsy Network
79 Main Street
North Kingston, RI, 02852
Toll free: 888-292-6522
Web site: http://narcolepsynetwork.org

National Adrenal Diseases Foundation
505 Northern Boulevard
Great Neck, NY, 11021
Telephone: 516-487-4992
Web site: http://www.nadf.us

National Alliance on Mental Illness
Colonial Place Three,
2107 Wilson Boulevard,
Suite 300
Arlington, VA, 22201-3042
Telephone: 703-524-7600
Web site: http://www.nami.org

The National Alliance on Mental Illness provides education, support, and advocacy for people with severe mental illnesses and for their families.

National Alopecia Areata Foundation
14 Mitchell Boulevard
San Rafael, CA, 94930
Telephone: 415-472-3780
Web site: http://www.naaf.org

National Aphasia Association
350 7th Avenue, Suite 902
New York, NY, 10001
Toll free: 800-922-4622
Web site: http://www.aphasia.org

National Association for Children of Alcoholics
11426 Rockville Pike, Suite 100
Rockville, MD, 20852
Toll free: 888-55-4COAS
Web site: http://www.nacoa.org

The National Association for Children of Alcoholics works on behalf of children affected by a parent's alcohol or drug abuse.

National Association for Colitis and Crohn's Disease
800 South Northwest Highway,
Suite 200
Barrington, IL, 60010
Toll free: 800-662-5874
Web site: http://www.nacc.org.uk

National Association for Down Syndrome
P.O. Box 206
Wilmette, IL, 60091
Telephone: 630-325-9112
Web site: http://www.nads.org

National Association of Anorexia Nervosa and Associated Disorders
P.O. Box 7
Highland Park, IL, 60035
Telephone: 847-831-3438
Web site: http://www.anad.org

National Association of Rescue Divers
P.O. Box 590474
Houston, TX, 77259-0474
Web site: http://www.rescuediver.
org/med/bends.htm

This organization's web site provides information on the medical history of the bends, as well as the condition, its symptoms, and treatment.

National Ataxia Foundation
2600 Fernbrook Lane, Suite 119
Minneapolis, MN, 55447
Toll free: 762-553-0167
Web site: http://www.ataxia.org

National Attention Deficit Disorder Association
9930 Johnnycake Ridge Road,
Suite 3E
Mentor, OH, 44060
Telephone: 440-350-9595
Web site: http://www.add.org

National Biological Information Infrastructure, USGS Biological Informatics Office
302 National Center
Reston, VA, 20192
Telephone: 703-648-4216
Web site: http://westnilevirus.nbii.gov

The National Biological Information Infrastructure provides information and statistical data on West Nile virus at its web site.

National Bone Marrow Transplant Link
29209 Northwestern Highway, Number 624
Southfield, MI, 48034
Toll free: 800-LINK-BMT
Web site: http://www.nbmtlink.org

National Brain Tumor Foundation
22 Battery Street, Suite 612
San Francisco, CA, 94111-5520
Toll free: 800-934-2873
Web site: http://www.braintumor.org

National Cancer Institute
Public Inquiries Office, 6116
Executive Boulevard, Room 3036A
Bethesda, MD, 20892-8322
Toll free: 800-4-CANCER
Web site: http://cancernet.nci.nih.gov

National Center for Biotechnology Information, National Library of Medicine
Building 38A
Bethesda, MD, 20894
Telephone: 301-496-2475
Web site: http://www.ncbi.nlm.nih.gov

The National Center for Biotechnology Information, a division of the National Library of Medicine, provides detailed information about genes and genetic diseases.

National Center for Complementary and Alternative Medicine
9000 Rockville Pike
Bethesda, MD, 20892
Toll free: 888-644-6226
Web site: http://www.nia.nih.gov

National Center for Environmental Health, Centers for Disease Control and Prevention
4770 Buford Highway NE
Atlanta, GA, 30341-3724

Toll free: 888-232-6789
Web site: http://www.cdc.gov/nceh

National Center for Injury Prevention and Control
4770 Buford Highway NE, Mailstop K65
Atlanta, GA, 30341-3724
Telephone: 770-488-1506
Web site: http://www.cdc.gov/ncipc

National Center for PTSD
215 North Main Street
White River Junction
VT, 05009
Toll free: 802-296-5132
Web site: http://www.ncptsd.org

National Center for Voice and Speech, Denver Center for the Performing Arts
1101 13th Street
Denver, CO, 80204
Telephone: 303-446-4834
Web site: http://www.ncvs.org

The National Center for Voice and Speech web site offers e-based learning for better vocal health.

National Clearinghouse for Alcohol and Drug Information
P.O. Box 2345
Rockville, MD, 20847-2345
Toll free: 800-729-6686
Web site: http://www.health.org

National Coalition for LGBT Health
1325 Massachusetts Avenue NW, Suite 705
Washington, DC, 20005
Telephone: 202-558-6828
Web site: http://www.lgbthealth.net

National Coalition for the Homeless
2201 P Street NW
Washington, DC, 20037
Telephone: 202-462-4822
Web site: http://www.nationalhomeless.org

The National Coalition for the Homeless is an advocacy network for homeless persons and providers of services to end homelessness.

National Council on Alcoholism and Drug Dependence
20 Exchange Place, Suite 2902
New York, NY, 10005
Toll free: 800-NCA-CALL
Web site: http://www.ncadd.org

National Digestive Diseases Information Clearinghouse (NDDIC)
2 Information Way
Bethesda, MD, 20892-3570
Toll free: 800-891-5389
Web site: http://digestive.niddk.nih.gov

The NDDIC is a service of the National Institute of Diabetes and Digestive and Kidney Diseases, National Institutes of Health.

National Dissemination Center for Children with Disabilities
P.O. Box 1492
Washington, DC, 20013
Toll free: 800-695-0285
Web site: http://www.nichcy.org

National Down Syndrome Society
666 Broadway, 8th Floor
New York, NY, 10012-2317
Toll free: 800-221-4602
Web site: http://www1.ndss.org

National Eating Disorders Association
603 Stewart Street, Suite 803
Seattle, WA, 98101
Toll free: 800-931-2237
Web site: http://www.nationaleatingdisorders.org

National Endocrine and Metabolic Diseases Information Service
6 Information Way
Bethesda, MD, 20892-3569
Toll free: 888-828-0904
Web site: http://www.endocrine.niddk.nih.gov

A division of the National Institute of Diabetes and Digestive and Kidney Diseases.

National Eye Institute
2020 Vision Place
Bethesda, MD, 20892-3655
Telephone: 301-496-5248
Web site: http://www.nei.nih.gov

National Federation of the Blind
1800 Johnson Street
Baltimore, MD, 21230
Telephone: 410-659-9314
Web site: http://www.nfb.org

National Foundation for Celiac Awareness
P.O. Box 544
Ambler, PA, 19002-0544
Telephone: 215-325-1306
Web site: http://www.CeliacCentral.org

National Fragile X Foundation
P.O. Box 37, 1615 Bonanza Street, Suite 202
Walnut Creek, CA, 94597
Toll free: 800-688-8765
Web site: http://www.fragilex.org

National Graves' Disease Foundation
P.O. Box 1969
Brevard, NC, 28712
Telephone: 828-877-5251
Web site: http://www.ngdf.org

National Headache Foundation
820 N. Orleans, Suite 217
Chicago, IL, 60610
Toll free: 888-643-5552
Web site: http://www.headaches.org

National Heart, Lung, and Blood Institute
P.O. Box 30105
Bethesda, MD, 20824-0105
Telephone: 301-592-8573
Web site: http://www.nhlbi.nih.gov
A division of the National Institutes of Health.

National Hemophilia Foundation
116 West 32nd Street, 11th Floor
New York, NY, 10001
Telephone: 212-328-3700
Web site: http://www.hemophilia.org

National Hopeline Network Crisis and Suicide Prevention Center
Kristin Brooks Hope Center,
1250 24th Street NW, Ste 300
Washington, DC, 20037
Toll free: 800-784-2433
Web site: http://www.hopeline.com
The National Hopeline Network Crisis and Suicide Prevention Center seeks to assist individuals in crisis and prevent suicide in doing so.

National Human Genome Research Institute
9000 Rockville Pike,
31 Center Drive, MSC 2152,
Building 31, Room 4B09
Bethesda, MD, 20892-2152
Telephone: 301-402-0911
Web site: http://www.genome.gov
The National Human Genome Research Institute is home to the Human Genome Project, an international research effort aimed at mapping the human genome.

National Institute for Occupational Safety and Health
1600 Clifton Road
Atlanta, GA, 30333
Toll free: 800-232-4636
Web site: http://www.cdc.gov/NIOSH
Part of the Centers for Disease Control and Prevention, the National Institute for Occupational Safety and Health is responsible for conducting research and making recommendations regarding the prevention of work-related injury and illness.

National Institute of Allergy and Infectious Diseases
Office of Communications and Public Liaison, 6610 Rockledge Drive, MSC 6612
Bethesda, MD, 20892-66123
Toll free: 866-284-4107
Web site: http://www3.niaid.nih.gov

National Institute of Arthritis and Musculoskeletal and Skin Diseases
1 AMS Circle
Bethesda, MD, 20892-3675

Toll free: 877-226-4267
Web site: http://www.niams.nih.gov

National Institute of Child Health and Human Development
P.O. Box 3006
Rockville, MD, 20847
Toll free: 800-370-2943
Web site: http://www.nichd.nih.gov

National Institute of Dental and Craniofacial Research
45 Center Drive, MSC 6400
Bethesda, MD, 20892
Telephone: 301-496-4261
Web site: http://www.nidcr.nih.gov/OralHealth

National Institute of Diabetes and Digestive and Kidney Diseases
Building 31, Room 9A06,
31 Center Drive, MSC 2560
Bethesda, MD, 20892-2560
Telephone: 301-496-2560
Web site: http://www2.niddk.nih.gov

National Institute of Environmental Health Sciences
P.O. Box 12233
Research Triangle Park, NC, 27709
Telephone: 919-541-3345
Web site: http://www.niehs.nih.gov

National Institute of General Medical Sciences
45 Center Drive, MSC 6200
Bethesda, MD, 20892-6200
Telephone: 301-496-7301
Web site: http://www.nih.gov/nigms

National Institute of Mental Health
Science Writing, Press, and Dissemination Branch,
6001 Executive Boulevard,
Room 8184, MSC 9663
Bethesda, MD, 20892-9663
Toll free: 866-615-6464
Web site: http://www.nimh.nih.gov

National Institute of Neurological Disorders and Stroke
P.O. Box 5801
Bethesda, MD, 20824
Web site: http://www.ninds.nih.gov

National Institute on Aging
31 Center Drive, MSC 2292,
Building 31, Room 5C27
Bethesda, MD, 20892
Telephone: 301-496-1752
Web site: http://www.nia.nih.gov

National Institute on Alcohol Abuse and Alcoholism
5635 Fishers Lane, MSC 9304
Bethesda, MD, 20892-9304
Telephone: 301-443-3860
Web site: http://www.niaaa.nih.gov

National Institute on Deafness and Other Communication Disorders, National Institutes of Health
31 Center Drive, MSC 2320
Bethesda, MD, 20892-2320
Telephone: 301-496-7243 (voice)
Telephone: 301-402-0252 (TTY)
Web site: http://www.nih.gov

National Institute on Drug Abuse
6001 Executive Boulevard,
Room 5213
Bethesda, MD, 20892-9651
Telephone: 301-443-1124
Web site: http://www.drugabuse.gov

National Institutes of Health
9000 Rockville Pike
Bethesda, MD, 20892
Telephone: 301-496-4000
Web site: http://www.nih.gov

National Institutes of Health Osteoporosis and Related Bone Diseases National Resource Center
2 AMS Circle
Bethesda, MD, 20892-3676
Toll free: 800-624-2663(BONE)
Web site: http://www.niams.nih.gov

National Kidney and Urologic Diseases Information Clearinghouse
3 Information Way
Bethesda, MD, 20892-3580
Toll free: 800-891-5390
Web site: http://kidney.niddk.nih.gov

National Kidney Disease Education Program
3 Kidney Information Way

Bethesda, MD, 20892
Toll free: 866-454-3639
Web site: http://nkdep.nih.gov

National Kidney Foundation
30 East Thirty-third Street
New York, NY, 10016
Toll free: 800-622-9010
Web site: http://www.kidney.org

National Lead Information Center
422 South Clinton Avenue
Rochester, NY, 14620
Toll free: 800-424-LEAD
Web site: http://www.epa.gov/lead
A federal clearinghouse for information on lead in paint, dust, and soil.

National Library of Medicine
8600 Rockville Pike
Bethesda, MD, 20894
Web site: http://www.nlm.nih.gov/medlineplus
The National Library of Medicine's MedlinePlus web site contains encyclopedia articles and directs users to medical journal articles and web sites on a wide range of diseases and their treatment.

National Lymphedema Network
Latham Square, 1611 Telegraph Avenue, Suite 1111
Oakland, CA, 94612-2138
Toll free: 800-541-3259
Web site: http://www.lymphnet.org

National Marfan Foundation
22 Manhasset Avenue
Port Washington, NY, 11050
Toll free: 800-862-7326
Web site: http://www.marfan.org

National Mental Health Association
2000 N. Beauregard Street,
6th Floor
Alexandria, VA, 22311
Toll free: 800-969-6642
Web site: http://www.nmha.org

National Mental Health Consumer Self Help Clearinghouse
1211 Chestnut Street, Suite 1207
Philadelphia, PA, 19107

Toll free: 800-553-4539
Web site: http://www.mhselfhelp.org

National Mental Health Information Center
P.O. Box 42557
Washington, DC, 20015
Toll free: 800-789-2647
Web site: http://mentalhealth.samhsa.gov

National Multiple Sclerosis Society
733 Third Avenue
New York, NY, 10017
Toll free: 800-344-4867
Web site: http://www.nmss.org

National Organization for Albinism and Hypopigmentation (NOAH)
P.O. Box 959
East Hampstead, NH, 03826-0959
Toll free: 800-473-2310
Web site: http://www.albinism.org

National Organization for Disorders of the Corpus Callosum
18032-C Lemon Drive
Yorba Linda, CA, 92886
Telephone: 714-747-0063
Web site: http://www.nodcc.org

National Organization for Rare Disorders
55 Kenosia Avenue, P.O. Box 1968
Danbury, CT, 06813-1968
Toll free: 800-999-6673
Web site: http://www.rarediseases.org

National Organization on Fetal Alcohol Syndrome
900 17th Street NW, Suite 910
Washington, DC, 20006
Toll free: 800-66-NOFAS
Web site: http://www.nofas.org

National Osteoporosis Foundation
1232 Twenty-second Street NW
Washington, DC, 20037-1292
Toll free: 800-231-4222
Web site: http://www.nof.org

National Ovarian Cancer Coalition
2501 Oak Lawn Avenue, Suite 435
Dallas, TX, 75219

Toll free: 888-682-7426
Web site: http://www.ovarian.org

National Pediculosis Association
P.O. Box 610189
Newton, MA, 02461
Toll free: 866-323-5465
Web site: http://www.headlice.org

National PKU News
6869 Woodlawn Avenue NE,
Suite 116
Seattle, WA, 98115-5469
Web site: http://www.pkunews.org

National Prion Disease Pathology Surveillance Center
Case Western Reserve University,
2085 Adelbert Road, Room 418
Cleveland, OH, 44106
Telephone: 216-368-0587
Web site: http://www.cjdsurv.com

National Psoriasis Foundation
6600 SW Ninety-second Avenue,
Suite 300
Portland, OR, 97223-7195
Telephone: 503-244-7404
Web site: http://www.psoriasis.org

National Reye's Syndrome Foundation
P.O. Box 829
Bryan, OH, 43506-0829
Toll free: 800-233-7393
Web site: http://www.reyessyndrome.org

National Rosacea Society
800 South Northwest Highway,
Suite 200
Barrington, IL, 60010
Toll free: 800-NO-BLUSH
Web site: http://www.rosacea.org

National Scoliosis Foundation
5 Cabot Place
Stoughton, MA, 02072
Toll free: 800-NSF-MYBACK
Web site: http://www.scoliosis.org

National Sexual Violence Resource Center
123 North Enola Drive
Enola, PA, 17025

Toll free: 877-739-3895
Web site: http://www.nsvrc.org
The National Sexual Violence Resource Center is a national information and resource hub relating to all aspects of sexual violence.

National Sleep Foundation
1522 K Street NW, Suite 500
Washington, DC, 20005
Telephone: 202-347-3472
Web site: http://sleepfoundation.org

National Spinal Cord Injury Association
1 Church Street #600
Rockville, MD, 20850
Toll free: 800-962-9629
Web site: http://www.spinalcord.org

National Stroke Association
96 Inverness Drive East, Suite I
Englewood, CO, 80112-5112
Toll free: 800-787-6537
Web site: http://www.stroke.org

National Stuttering Association
119 W. 40th Street, 14th Floor
New York, NY, 10018
Toll free: 800-937-8888
Web site: http://www.nsastutter.org

National Sudden Infant Death Resource Center
2115 Wisconsin Ave., NW
Washington, DC, 20007
Toll free: 866-866-7437
Web site: http://www.sidscenter.org

National Tay-Sachs and Allied Diseases Association
2001 Beacon Street, Suite 204
Brookline, MA, 02146
Toll free: 800-906-8723
Web site: http://www.ntsad.org

National Toxicology Program
P.O. Box 12233, MD, K2-03,
111 T. W. Alexander Drive
Durham, NC, 27713
Telephone: 919-541-0530
Web site: http://ntp.niehs.nih.gov
The National Toxicology Program evaluates a wide range of chemicals found in food products, medicines, and the

environment for possible harmful effects on human health.

National Vitiligo Foundation
P.O. Box 23226
Cincinnati, OH, 45223
Telephone: 513-541-3903
Web site: http://www.nvfi.org

National Weather Service, Office of Climate, Water, and Weather Services
1325 East West Highway
Silver Spring, MD, 20910
Web site: http://www.nws.noaa.gov/om/brochures/heat_wave.shtml
The National Weather Service offers information on the heat index as well as heat-related disorders on its web site.

National Women's Health Information Center
8270 Willow Oaks Corporate Drive
Fairfax, VA, 22031
Toll free: 800-994-9662
Web site: http://www.4woman.gov
Web site: http://www.womenshealth.gov
A service of the Office on Women's Health in the Department of Health and Human Services.

Nemours Center for Children's Health Media, Alfred I. Dupont Hospital for Children
1600 Rockland Road
Wilmington, DE, 19803
Web site: http://www.KidsHealth.org
This organization is dedicated to issues of children's health and produces the KidsHealth web site.

Nephron Information Center
Web site: http://www.nephron.org
The Nephron Information Center is a gateway site with many links to information and current research.

Neuroscience for Kids
Web site: http://faculty.washington.edu/chudler/alz.html

A web site maintained by Eric Chudler at the University of Washington, Seattle. It features easy-to-understand information on a range of topics related to the brain and nervous system. The web site gives an extensive bibliography of readings for children and teens.

New York State Department of Health
Corning Tower, Empire State Plaza
Albany, NY, 12237
Web site: http://www.health.state.ny.us
The New York State Department of Health posts information on various health issues on its web site.

New York Thyroid Center, Herbert Irving Pavilion
161 Fort Washington Avenue,
8th Floor
New York, NY, 10032
Telephone: 212-305-0442
Web site: http://cpmcnet.columbia.edu/dept/thyroid
The New York Thyroid Center, part of the Columbia University Medical Center Department of Surgery, posts information on thyroid diseases and their treatment at its web site.

New York University Langone Medical Center
550 First Avenue
New York, NY, 10016
Telephone: 212-263-7300
Web site: http://www.med.nyu.edu/patientcare/library
The Langone Medical Center of New York University posts illustrated information about various diseases at its web site.

New Zealand Dermatological Society
c/o Tristram Clinic, 6 Knox Street
Hamilton, New Zealand
Web site: http://www.dermnetnz.org

NHS Direct
Riverside House, 2a Southwark Bridge Road
London, UK, SE1 9HA
Web site: http://www.nhsdirect.nhs.uk
Britain's NHS Direct provides information on various health issues at its web site.

NLD on the Web!
Web site: http://www.nldontheweb.org
NLD on the Web! is a web site that provides information about nonverbal learning disabilities.

Nobel Web AB
Sturegatan 14
Stockholm Sweden
Web site: http://nobelprize.org/educational_games/medicine/immunity
The official web site of the Nobel Foundation, Nobel Web AB posts information on the immune system, including an interactive game and several articles written for children.

North American Menopause Society
5900 Landerbrook Drive, Suite 390
Mayfield Heights, OH, 44124
Telephone: 440-442-7550
Web site: http://www.menopause.org

O

Obsessive-Compulsive Foundation
P.O. Box 961029
Boston, MA, 02196
Telephone: 617-973-5801
Web site: http://www.ocfoundation.org

Occupational Safety and Health Administration
200 Constitution Avenue NW
Washington, DC, 20210
Web site: http://www.osha.gov
Part of the Department of Labor, the Occupational Safety and Health Administration helps to ensure safe and healthy working conditions.

Office of the Surgeon General
5600 Fishers Lane, Room 18-66
Rockville, MD, 20857
Telephone: 301-443-4000
Web site: http://www.surgeongeneral.gov
A part of the federal Office of Public Health and Science.

The Ohio State University Medical Center
410 W. 10th Avenue
Columbus, OH, 43210
Toll free: 800-293-5123
Web site: http://medicalcenter.osu.edu/patientcare
The OSU Medical Center posts information on many diseases at its web site.

Online Asperger's Syndrome Information and Support (OASIS)
Web site: http://www.udel.edu/bkirby/asperger

Operation Smile
6435 Tidewater Dr.
Norfolk, VA, 23509
Telephone: 757-321-7645.
Web site: http://www.operationsmile.org
Operation Smile provides cleft palate/lip surgeries for children without access to medical care in many countries.

Optometrists Network
93 Bedford Street, Suite 5D
New York, NY, 10014
Web site: http://www.optometrists.org

Oral Cancer Foundation
3419 Via Lido, #205
Newport Beach, CA, 92663
Telephone: 949-646-8000
Web site: http://www.oralcancerfoundation.org

Osteogenesis Imperfecta Foundation
804 W. Diamond Ave, Suite 210
Gaithersburg, MD, 20878
Toll free: 800-981-2663
Web site: http://www.oif.org

Outdoor Action Program, Princeton University
350 Alexander Street
Princeton, NJ, 08540

Telephone: 609-258-3552
Web site: http://www.princeton.
edu/~oa/safety/hypocold.shtml
The Outdoor Action Program at Princeton University posts the Outdoor Action Guide to Hypothermia And Cold Weather Injuries at its web site.

Ovarian Cancer National Alliance
910 17th Street NW, Suite 1190
Washington, DC, 20006
Toll free: 866-399-6262
Web site: http://www.
ovariancancer.org

Overeaters Anonymous
P.O. Box 44020
Rio Rancho, NM, 87174
Telephone: 505-891-2664
Web site: http://www.
overeatersanonymous.org

Overeaters Anonymous is a support organization that deals specifically with recovery from excessive eating.

P

Pan American Health Organization
525 23rd Street NW
Washington, DC, 20037
Telephone: 202-974-3000
Web site: http://www.paho.org

The Pan American Health Organization provides information about travel medicine in the western hemisphere on its web site.

Parents of Galactosemic Children
P.O. Box 2401
Mandeville, LA, 70470-2401
Toll free: 866-900-PGC1
Web site: http://www.galactosemia.org

Patient Power
9220 SE 68th Street
Mercer Island, WA, 98040-5135
Web site: http://www.patientpower.
info

Patient Power offers a webcast series called "Living with PKU." Approaches to managing PKU, including information about a phenylalanine-restricted diet, is available from its web site.

Penn State Milton S. Hershey Medical Center
500 University Drive
Hershey, PA, 17033
Toll free: 800-243-1455
Web site: http://www.hmc.psu.edu/
healthinfo

The Penn State College of Medicine posts health information on its web site.

Pennsylvania Coalition Against Rape
125 N. Enola Drive
Enola, PA, 17025
Telephone: 717-728-9764
Web site: http://www.pcar.com

PFLAG (Parents, Families & Friends of Lesbians and Gays)
1101 14th Street NW, Suite 1030
Washington, DC, 20005
Telephone: 202-638-4200
Web site: http://www.pflag.org

PFLAG is a national organization promoting tolerance and acceptance among gay, lesbian, and bisexual persons and their family and friends.

Pituitary Disorders Education & Support
P.O. BOX 571
Brighton, MI, 48116
Telephone: 810-923-3379
Web site: http://www.
pituitarydisorder.net/index.html

Pituitary Network Association
P.O. Box 1958
Thousand Oaks, CA, 91358
Telephone: 805-499-9973
Web site: http://www.pituitary.org

Postpartum Education for Parents
P.O. Box 6154
Santa Barbara, CA, 93160
Toll free: 805-564-3888
Web site: http://www.sbpep.org

Postpartum Support International
P.O. Box 60931
Santa Barbara, CA, 93160

Toll free: 800-994-4PPD
Web site: http://postpartum.net

Prader-Willi Syndrome Association
8588 Potter Park Drive, Suite 500
Sarasota, FL, 34238
Toll free: 800-926-4797
Web site: http://www.pwsausa.org

Psychology Today
115 East 23rd Street, 9th Floor
New York, NY, 10010
Web site: http://www.psychologytoday.
com

The web site of the magazine Psychology Today *provides information on various psychological conditions.*

Q

QuitNet
Web site: http://www.quitnet.org

This site helps smokers quit smoking and provides news and resources related to smoking cessation.

R

Rape, Abuse, and Incest National Network
635-B Pennsylvania Avenue SE
Washington, DC, 20003
Toll free: 800-656-HOPE
Web site: http://www.rainn.org

Raynaud's Association
94 Mercer Avenue
Hartsdale, NY, 10530
Toll free: 800-280-8055
Web site: http://www.raynauds.org

Reach Out for Youth with Ileitis and Colitis
84 Northgate Circle
Melville, NY, 11747
Telephone: 631-293-3102
Web site: http://www.
reachoutforyouth.org

Research to Prevent Blindness
645 Madison Avenue, Floor 21
New York, NY, 10022-1010

Toll free: 800-621-0026
Web site: http://www.rpbusa.org

RESOLVE, The National Infertility Association
1310 Broadway
Somerville, MA, 02144
Telephone: 617-623-0744
Web site: http://www.resolve.org

Royal Adelaide Hospital
275 North Terrace, First Floor
Adelaide, SA, 5000, Australia
Telephone: +61 (8) 8222 5075
Web site: http://www.stdservices.
on.net/std/nsu/facts.htm

The Royal Adelaide Hospital web site contains information on many diseases.

S

Sarcoma Foundation of American
9884 Main Street, P.O. Box 458
Damascus, MD, 20872
Toll free: 212/668-1000
Web site: http://www.curesarcoma.
org/aboutSarcoma.htm

Scleroderma Foundation
300 Rosewood Drive, Suite 105
Danvers, MA, 01923
Toll free: 800-722-4673
Web site: http://www.scleroderma.org

Seasonal Affective Disorder Association
P.O. Box 989
Steyning, England, BN44 3HG
Web site: http://www.sada.org.uk

Seeing Eye Inc.
P.O. Box 375
Morristown, NJ, 07963-0375
Telephone: 973-539-4425
Web site: http://www.seeingeye.org

Seeing Eye Inc. is the pioneer guide dog school in the United States. Its web site provides an excellent overview of its history and of guide-dog training.

Selective Mutism Foundation
P.O. Box 13133
Sissonville, WV, 25360

Web site: http://www.
selectivemutismfoundation.org

Selective Mutism Group
30 South J Street, 3A
Lake Worth, FL, 33460
Web site: http://www.
selectivemutism.org

Sexual Medicine Society of North America
1100 E. Woodfield Road, Suite 520
Schaumburg, IL, 60173
Telephone: 847-517-7225
Web site: http://www.smsna.org

The Sexual Medicine Society of North America aims to promote, encourage, and support the highest standards of practice, research, education, and ethics in the study of the anatomy, physiology, pathology, diagnosis, and treatment of human sexual function and dysfunction.

Shape Up America!
6707 Democracy Boulevard, Suite 306
Bethesda, MD, 20817
Web site: http://www.shapeup.org

Shape Up America! offers up-to-date information about healthy weight and increased exercise.

Sickle Cell Disease Association of America
231 East Baltimore Street, Suite 800
Baltimore, MD, 21202
Toll free: 800-421-8453
Web site: http://www.
sicklecelldisease.org

Sickle Cell Information Center
Grady Memorial Hospital,
P.O. Box 109
Atlanta, GA, 30303
Web site: http://www.scinfo.org

Sight and Hearing Association
1246 University Ave. W., Suite 226
St. Paul, MN, 55104-4125
Toll free: 800-992-0424
Web site: http://www.
sightandhearing.org

Sjögren's Syndrome Foundation
6707 Democracy Boulevard, Suite 325
Bethesda, MD, 20817
Toll free: 800-475-6473
Web site: http://www.sjogrens.com

Skin Cancer Foundation
149 Madison Avenue, Suite 901
New York, NY, 10016
Telephone: 212-725-5176
Web site: http://www.skincancer.org

Smoke-Free.gov
Web site: http://www.smokefree.gov
This federal web site offers resources to help people quit smoking.

Social Phobia/Social Anxiety Association
2058 E. Topeka Drive
Phoenix, AZ, 85024
Web site: http://www.socialphobia.org

Social Security Administration Office of Public Inquiries
Windsor Park Building,
6401 Security Boulevard
Baltimore, MD, 21235
Toll free: 800-772-1213
Web site: http://www.ssa.gov/
disability
The Social Security Administration maintains a web site called Social Security Online, which provides information about benefits available for people with disabilities.

Society for Adolescent Medicine
1916 Copper Oaks Circle
Blue Springs, MO, 64015
Telephone: 816-224-8010
Web site: http://www.
adolescenthealth.org
The Society for Adolescent Medicine is committed to improving the health care of adolescents, including reproductive health issues.

Southern California Orthopedic Institute
6815 Noble Avenue
Van Nuys, CA, 91405
Telephone: 818-901-6600

Organizations

Web site: http://www.scoi.com/scoilio.htm

Spina Bifida Association
4590 MacArthur Boulevard, NW
Washington, DC, 20007
Toll free: 800-621-3141
Web site: http://www.sbaa.org

Spine-health.com
790 Estate Drive
Deerfield, IL, 60015
Telephone: 312-224-4150
Web site: http://www.spine-health.com

Stuttering Foundation of America
P.O. Box 11749, 3100 Walnut
Grove Road, Suite 603
Memphis, TN, 38111-0749
Toll free: 800-992-9392
Web site: http://www.stutteringhelp.org

Substance Abuse and Mental Health Services Administration
1 Choke Cherry Road
Rockville, MD, 20857
Toll free: 877-SAMHSA-7
Web site: http://www.homeless.samhsa.gov

A part of the Department of Health and Human Services, the Substance Abuse and Mental Health Services Administration provides links to numerous articles about homelessness at its Homelessness Resource Center web site.

Sudden Infant Death Syndrome Network, Inc.
PO Box 520
Ledyard, CT, 06339
Web site: http://www.sids-network.org

T

ThyCa: Thyroid Cancer Survivors' Association
P.O. Box 1545
New York, NY, 10159
Toll free: 877-588-7904
Web site: http://www.thyca.org

1904

TMJ Association
P.O. Box 26770
Milwaukee, WI, 53226-0770
Telephone: 262-432-0350
Web site: http://www.tmj.org

TOPS Club
4575 South 5th Street
Milwaukee, WI, 53207-0360
Toll free: 800-932-8677
Web site: http://www.tops.org

TOPS Club is designed for people of all ages who are trying to Take Off Pounds Sensibly (hence, the name).

Tourette Syndrome Association
42-40 Bell Boulevard, Suite 205
Bayside, NY, 11361
Toll free: 800-237-0717
Web site: http://www.tsa-usa.org

Trichotillomania Learning Center
207 McPherson Street, Suite H
Santa Cruz, CA, 95060-5863
Telephone: 831-457-1004
Web site: http://www.trich.org

TSS Information Service
P.O. Box 450
Godalming Surrey GU7 1GR UK
Web site: http://www.toxicshock.com

Turner Syndrome Society of the United States
10960 Millridge North Drive, No. 214A
Houston, TX, 77070
Toll free: 800-365-9944
Web site: http://www.turnersyndrome.org/index.php

U

UNAIDS
20 Avenue Appia
CH - 1211 Geneva 27, Switzerland,
Telephone: 41-22-791-3666
Web site: http://www.unaids.org/en

UNAIDS is the Joint United Nations Program on HIV/AIDS, which works globally to fight the epidemic.

Union of Concerned Scientists
1600 Clifton Road
Atlanta, GA, 30333
Toll free: 800-311-3435
Web site: http://www.ucsusa.org

A science-based, nonprofit organization that combines independent scientific research and citizen action to work toward a healthy environment and a safer world.

United Cerebral Palsy
1660 L Street NW, Suite 700
Washington, DC, 20036
Toll free: 800-872-5827
Web site: http://www.ucp.org

United Ostomy Association
19772 MacArthur Boulevard
Irvine, CA, 92612-2405
Toll free: 800-826-0826
Web site: http://www.uoa.org

University of California, San Francisco Memory and Aging Center
400 Parnassus Avenue
San Francisco, CA, 94143
Telephone: 415-476-6880
Web site: http://www.ucsfhealth.org

University of Iowa Hospitals and Clinics
200 Hawkins Drive
Iowa City, IA, 52242
Web site: http://www.uihealthcare.com

The University of Iowa Hospitals and Clinics posts information on a variety of diseases at its web site.

University of Maryland Medical Center
22 S. Greene Street
Baltimore, MD, 21201-1595
Telephone: 410-328-8667
Web site: http://www.umm.edu/ency

The University of Maryland Medical Center publishes information on various conditions at its web site.

University of Michigan Health System
1500 E. Medical Center Drive
Ann Arbor, MI, 48109

Telephone: 734-936-4000

Web site: http://www.med.umich.edu

The University of Michigan Health System posts information on various conditions as part of its web-based Health Advisors.

University of Texas M. D. Anderson Cancer Center

1515 Holcombe Boulevard

Houston, TX, 77030

Toll free: 800-392-1611

Web site: http://www.mdanderson. org/diseases/braincancer

The M. D. Anderson Cancer Center provides a section on brain tumors at its web site.

University of Virginia Health System

P.O. Box 800224

Charlottesville, VA, 22908

Telephone: 434-924-3627

Web site: https://www.med.virginia. edu/uvahealth

The University of Virginia posts information about many health issues on its web site.

V

Vanderbilt University Medical Center, Delirium and Cognitive Impairment Study Group, Center for Health Services Research

1215 21st Avenue S., 6th Floor

Medical Center East, Suite 6000

Nashville, TN, 37232-8300

Telephone: 615-936-1010

Web site: http://www.icudelirium. org/delirium

Vanderbilt University Medical Center and Veterans Administration sponsor a web site that provides information regarding the identification and treatment of delirium among intensive

care patients. The introductory sections on delirium are particularly good.

Vascular Disease Foundation

1075 S. Yukon, Suite 320

Lakewood, CO, 80226

Telephone: 303-989-0500

Web site: http://www.vdf.org

Vestibular Disorders Association

P.O. Box 13305

Portland, OR, 97213-0305

Web site: http://www.vestibular.org

W

Wake Forest Institute for Regenerative Medicine

Richard H. Dean Biomedical Research Building, 391 Technology Way

Winston-Salem, NC, 27157

Telephone: 336-713-7293

Web site: http://www.wfirm.org

The Wake Forest Institute for Regenerative Medicine was in 2009 focused on tissue engineering as a way to treat battlefield injuries as well as solve the problem of the shortage of donors for organ transplantation.

WE MOVE

204 West 84th Street

New York, NY, 10024

Toll free: 800-437-MOV2

Web site: http://www.wemove.org

WE MOVE is dedicated to educating and informing patients, professionals and the public about the latest clinical advances, management, and treatment options for neurologic movement disorders.

Weight-control Information Network

1 WIN Way

Bethesda, MD, 20892-3665

Toll free: 877-946-4627

Web site: http://win.niddk.nih.gov

The Weight-control Information Network is a federally supported web site dealing with obesity and weight control

White Ribbon Campaign

365 Bloor Street East, Suite 203

Toronto, Ontario,

Canada, M4W 3L4,

Telephone: 416-920-6684

Web site: http://www.whiteribbon.ca

A nonprofit organization focusing on men working to end men's violence against women.

Williams Syndrome Association

P.O. Box 297

Clawson, MI, 48017

Toll free: 800-806-1871

Web site: http://www. williams-syndrome.org

World Health Organization

Avenue Appia 20

1211 Geneva 27, Switzerland

Web site: http://www.who.int

World Organization for Animal Health

12 rue de Prony

Paris, France, 75017

Telephone: +33 (0)1 44 15 18 88

Web site: http://www.oie.int

The World Organization for Animal Health provides information on diseases that affect animals, including avian influenza.

Y

Yale Child Study Center

230 South Frontage Rd.

New Haven, CT, 06520

Telephone: 203-785-2540

Web site: http://www.med.yale.edu/ chldstdy

The Yale Child Study Center has been committed to research, treatment, and training related to children and their families for nearly 100 years.

Index

This index is sorted word-by-word. References to individual volumes are listed before colons; numbers following a colon refer to specific page numbers within that particular volume. Page numbers referring to main essays are in **bold** type. Page numbers referring to illustrations are in *italic* type.

A

E

Glandular fever. *See* Mononucleosis, infectious
Glandular tularemia, 4:1732
Glasgow coma scale, 4:1607
The Glass Menagerie (Williams), 3:1307
Glaucoma, 1:232, 2:*714*, **714–16**
    Marfan syndrome, 3:1066
    medical marijuana, 4:1615
Glial-cell cancers (gliomas), 1:248–49, 250, 252, 268
Glioblastomas, 1:249, 252
Global amnesia, 3:1075
Global aphasia, 4:1557
Global Initiative for Chronic Lung Disease (GOLD), 1:375
Global warming. *See* Climate change
Glomerlular membrane, 3:1167, 1168, 1170
Glomeruli, 2:*718*, 718–19, 3:972–73, 974
    nephrotic syndrome, 3:1168, 1169–70
Glomerulonephritis, 2:**717–20,** *718*, 3:974
    nephrotic syndrome, 3:1169
    strep throat and, 2:717, 4:1552
Glucagon, 2:840–41, 843, 866, 867, 3:1251, 1253
Glucagonomas, 2:841, 843, 844
Glucocorticoid-based medications. *See* Corticosteroids; Steroids
Glucose, 2:866
    alcohol consumption, 2:756
    brain energy, 1:169
    diabetes, 2:511, *512*, 513–14, 516, 517
    glycogen storage diseases, 2:720–26, 3:1114–15
    hypoglycemia, 2:866–68
    from lactose, 3:985, 986
    pancreatic tumors, 2:840–41, 843
    regulation, 3:1110, 1252
    testing, 2:514, 515, 516, 517, 523, 868, 3:1122
Glucose-6-phosphatase, 3:1114–15
Glutamic acid, 3:1363
Glutamine, 4:1500
Gluten intolerance, 1:329–32, 3:1052, 1054
Glycogen
    blood sugar regulation, 3:1110, 1253

hangover, 2:756
hypoglycemia, 2:866, 868
Glycogen storage diseases, 2:**720–26,** 3:1114–15
Glycogen synthetase deficiency, 2:724
Glycoproteins, 4:*1477*
Goats
    anthrax, 1:118
    scrapie, 1:448, 3:1348, 1351
Goiter, 2:540, 4:1667, 1668, *1668,* 1669
    See also Thyroid disease
Goldberger, Joseph, 2:538
Golden staph. *See* Staphylococcus aureus bacteria
Gonadotropin, 2:840, 844, 4:1486
Gonadotropin-releasing hormone, 3:1092, 1093
Gonococcal ophthalmia, 1:419
Gonorrhea, 2:**727–30,** 4:1492
    congenital infection, 1:416, 419, 422, 424–25, 433, 434, 2:728, 729
    pelvic inflammatory disease (PID), 3:1274, 1276, 1277
Good cholesterol. *See* HDL cholesterol
Goodpasture's syndrome, 2:719
Gout, 1:143–44, 2:**730–33,** 3:977, 1191
Graafian follicle cysts, 3:1237
Grades, academic, 4:1652
    See also School failure
Gradual-onset lymphedema, 3:1037, 1039, 4:1775
Graduate Record Exam (GRE), 4:1648, 1652
Grafts
    aneurism repair, 1:101, 3:1066–67, 4:1771
    bone, 2:620, 3:1221
    dura matter, 1:448, 3:1352
    heart bypass surgery, 4:1769, 1770
    skin, 1:293, 2:667, 4:1788
Gram staining, 2:522
Grand mal seizures, 2:609, 4:1469
Grandin, Temple, 1:175
Grandiose delusions, 2:489, 3:1286
Graves' disease, 4:1667, 1668
    exophthalmos, 4:*1667*
    ophthalmoplegia, 3:1203
    See also Hyperthyroidism; Thyroid disease

Great pox. *See* Syphilis
Greece. *See* Ancient Greece; Greek language roots; Mythological roots
Greek language roots
    agoraphobia, 1:33
    anthrax, 1:119
    asthma, 1:157
    autism, 3:1292
    cataplexy, 3:1162
    chorea, 2:850
    diabetes, 2:512
    dyslexia, 2:562
    dyspepsia (heartburn), 2:788
    dystrophy, 3:1144
    hydrocephalus, 2:852
    leukemia, 3:1011
    menstrual terms, 3:1097
    myopia, 3:1166
    panic, 3:1256
    pedophilia, 3:1269
    pneumoconiosis, 3:1308
    porphyria, 3:1322
    prefixes, 2:512, 655, 658, 3:1097
    psoriasis, 3:1359
    schizophrenia, 2:551
    sclerosis, 3:1131
    scoliosis, 4:1460
    soma, 4:1547
    sphygmomanometer, 2:860
    staphylococci, 4:1699
    strabismus, 4:1582
    trichotillomania, 4:1720
    typhus, 4:1743
    See also Mythological roots
Greenstick fractures, 1:278
Grief, 2:481, 482
    See also Death and dying
Groin pulls, 4:1585
Ground Zero lung, 2:602, 3:1309, 4:*1694*
Group A streptococcus (GAS) infections, 4:1589–91
    abscesses, 1:2, 4:1511
    rheumatic fever, 3:1408–11
    scarlet fever, 4:1437–39, 1589
    strep throat, 4:1550–52, 1589
Group B streptococcus (GBS) infections, 4:1589, 1591–92
    congenital infection, 1:416, 417, 421, 423, 425, 4:1475, 1591–92
    prevention, 1:425, 4:1476–77

Index

U

U-238, 1:221–22, 313
Uganda, Ebola hemorrhagic fever, 2:576–77, *578, 579*
Ukraine, Chernobyl accident (1986), 3:1383
Ulcerative colitis. *See* Inflammatory bowel disease
Ulcerative proctitis, 2:906
Ulceroglandular tularemia, 4:1732
Ulcers
  anemia cause, 1:92
  bedsores, 1:193–94
  canker sores (aphthous ulcers), 1:316–17, 2:825, 3:1212–13
  Crohn's disease, 1:452, 453
  Helicobacter pylori infection, 2:794–97, 3:1201, 1278–79, 1280
  Mycobacterium marinum infection, 3:1151
  Mycobacterium ulcerans infection, 3:1151–52
  peptic, 3:1277–81, *1278*
  tularemia, 4:*1732,* 1732–34
Ultra-fast computed tomography, 2:775
Ultrasound imaging, 2:528
  birth defects, 1:223, 385, 4:1559
  cancer, 1:226
  congenital infections, 1:421–22, 423
  ectopic pregnancy, 3:1340
  fetal heartbeats/images, 1:430, 2:528, 3:*1337*
  menstrual disorders, 2:598, 3:1097
  ovarian cysts, 3:1236, 1239, 1240, 1241, 1242
Ultraviolet light therapy, 3:1360, 4:1524, 1788
Ultraviolet radiation, 3:1056, 1057, 1058, 1061, 4:1516, 1517, 1518
Umbilical hernia, 2:*821,* 821, 822
Unconsciousness. *See* Consciousness; Stupor and coma
Unipolar depression. *See* Depressive disorders
United Kingdom
  insanity defense rules, 3:1368
  Mad cow disease, 1:448, 449, 3:1349, 1352
  neural tube defects, 1:98, 3:1172
  pertussis vaccinations, 4:1760

royal line, and hemophilia, 1:87
  sheep cloning, 3:1392, 1398
United States and the world, comparisons
  AIDS/HIV, 1:40–41
  albinism, 1:49
  amebiasis, 1:78
  arthritis, 1:143
  ascariasis, 1:149
  birth defects, 1:222
  blindness, 1:233
  breast cancer, 1:272
  breastfeeding, 2:646
  cancer, 1:307
  cholera, 1:358
  cleft palate, 1:382
  coccidioidomycosis, 1:387
  diabetes, 2:518
  encephalitis, 2:588
  epilepsy, 2:607
  heart disease, 2:770, 773
  hepatitis, 2:817
  hookworm, 2:837
  hypertension, 2:859
  malignant melanoma, 3:1056
  multiple sclerosis, 3:1133
  pelvic inflammatory disease (PID), 3:1276
  pneumonia, 3:1313
  schistosomiasis, 4:1441
  stroke, 4:1602
  substance abuse, 4:1614
  trypanosomiasis, 4:1723
  tuberculosis, 4:1727
  typhoid fever, 4:1739
United States Army, 4:1806
University of Pennsylvania Smell Identification Test (UPSIT), 1:117
Updike, John, 3:1359
Upper GI series, 1:453, 2:945, 3:1280, 4:1580
Upset stomach. *See* Gastroenteritis
Ureaplasma urealyticum, 3:1153–54, 1155, 1156
Uremia, lupus, 3:1030
Urethra
  nonspecific urethritis, 3:1182–84, 4:1490, 1745
  trichomoniasis, 4:1717–19
  urinary tract infections, 4:1745, 1746

Urge incontinence. *See* Overactive bladder
Uric acid
  glycogen storage diseases, 2:721, 723
  gout, 1:143, 2:730, 731–33
  kidney stones, 3:977
Uricosuric drugs, 2:733
Urinary system, 1:*225,* 2:*896,* 3:969, 973, *1182, 1243,* 4:*1745*
  kidney stones, 3:*976,* 976–77, 977–78
  metabolic diseases, 3:1109
Urinary tract infections, 4:**1745–48**
  group B strep, 4:1475, 1591
  mycoplasmas, 3:1153–54, 1155–56, 4:1745
  nonspecific urethritis, 3:1182–84, 4:1490, 1745
  risk factors, 2:881
  testing, 2:523
  tuberculosis, 4:1728
Urinary urgency, 3:1243–46
Urine tests, 2:523
  diabetes, 2:514, 516
  electrolyte disorders, 2:673
  kidney disease, 3:975
  mercury poisoning, 3:1101
  nephrotic syndrome, 3:1168, 1170
  overactive bladder, 3:1245
  phenylketonuria (PKU) discovery, 3:1112, 1295
  porphyria, 3:1115
  stupor and coma, 4:1607
  urinary tract infections, 3:1183, 4:1746–47
Urine/urination
  alcohol consumption, 2:756
  diabetes, 2:511, 513–14
  glomerulonephritis, 2:717–18, 719
  glycogen storage diseases, 2:724, 725
  hepatitis, 2:818
  incontinence, 2:895–96
  jaundice, 3:964
  liver cancer, 3:1020
  metabolic diseases, 3:1109, 1111–13, 1115, 1295
  nephrotic syndrome, 3:1168, 1170
  nonspecific urethritis, 3:1183
  overactive bladder, 3:1243–46
  porphyria, 3:1113, 1115, 1323